Molecular Biology, Pathogenicity, and Ecology of Bacterial Plasmids

Molecular Biology, Pathogenicity, and Ecology of Bacterial Plasmids

Edited by

STUART B. LEVY
Tufts University School of Medicine
Boston, Massachusetts

ROYSTON C. CLOWES
The University of Texas at Dallas
Richardson, Texas

and

ELLEN L. KOENIG
Universidad Nacional Pedro Henriquez Urena
Santo Domingo, Dominican Republic

PLENUM PRESS • NEW YORK AND LONDON

Library of Congress Cataloging in Publication Data

Main entry under title:

Molecular biology, pathogenicity, and ecology of bacterial plasmids.

"This book resulted from presentations at an international conference on
bacterial plasmids, held January 5-9, 1981, in Santo Domingo, Dominican
Republic"—Pref.
  Bibliography: p.
  Includes index.
  1. Plasmids—Congresses. 2. Drug resistance in microorganisms—Congresses.
3. Bacterial diseases—Congresses. I. Levy, Stuart B. II. Clowes, Royston
C., 1921—   .III. Koenig, Ellen L.
QR76.6.M64   616'.014   81-8692
ISBN 0-306-40753-1   AACR2

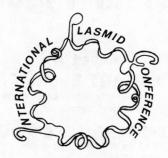

Proceedings of the International Plasmid Conference on
Molecular Biology, Pathogenicity, and Ecology of Bacterial
Plasmids, held January 5-9, 1981, in Santo Domingo,
Dominican Republic

© 1981 Plenum Press, New York
A Division of Plenum Publishing Corporation
233 Spring Street, New York, N.Y. 10013

Printed in the United States of America

This book resulted from presentations at an international conference on bacterial plasmids held January 5-9, 1981 in Santo Domingo, Dominican Republic. This was the first meeting of its kind in the Southern Hemisphere. The meeting place was selected for its relaxed and comfortable climate, conducive to interactions among participants. More importantly the locale facilitated the participation of nearby Latin American clinical and research scientists who deal directly with the health manifestations of pathogenic plasmids. Diseases and socio-economic practices of developing countries exist in the Dominican Republic whose scientific community could directly benefit from having the meeting there.

The book includes the talks as well as extended abstracts of poster presentations from the meeting. This combination, which provides readers with reviews as well as recent findings, captures the full scientific exchange which took place during the 5-day meeting.

As one indication of pathogenicity related to plasmids, the conferees were surveyed for gastro-intestinal problems during and after their stay in the Dominican Republic. The results are summarized at the end of this book.

Stuart B. Levy
Royston C. Clowes
Ellen L. Koenig

ACKNOWLEDGMENT

The organizers thank the host Universities, friends and colleagues who helped in setting up the meeting from which this book evolved. We recognize, in particular, the medical students of Universidad Pedro Henriquez Urena who worked tirelessly during the entire conference period, and A. Ryan whose concerned efforts towards the meeting and book are appreciated. We are grateful to R. Saltzberg-Brown of Great Escape in Waltham, Massachusetts for her diligent handling and understanding of the travel needs of the participants. The meeting would not have been possible without the generous support of the following organizations and industries:

Fogarty International Center,
 U.S. National Institute of Health
U.S. Environmental Protection
 Agency
World Health Organization
Canadian Biochemical Society
Office of Congressman
 Thomas B. Evans (Delaware)
Tufts University School of
 Medicine
Universidad Nacional Pedro
 Henriquez Urena

Abbott Laboratories
Albo CxA
Burroughs Wellcome Company
Cetus Corporation
Ciba-Geigy Company
Dow Chemical Company
E. I. DuPont de Nemours and
 Co., Inc.
Hoffman LaRoche, Inc.
Merck, Sharp and Dohme
 Laboratories
Rosario Dominicana
Sandoz Company
Schering-Plough Corporation
Smith, Kline and French
 Laboratories
Upjohn Company

CONTENTS

IV. TRANSFER AND MOBILIZATION OF PLASMIDS

V. PLASMID REPLICATION, MAINTENANCE AND INCOMPATIBILITY

VI.   TRANSPOSITION AND GENETIC REARRANGEMENTS

VII. MEDICAL, PUBLIC HEALTH AND INDUSTRIAL APPLICATIONS OF PLASMIDS

VIII.   EFFECTS OF ANTIBIOTIC USAGE ON ANTIBIOTIC RESISTANCE
                    IN MAN AND ANIMALS

IX.   BRIEF REPORTS ON ALL TOPICS   575

EVOLUTION AMONG ANTIBIOTIC RESISTANCE

PLASMIDS IN THE HOSPITAL ENVIRONMENT

W. Edmund Farrar, Jr.

Infectious Diseases Division
Medical University of South Carolina
Charleston, South Carolina   29405

Plasmid mediated resistance to antibiotics was first discovered about 25 years ago in Japan because of the unexpected appearance of multiple drug resistance during an outbreak of bacillary dysentery (1). Ever since this time the unexpected appearance of a new or unusual drug resistance marker or an unusual pattern of multiple drug resistance has been a clue that plasmids might be involved as carriers of the resistance genes, and in many cases the 'epidemic strain' of the pathogen involved in the outbreak has been found to contain one or more resistance plasmids. Spectacular examples of this are the extensive epidemic of bacillary dysentery due to Shigella dysenteriae Type I in Central America and southern Mexico during 1969-70, investigated by Mata, et al. (2) and the somewhat smaller but still dramatic epidemic of typhoid fever which occurred in and around Mexico City in 1972, investigated by Olarte et al. (3). In both instances the epidemic strain was found to contain a plasmid which conferred resistance to multiple antibiotics. On a smaller scale, many outbreaks of hospital-associated infection have been shown to be due to a particular strain of a gram-negative organism which contains one or more plasmids.

More recently, within the last four or five years, with the simplification of some of the methods of molecular biology which can be used to investigate plasmids as physical entities, it has become possible for individuals whose interests and backgrounds lie primarily in the clinical and epidemiological aspects of antibiotic resistance, and who are not card-carrying molecular biologists, to investigate plasmids more directly, and to adequately compare plasmids isolated in clinical surroundings with one another. During this time there have been several well-

1

documented cases in which outbreaks of infection in hospitals have
been shown to be due to two or more different species of gram-
negative bacilli harboring a common resistance plasmid. Examples
of this are the finding by Elwell et al. (4) at Seattle of a
plasmid conferring resistance to tobramycin and other antibiotics
in both Klebsiella pneumoniae and Enterobacter cloacae in a burn
unit, and the finding by Sadowski et al. (5) at Minneapolis of a
plasmid conferring resistance to gentamicin in four different
species of gram-negative bacilli. In this outbreak one patient
was found to be inhabited by three different species of
microorganism harboring this plasmid, strongly suggesting that
transmission of the plasmid from one bacterial species to another
occurred in vivo. In Boston, O'Brien et al. (6) have found a
plasmid conferring resistance to gentamicin and other antibiotics
in six different species of gram-negative bacilli at the Peter
Bent Brigham Hospital, and again at Seattle Tompkins et al. (7)
have also found a common resistance plasmid in six species of
gram-negative pathogens at one hospital. In these instances it is
appropriate to speak of an 'epidemic plasmid' rather than an
'epidemic strain'.

We have recently had the opportunity to investigate an
extensive outbreak of hospital-associated infections due to
gentamicin-resistant organisms in which the common element
appeared to be a transposable DNA sequence carrying the gentamicin
resistance gene, which moved from one plasmid to another, these
plasmids in turn spreading among several bacterial species. The
molecular biological studies were carried out in my laboratory at
the Medical University of South Carolina, primarily by Craig
Rubens, as part of a doctoral research project. The epidemiological aspects of the study were performed by Zell McGee and
William Schaffner at Vanderbilt University, where this outbreak
took place.

Beginning in late 1973, an increase in hospital-associated
infections due to gentamicin-resistant organisms was seen at
Vanderbilt University Medical Center (Figure 1). At this time
most of these infections were due to Serratia marcescens and
Pseudomonas aeruginosa. Later, in 1976, an increase in infections
due to getamicin-resistant strains of Klebsiella pneumoniae was
observed, with a few cases caused by gentamicin-resistant strains
of Enterobacter cloacae. No increase in infections due to
Escherichia coli was seen. The outbreak eventually involved four
hospitals in the Nashville area, interhospital spread apparently
taking place on the hands of the medical staff (8). At one
hospital an outbreak of infections due to Serratia marcescens was
immediately followed by an upsurge of cases due to Klebsiella
pneumoniae resistant to the same group of antibiotics (9).

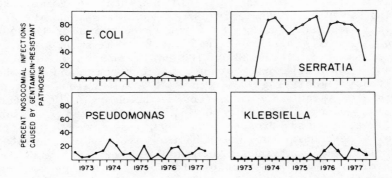

Figure 1. Per cent of nosocomial infections caused
by gentamicin-resistant pathogens at
Vanderbilt University Medical Center,
1973 - 1977.

From the several hundred strains isolated during this outbreak, a group of 25 strains was selected which represented each of the different species of bacteria involved, different times during the five-year period, and different hospitals and wards where infections with gentamicin-resistant bacteria were occurring (Table 1). These strains were examined for plasmid DNA content, antibiotic resistance markers, and presence of aminoglycoside modifying enzymes. (The enzyme studies were kindly performed by Kenneth Price and Peter Kressel at Bristol Laboratories). Gentamicin-resistant strains of Pseudomonas aeruginosa all contained a single 9.8 Md plasmid, and were also resistant to most other commonly used antibiotics with the exception of amikacin. They produced an aminoglycoside acetyltransferase (either AAC 3-1 or AAC 3-3) and the aminoglycoside phosphotransferase APH 3-1. Gentamicin-sensitive strains of P. aeruginosa lacked this plasmid, were sensitive to gentamicin and tobramycin, and did not contain aminoglycoside-modifying enzymes. Gentamicin-resistant strains of Serratia marcescens isolated during the first three years of the outbreak (Groups I and II) also contained a 9.8 Md plasmid, plus another larger plasmid of either 80 or 100 Md. These strains were also resistant to numerous other antibiotics and elaborated aminoglycoside-modifying enzymes. A single strain of gentamicin-resistant S. marcescens isolated in 1976 (Group III) contained a single 105 Md plasmid, but exhibited resistance to aminoglycosides and produced the AAC 3-3 enzyme. Strains of Klebsiella pneumoniae and Enterobacter cloacae, all isolated late in the outbreak, contained plasmids of either 105 or 110 Md, were resistant to multiple antibiotics including gentamicin and tobramycin, and were found to possess aminoglycoside modifying enzymes. Thus, a preliminary assessment indicated that gentamicin-resistant strains of all species contained either a small 9.8 Md plasmid, or a very large plasmid of 105 Md or larger.

In order to separate the different plasmids from one another, we took advantage of the fact that small plasmids (approximately 10 Md or less) are likely to be nonself-transmissible, but readily transform $CaCl_2$ treated E. coli, whereas larger plasmids (approximately 30 Md or larger) are likely to be self-transmissible but not readily taken up by $CaCl_2$ treated E. coli. Table 2 shows the results of transformation experiments with $CaCl_2$ treated E. coli C600. In every case it was possible to obtain transformants containing the small 9.8 Md plasmid. As seen in this table, this plasmid conferred resistance to β-lactam antibiotics and to the aminoglycosides, along with the ability to produce aminoglycoside-modifying enzymes. Table 3 shows the results of conjugation experiments between gentamicin-resistant strains containing large plasmids and rif[r] E. coli SF186. Plasmids of 80 Md and 100 Md size do not confer resistance to aminoglycoside antibiotics nor ability to elaborate

Table 1. Antibiotic Resistance Patterns, Plasmid DNA Content and Aminoglycoside-modifying Enzymes of Representative Gram-negative Bacilli from Nosocomial Infections.

Organism	No. Tested	Antibiotic Resistance Markers[a]											Plasmid DNA (Mass)	Aminoglycoside Modifying Enzymes
		Ap	Cb	Cd	Tc	Sm	Cm	Su	Gm	Tb	Km	Ak		
P. aeruginosa	5	+	+	+	+	+	+	+	+	+	+	-	9.8 Md	AAC 3-1 or AAC 3-3 & APH 3-1
S. marcescens														
Group I	5	+	+	+	+	+	-	-	+	+	+	-	80 Md & 9.8 Md	AAC 3-1 or AAC 3-3 & APH 3-1
Group II	8	+	+	+	+	+	+	+	+	+	+	-	100 Md & 9.8 Md	AAC 3-1, AAC 3-3, AAC 6'-2 & APH 3-1
Group III	1	+	+	+	+	+	+	+	+	+	+	-	105 Md	AAC 3-3
K. pneumoniae	4	+	+	+	+	+	+	+	+	+	+	-	105 Md	AAC 3-1 or AAC 3-3
E. cloacae	2	+	+	+	+	+	+	+	+	+	+	-	110 Md	AAC 3-1 or AAC 3-3 & APH 3-1

a) Ampicillin (Ap), Carbenicillin (Cb), Cephaloridine (Cd), Tetracycline (Tc), Streptomycin (Sm), Chloramphenicol (Cm), Sulfamethoxazole (Su), Gentamicin (Gm), Tobramycin (Tb), Kanamycin (Km), Amikacin (Ak). (+) Denotes presence of the resistance marker.

Table 2. Transformation of E. coli C600 by Plasmid DNA from Gentamicin-resistant Epidemic Strains.

Plasmid DNA From	Mass of Plasmid Transformed into Recipient E. coli	Antibiotic Resistance Transformed into E. coli										Aminoglycoside-Modifying Enzymes Transformed into E. coli
		Ap	Cb	Cd	Tc	Sm	Cm	Su	Cm	Tb	Km	
P. aeruginosa	9.8 Md	+	+	+	-	'	-	-	+	Iᵃ	+	AAC 3-1 & APH 3-1
		+	+	+	-	-	-	-	+	+	+	AAC 3-3 & APH 3-1
S. marcescens												
Group I	9.8 Md	+	+	+	-	-	-	-	+	I	+	AAC 3-1 & APH 3-1
Group II	9.8 Md	+	+	+	-	-	-	-	+	I	+	AAC 3-1 & APH 3-1
	9.8 Md	+	+	+	-	-	-	-	+	+	+	AAC 3-3 or AAC 6'-2 & APH 3-1

a) AAC 3-1 mediates intermediate tobramycin resistance (MIC 4-16 µg/ml) in E. coli

Table 3. Conjugation Experiments Between Gentamicin-resistant Epidemic Strains and Recipient rif^r E. coli SF186.

Donor	Mass of Plasmid Transferred	Antibiotic Resistance Transferred into SF186										Aminoglycoside-Modifying Enzyme
		Ap	Cb	Cd	Te	Sm	Cm	Su	Gm	Tb	Km	
S. marcescens												
Group I	80 Md	+	+	+	+	+	-	-	-	-	-	None
Group II	100 Md	+	+	+	+	+	+	+	-	-	-	None
Group III	105 Md	+	+	+	+	+	+	+	+	+	+	AAC 3-3
K. pneumoniae	105 Md	+	+	+	+	+	+	+	+	I[a]	-	AAC 3-1
	105 Md	+	+	+	+	+	+	+	+	+	+	AAC 3-3
E. cloacae	110 Md	+	+	+	+	+	+	+	+	I	-	AAC 3-1 & APH 3-1
	110 Md	+	+	+	+	+	+	+	+	+	+	AAC 3-3 & APH 3-1

a) AAC 3-1 mediates intermediate tobramycin resistance (4-16 μg/ml) in E. coli

aminoglycoside-modifying enzymes, whereas plasmids of 105 Md or 110 Md confer aminoglycoside resistance along with ability to elaborate enzymes which modify these agents.

We next looked for evidence of relatedness among the various plasmids found in these strains. Digests were prepared from 9.8 Md plasmids obtained from five different strains, using the restriction endonuclease Hinc II. These included three strains of S. marcescens and two of P. aeruginosa. Agarose gel electrophoresis revealed that the pattern of fragments produced was the same in all of these plasmids. When large plasmids (80 to 110 Md) were cleaved with Hind III, many common fragments were observed, with the largest number of fragments produced from the 110 Md plasmids. Similar results were obtained with Bam HI. DNA-DNA hybridization studies also revealed a high degree of DNA base sequence homology among these large plasmids (Table 4). When plasmids of the same molecular size were hybridized, essentially complete homology was found.

These findings led us to believe that a transposable DNA sequence containing the genes for aminoglycoside resistance, originally present on the 9.8 Md plasmid, had been translocated to a larger (probably 100 Md) plasmid, resulting in the formation of a composite plasmid containing all the resistance markers observed in the strains isolated from this outbreak. Experiments to test this hypothesis were performed and have been described previously (10). Briefly, a 105 Md plasmid from a strain of S. marcescens was put into E. coli containing the small plasmid pMB8. Hybrid plasmids were found in these cells, which appeared to represent concatameric forms of pMB8 into which was inserted a transposon corresponding to a molecular size of 6.2 Md, containing genes for resistance to aminoglycosides and β-lactam antibiotics. Heteroduplex analysis confirmed this interpretation. The transposition event was shown to be independent of the rec A system. Similar experiments were done with a 105 Md plasmid from a strain of K. pneumoniae, with identical results. Finally, heteroduplex analysis using pBM8::6.2 Md transposon and a 9.8 Md plasmid from S. marcescens revealed that these two plasmids shared a contiguous 6.2 Md region. The findings thus indicate that not only do the 105 Md plasmids contain a transposon carrying the genes for gentamicin resistance, but that this transposable sequence originated on the 9.8 Md plasmids found in strains isolated in the early stages of the outbreak.

It is interesting to view these events from the perspective of a selfish gentamicin resistance gene. As long as this gene was restricted to a small non-conjugative plasmid, its horizon was quite limited. An opportunity to enter a new bacterial species

Table 4. Hybridization between ^{3}H-labeled Plasmid DNA and Unlabeled DNA.

Source of Unlabeled DNA	Molecular Weight of Plasmid (Md)	Relative DNA Sequence Homology				
		^{3}H-SM80	^{3}H-SM100	^{3}H-SM105	^{3}H-KP105	^{3}H-EC110
S. marcescens	80	100	84	77	77	62
S. marcescens	100	100	100	80	82	78
S. marcescens	105	99	77	100	95	88
K. pneumoniae	105	100	92	96	100	91
E. cloacae	110	100	100	100	100	100

would arise only if a large, conjugative plasmid happened to enter the cell in which it was residing. This might result in its mobilization and transfer into a new bacterial host. However, when the DNA sequence of which it is a part underwent transposition to a larger conjugative plasmid, it acquired the ability to spread to additional bacterial species, with opportunity to inhabit a greater variety of patients and a wider diversity of niches within the hospital environment.

1.   Watanabe, T.: Infective heredity of multiple drug
        resistance in bacteria. Bacteriol. Rev. 27:87-115,
        1963.
2.   Mata, L.J., Gangarosa, E.J., Caceres, A., Perera, D.R.,
        and Mejicanos, M.L.: Epidemic Shiga bacillus dysentery
        in Central America. I. Etiologic investigations in
        Guatemala, 1969. J. Infect. Dis. 122:170-180, 1970.
3.   Olarte, J. and Galindo, E.: Salmonella typhi resistant
        to chloramphenicol, ampicillin and other anti-microbial
        agents: strains isolated during an extensive typhoid
        fever epidemic in Mexico. Antimicrob. Agents Chemother.
        4:597-601, 1972.
4.   Elwell, L.P., Inamine, J.M., and Minshew, B.H.: Common
        plasmid specifying tobramycin resistance in two enteric
        bacteria isolated from burn patients. Antimicrob. Agents
        Chemother. 13:312-317, 1978.
5.   Sadowski, P.L., Peterson, B.C., Gerding, D.N., Cleary,
        P.P.: Physical characterization of ten R plasmids
        obtained from an outbreak of nosocomial Klebsiella
        pneumoniae infections. Antimicrob. Agents Chemother.
        15:616-624, 1979.
6.   O'Brien, T.F., Ross, D.G., Guzman, M.A., Medeiros,
        A.A., Hedges, R.W., Botstein, D.: Dissemination of an
        antibiotic resistance plasmid in hospital patient flora.
        Antimicrob. Agents Chemother. 17:537-543, 1980.
7.   Tompkins, L.S., Plorde, J.J., Falkow, S.: Molecular
        analysis of R-factors from multiresistant nosocomial
        isolates. J. Infect. Dis. 141:625-636, 1980.
8.   Schaberg, D.R., Alford, R.H., Anderson, R.A., Melly,
        M.A., Schaffner, W.: An outbreak of nosocomial
        infection due to multiply-resistant Serratia marcescens:
        evidence of interhospital spread. J. Infect. Dis.
        134:181-186, 1976.
9.   Thomas, F.E., Jackson, R.T., Melly, M.A., and Alford,
        R.H.: Sequential hospitalwide outbreaks of resistant
        Serratia and Klebsiella infections. Arch. Intern. Med.
        137:581-584, 1977.
10. Rubens, C.E., McNeill, W.F., Farrar, W.E.: Evolution
        of multiple antibiotic resistance plasmids mediated
        by transposable plasmid deoxyribonucleic acid
        sequences. J. Bacteriol. 140:713-719, 1979.

R FACTORS PRESENT IN EPIDEMIC STRAINS OF <u>SHIGELLA</u> AND <u>SALMONELLA</u> SPECIES FOUND IN MEXICO

Jorge Olarte

Laboratorio de Bacteriologia Intestinal
Hospital Infantil de Mexico
Mexico 7, D.F., Mexico

The appearance of <u>Shigella flexneri</u> resistant to common antibiotics (tetracycline, chloramphenicol and streptomycin) was detected in Mexico as early as 1955 (1,2). Of particular importance was the clinical failure observed in the treatment with tetracycline of children with acute dysentery caused by strains of <u>S. flexneri</u> resistant in vitro to this antibiotic. After the discovery of R plasmids in Japan, we tested our culture collection of <u>Shigella</u>, <u>Salmonella</u> and <u>Escherichia coli</u>, including strains which were isolated between the years 1955 and 1969, and found that a large proportion of the resistances observed in these cultures was transmisible to <u>E. coli</u> K-12 (3).

The proportion of the number of multiple resistant strains increased during the following years, particularly in the <u>Shigella</u> group (Table 1). However, the process has not been steady showing ups and downs. Shortly after the introduction of new antibiotics such as ampicillin, aminoglycosides and cephalosporins, strains resistant to them also appeared.

<u>SHIGELLA</u> <u>DYSENTERIAE</u> TYPE 1 EPIDEMICS

In spite of the fact that the clinicians became concerned about the negative repercussions observed in the treatment of infections caused by multiple resistant strains of enteropathogenic bacteria, if was not until 1969-1970 when the true epidemic importance of this kind of resistance became evident due to the dysentery outbreak originated by a multiple resistant strain of <u>S. dysenteriae</u> type 1 which spread through Central America and Mexico (4,5). The organism showed a uniform and persistent resistance pattern representing a single clone.

Table 1.   Shigella Strains Isolated in Mexico City from 1953 to 1976,
           Resistant to Various Antibiotics [a]

Year of isolation	No. of strains tested	Per cent resistant to 10 mcg/ml or more [b]			
		T	C	S	A
1953	31	0	0	74	
1955	26	19	8	50	
1956	41	34	7	39	
1957	33	39	3	39	
1959	71	38	21	63	
1960	44	43	20	73	0
1961	41	34	27	41	
1962-1964	53	36	32	53	3
1965	57	30	19	61	7
1967	55	35	35	58	
1971	42	48	36	100	14
1975	69	52	16	99	7
1976	25	76	36	96	56

[a] Source: Olarte, J. 1978 Bol.Med. Hosp.Infant. Mex., 35:295-309.
[b] T: tetracycline, C: chloramphenicol, S: streptomycin, A: ampicillin

As seen in Table 2, it was found that the R factors conferring
resistance to chloramphenicol, streptomycin, tetracycline, and sulfonamides, present in all samples tested of the epidemic strain of
Shiga 1 belonged to the incompatibility group O plasmid (6). This
incompatibility group was described by Hedges, Datta et al. (7), and
was originally found in two strains of enteropathogenic Escherichia
coli, serotypes O86:B7 and O126:B16, isolated in our Hospital from
babies with acute diarrhea in 1956; it was of interest since it confers resistance to ampicillin, yet its host strains were isolated
before ampicillin was ever used. The corresponding beta-lactamases
were studied at the laboratory of Stanley Falkow (8). Group O plasmids
have been also found in S. flexneri and are apparently common in Central America and Mexico (6). The Shiga 1 epidemic, which extended from
1968 to 1970 attacking over 100,000 persons, almost entirely subsided
during the following years.

In Mexico City on June 1972 (Table 2), an outbreak of dysentery
due to S. dysenteriae type 1 took place in a hospital ward lodging
children under treatment for tuberculosis. This time the causative
organism was resistant to ampicillin, in addition to chloramphenicol,
tetracycline, streptomycin, and sulfonamides. The ampicillin resistance could be transferred independently from the other drug resis-

Table 2. R Factors Found in Shigella dysenteriae 1 and
Escherichia coli

ORGANISM	STRAIN	ORIGIN	RESISTANCE[a]	TRANSFERRED	COMPATIBILITY GROUP
S. DYSENTERIAE 1	EPIDEMIC (SEVERAL HUNDRED ISOLATED)	CENTRAL AMERICA AND MEXICO 1968 - 1970	C S T Su	C S T Su	O
E. COLI 086 : B7	SPORADIC CASE (E - 997)	MEXICO CITY, 1956	A S T Su	A S T Su	Iω AND O
E. COLI 0126 : B16	SPORADIC CASE (E - 1235)	MEXICO CITY, 1956	A C S T Su	A C S T Su	Iω AND O
S. DYSENTERIAE 1	HOSPITAL OUTBREAK (5 STRAINS)	MEXICO CITY, 1972	A C S T Su	C S T Su[b] A[c]	O
S. DYSENTERIAE 1	COMMUNITY OUT- BREAK (762)	COSTA RICA, 1974	A C S T Su	C S T Su[b] A[c]	
S. DYSENTERIAE 1	COMMUNITY OUT- BREAK (6986)	BANGLA DESH, 1972 - 1973	A C S T Su	A C S T Su A[c]	

a   C: CHLORAMPHENICOL,   S: STREPTOMYCIN,   T: TETRACYCLINE,   Su: SULFONAMIDES,   A: AMPICILLIN
b   80 - MDAL CONJUGATIVE   R - PLASMID
c   5.5 - MDAL NONCONJUGATIVE   PLASMID
SOURCE: COMPILED FROM REFS. 6, 9, 10

tances from five recovered strains of S. dysenteriae type 1 to E. coli
K-12 (9). It was found that these strains were carrying two different
plasmids, the O 80 megadaltons plasmid detected in the former epidemic
strain, and a 5.5 megadaltons plasmid which contained the ampicillin
transposon (TnA) sequences and was nonconjugative (10). It is interesting that strains of Shiga bacillus with the same resistance pattern
coded by identical plasmids were also isolated in Costa Rica, and
strains of Shiga with the same ampicillin 5.5 megadaltons plasmid
were simultaneously found in Bangla Desh. The ubiquity of this small
ampicillin plasmid is noteworthy.

The practical implications of such resistant strains have been
previously emphasized (9,10).

TYPHOID FEVER EPIDEMIC

Though strains of Salmonella typhi resistant to chloramphenicol
were found in different parts of the world since the early sixties
(11), it was until 1972 when a strain resistant to multiple antibiotics, including chloramphenicol, caused a large and rapid spreading
epidemic of typhoid fever in Mexico City, Pachuca and other communities of Mexico. Over 10,000 cases were seen (12).

As shown in Table 3, all chloramphenicol resistant strains of
S. typhi isolated during the outbreak, which were studied in various

laboratories in Mexico (12,13), the United States (14), and England (6,11), were uniformly resistant to chloramphenicol, streptomycin, tetracicline, and sulfonamides, and had the same phage sensitivity pattern, representing a single clone. The resistance was caused by a transmissible plasmid of the incompatibility group H. Considering that the outbreak of typhoid fever in Mexico followed the severe epidemic of bacillary dysentery in Central America, already mentioned, in which the causative organism was resistant to the same four drugs, the question was raised of whether the same plasmid was present in both epidemic pathogens (15). However, the studies accomplished indicate that each organism carried a phylogenetically distinct plasmid, H and O incompatibility group, respectively (6,14).

In the course of the typhoid outbreak seven strains of S. typhi were isolated in different localities, which were resistant to ampicillin in addition to chloramphenicol, streptomycin, tetracycline, and sulfonamides (Table 3). One of these (H-185), was also resistant to kanamycin. All seven strains were infected with the H plasmid conferring resistance to the four drugs to which the epidemic strain was resistant, but in addition were carrying several different R plasmids. In four strains (H-185, La Raza 2, LA, and JM) the ampicillin resistance plasmid was nonconjugative, but was mobilized by the

Table 3. R Factors Found in Salmonella typhi
in Mexico - 1972

STRAIN	ORIGIN	RESISTANCE	TRANSFERRED	COMPATIBILITY GROUP	PHAGE TYPE [a]
EPIDEMIC (MORE THAN 10 000 CASES)	MEXICO-CENTRAL STATES AND WEST COST	C S T Su	C S T Su	H	D V S - 2 [b]
SPORADIC CASES:					
H - 185	MEXICO CITY	A K C S T Su	K A K [c] C S T Su	Iω AND O — H	D V S - 10
LA RAZA 1	MEXICO CITY	A C S T Su	A C S (K) C S T Su	A AND C H	D V S - 11
PUEBLA 12	PUEBLA	A C S T Su	A S C S T Su	Iᴧ H	D V S - 2 [b]
J R R	ACAPULCO	A C S T Su	A C S T Su	Iδ H	Vi NEGATIVE
LA RAZA 2	MEXICO CITY	A C S T Su	C S T Su A C S T Su [c]	H —	
L A	MEXICO CITY	A C S T Su	C S T Su A C S T Su [c]	H —	D V S - 10
J M	TULANCINGO	A C S T Su	C S T Su A C S T Su [c]	H —	D V S - 2 [b]

[a]   ACCORDING TO E. S. ANDERSON - LONDON (PERSONAL COMMUNICATION)
[b]   EPIDEMIC STRAIN (Vi DEGRADED APPROACHING GROUP A - ACCORDING TO CDC)
[c]   THE A RESISTANCE WAS NOT SELF-TRANSMISSIBLE, BUT MOBILIZED BY ACCOMPANYING PLASMID
SOURCE: COMPILED FROM REFS. 6, 12

accompanying transmissible plasmid. The other three strains had
conjugative ampicillin resistance plasmids, all different from one
another in compatibility (A and C in strain La Raza 1, I∢in strain
Puebla 12, and I&in strain JRR). The kanamycin resistance in strain
H-125 was plasmid determined and transmissible, coded by incompatibility group Iω and O (6).

The epidemic strain of S. typhi was of a Vi degraded phage type.
Two ampicillin resistant strains (Puebla 12 and JM) were of the same
phage type of the epidemic strain, one (JRR) was Vi negative, another
(La Raza 2) was not phage typed. The remaining three ampicillin resistant strains (H-185, La Raza 1, and LA) showed different phage sensitivities. According to E.D. Anderson the epidemic strain and these
three strains correspond to new phage types to be described (personal
communication).

These findings show that the carrying of the H plasmid of the
epidemic strain did not prevent the acquisition of other R factors
by the same strain. This was also true in the case of the O plasmid
of the epidemic strain of Shiga bacillus. There is the possibility
that the acquisition of some R factors could influence in some way
the phage sensitivity of S. typhi; however, Alfaro, Martuscelli and
Mendoza (16), have obtained some experimental results contrary to
this hypothesis.

The typhoid outbreak was apparently a self-limited event. Typhoid
fever has been endemic in Mexico City for a long time, but its ocurren
ce in epidemic form has been rather unusual for the last 30 years. The
explosive outbreak began in early 1972, reached a peak by the middle
of the year and then declined to almost disappear in 1973. It is not
clear how the epidemic started, but it is even more difficult to
understand why it did not spread to the whole country and Central and
South America, considering the large number of residual carriers that
would be expected from such a large number of cases, combined with
epidemiological conditions over this large area propicious for its
propagation.

As seen in Table 4, the proportion of S. typhi chloramphenicol
resistant strains isolated in Mexico City was very high (94.7 %) in
1972, decreased through 1973, and then, with the exception of 1975
(23.5 %), it has declined dramatically. It is not known when the
resistant strain first make its appearance in Mexico. We detected
it at the time the outbreak was obvious, but the search for resistant
strains during the years immediately before the outbreak was neglected, since we become complacent, believing that the susceptibility
of the organism to chloramphenicol was very stable.

The decreasing incidence of the resistant strain could be due
to either genetic, ecological, or epidemiological causes, or a
combination of them. Unfortunately, we can not place too much trust

Table 4. Decreased Incidence of S. typhi Resistant to Chloramphenicol,
         Mexico City - 1972 to 1980

Year		Number of strains	Per cent resistant
1972 [a]		226	94.7
1973	Jan-Jun	604	60.7
	Jul-Dec	179	41.3
1974 [b]		109	3.5
1975 [b]		230	23.5
1976 [b]		142	4.9
1977 [b]		89	6.2
1978 [b]		60	3.6
1979 [b]		95	0.0
1980 [b]		108	3.7

[a] From Ref. 13.   [b] Data provided by J. Martuscelli, UNAM, Mexico.

in the epidemiological data collected during the outbreak. The
behavior of resistant strains in nature is not well understood.

SALMONELLOSIS OTHER THAN TYPHOID FEVER

Regarding the infections caused by species of Salmonella called
of animal origin, strains resistant to multiple drugs have been
detected in Mexico for many years (3). From time to time we have
observed outbreaks of limited importance which mainly affect young
children. No doubt that these outbreaks have spread through the
community in general; however, they have been only studied in pediatric hospitals. The extension that these organisms have affected
different animal species in Mexico is not well known.

As shown in Table 5, a strain of S. poona resistant to nine.
drugs was isolated from 154 children with acute gastroenteritis
attending the Hospital Infantil de Mexico, from May to July, 1976.
Twenty-three had septicemia, and nine septicemia and meningitis;
seven of the latter died (17). From June, 1979 to May, 1980, a strain
of S. newport resistant to eight drugs was isolated in the same Hospital from 51 children with acute gastroenteritis. Five had septicemia and two septicemia and meningitis. In both outbreaks some of
the children were already infected with the salmonella at the time
of admission, whereas others acquired the salmonella in the hospital

Table 5. Salmonellosis in Children Caused by Multiple
         Resistant Strains of S. poona and S. newport,
         Hospital Infantil de Mexico

ORGANISM	ILLNESS		RESISTANCE
S. POONA (MAY - JULY, 1976)	GASTROENTERITIS	122 CASES	AMPICILLIN, CHLORAMPHENICOL, TETRACYCLINES, CEPHALOTHIN,
	GASTROENTERITIS COMPLI-CATED WITH SEPTICEMIA	23 CASES	KANAMYCIN, STREPTOMYCIN,
(From Ref.17)	GASTROENTERITIS COMPLI-CATED WITH SEPTICEMIA AND MENINGITIS	9 CASES	GENTAMICIN, CARBENICILLIN, SULFANOMIDES
S. NEWPORT (JUNE 1959 - MAY 1980)	GASTROENTERITIS	44 CASES	AMPICILLIN, CHLORAMPHENICOL, CEPHALOTHIN, STREPTOMYCIN,
	GASTROENTERITIS COMPLI-CATED WITH SEPTICEMIA	5 CASES	KANAMYCIN, GENTAMICIN,
	GASTROENTERITIS COMPLI-CATED WITH SEPTICEMIA AND MENINGITIS	2 CASES	SULFONAMIDES

as a result of cross infection. The resistance present in both strains
of Salmonella is transmissible; the R factors involved are under study.

Similar outbreaks of gastroenteritis caused by multiresistant
Salmonella serotypes of animal origin have been reported in various
regions. Of particular importance have been certain strains of S.
wien which have spread through various countries in Southern Europe
and North Africa (18), and S. typhimurium in South America (19), the
Middle East and Great Britain (18,20).

The possibility that epidemic multiresistant strains of enteropathogenic bacteria possess, in addition to the R factors, an enhanced
virulence or a factor which facilitates its transmissibility, has
been the subjet of much speculation and remains to be resolved.

The data presented in this review are a good example of what
likely could occur in any country that, like Mexico, meets the conditions for the propagation of enteric infections, together with its
high incidence and the indiscriminate use of antimicrobial drugs.

REFERENCES

1. Olarte, J., De la Torre, J. Resistance of Shigella flexneri to
   tetracyclines, chloramphenicol and streptomycin. A study of 131
   freshly isolated strains. Am. J. Trop. Med. Hyg. 8:324-326, 1959.
2. Olarte, J., Galindo, E., Joachin, A. Sensitivity of Salmonella,
   Shigella, and enteropathogenic Escherichia coli species to cephalothin, ampicillin, chloramphenicol, and tetracycline. Antimicrobial Agents and Chemotherapy-1962, p. 787-793.
3. Olarte, J., Galindo, E. Factores de resistencia a los antibioti-
   cos encontrados en bacterias enteropatogenas aisladas en la ciu-
   dad de México. Rev. Lat-Amer. Microbiol. 12: 173-179, 1970.
4. Mata, L. J., Gangarosa, E. J., Cáceres, A., Perera, D. R., Meji-
   canos, M. L. Epidemic Shiga bacillus dysentery in Central America.
   I. Etiologic investigation in Guatemala, 1969. J. Infect. Dis.
   122: 170-180, 1970.
5. Olarte, J., Varela, G., Galindo, E. Infeccion por Shigella dysenteriae 1 (Bacilo de Shiga) en Mexico. Bol. Med. Hosp. Infant. Mex.
   28: 605-612, 1971.
6. Datta, N., Olarte, J. R factors in strains of Salmonella typhi
   and Shigella dysenteriae 1 isolated during epidemics in Mexico:
   classification by compatibility. Antimicrob. Ag. Chemother. 5:
   310-317, 1974.
7. Hedges, R. W., Datta, N., Kontomichalou, P., Smith, J. T. Molecular specificities of R factor-determined beta-lactamases: correlation with plasmid compatibility. J. Bacteriol. 117: 56-62, 1974.
8. Evans, J., Galindo, E., Olarte, J., Falkow, S. Beta-lactamase of
   R factors. J. Bacteriol. 96: 1441-1442, 1968.
9. Olarte, J., Filloy, L., Galindo, E. Resistance of Shigella dysenteriae type 1 to ampicillin and other antimicrobial agents:
   strains isolated during a dysentery outbreak in a hospital in
   Mexico City. J. Infect. Dis. 133: 572-575, 1976.
10. Crosa, J. H., Olarte, J., Mata, L. J., Lattropp, L. K., Peñaranda,
    M. E. Characterization of an R-plasmid associated with ampicillin
    resistance in Shigella dysenteriae type 1 isolated from epidemics.
    Antimicrob. Ag. Chemoth. 11: 553-558, 1977.
11. Anderson,E. S., Smith, H. R. Chloramphenicol resistance in the
    typhoid bacillus. Brit. Med. J. 3: 329-331, 1972.
12. Olarte, J., Galindo, E. Salmonella typhi resistant to chloramphe-
    nicol, ampicillin, and other antimicrobial agents: strains isola-
    ted during an extensive typhoid fever epidemic in Mexico. Antimi-
    crob. Ag. Chemother. 4: 597-601, 1973.
13. Bessudo, D. M., Olarte, J., Mendoza-Hernandez, P., Galindo, E.,
    Carrillo, J., Gutierrez-Trujillo, Kumate, J. Aislamiento de S.
    typhi resistente a altas concentraciones de cloranfenicol. Bol.
    Ofic. Sanit. Panamer. 64: 1-6, 1973.
14. Thorne, G. M., Farrar, W. E. Genetic properties of R factors
    associated with epidemic strains of Shigella dysenteriae type 1
    from Central America and Salmonella typhi from Mexico. J. Infect.
    Dis. 128: 132-136, 1973.

15. Gangarosa, E. J., Bennett, J. V., Wyatt, C., P.E. Pierce, Olarte, J., Mendoza-Hernandez, P., Vazquez, V. An epidemic-associated episome? J. Infect. Dis. 126: 215-218, 1972.
16. Alfaro, G., Martuscelli, J., Mendoza-Hernandez, P. Antibiotic resistance and phage-types of Salmonella typhi strains isolated in Mexico City. Rev. Lat-Amer. Microbiol. 20: 5-11, 1978.
17. Filloy, L., Borjas-Garcia, E. Epidemia por Salmonella poona (del Grupo G.) resistente a altas concentraciones de ampicilina, cloranfenicol y otros agentes antimicrobianos. Bol. Med. Hosp. Infant. 35: 355-359, 1978.
18. McConnell, M. M., Smith, H. R., Leonardopoulos, J., Anderson, E.S. The value of plasmid studies in the epidemiology of infections due to drug-resistant Salmonella wien. J. Infect. Dis. 139: 178-190, 1979.
19. Peluffo, C.A., Irino, K., Mello, S. Virulencia y multirresistencia a drogas de cepas epidemicas de S. typhimurium aisladas en hospitales infantiles de Sudamerica. Mem. Inst. Butantan. 38: 1-12, 1974.
20. Threlfall, E. J., Ward, L. R., Rowe, B. Spread of multiresistant strains of Salmonella typhimurium phage types 204 and 193 in Britain. Brit. Med. J. 2: 997, 1978.

TRIMETHOPRIM-RESISTANT BACTERIA IN HOSPITAL AND IN

THE COMMUNITY: SPREAD OF PLASMIDS AND TRANSPOSONS

Naomi Datta and Hilary Richards

Department of Bacteriology
Royal Postgraduate Medical School
Du Cane Road, London W12 0HS, England

INTRODUCTION

Trimethoprim is a very effective synthetic antibacterial drug
that was introduced for use in human and veterinary medicine about
10 years ago in Europe (7 years in the US). Until recently it has
been used always in conjunction with a sulfonamide. Trimethoprim
and sulfonamides act synergistically, at different points upon the
folic acid cycle of bacteria and using both drugs together should
prevent the emergence of resistant mutants[1]. Trimethoprim-sulfonamide preparations are effective against a wide range of bacteria
and have been extensively used in treating urinary, respiratory and,
to a lesser extent, gastrointestinal infections in hospitals and in
the community.

Combining trimethoprim with sulfonamide could not entirely
prevent the emergence of trimethoprim-resistance since resistance
to sulfonamides, often plasmid-determined[2] was already common.
Using trimethoprim-sulfonamide to treat infection caused by bacteria
highly resistant to sulfonamide is equivalent to treating the
infection with trimethoprim alone[3]. Laboratory-selected trimethoprim-resistant mutants are frequently thymine-requiring. Some
clinical isolates are of this kind while others show quantitative
or qualitative alterations in dihydrofolate reductase activity[4].

Although most published reports on trimethoprim resistance
refer to members of the Enterobacteriaceae, resistance in Staphylococcus aureus[5], S. albus[6], Streptococcus faecalis[5] and in occasional
strains of Haemophilus influenzae[7] has been noted.

Plasmids determining trimethoprim resistance were first

identified in 1972[8] and plasmid-mediated resistance permits normal
bacterial growth at high concentrations of trimethoprim. The
plasmids determine production of trimethoprim-insensitive dihydrofolate reductase (DHFR) that the bacterium uses when its native
enzyme is inhibited by the drug[9],[10]. Two types of plasmid-determined DHFR have been identified[11] and sometimes plasmid DHFR is
encoded by transposable DNA sequences[12],[13]. We have collected
bacteria from various sources and characterised trimethoprim-
resistance plasmids and transposons, the aim being to gain understanding of the routes of dissemination of the resistance genes.

MATERIALS AND METHODS

Sources of bacterial strains

     Three sets of urinary isolates of Escherichia coli were
tested: 1) 93 from schoolgirls taking part in a long-term study
of bacteriuria in schoolgirls, 1979-80[14]; 2) 187 from specimens
sent by general practitioners to the diagnostic laboratory,
Department of Bacteriology, Royal Postgraduate Medical School,
January-August 1980; and 3) 269 from inpatients in Hammersmith
Hospital, London, July and August 1980.

     The strains were identified by conventional biochemical methods
and tested for sensitivity using a disc diffusion method[15].

Plasmid transfer and characterization

     These were as described previously using E. coli Kl2 strain
J62-2 as primary recipient and the recA strains PB1150 and HH26[16],[17].

Tests for transposition of trimethoprim resistance

     1) Genetic analysis. Transposition was indicated if trimetho-
prim resistance was retained in E. coli Kl2 after a plasmid that
had carried it was eliminated during incompatibility tests or in
"curing" experiments. If the new locus was in the chromosome, this
was indicated by non-transmissibility of the resistance and lack of
plasmid bands after gel electrophoresis of lysates. A second transposition event could then be shown by introducing a conjugative
plasmid (without trimethoprim resistance) and retesting for transfer
of trimethoprim resistance. Transpostion to another plasmid, at the
first or second transposition event, was shown by linkage in transfer
experiments and by DNA analysis. Serial transfer from plasmid to
chromosome, chromosome to plasmid or plasmid to plasmid was looked
for in Rec+ or recA hosts.

     2) Restriction enzyme analysis. Having identified a transposon,
its mass was determined (from the increase in molecular weight upon

its acquisition by another plasmid) and its susceptibility to cutting by restriction enzymes (from the altered restriction pattern yielded by a plasmid upon its acquisition). Enzymes used were EcoR1 and HindIII, from BRI Inc. When Tn7 is digested with HindIII, two characteristic internal fragments (Fig. 1) can be recognised by their migration in gel electrophoresis.

For the purposes of this paper, we took transposition of trimethoprim-streptomycin/spectinomycin resistance, mass of DNA transposed and identification of the characteristic HindIII fragments, as evidence for the presence of Tn7 or a closely similar transposon, without testing each example for transpostion in a recA host. Methods for DNA extraction, digestion with enzymes and gel electrophoresis were as described by Datta et al[18].

Figure 1   Map of Tn7

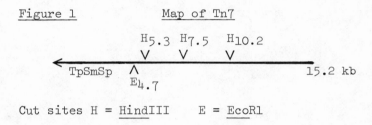

Cut sites H = HindIII   E = EcoR1

RESULTS

The incidence of trimethoprim-resistance in enterobacteria

1) In the community. Strains of E. coli isolated from urinary tract infections outside hospital are rarely trimethoprim-resistant. Table 1 shows our latest results of tests for sensitivity to ampicillin, sulfonamide and trimethoprim on E. coli strains from two groups of non-hospitalized people. Table 2 shows the trend over the last 2 decades for the sensitivity of comparable bacteria to ampicillin and trimethoprim.

Table 1.   Resistance to trimethoprim (Tp), sulfonamide (Su), and
           ampicillin (Ap) in urinary isolates of E. coli

Total resistant to	Numbers (%) from		
	Schoolgirls (Cardiff) 1979-80	General practice (Hammersmith) Jan-Aug 1980	Inpatients (Hammersmith) July-Aug 1980
Tp	0	3 (1.6)	27 (10.0)
Su	12 (12.9)	42 (22.5)	81 (30.1)
Ap	16 (17.2)	47 (25.1)	73 (27.1)
Sensitive to Tp Su Ap	75 (80.6)	122 (65.2)	157 (58.4)
Total	93 (100)	187 (100)	269 (100)
Combinations of resistance			
Tp	0	1 (0.5)	2 (0.7)
Su	2 (2.2)	17 (9.1)	31 (11.5)
Ap	6 (6.5)	22 (11.8)	25 (9.3)
SuTp	0	0	6 (2.2)
ApTpSu	0	2 (1.1)	15 (5.6)
ApTp	0	0	5 (1.5)
ApSu	10 (10.8)	23 (12.3)	29 (10.8)

All Tp-resistant strains, but not all Tp-sensitive ones, were
tested for sensitivity to a wide range of antibacterial drugs, not
shown here.

        2) In hospital. Trimethoprim resistance has been increasing
in frequency in hospital infections. Table 1 shows our results
for E. coli from urinary infections. When all enterobacteria from
all infected sites are included, the incidence of trimethoprim
resistance in the same hospital was 20%.

Table 2.   E. coli from urinary-tract infections in the
community

	Percentage resistant to:	
Year	ampicillin	trimethoprim
1960	0	0
1970	5	1
1980	25	1

Data, from refs. 19,20 and 21 and this paper, summarize
findings in several groups of patients in England and
Wales.

Trimethoprim-resistance plasmids

The first trimethoprim resistance plasmids were very uniform,
though found in a variety of bacterial species. They were of
incompatibility group W (IncW), had molecular masses of about 25
Md and determined resistance to sulfonamides(Su) and trimethoprim
(Tp) (example, R388). In a collection of trimethoprim-resistant
bacteria made in 1972 these were the only trimethoprim resistance
plasmids found. They were found only in bacteria isolated in London
hospitals: no trimethoprim resistance plasmids were detected in
isolates from other parts of England and Wales[22]. In several later
studies, plasmids of many different incompatibility groups carried
trimethoprim resistance (Table 3) and the resistance patterns were
different from the original TpSu. Bacteria carrying these plasmids
were nearly always sulfonamide-resistant but sulfonamide resistance
genes were not necessarily determined by the trimethoprim resistance
plasmids. Some plasmids, e.g. R751, carried no resistance except to
trimethoprim[24], others carried multiresistance e.g. pTH1[18].

Table 3.   Trimethoprim resistance plasmids: range of
Incompatibility (Inc) Groups

Year	Inc Groups found
1972	W
1980	W B C D I FII N P X

Data in refs. 16, 18, 22 and 23 and unpublished results.

Trimethoprim-resistance plasmids have usually been identified
in bacteria from environments where the drug is most used i.e. from
hospital patients and farm animals. Of the 27 trimethoprim E. coli
strains from hospital infections, listed in Table 1, 24 carried
trimethoprim resistance plasmids. Although resistance to trimethoprim is unusual in bacteria causing human infections outside hospital, when it does occur it is often plasmid-determined. From
urinary tract infections in the community, we had only 3 trimethoprim-resistant E. coli from a total of 280 (Table 1). In 2 of
the 3, the resistance was plasmid-borne.

Trimethoprim-resistance transposons

Two transposons carrying trimethoprim-resistance genes are
known, Tn7[12] and Tn402[13].

Tn7 determines a low level of resistance to streptomycin/
spectinomycin and a high level of trimethoprim resistance. It is
approximately 15 kilobases (kb) and a restriction map of it is
shown in Fig. 1. It transposes very readily e.g. if a plasmid
carrying Tn7 is transferred to E. coli K12 and then eliminated, a
high proportion (between 1% and 50%) of the "cured" clones still
carry the transposon, now integrated into the chromosome.

We have identified Tn7 in plasmids and chromosomes of many
naturally-occurring bacteria, isolated from man and animals. The
first example[12] came from E. coli from a calf that had been fed
large. doses of a trimethoprim-sulfonamide combination for experimental purposes. Later examples from farm animals were in E. coli[17]
and Salmonella[25]. Trimethoprim-sulfonamide combinations have been
extensively used in animals in England for both therapy and prophylactic purposes. Smith[26] has shown that an increasing proportion
of faecal E. coli from healthy market pigs carry trimethoprim resistance plasmids. We have examined 15 such plasmids (received from
H. W. Smith) and have positively identified Tn7 in 6 of them.

In hospital infections, Tn7 has been found in plasmids of
different genera[16,18] and also in the chromosomes of infecting
bacteria[18]. Of the 27 trimethoprim E. coli strains from hospital
infections (Table 1) trimethoprim resistance plasmids were identified
in 24 strains and 18 of these carried Tn7-like sequences.

In the two cases of plasmid-determined resistance in community
infections, Tn7 was identified in both. There was no epidemiological
connexion between the patients and the Tn7-bearing plasmids were
different in their resistance patterns and molecular masses.

Tn7 determines DHFR type I of Pattishall et al[11]. Tn402,
identified in plasmid R751[13,24], determines DHFR type II[27]. Tn402
transposes at a frequency too low to be detected in our studies,

but DHFR II is carried by naturally occurring plasmids of at least
four incompatibility groups[27], indirect evidence for the spread of
Tn402 in nature.

DISCUSSION

     Despite widespread use of trimethoprim-sulfonamide combinations,
trimethoprim-resistance is still uncommon (frequency 1%) in strains
of E. coli isolated from urinary tract infections in the community
outside hospitals. This is our finding in the new isolates described here; it confirms the experience of others[21],[28]. In the
same strains, the incidence of resistance to sulfonamides and to
ampicillin is higher (Table 1). The frequency of acquired resistance
to any antibacterial drug evidently depends upon various factors
among which are: 1) the ability of the bacteria to become resistant
by mutation, 2) access to a pool of resistance genes that may be
transferred from one bacterium to another and 3) the degree of
selection for resistance in the environment.

     In the case of trimethoprim, acquisition of resistance, by
mutation can be demonstrated in the laboratory[1] but during short
courses of therapy in man, infecting or commensal enterobacteria do
not commonly mutate to resistance. Lacey et al[6] studied the effects
of 5-day courses of trimethoprim-sulfonamide or of trimethoprim
alone upon the bacteria carried by 279 patients and found no trimethoprim-resistant Enterobacteriaceae. Resistant mutants of
Streptococcus faecalis, however, readily appear on exposure to
trimethoprim[5].

     During the use of long-term co-trimoxazole for the control of
intractable urinary infections, some strains of E. coli were found
that had become trimethoprim-resistant by mutation[29].

     Our research is concerned with the second factor determining
the incidence of resistance, the availability of a pool of plasmid
genes that may be acquired by contact with other, already-resistant
bacteria. The low incidence of trimethoprim-resistant E. coli in
urinary infections in the community indicates that this pool, in
the intestinal bacteria of people outside hospitals, is still small.
Had it been greater, resistant Enterobacteriaceae might have been
isolated from the patients studied by Lacey et al[6] after short-term
courses of therapy. From patients on long-term prophylaxis studied
by Pearson et al[29], strains of Enterobacteriaceae carrying trimethoprim resistance plasmids were isolated in a few cases. Here the
third factor was operative, there being strong selection for resistance when trimethoprim was taken for months rather than days.

     We have found transposons resembling, or identical with, Tn7
in plasmids of many incompatibility groups in bacteria of various
genera in a variety of environments in England i.e. in hospital

infections, in E. coli from urinary infections in the community, in salmonella from man and animals and in the normal intestinal E. coli of market pigs. Tn7 has been found in the chromosomes of naturally-occurring bacteria from which loci it transposes very readily, in the laboratory, to plasmids that did not previously carry trimethoprim-resistance. Tn402, though it does not transpose so readily in laboratory experiments, is found on a variety of naturally-occurring plasmids. These transposons possess a potential for world-wide dissemination. Such a thing has already happened with Tn1 and related transposons that determine resistance to penicillins, including ampicillin and carbenicillin, mediated by the TEM β-lactamase[30]. Tn1-related genes are carried by plasmids of many types and are now common in bacteria, isolated in all continents, and of many genera including all the Enterobacteriaceae, Pseudomonas aeruginosa, Haemophilus influenzae and Neisseria gonorrhoeae. The spread of Tn1-determined β-lactamase genes is largely responsible for the high incidence of ampicillin resistance in E. coli and other Enterobacteriaceae both in and out of hospitals (Tables 1 and 2). The very successful spread of this DNA element can be related to its facility in transposition and by heavy use of ampicillin in the treatment of many kinds of infections, trivial or severe. Trimethoprim resembles ampicillin in its wide spectrum of activity, low toxicity and convenient oral dosage. Until recently it has been used in combination with a sulfonamide but it is now available for use alone, in which form it is more acceptable to patients, having fewer unpleasant side-effects. Since neither Tn7 nor Tn402 determines sulfonamide resistance their dissemination may be favoured by use of trimethoprim alone.

The frequency of resistance acquired by gene transfer depends upon the extent of the pool of transmissible or transposable resistance genes and the selection of resistant bacteria depends upon use of the drug. With the use of trimethoprim alone, we should look for changes in these variables.

REFERENCES

1. S. R. M. Bushby, Combined antibacterial action in vitro of trimethoprim and sulfonamides. Postgrad. Med. J. 45:(Suppl) 10-16 (1969).

2. N. Datta, Drug resistance and R factors in the bowel bacteria of London patients before and after admission to hospital, Brit. med. J. 2:407-411 (1969).

3. R. N. Grüneberg, The use of co-trimoxazole in sulfonamide resistant Escherichia coli urinary tract infection, J. antimicrob. Chemother. 1:305-310 (1975).

4. J. M. T. Hamilton-Miller, Mechanisms and distribution of bacterial resistance to diaminopyrimidines and sulfonamides, J. antimicrob. Chemother. 5:(suppl. B) 61-73 (1979).

5. E. L. Lewis, and R. W. Lacey, Present significance of resistance
    to trimethoprim and sulfonamides in coliforms, Staphylo-
    coccus aureus and Streptococcus faecalis, J. Clin. Path.
    26:175-180 (1972).

6. R. W. Lacey, V. L. Lord, H. K. W. Gunasekera, P. J. Lieberman,
    and D. E. A. Luxton, Comparison of trimethoprim alone with
    trimethoprim-sulfamethoxazole in the treatment of respira-
    tory and urinary infections with particular reference to
    selection of trimethoprim resistance, Lancet 1:1270-1273
    (1980).

7. A. J. Howard, C. J. Hince, and J. D. Williams, Antibiotic
    resistance in Streptococcus pneumoniae and Haemophilus
    influenzae. Report of a study group on bacterial resis-
    tance, Brit. med. J. 1:1657-1660 (1978).

8. M. P. Fleming, N. Datta, and R. N. Grüneberg, Trimethoprim
    resistance determined by R factors, Brit. med. J. 1:726-
    728 (1972).

9. S. G. B. Amyes, and J. T. Smith, R-factor trimethoprim resis-
    tance mechanism: an insusceptible target site, Biochem.
    Biophys. Res. Commn. 58:412-418 (1974).

10. O. Sköld, and A. Widh, A new dihydrofolate reductase with low
    trimethoprim sensitivity induced by an R factor mediating
    high resistance to trimethoprim, J. biol. Chem. 249:4324-
    4325 (1974).

11. K. H. Pattishall, J. Acar, J. J. Burchall, F. W. Goldstein,
    and R. J. Harvey, Two distinct types of trimethoprim-resis-
    tant dihydrofolate reductase specified by R plasmids of
    different compatibility groups, J. biol. Chem. 252:2319-
    2323 (1977).

12. P. T. Barth, N. Datta, R. W. Hedges, and N. J. Grinter,
    Transposition of a deoxyribonucleic acid sequence encoding
    trimethoprim and streptomycin resistance from R483 to other
    replicons, J. Bact. 125:800-810 (1976).

13. J. A. Shapiro, and P. Sporn, Transposon Tn402: a new trans-
    posable element determining trimethoprim resistance that
    inserts into bacteriophage lambda, J. Bact. 129:1632-1635
    (1977).

14. A. W. Asscher, E. R. Verrier-Jones, K. Verrier-Jones,
    R. Mackenzie, and L. A. Williams, Bacteriologic follow-up
    of schoolgirls with untreated covert bacteruria, Kidney
    International 16:92 (1979).

15. E. J. Stokes, and P. M. Waterworth, Antibiotic sensitivity
    tests by diffusion methods, Association of Clinical
    Pathologists Broadsheet, 55:1-12, British Medical
    Association, London (1972).

16. N. Datta, S. Dacey, V. Hughes, S. Knight, H. Richards,
    G. Williams, M. Casewell, and K. P. Shannon, Distribution
    of genes for trimethoprim and gentamicin resistance in
    bacteria and their plasmids in a general hospital, J. gen.
    Microbiol. 118:495-508 (1980).

17. P. T. Barth, and N. Datta, Two naturally occurring transposons
     indistinguishable from Tn7, J. gen. Microbiol. 102:129-134
     (1977).
18. N. Datta, V. M. Hughes, M. E. Nugent, and H. Richards, Plasmids
     and transposons and their stability and mutability in bacteria
     isolated during an outbreak of hospital infection, Plasmid 2:
     182-196 (1979).
19. J. L. Harkness, F. M. Anderson, and N. Datta, R factors in
     urinary tract infection, Kidney International 8:S130-S133
     (1975).
20. R. N. Grüneberg, Susceptibility of urinary pathogens to various
     antimicrobial substances: a four year study, J. Clin. Path.
     29:292-295 (1976).
21. R. N. Grüneberg, Antibiotic sensitivities of urinary pathogens
     1971-1978, J. Clin. Path. 33:853-856 (1980).
22. N. Datta, and R. W. Hedges, Trimethoprim resistance conferred
     by W plasmids in Enterobacteriaceae, J. gen. Microbiol.
     72:349-356 (1972).
23. N. Datta, M. Nugent, S. G. B. Amyes, and P. McNeilly, Multiple
     mechanisms of trimethoprim resistance in strains of
     Escherichia coli from a patient treated with long-term
     co-trimoxazole, J. antimicrob. Chemother. 5:399-406 (1979).
24. R. S. Jobanputra, and N. Datta, Trimethoprim resistance factors
     in enterobacteria from clinical specimens, J. med. Microbiol.
     7:169-177 (1974).
25. H. Richards, N. Datta, C. Wray, and W. J. Sojka, Trimethoprim
     resistance plasmids and transposons in Salmonella, Lancet
     2:1194-1195 (1978).
26. H. W. Smith, Antibiotic-resistant Escherichia coli in market
     pigs in 1956-1979; the emergence of organisms with plasmid-
     borne trimethoprim resistance, J. Hyg., Camb. 84:467-477
     (1980).
27. M. E. Fling, and L. P. Elwell, Protein expression in Escherichia
     coli minicells containing recombinant plasmids specifying
     trimethoprim-resistant dihydrofolate reductase, J. Bact.
     141:779-785 (1980).
28. Anonymous, Bacterial resistance to trimethoprim, Brit. med. J.
     281:571-572 (1980).
29. N. J. Pearson, K. J. Towner, A. M. McSherry, W. R. Cattell,
     and F. O'Grady, Emergence of trimethoprim-resistant entero-
     bacteria in patients receiving long-term co-trimoxazole for
     the control of intractable urinary tract infection, Lancet
     2:1205-1209 (1979).
30. M. P. Calos, and J. H. Miller, Transposable elements: review,
     Cell 20:579-595 (1980).

ECOLOGICAL FACTORS THAT AFFECT THE SURVIVAL, ESTABLISHMENT, GROWTH

AND GENETIC RECOMBINATION OF MICROBES IN NATURAL HABITATS

G. Stotzky and V.N. Krasovsky

Department of Biology
New York University
New York, N.Y. 10003

Despite the remarkable advances in the isolation, analysis, reconstruction,and methods of introducing new genes into organisms, the ultimate fate of natural and manipulated genetic material is dependent on the survival, establishment, and growth of the organismal vectors (usually microbes) that house the genetic material in the natural habitats into which the vectors are introduced. Survival, establishment, and growth are, in turn, dependent on the genetic constitution of the microbes and on the physical (temperature, pressure, electromagnetic radiation, surfaces, spatial relations), chemical (carbonaceous substrates, ironganic nutrients, growth factors, ionic composition, available water, pH, oxidation-reduction potential, gaseous composition, toxicants), and biological (characteristics of and positive and negative interactions between microbes) factors of the various habitats (Fig. 1). Limitations of space preclude a detailed discussion of and an extensive bibliography to these ecological factors and to the genetical aspects of this report. Consequently, reference is made to reviews wherever possible.

The relative influence of these individual ecological factors differs with the recipient habitat and is usually greater on introduced than on indigenous microbes. Furthermore, none of these factors operates individually but in concert with numerous other factors, and although one or a few factors may be dominant in a specific habitat, their influences may have indirect, but cascading, effects on other characteristics. Consequently, an alteration in one environmental factor may result in simultaneous or subsequent changes in other factors, and ultimately, the habitat and the ability of both introduced microbes and of portions

HABITAT \ FACTOR	SUBSTRATES (carbon)	INORGANIC NUTRIENTS	GROWTH FACTORS	IONIC COMPOSITION	WATER	TEMPERATURE	PRESSURE	RADIATION (e-m spectrum)	GASEOUS COMPOSITION	pH	Eh (redox potential)	SURFACES (particulates)	SPATIAL RELATIONS	MAGNETIC FIELDS	TOXICANTS	CHARACTERISTICS OF ORGANISMS	POSITIVE INTERACTIONS	NEGATIVE INTERACTIONS	OTHERS
SOILS	x				x							x							
PLANTS		x						x											
ATMOSPHERE					x			x								x			
FRESH WATERS		x												x					
SALT WATERS							x	x											
ESTUARIES & SEASHORES				x					x										
WASTE WATERS (sewage)											x				x				
RUMEN & CECUM									x										
GASTROINTESTINAL TRACT											x	x							
GENITOURINARY TRACT											x								
RESPIRATORY TRACT																x			
ORAL CAVITY												x							
SKIN				x	x													x	
INSECTS & OTHER INVERTEBRATES									x										
FOODS						x			x										
PETROLEUM																			
MATÉRIELS					x														
INDUSTRIAL FERMENTATIONS									x	x						x			
LABORATORY					x											x			
OTHERS																			

Fig. 1.   Physical, chemical, and biological factors that affect the ecology of microorganisms in various habitats. For illustrative purposes, some of the dominant factors in some habitats have been indicated.

of the indigenous microbiota to survive are changed. Inasmuch
as the possible permutations of interactions between these environmental factors are essentially unlimited, the relative success of
microbes containing new genetic information to survive, establish
and grow in these natural habitats cannot be easily predicted.

The heightened activity in recombinant DNA technology increases
the probability that genetically engineered microbes will eventually
be introduced - either accidentally or deliberately - into natural
habitats, such as soils, waters, and sediments, which are the
major final repositories for all microbes. Inasmuch as such
microbes will contain new DNA sequences - some inadvertently inserted along with desired and, presumably, harmless sequences -
there are potential dangers to the health of plants and animals,
including humans, and to other aspects in the biosphere, especially
if such microbes are able to grow better in the recipient environment than the indigenous microbiota or the experimental parental
strains (1-5)and as even minor changes in a single biosynthetic
capability can apparently result in significantly increased growth
rates (6) and, hence, presumably in greater survival and colonization by introduced microbes. For example, will bacteria with an
acquired ability to fix N_2, coupled with existing capabilities
for rapid growth, efficient metabolism, and survival value in
natural habitats, reduce the N_2 content of the atmosphere, enhance
pollution of ground-waters with NO_3^-, and deplete the ozone layer
due to formation of NO_x from NO_3^- ? Will organisms engineered to
destroy oil-spills remain restricted to these spills or will they
spread and eventually also degrade petroleum products in the
refinery and the gas station, especially if they also acquired
other genes that will enhance their ability to survive in these
habitats?

The survival value of manipulated microbes in natural habitats
is presumably low and there should, therefore, be little danger of
their establishment and proliferation in natural habitats, and
some "constructed" host organisms are so auxotrophic and debilitated that they should "self-destruct" outside of enriched laboratory media (7). However, there have been few studies on the
survival of such microbes in natural habitats and on the ability
of debilitated recipients to acquire the genes from the natural
habitat into which they may be deposited that will reduce their
degree of auxotrophy and enhance their survival. There have
apparently been no studies on the influence of the physicochemical
characteristics of the recipient environment on the survival of
and the acquisition of genes by these microbes. These characteristics have major roles in determining the survival, establishment, and growth of both indigenous and introduced microorganisms
in natural habitats (8).

Most studies on genetic recombination in bacteria have been
conducted in vitro, and there are few data showing that gene
transfer occurs in situ. A few in vivo studies have been conducted with zxenic animals or with animals in which the normal
biota, usually of the intestinal tract, had been greatly reduced
or eliminated by antibiotic pretreatment, and these have focused
on conjugation, primarily R-factor transfer, as the mechanism of
gene transfer (9-32).

A few studies have investigated the transfer of R-factors in
non-animal habitats. Smith (33) showed that 373 strains from
435 strains of Escherichia coli that were isolated from 90 river
water samples in Great Britain and were resistant to chloramphenicol could transfer this resistance to F⁻ strains of E. coli K12,
and 179 of these strains were resistant to five or more antibiotics. Furthermore, 208 of these strains could also transfer
the resistance to chloramphenicol to Salmonella typhimurium.
Antibiotic-resistant bacteria containing conjugative R-factor
plasmids have also been isolated in sewage-impacted waters in
the United States (e.g., in the Hudson River, the new York Bight
(34,35(, and in Chesapeake Bay (36). Many of these strains contained plasmids that conferred resistance not only to antibiotics
but also to heavy metals (37) and to other antibacterial agents,
such as the algal product, chlorellin (38).

Transfer of R-factor genes by transduction has been demonstrated in Staphylococcus aureus (39-42) and in Pseudomonas
aeruginosa (43). Certain soil-borne bacteria (e.g., species of
Pseudomonas, Arthrobacter, and Acinetobacter) and some non-soil
bacteria (e.g., species of Klebsiella and Serratia) appear to be
evolving genetic competence, via plasmid transfer, for the utilization of a spectrum of aromatic hydrocarbons that were assumed
to be not only recalcitrant but also toxic to these organisms
(44-46). Furthermore, conjugation in vitro in soil-borne bacteria,
such as pseudomonads, has been demonstrated (47-49).

Although there is empirical evidence (i.e., increase in nosocomial infections by drug-resistant bacteria) to indicate that the
transfer of genes conferring resistance to antibiotics and heavy
metals occurs in natural habitats, there is little experimental
evidence to verify this, as most of these studies have been restricted to either isolating such resistant bacteria from natural
habitats or demonstrating the transfer and expression of such
genetic material under controlled laboratory conditions. Essentially no studies have attempted to bridge these experimental
extremes, probably because of the lack of both techniques to study
genetic recombination in natural habitats and interest on the part
of scientists trained in microbial genetics.

Both auxotrophic and prototrophic strains of E. coli K12 can survive, multiply, and conjugate in sterile soils (50). The presence of clay minerals, especially montmorillonite, increased the frequency of recombination, probably because clays enhance bacterial growth. This enhancement is due, in great part, to the ability of clays to buffer soils against changes in pH, which, in turn, is a function of the cation exchange capacity of the clays. Many of the mechanisms whereby clay minerals affect the survival, establishment, growth, and metabolic activities of microbes in natural habitats have been defined (8,51). Preliminary studies on conjugation in non-sterile soils have indicated that the frequency of recombination is significantly less than in sterile soils (Krasovsky and Stotzky, unpublished).

The decrease in frequency of recombination in non-sterile soils supports results obtained with the transfer of drug-resistance plasmids in an animal system (21,22). The frequency of transfer of a multiple drug-resistance plasmid from Salmonella typhosa to E. coli in the bladder of healthy rabbits was as high (and, in some instances, higher) as in in vitro systems containing either sterile urine or synthetic mating media. However, in the presence of other bacteria (exogens; i.e., Proteus mirabilis and non-conjugative E. coli), the frequency of transfer decreased significantly (Fig. 2). This decrease was not the result of a physical (i.e., steric) interference of the exogens in the conjugation process, as polystyrene latex particles of the same size and at the same concentration as the exogens had essentially no effect on the frequency of plasmid transfer, suggesting that the exogens caused a chemical interference with conjugation. Whether such interference was responsible for the lower frequencies of conjugation in non-sterile than in sterile soils is not known, but as a variety of species may be in close proximity in various natural microbial habitats (52-54), such interference could be possible.

The studies of conjugation in sterile soil also indicated that bacteria auxotrophic for different nutrients could co-exist, both in soil and on replica-plated agar media, by cross-feeding (syntrophism), rather than by having undergone genetic recombination (50). This observation emphasizes the need to investigate carefully both claims for apparent genetic recombination in natural habitats and the possibility that auxotrophs can survive in natural habitats, despite their apparent fragility and debilitation, if other microbes in the same habitat serve as commensals to provide the nutrients that the auxotrophs are incapable of synthesizing. Sagik and Sorber (55) indicated that such auxotrophs (e.g., the EK2 host, DP50supF) can survive in a nutrient-rich environment (i.e., a model sewage treatment plant). This survival appeared to be associated with the solid portion of the waste stream, again indicating that particulates and the resultant

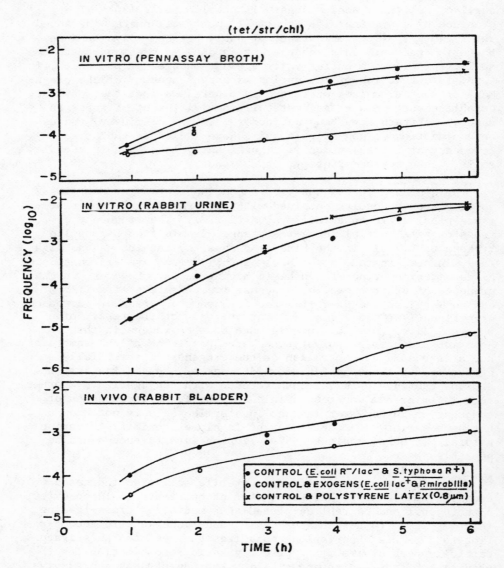

Fig. 2.   Frequency of transfer of a plasmid conferring resistance
          to tetracycline, streptomycin, and chloramphemicol from
          Escherichia coli to Salmonella typhosa in vivo and in
          vitro, in the presence and absence of Proteus mirabilis
          and a non-conjugative E. coli or polystyrene latex parti-
          cles (ref. 21,22).

increases in surface area enhance the growth and survival of bacteria (8,51). Furthermore, cometabolism or "shared" detoxification" of inhibitors can contribute to the survival of toxin-sensitive microbes in the absence of any genetic recombination (54,56,57,58).

There is little documentation that transformation occurs in natural microbial habitats (4,5,59,60). Although this lack of information is a reflection primarily of the paucity of studies on transformation in situ, it may also reflect an unsubstantiated concept; namely, that "naked" DNA is very susceptible to enzymic degradation in natural habitats. However, Greaves and Wilson (61,62) have indicated that nucleic acids adsorb to clay minerals in soil, especially to montmorillonite, and that this sorption provides protection to the nucleic acids against enzymic degradation. Similarly, viruses, proteins, peptides, and amino acids adsorbed to clays are protected to various degrees against microbial degradation (8,51). Consequently, both naked DNA (involved in transduction) may persist in natural habitats in the absence of an appropriate host.

This apparent protection against degradation of soluble organics and of viruses as a result of adsorption to clay minerals is an important consideration in any potential genetic exchange in habitats containing clays and, probably, other surface-active particulates. It might be expected that transforming DNA and transducing viruses would not long survive in natural habitats in the absence of hosts and be rapidly degraded by the indigenous microbiota, as nucleic acids and viruses should be ideal substrates for non-host microbes (i.e., they contain C, N, and P and, in the case of viruses, also S). However, evidence is accumulating that DNA and viruses persist in natural habitats as a result of being adsorbed to clay minerals, which protects against both physicochemical and biological inactivation. Furthermore, this adsorption does not reduce the catalytic activity of enzymes (in fact, it may increase it (8); or the ability of viruses to infect their hosts (51,63-65). Consequently, if viruses and transforming DNA (no studies have apparently been conducted on the transforming ability of adsorbed DNA) persist in natural habitats, it is possible that their genetic information could eventually be transmitted to any suitable host that may be introduced, inadvertently or deliberately, into these habitats.

The survival and subsequent establishment of microbes that are not inhabitants of a particular habitat have been sporadically studied; e.g., the survival of enteric bacteria (including E. coli, Salmonella sp., Shigella sp) that could be introduced into soils and waters by wastewater or sludge applications (66-68) and of Listeria monocytogenes (69) and Clostridium botulinum (70).

These studies have generally indicated that soil and natural
waters are not particularly hospitable habitats for these microbes,
although there are reports of some exceptions, especially when
these habitats have been carefully examined (71). Although many
of the bacterial species currently used in recombinant DNA technology are not normal inhabitants of soil and water and, therefore, do not survive long in these habitats, the spectrum of
organisms that are increasingly being used include species that
are indigenous to these habitats. No data are apparently available
on the ability of introduced microbes to transfer genetic information to indigenous microbes in various natural habitats and vice
versa, although this is, obviously, a very important consideration
in the survival of genetically manipulated microbes and of their
genetic informati-n in such habitats.

When survival, establishment, and subsequent growth of introduced microbes have occurred, some physiochemical factor has
usually been implicated. For example, the establishment of
Fusarium oxysporum f. cubense, the causal agent of Fusarium wilt
of banana, in soils (more than 140) throughout the banana growing
areas of the world was correlated with the absence in these soils
of a specific clay jineral that had the characteristics of montmorillonite. Similarly, Histoplasma capsulatum, a fungus pathogenic to humans and which has a discrete geographic distribution,
was isolated essentially only from soils (131 from 134 soils)
that did not contain this clay mineral. Preliminary studies
with some other fungal pathogens of humans (e.g., Cryptococcus
neoformans, Blastomyces dermatitidis) showed similar patterns,
although the geographic distribution of Coccidioides immitis
appeared not to be correlated with the clay mineralogy but
rather with the salinity of the soils (8). Introduction of these
fungi into the habitat was not the limiting factor for their subsequent growth and survival (e.g., healthy banana plantations
were routinely irrigated with surplus waters from diseased plantations; birds and bats, the presumed spreading vectors of H.
capsulatum, defecate everywhere), but rather, the limiting factor
was their establishment as members of the soil microbiota.

Studies on various levels of experimental complexity have
shown that clay minerals affect the establishment and growth of
fungi in soil primarily by influencing the activities of indigenous bacteria, which, in turn, exert a biological control on
the fungi (8). Furthermore, competition between bacteria and
fungi in soil and other habitats is mediated by pH, osmotic
pressure, nutrient levels, oxygen content, and toxicants, and
the types of clay minerals present modulate the effects of these
physicochemical factors (8,37,51,72,73).

Consequently, clay minerals, as only one example of an

ecological factor, have a major role in the establishment and
growth of microbes, in the survival of viruses, in the persistence
of readily degradable organics, and in the genetic recombination
in bacteria in habitats that contain clays. The pH, which is an
important factor in genetic recombination _in vitro_ (74-77), also
appears to affect genetic recombination in soil (Fig. 3), and the
effect of pH, in turn, is modified by the buffering capacity of
different clays (8).

These interactions are indicative of how individual ecological
factors can influence other factors, which, in turn, can affect
a spectrum of microbial events in natural habitats.

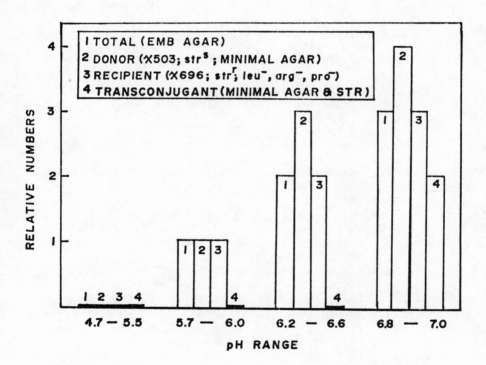

Fig. 3.   Effect of pH on survival and growth of auxotrophic and
          prototrophic strains of _Escherichia coli_ and on their
          conjugation in soil (Krasovsky and Stotzky, unpublished).

REFERENCES

1. Harder, W., Kuenen, J.G., and Matin, A., 1977, J. Appl. Bacteriol., 43: 1-24.
2. Veldkamp, H., and Jannasch, H.W., 1972, J. Appl. Chem. Biotech., 22: 105-123.
3. Konings, W.N., and Veldkamp, H., 1980, in: "Contemporary Microbial Ecology," D.C. Ellwood, J.N. Hedger, M.J. Latham, J.M. Lynch, and J.H. Slater, eds., Academic Press, London, pp. 161-191.
4. Graham, J.B., and Istock, C.A., 1978, Molec. Gen. Genet., 166: 287-290.
5. Graham, J.B., and Istock, C.A., 1979, Science, 204: 637-639.
6. Mason, T.G., and Slater, J.H., 1979, Antonie van Leeuwenhoek J. Microbiol. Serol., 45: 253-263.
7. Curtiss, R., Inoue, M., Pereira, D., Hsu, J.C., Alexander, L., and Rock, L., 1977, in: "Molecular Cloning of Recombinant DNA", W.A. Scott, and R. Werner, Eds., Academic Press, New York, pp. 99-114.
8. Stotzky, G., 1972, Crit. Rev. Microbiol., 2: 59-137.
9. Schneider, H., Formal, S.B., and Baron, L.S., 1961, J. Exp. Med. 114: 141-148.
10. Ottolenghi, E., and Macleod, C.M., 1963, Proc. Natl. Acad. Sci. U.S., 50: 417-419.
11. Kasuya, M., 1964, J. Bacteriol., 88: 322-328.
12. Guinee, P.A.M., 1965, Antonie van Leeuwenhoek J. Microbiol. Serol., 31: 314-321.
13. Walton, J.R., 1966, Nature, 211: 312-313.
14. Anderson, E.S., 1968, Annu. Rev. Microbiol., 22: 131-180.
15. Anderson, E.S., 1975, Nature 255: 502-504.
16. Salzman, T.C., and Klemm, L. 1968, Proc. Soc. Exp. Biol. Med., 128: 392-394.
17. Jones, R.T., nad Curtiss, R., 1969, Bacteriol. Proc., 66-67.
18. Reed, N.D., Siekman, D.G., and Georgi, C.E., 1969, J. Bacteriol., 100: 22-26.
19. Jarolmen, H., and Kemp, G., 1969, J. Bacteriol., 99: 487-490.
20. Jarolmen, H., 1971, Ann. N.Y. Acad. Sci., 182: 72-79.
21. Richter, M.W., Stotzky, G., and Amsterdam, D., 1973a, Abstr. Ann. Mtng. Amer. Soc. Microbiol., p. 85.
22. Richter, M.W., Stotzky, G., and Amsterdam, D., 1973b, Proc. 1st Internatl. Cong. Bacteriol., Jerusalem, p. 275.
23. Smith, H.W., 1971, Ann. N.Y. Acad. Sci., 182: 80-90.
24. Smith, H.W., 1975, Nature, 255: 500-502.
25. Anderson, J.D., 1973, J. Med. Microbiol., 6: xix.
26. Smith, M.G., 1975, J. Hyg., 75: 363-370.
27. Smith, M.G., 1976, Nature, 261: 348.
28. Falkow, S., 1975, "Infectious Multiple Drug Resistance", Pion Ltd., London.
29. Reanney, D., 1976, Bacteriol. Rev., 40: 552-590.
30. Reanney, D., 1977, Bioscience, 27: 340-344.

31. Reanney, D., 1978, in: "Genetic Interaction and Gene Transfer", Brookhaven Symp. Biol., 39: 248-271.
32. Gyles, C., Falkow, S., & Robbins, L., 1978, Am. J. Vet. Res., 39: 1438-1441.
33. Smith, H.W., 1970, Nature 228: 1286-1288.
34. Sturtevant, A.B., Jr., and Feary, T., 1968, Appl. Microbiol, 18: 918-924.
35. Timoney, J.R., Port, J., Giles, J., and Spanier, J., 1978, Appl. Environ. Microbiol., 36: 465-472.
36. Austin, B., Allen, D.A., Mills, A.L., and Colwell, R.R., 1977, Can. J. Microbiol., 23: 282-288.
37. Babich, H., and Stotzky, G., 1980, Crit. Rev. Microbiol., 8: 99-145.
38. Grabow, W.O.R., Middendorf, I.G., and Prozeksy, O.W., 1973, Water Res., 7: 1589-1597.
39. Novick, R.P., 1963, J. Gen Microbiol. 33: 121-136.
40. Novick, R.P., and Bouanchaud, D., 1971, Ann. N.Y. Acad. Sci., 182: 279-294.
41. Novick, R.P., and Morse, S.I., 1967, J. Exp. Med., 125: 45-59.
42. Novick, R.P., and Roth, C., 1968, Bacteriol. Proc., A12.
43. Morrison, W.D., Miller, R.V. and Sayler, G.S., 1978, Appl. Environ. Microbiol., 36: 724-730.
44. Chakrabarty, A.M., 1976, Annu. Rev. Genet., 10: 7-30.
45. Chakrabarty, A.M., 1978, ASM News, 44: 687-690.
46. Jacoby, G.A., Rogers, J.E., Jacob, A.E., and Hedges, R.W., 1978, Nature, 274: 179-180.
47. Holloway, B.W., 1969, Bacteriol. Rev., 33: 419-443.
48. Holloway, B.W., 1979, Plasmid, 2: 1-19.
49. Hedges, R.W., and Jacob, A.E., 1977, Fed. Europ. Microbiol. Soc. Microbiol. Letters, 2: 15-19.
50. Weinberg, S.R., and Stotzky, G., 1972, Soil Biol. Biochem. 4: 171-180.
51. Stotzky, G., 1981, in: "Microbial Adhesion to Surfaces", P.R. Rutter, ed., Harwood, London (in press).
52. Meers, J.L., 1973, Crit. Rev. Microbiol., 2: 139-184.
53. Slater, J.H., and Bull, A.T., 1978, in:"Companion to Microbiology", A.T. Bull and P.M. Meadow, eds., Longmans, London, pp. 181-201.
54. Slater, J.H., and Godwin, D., 1980, in: "Contemporary Microbial Ecology", D.C. Ellwood, J.N. Hedger, M.J. Latham, J.M. Lynch, and J.H. Slater, eds., Academic Press, London pp. 137-161.
55. Sagik, B., and Sorber, C.A., 1979, Recombinant DNA Bull, 2: 55-61. (also 1978 report).
56. Senior, E., Bull, A.T., and Slater, J.H., 1976, Nature 263: 476-479.
57. Daughton, C.G., and Hsieh, D.P.H., 1977, Appl. Environ. Microbiol., 34: 175-184.

58. Slater, J.H., and Somerville, H.J., 1979, in: "Microbial
     Technology: Current Status and Future Prospects, A.T. Bull,
     C.R. Ratledge, and D.C. Ellwood, eds., Cambridge University
     Press, pp. 221-261.
59. Conant, J.E., and Sawyer, W.D., 1967, J. Bacteriol., 93:
     1869-1875.
60. Saunders, J.R., 1979, Nature, 278: 601-602.
61. Greaves, M.P., and Wilson, M.J., 1970, Soil Biol. Biochem.
     2: 257-268.
62. Greaves, M.P., and Wilson, M.J., 1973, Soil Biol. Biochem.
     5: 275-276.
63. Bystricky, V., Stotzky, G., and Schiffenbauer, M., 1975, Can.
     J. Microbiol., 21: 1278-1282.
64. Duboise, S.M., Moore, B.E., Sorber, C.A., and Sagik, B.P.,
     1979, Crit. Rev. Microbiol., 7: 245-285.
65. Stotzky, G., Schiffenbauer, M., Lipson, S.M., and Yu, B.H.,
     1981, in: "Viruses and Wastewater Treatment", M. Goddard
     and M. Butler, eds., Pergamon Press, Oxford (in press).
66. Rudolfs, W., Falk, L.L., and Rogotzkie, R.A., 1950, Sewage
     Ind. Wastes, 22: 1261-1281.
67. Glathe, H., Knoll, K.H., and Makawi, A.A.M., 1963a, Z.
     Pflanz. Dung. Bodenk., 100: 142-147.
68. Glathe, H., Knoll, K.H., and Makawi, A.A.M., 1963b, Z.
     Pflanz. Dung. Bodenk., 100: 224-229.
69. Welshimer, H.J., 1960, J. Bacteriol., 80: 316-321.
70. Wentz, M.W., Scott, R.A., and Wennes, J.W., 1967. Science
     155: 89.
71. Alexander, M., 1971, "Microbial Ecology", Wiley, New York.
72. Rosenzweig, W.D., and Stotzky, G., 1979, Appl. Environ.
     Microbiol., 38: 1120-1126.
73. Rosenzweig, W.D., and Stotzky, G., 1980, Appl. Environ.
     Microbiol., 39: 354-360.
74. Jacob, F., Brenner, S., and Cuzin, F., 1963, Cold Spring
     Harbor Symp. Quant. Biol., 28: 329-348.
75. Wollman, E.L., Jacob, F., and Hayes, W., 1962, Cold Spring
     Harbor Symp. Quant. Biol., 21: 141-162.
76. Curtiss, R., 1969, Annu. Rev. Microbiol., 23: 69-136.
77. Curtiss, R., Charamella, L.J., Stallions, D.R., and Mays,
     J.A., 1968, Bacteriol. Rev., 32: 320-348.

EPIDEMIOLOGY AND GENETICS OF HEMOLYSIN FORMATION IN ESCHERICHIA COLI

Werner Goebel, Angelica Noegel, Ursula Rdest, Dorothee Müller and Colin Hughes

Institut fur Genetik und Mikrobiologie der Universität Würzburg
West Germany

Hemolysins or cytolysins are extracellular toxic proteins that disrupt the membranes of erythrocytes and other differentiated eucaryotic cells.[1] Most hemolysins seem to have little or no effect on procaryotic cells. The hemolytic phenotype is frequently associated with pathogenic strains of a given bacterial species. There is clear evidence for the involvement in pathogenesis for cytolysins in Gram-positive pathogenic bacteria, such as streptolysins produced by Streptococcus pyogenes, α-, β-, γ- and δ-toxins from Staphylococcus aureus, θ-toxin from Clostridium perfringens, listeriolysins from Listeria monocytogenes and others.[1] These toxins all of which can be considered as hemolysins disrupt eucaryotic membranes by different modes of action, which are only partially understood. Whereas some cytolysins act as enzymes, like the staphylococcal β-toxin which is a sphingomyelinase,[2] others like the "SH-activated cytotoxins" including streptolysin O, C. perfringens θ-toxin, cereolysin (Bacillus cereus) and listeriolysin disrupt eucaryotic membranes by a non-enzymatic mode of action, using probably cholesterol as receptor.[3]

Hemolytic strains are also found in Gram-negative bacteria, especially in Escherichia coli, Proteus morganii and Pseudomonas aeruginosa. The significance of these hemolysins in pathogenesis, however, is still controversial and based on more circumstantial evidence.[4-6] Whereas only a small percentage of E. coli strains isolated from the intestines of healthy individuals or patients suffering from acute diarrhoea are hemolytic, E. coli strains with the capability of producing hemolysin are frequently occurring in extra-intestinal infections. E. coli strains are frequently causing urinary tract infections and a high percentage of these E. coli

strains are hemolytic as already observed by Dudgeon in 1921 and
reconfirmed by several other groups (Table 1). There is still some
debate whether or not there is a correspondence between faecal E.
coli strains and E. coli strains found in urinary tract infections.
It appears, however, that certain E. coli 0-serotypes, especially
04 and 06 are more frequently encountered in urinary tract infections than others and again most 04 and 06 E. coli isolates are
hemolytic.[6] This seems to support the suggestion that these two
serotypes may be especially pathogenic for the urinary tract and
that hemolysin may be a special virulence factor. Hemolytic E.
coli strains are also frequently occurring in other extra-intestinal
infections, such as peritonitis, appendicitis or bacteremias.[6,7]
No correlation, on the other hand, has been found between hemolysin
and enterotoxin production and there is no evidence for an association of hemolysin production and colonization factors, such as CFAI
or II.[8,9] Transmissible plasmids have been found to determine
hemolysin production in many faecal hemolytic E. coli strains from
human and animal sources. On the contrary, most hemolytic E. coli
strains from extra-intestinal infections do not seem to carry
plasmids connected to hemolysin production. A large number of Hly-
plasmids have been isolated and characterized.[10-14] Their molecular
weights range from 40 to 93 x 10^6 daltons; they are transmissible
and most of them belong to rather rare incompatibility groups, such
as incI2, incFIII, IV and VI (Table 2). There is circumstantial
evidence that the Hly determinant may move between various plasmids
residing in the same bacterial cell and, as shown later, there are
Hly plasmids which share only the hemolysin determinant as common
sequence.

Table 1. Frequency of Occurrence of Hemolytic E. coli

Origin	No. Hemolytic/ No. Tested	%	Reference
Stool	8/100	7.3	DeBoy et al.(1980)
Blood	7/ 14	50.0	"
Urine	4/ 20	35.0	"
Misc. Wounds	8/ 23	34.8	"
Blood	18/ 51	35.0	Minshew et al.(1978)
Urine	29/ 59	49.0	"
Sputum	2/ 5	40.0	"
Miscellaneous	16/ 27	59.0	"
Stool			
EEC	0/ 9	0	"
Normal	1/ 20	5.0	"
Urine	26/59	44.4	our data
Stool	2/39	5.0	"

Plasmid-determined hemolysin of E. coli is secreted apparently
through both membranes since most of it appears in the mid-
logarithmic growth phase in the supernatant from where it can be
isolated as a protein with a molecular weight of about 60,000
daltons. In addition, internal active hemolysin is found which can
be chased into the extracellular pool[15] suggesting that it represents hemolysin en route to secretion.

By mutagenizing hemolytic E. coli cells with nitrosoguanidine,
we obtained two types of hemolysis-negative mutants, those which do
not synthesize any active hemolysin and those which still produce
active internal hemolysin that is not secreted. Similar mutants
were obtained by transposon mutagenesis with the ampicillin transposon Tn3. These mutations have been mapped on the Hly plasmid
pHly152.[16] Tn3 insertions leading to a complete loss of hemolysin
activity map within a region of about 3500 bp (Fig. 1), whereas
insertions causing a defect of the extracellular transport of
hemolysin map immediately to the right in a region of about 1500 bp
(Fig. 1). Recombinant plasmids with either EcoRI-F or HindIII-E
inserted into pACYC184 are able to complement hemolysin-negative
Tn3 mutants with Tn3 insertions located in the first 500 bp of the
5000 bp region. Both of these restriction fragments cover the left
part of the hemolysis region (Fig. 1). Tn3 mutants with impaired
transport functions for hemolysin, all of which carry the Tn3
insertions in the right 1500 bp region covered by EcoRI-G, can be
complemented to full extracellular hemolysin production by a recombinant DNA carrying this fragment. The other hemolysin-negative
mutants with Tn3 insertions in the middle 3000 bp part of the
hemolysis region are complemented by recombinant DNA carrying a
Bam-Sal fragment, which includes a large part of the whole hemolysis region. Cloning of this part of the hemolysis determinant
proved to be difficult and was only possible with the aid of the
vector plasmid p31 (J. Hedgpeth, personal communication) which
allows the insertion of the Bam-Sal fragment into a site of very

Table 2.   Plasmids from Hemolytic E. coli Strains

Plasmid	M.W. (x10^6 dalton)	Inc Group	Source	Reference
pHly152	40	I2	Mouse	Goebel et al.(1974)
pHly167	40	I2	Pig	"
pHly20	42	I2	Pig	"
pHly-P212	ND	FVI	Pig	Monti-Bragadin (1975)
MIP240	ND	FIII	Human	LeMinor et al.(1976)
MIP241	ND	I2	Human	"
pSU316	48	FIII/IV	Human	DelaCruz et al.(1980)
pSU5	93	Iα/I2	Pig	"
pSU105	77	FVI	Pig	"
pSU233	60	?	Pig	"

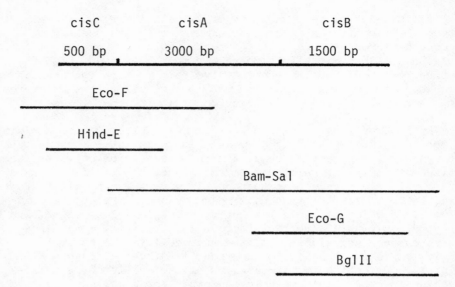

Fig. 1.   Schematic presentation of the hemolysis region which con-
          sists of three cistrons, C, A and B.   These cistrons are
          defined by Tn3 insertions leading to different hemolysis-
          negative mutants and their complementation be recombinant
          plasmids carrying the restriction fragments listed below.

low transcription activity (Fig. 2).   Increased gene expression of
this part of the hemolysis region is lethal to the cell as demonstrated by the following experiment.   A BglII fragment carrying the
λcI_{857} gene together with the left (P_L) and the right (P_R) promoters
of phage λ was inserted in front of the Bam-Sal fragment (Fig. 3)
of the recombinant DNA p31-2, thus allowing an induced transcription
of the genetic information of the inserted Bam-Sal fragment at
elevated temperature (42°C).   Whereas E. coli cells carrying this
new recombinant plasmid (p31-2cI) grow normally at 30-35°C, no
growth occurs anymore upon a shift of the temperature to 42°C.   The
rate of survivors after 1 hr treatment of these cells at 42°C is
less than one in 10^5 cells.   The removal of the right part of the
Bam-Sal fragment by deleting the BglII fragment of p31-2cI (Fig. 3)
does not eliminate the killing activity at 42°C, indicating that
the region between the Bam and the BglII site is responsible for
the lethal effect.   Whereas neither p31-2cI nor p31-2cI BglII$_{del}$
determine extracellular hemolysin (intracellular hemolysin activity
is, however, observed in E. coli cells harboring these plasmids),
extracellular hemolysin is secreted when cells carrying the plasmid
p31-2cI are complemented with recombinant DNAs having either EcoRI-F
or HindIII-E inserted into pACYC184.   Cells carrying this combination

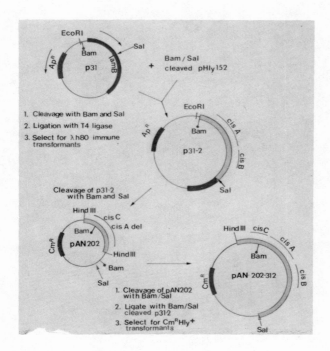

Fig. 2. Construction of recombinant plasmids carrying either cisA
and cisB (p31-2) or the whole hemolysis determinant, i.e.
cisC, cisA and cisB (pAN202-312).

of plasmids are still killed at 42°C. Under these conditions a
large amount of extracellular hemolysin is produced.

The complementation data described suggest that the hemolysis
region consists of three cistrons (Fig. 1), which are determining
synthesis and transport of hemolysin. Recently we succeeded in the
construction of a recombinant plasmid, which carries the whole
hemolysis determinant inserted into pACYC184 (Fig. 3). In spite of
the high copy number of this plasmid, pAN202-312, cells harboring
it synthesize and secrete roughly the same amount of external and
internal hemolysin as cells carrying the single copy wild-type
plasmid pHly152. This may indicate a rather tight control of the
expression of the hemolysis determinant, which seems to occur from
a single promoter transcribing all three cistrons from left to
right (i.e. cisC → cisB).

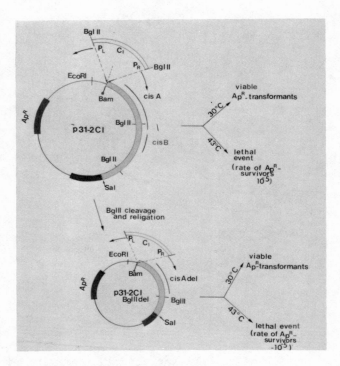

Fig. 3.   Construction of recombinant plasmids which carry the
          promoter P_R and P_L together with the cI gene of phage λ
          in front of cisA.

        Hemolysis is not a very specific reaction and it is conceivable
that different extracellular proteins may be causing the hemolytic
phenotype in hemolytic E. coli strains.   There are reports on
different hemolysins in E. coli.[4] We therefore carried out hybridization studies with the cloned hemolysis determinant of plasmid
pHly152 and various Hly plasmids of faecal hemolytic E. coli strains
and the chromosomal DNA of hemolytic E. coli strains from extra-
intestinal infections.   All plasmids tested hybridize well with
radioactive DNA probes carrying cisC, A or B of pHly152, indicating
that these plasmid-inherited hemolysin determinants are alike if
not identical.   There are, however, remarkable differences in the
overall hybridization between the standard Hly plasmid pHly152 and
the other Hly plasmids (Table 3).   Four Hly plasmids all of which
belong to the incompatibility group incI2 share sequence homologies
extending far beyond the hemolysis determinant.   Others have only
little sequence homologies besides the common hemolysis determinant
(Table 3).   There appears to be a rather defined right end of the

hemolysis determinant (at the cisB side) in all Hly plasmids, whereas the left end (at the cisC side) varies to a much larger extent in these plasmids.[17]

Chromosomally determined hemolysin from extra-intestinal E. coli isolates has similar biochemical properties as the plasmid-determined hemolysin from faecal strains. Besides, similar hemolysis-negative mutants can be isolated from these hemolytic E. coli strains, i.e. those that produce no active hemolysin and those that produce internal hemolysin only. This suggests that the chromosomal Hly determinant has a similar genetic complexity as the plasmid Hly determinant. Hybridization of chromosomal DNA from three such hemolytic strains with the plasmid Hly determinant is considerably lower than that of total DNA from plasmid-determined hemolytic strains with the same probe. A more detailed hybridization study indicates that a fragment carrying cisB of plasmid-encoded Hly determinant shows strong hybridization, one with cisC still shows some hybridization, but a fragment with cisA shows little or no hybridization with DNA of hemolytic E. coli possessing chromosomal Hly determinants. The hybridization data are supported by the recent observation that the chromosomal Hly determinant can complement plasmid-coded cisC and cisB but not cisA mutants. Thus it appears that plasmid- and chromosome-inherited Hly determinants may share two common cistrons (cisB and cisC), but cisA which seems to code for the hemolysin protein itself is entirely different in both determinants suggesting possibly different functions of these two types of hemolysins.

Table 3. Hybridization of different Hly Plasmids with the Hly-Determinant of pHly152

Plasmid	Hybridization with cisC	cisA	cisB	Hybridization Outside of the Hly Determinant
pHly167 incI2	+	+	+	100%
pHly20 incI2	+	+	+	>90%
pHly124 incI2	+	+	+	~70%
pSU5 incI2/Iα	+	+	+	~50%
pSU233 —	+	+	+	~15%
pSU105 incFVI	+	+	+	~ 8%
pSU316 incFIII/IV	+	+	+	< 5%

References

1. T. Wadstrom, in: "Bacterial Toxins and Cell Membranes," J.
    Jeljaszewicz and T. Wadström, eds., Academic Press, London
    (1978).
2. M. Rogolsky, Microbiol. Rev. 43:320 (1978).
3. C.J. Smyth and J.L. Duncan, in: "Bacterial Toxins and Cell
    Membranes," J. Jeljaszewicz and T. Wadstrom, eds., Academic
    Press, London (1978).
4. J. Jorgensen et al., J. Med. Microbiol. 9:173 (1976).
5. B.H. Minshew, J. Jorgensen, G.W. Counts, and S. Falkow, Infect.
    Immun. 20:50 (1978).
6. J.M. DeBoy, J.K. Wachsmuth, and B.R. Davis, J. Clin. Microbiol.
    12:193 (1980).
7. E.M. Cooke, J. Path. Bacteriol. 95:101 (1968).
8. D.G. Evans, D.J. Evans, W.S. Tjoa, and H.L. DuPont, Infect.
    Immun. 19:727 (1978).
9. D.G. Evans and D.J. Evans, Infect. Immun. 21:638 (1978).
10. W. Goebel and H. Schrempf, J. Bacteriol. 106:311 (1971).
11. W. Goebel, B. Royer-Pokora, W. Lindenmaier, and H. Bujard, J.
    Bacteriol. 118:964 (1974).
12. S. LeMinor and E. LeCoueffic, Ann. Microbiol. (Paris) 126:313
    (1975).
13. C. Monti-Bragadin, L. Samer, G.D. Rottini, and B. Pani, J. Gen.
    Microbiol. 86:367 (1975).
14. F. De la Cruz, J.C. Zabala, and J.M. Ortiz, Plasmid 2:507
    (1979).
15. W. Springer and W. Goebel, J. Bacteriol. 144:53 (1980).
16. A. Noegel, U. Rdest, and W. Goebel, J. Bacteriol. (in press).
17. F. De la Cruz, D. Müller, J.M. Ortiz, and W. Goebel, J.
    Bacteriol. 143:825 (1980).

CHROMOSOMAL AND PLASMID-MEDIATED TRANSFER OF CLINDAMYCIN RESISTANCE

IN BACTEROIDES FRAGILIS

F.P. Tally[1], M.J. Shimell[1], G.R. Carson[2] and M.H. Malamy[2]

[1]Department of Medicine and [2]Department of Molecular
Biology and Microbiology, Tufts University School of
Medicine, Boston, MA 02111

ABSTRACT

The characteristics of the clindamycin-erythromycin (clin[r])
resistance transfer factor from Bacteroides fragilis TMP 10 are
presented. Transfer ability and the determinant for clin[r] are
found on a 15.6 kilobase plasmid named $_p$BFTM 10. Recent clindamycin and tetracycline resistant strains of Bacteroides fragilis
have been isolated in Chicago. The Chicago tet[r] isolate, TMP 230,
transfers both clin[r] and tet[r], but appears to be plasmid free when
tested by standard methods. Homology between the clin[r] transfer
factor pBFTM 10 and the chromosome of the TMP 230 could be demonstrated by the Southern hybridization technique. The location of
the clin[r] determinant on the chromosome and mode of transfer are
under invistigation.

Anaerobic bacteria are prominent members of the normal flora
of man; in the colon anaerobic organisms including Bacteroides,
Clostridia and non-sporing, gram-positive bacilli outnumber facul-
tative bacteria such as E. coli and Streptococcus fecaelis by
about 1000:1 (1). Over the past 20-25 years anaerobic bacteria
have been increasingly recognized as important pathogens in human
suppurative infections (2). Bacteroides fragilis emerges as the
most important anaerobic bacterium in abdominal, surgical and
gynecological infections because it most frequently invades the
bloodstream in this setting. Most B. fragilis strains are resistant to intermediate levels of penicillin G and cephalosporins;
they are uniformly resistant to the aminoglycoside antibiotics,
and in the 1960's it was noted that there was the emergence of
widespread resistance to tetracycline (3,4). This latter resistance was important because tetracycline was the agent of choice

51

in treating infections involving B. fragilis in the 1950's. More
recently there have been reports of the increasing incidence of
high-level penicillin resistance and scattered reports of resistance to chloramphenicol, clindamycin, cefoxitin, and metronidazole
(5-9). Clindamycin resistance is important because this drug has
currently been the prime agent for treating bacteroides infections.

Because of the widespread resistance in Bacteroides fragilis
and closely related species, numerous attempts have been made to
transfer the penicillin or tetracycline resistance (tet^r) determinants both within B. fragilis and from B. fragilis to E. coli
(10,11). Until the late 1970's the only documented successful
transfer of tetracycline resistance was from B. fragilis to E. coli
by an undescribed mechanism by Mancini and Behme (12). There is
one report of the transfer of ampicillin resistance from E. coli
to B. fragilis and a fusobacterium, but the ampicillin resistance
was unstable (13). Transformation of E. coli to ampicillin resistance was reported with DNA from B. fragilis; however, the
plasmid used to transform could not be visualized in the E. coli
(15). In 1979, three laboratories concurrently reported the transfer of clindamycin resistance determinants within the genus Bacteroides, Privitera et al. at the Pasteur Institute, Welch and Macrina
in Richmond, Virginia, and our own studies (15,16,17).

Investigations at the Pasteur Institute disclosed the transfer
of both clindamycin (clin^r) and tetracycline resistance (tet^r) from
a strain of B. fragilis isolated in France to another B. fragilis
strain. They showed that erythromycin and streptogramin resistance
were transferred with the clin^r, and these resistances were spontaneously curable. Further work by the French group demonstrated that
transfer of tet^r in B. fragilis could be induced to a higher frequency by pretreatment of the donor culture with subinhibitory
levels of tetracycline (18). Welch and Macrina working with the
isolate from the Pasteur Institute demonstrated that the transfer
of clindamycin, erythromycin and streptogramin resistance was
associated with a 27 megadalton plasmid (16). Our laboratory was
working with a different strain of Bacteroides fragilis, isolated
in California, that was highly resistant to clindamycin and erythromycin and possessed a different plasmid associated with the transfer
of the clindamycin resistance. This paper describes the characterization of our clindamycin resistance transfer factor.

Standard anaerobic techniques in an anaerobic glovebox were
employed, and the matings were carried out utilizing Nalgene
filters (17). DNA was analyzed by agarose gel electrophoresis,
and cells were lysed by a number of different procedures. DNA-DNA
hybridization studies were carried out by a modification of the
Southern technique (19,20,21,22,23).

Table 1.   Characteristics of the Donor and Recipient Strains
of B. fragilis[a]

Organisms	Phenotypic Characteristics
DONORS	
B. fragilis TMP 10	clin^r,tet^r,rif^s,nal^s,phage^r
B. fragilis TMP 230	clin^r,tet^r,rif^s.nal^s,phage^s
RECIPIENTS	
B. fragilis TM 2000	clin^s,tet^r,rif^r,nal^s,phage^s
B. fragilis TM 4000	clin^s,tet^s,rif^r,nal^s,phage^s
B. fragilis TM 4500	clin^s,tet^s,rif^r,nal^r,phage^s
B. fragilis JC 101	clin^s,tet^s,rif^r,nal^s,phage^s,his$^-$, arg$^-$
B. thetaiotaomicron TM 5000	clin^s,tet^r,rif^s,nal^s,phage^r,rham$^+$, ara$^+$

[a]
   Abbreviations: clin-clindamycin-erythromycin, tet-
   tetracycline, rif-rifampicin, nal-nalidixic acid, phage-
   phage susceptibility, arg$^-$,his$^-$ requires arginine or
   histidine to grow on minimal medium, rham$^+$ ara$^+$ – grows on
   minimal medium with rhamnose or arabinose as only carbon
   source.

Bacteroides fragilis TMP 10 was mated with B. fragilis TM
2000 for clin^r-rif^r isolates, and a low number of transicpients
were obtained which were confirmed as transcipients by their phage
patterns. Transcipient strains were tested for retransfer of clin^r
to Bacteroides thetaiotaomicron. Clin^r, ara$^+$ isolates were confirmed
by checking for rham$^+$. In all instances erythromycin resistance was
transferred with clindamycin resistance. Thus, these studies plus
the studies by the French group and the Richmond Virginia group show
that there is intra-and interspecies transfer of resistance determinants within the genus Bacteroides.

Analysis of the extrachromosomal DNA in a number of our transcipients is shown in Figure 1 (17). In lane 1 is the original recipient, TM 2000, and in lanes 7 & 8 are the original donor, TMP 10.
In lane 2 is a strain which was originally isolated as clin^r but
subsequently was found to have spontaneously lost clin^r; it posseses a 2.8 kb plasmid shown in two molecular forms (covalently closed
circle and open circle). In lane 3 is a strain which has retained
its clin^r, and the only additional plasmid is the high molecular
weight one. Thus, the minimal requirements for the transfer of the
clin^r that we originally described were the presence of these two
plasmids (17).

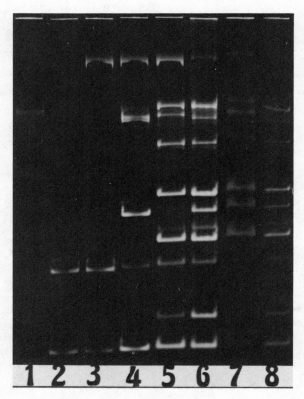

Figure 1. Agarose gel analysis of DNA in parental and transcipient strains of Bacteroides. Each gel slot contained 5-25µl
of DNA purified by the CsCl-EtEr (cesium chloride-ethidium
bromide) method (lanes 2-8) or phenol-extracted cleared lysates
(lane 1). Samples were obtained from: (1) <u>Bacteroides fragilis</u>
strain TM2000; (2) <u>B. fragilis</u> TM2010; (3) <u>B. fragilis</u> TM2006;
(4) <u>B. fragilis</u> TM2008; (5) <u>B. fragilis</u> TM2002; (6) <u>B. fragilis</u>
TM2001; (7) B. fragilis TMP10, preparation A; (8) <u>B. fragilis</u>
TMP10, preparation B (obtained on a different day from preparation A).

     At this point, Privitera published his studies on the induc-
ibility of tetracycline resistance transfer in <u>B. fragilis</u> (18).
This prompted us to re-examine our strains since the original donor
TMP 10 and recipient TM 2000 were known to be tet^r. Utilizing a
plasmid-free recipient strain TM 4000 kindly supplied by Dr. Sebald
from the Pasteur Institute we studied the transfer of both clin^r
and tet^r from TMP 10 to a nalidixic acid resistant (nal^r) derivative of the Sebald strain called TM 4500. The original donor was
mated under 3 conditions, uninduced, induced with tetracycline, and
induced with clindamycin (Table 2).

Table 2. Effect of Antibiotic Pretreatment on Resistance Transfer
Frequency from B. fragilis TMP 10 to B. fragilis TM 4500

| Condition | (Mating Frequency per donor input) | |
	Tet Transfer*	Clin Transfer**
Untreated	10^{-7}	10^{-8}
Clindamycin	10^{-5}	10^{-6}
Tetracycline	10^{-3}	10^{-4}

*Primary selection on tet rif plates, secondary character phage[s]
nal[r]
**Primary selection on clin rif plates

In the uninduced mating there was low level transfer of both clin[r]
and tet[r]; however, with tetracycline or clindamycin induction there
was a 2-4 log increase in the frequency of transfer. The transfer
of tet[r] was not associated with a detectable extrachromosomal
element (25).

In order to properly characterize our clindamycin resistance
transfer factor it was necessary to isolate it in a plasmid-free
tetracycline susceptible background. Bacteroides fragilis TMP 10
was mated with strain TM 4000, selecting for clin[r]-rif[r] and checking for tet[s] and phage[s]. Several tet[s]-clin[r] transconjugants were
isolated, and they could retransfer clin[r] to a TM 4500.

Several isolates were analyzed for extra chromosomal DNA; some
strains contained one plasmid. The plasmid DNA from strain TM 4003
was isolated and designated pBFTM 10. pBFTM 10 measures 15.6 kb
when compared to pBR322 by electron microscopy. This plasmid was
also sized by specific restriction endonucleases including Eco R1,
Hind III and Pvu II. A preliminary restriction map of pBFTM 10
is illustrated (Figure 2). A spontaneous clindamycin susceptible
derivative of TM 4003 possesses a plasmid with a 4.5 kb deletion of
pBFTM 10. For this reason, the 4.5 kb fragment of pBFTM 10 is
believed to carry clin[r].

Close cell-to-cell contact is required for transfer. The
process is resistant to DNAase treatment of the donor and recipient
cells, and supernatants of chloroform-treated donor cells do not
transfer. Finally, there is no increased frequency of transfer by
pretreatment with clindamycin when the donor and recipient are in
a tetracycline susceptible background. Despite the small size we
feel that pBFTM 10 is a self-transferable plasmid, but we cannot rule
out the possible requirement for host chromosomal functions to affect
the transfer. It has been used to mobilize penicillin/ampicellin
resistance from another strain of B. fragilis (26).

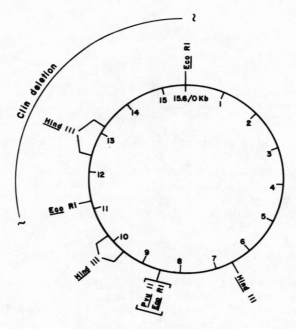

Figure 2.   Preliminary Restriction Map of pBFTM 10.

     The clindamycin transfer factor, pBFTM 10, can also be used
as a probe to investigate other clin^r bacteroides, and was employed as such to study strains from a recent outbreak of clin^r
bacteroides on the surgical wards of the University of Illinois
Hospital in Chicago.

     B. fragilis TMP 230, a clin^r and tet^r isolate from Chicago
which is known to be rif^s and nal^s, was mated with a laboratory
derivative of strain TM 4000 called JC 101 (clin^s,tet^s,rif^r,nal^s,
arg$^-$,his$^-$) using filter mating techniques with and without tetracycline induction of the donor. There was no transfer of tet^r or
clin^r without tetracycline induction. However, with tetracycline
induction transfer of both tet^r and clin^r occurred. The frequency
of tetracycline transfer was 5 X 10^{-4} and clindamycin 1 X 10^{-5}.
All clindamycin resistant isolates were also tetracycline resistant

while one-third of the tetracycline resistant transconjugants were clindamycin resistant.

Analysis of the donor and transcipient strains for extra-chromosomal DNA failed to reveal the existence of closed circular molecules. Based on the assumption that the clindamycin resistant determinant in strain TMP 230 may be related to the previously des-cribed clindamycin transfer factor pBFTM 10, an Eco Rl digest of the chromosome of TMP 230 was probed with nick-translated ^{32}P DNA from pBFTM 10 utilizing a modification of the Southern hybridiz-ation technique (23); the uncleaved chromosome of TMP 230 possesses some homology with pBFTM 10, and this homology has been localized in 3 Eco Rl fragments of the chromosome.

TMP 230 was mated with JC 101 and the chromosome of 2 trans-conjugants were probed with ^{32}P-labelled pBFTM 10 as described above. The homology with pBFTM 10 was strongest in the donor but was clearly evident in both the transcipients. These data indicate that there was transfer of clindamycin resistance determinants similar to that found on pBFTM 10 from the chromosome of strain TMP 230 to the chromosome of the recipient JC 101 by a yet un-disclosed mechanism. Probing of Eco Rl and Pvu II digests of the TMP 230 and its transcipients reveals that there are different amounts of DNA being acquired in the transcipients and that the sites of insertion in each transconjugant are changed from the donor. This supports our belief that the DNA coding the resistance is inserted into the chromosome rather than residing on a large plasmid which was not detected. The mechanism of chromosomal transfer is not presently understood. It may be similar to the "conjugal transposon"-mediated tetracycline resistance transfer in Streptococcus fecaelis as reported by Clewell and his associates (27).

In conclusion, we have presented data from our laboratory showing that clindamycin resistance transfer in our strain of Bacteroides fragilis TMP 10 is associated with a 15.6 kilobase plasmid called pBFTM 10. This clindamycin transfer factor can be used as a prob for the location of clindamcyin resistance deter-minants in other resistant bacteroides. Clindamycin transfer may be independent or associated with a tetracycline transfer element located in the chromosome.

1. S.M. Finegold, D.J. Flora, H.R. Attebery, et al., Fecal bacteriology of colonic polyp patients and control patients, Cancer Res. 35:3407-3417 (1975).
2. S.L. Gorbach and J.G. Bartlett, Anaerobic infections, N. Engl. J. Med. 290:1177-1184, 1237-1245, 1289-1294 (1974).
3. W.J. Martin, M. Gardner, J.A. Washington II, In vitro antimicro-bial susceptibility of anaerobic bacteria isolated from clinical specimens, Antimicrob. Agents Chemother. 1:148-158 (1972)

4. V.L. Sutter, Y.Y. Kwok and S.M. Finegold, Standardized anti-
    microbial disc susceptibility testing of anaerobic bacteria.
    I. Susceptibility of Bacteroides fragilis to tetracycline,
    Appl. Microbiol. 23:268-275 (1972).

5. F.P. Tally, N.V. Jacobus, J. G. Bartlett and S.L. Gorbach,
    Susceptibility of anaerobes to cefoxitin and other cephalo-
    sporin antibiotics, Antimicrob. Ag. Chemother. 7:128-132 (1975)

6. J.S. Salaki, R. Black, F.P. Tally, et al., Bacteroides fragilis
    resistant to the administration of clindamycin, Amer. J. Med.
    60:426-428 (1976).

7. R.E. Bawdon, E. Rozmiej, S. Palchaudhuri and J. Krakowiak,
    Variability in the susceptibility pattern of Bacteroides
    fragilis in four Detroit area hospitals, Antimicrob. Ag.
    Chemother. 16:664-666 (1979).

8. B. Olsson, K. Dornbusch and C.E. Nord, Factors contributing to
    resistance to beta-lactam antibiotics in Bacteroides fragilis,
    Antimicrob. Ag. Chemother. 15:263-268 (1979).

9. J.R. Ingham, S. Eaton, C. W. Venables, et al., Bacteroides
    fragilis resistant to metronidazole after long-term therapy,
    Lancet 1:214 (1978).

10. J.D. Anderson and R.B. Sykes, Characterization of a beta-
    lactamase obtained from a strain of Bacteroides, J. Med.
    Microbiol. 6:201-206 (1973).

11. A.E. Weinrich and V.E. Del bene, Beta-lactamase activity in
    anaerobic bacteria, Antimicrob. Ag. Chemother. 10:106-111
    (1976).

12. C. Mancini and R.J. Behme, Transfer of multiple antibiotic re-
    sistance from Bacteroides fragilis to Escherichia coli, J.
    Infect. Dis. 136:597-600 (1977).

13. S.J. Burt and D.R. Woods, R factor transfer to obligate an-
    aerobes from Escherichia coli, J. Gen. Microbiol. 93:405-409
    (1976).

14. F.E. Young and L. Mayer, Genetic determinants of microbial
    resistance in antibiotics, Rev. Infect. Dis. 1:55-62 (1979).

15. G. Privitera, A. Dublanchet and M. Sebald, Transfer of multiple
    antibiotic resistance between subspecies of Bacteroides
    fragilis, J. Infect. Dis. 139:97-101 (1979).

16. R.A. Welch, K.R. Jones and F.L. Macrina, Plasmid-mediated
    transfer of lincosamide macrolide and tetracycline resist-
    ance in Bacteroides, Plasmid 2:261-268 (1979).

17. F.P. Tally, D.R. Snydman, S.L. Gorbach, et al., Plasmid-mediated
    transferable resistance to clindamycin and erythromycin in
    Bacteroides fragilis, J. Infect. Dis. 139:83-89 (1979).

18. G. Privitera, M. Sebald and F. Fayolle, Common regulatory
    mechanism of expression and conjugate ability of a tetra-
    cycline resistance plasmid in Bacteroides fragilis, Nature
    278:657-659 (1979).

19. D.B. Clewell and D.R. Helinski, Supercoiled circular DNA-protein
    complex in Escherichia coli:purification and induced con-
    version to an open circular DNA form, Proc. Natl. Acad. Sci.,
    USA (1969).

20. J.A. Meyers, D. Sanchez, L.P. Ewell and S. Falkow, Simple
     agarose gel electrophoretic method for the identification and
     characterization of plasmid deoxyribonucleic acid, J. Bacteriol.
     127:1529-1537 (1976).
21. T. Eckhardt, A rpaid method for the identification of plasmid
     deoxyribonucleic acid in bacteria, Plasmid 1:584-588 (1978).
22. R. Davis, J. Roth and D. Botstein , "Advanced Bacterial Gen-
     etics Laboratory Manual",Cold Spring Harbor, NY (1980).
23. E. Southern, Detection of specific sequences among DNA frag-
     ments separated by gel electrophoresis. J. Mol. Biol. 98:
     503-517 (1975).
24. A.E. Franke and D.B. Clewell, Evidence for a chromosome-
     borne resistance transposon (Tn 916) in Streptococcus fecaelis
     that is capable of "conjugal" transfer in the absence of a
     conjugative plasmid, J. Bacteriol. 145:494-502 (1981).
25. D.R. Snydman, F.P. Tally, M.J. Shimell, S.L. Gorbach and M.H.
     Malamy, Transferable tetracycline resistance B. fragilis, 19th
     Interscience Conference on Antimicrob. Ag. and Chemother.
     Boston, MA (1979).
26. T. Butler, F.P. Tally, S.L. Gorbach, M. Malamy, Transferable
     ampicillin resistance in B. fragilis. Clinical Research 28:
     365, 1980.
27. D. Clewell, Conjugation in gram-positive bacteria, International
     Plasmid Meeting, Sano Domingo, 1981.

Acknowlegement

    The work on transferable resistance in our laboratory has
been supported by an NIH grant from the National Institutes of
Allergy and Infectious Disease, Grant #1-R01-AI-15389-01A1BM.

CAMPYLOBACTER JEJUNI: CHARACTERISTIC FEATURES OF THE ORGANISM AND
IDENTIFICATION OF TRANSMISSIBLE PLASMIDS IN TETRACYCLINE-RESISTANT
CLINICAL ISOLATES

Diane E. Taylor*

Research Institute and Department of Bacteriology,
The Hospital for Sick Children, Toronto, Canada M5G 1X8

INTRODUCTION

In recent years Campylobacter jejuni has been recognized[1,2]
throughout the world as a common cause of bacterial diarrhea.
The organism is microaerophilic, and therefore requires special
conditions for selection and growth. Methods developed by Butzler
and colleagues[3,4] in Belgium and Skirrow[5] in the United Kingdom
have enabled many microbiological laboratories to isolate this organism from stools and have led to its recognition as a significant
enteric pathogen. The relative frequencies of organisms causing
gastroenteritis isolated during 1978 and 1979 at the Hospital for
Sick Children, Toronto are shown in Table 1. Among pediatric patients reporting with diarrhea, C. jejuni was isolated almost as
often as non-typhoidal salmonella. Other enteric pathogens were
isolated much less frequently. The most common clinical features
of campylobacter enteritis are diarrhea, often accompanied by blood
in the stools, and abdominal pain[2]. Several excellent review ar-
ticles have been published recently, dealing with both the disease
and the causative organism[1,2,6,7,8]. The reader is referred to
them for more detailed information. In this article, I will describe the significant features of campylobacters, including their
morphology, growth requirements and resistance to antibiotics.
I will then discuss recent work on transmissible plasmids that mediate tetracycline resistance in C. jejuni, a preliminary report
of which has been published[9].

―――――――
*Present address: Department of Medical Bacteriology, The University
                  of Alberta, Edmonton, Alberta, Canada T6G 2H7.

Table 1.   Relative Frequency of Different Enteric Pathogens
            Isolated at The Hospital for Sick Children, Toronto[a]

| | Number of Cases | |
Pathogen	1978	1979
Campylobacter jejuni	103	100
Salmonella spp. (non-typhoidal)	129	105
Salmonella typhi	6	6
Shigella spp.	22	15
Yersinia enterocolitica	12	17
Enteropathogenic Escherichia coli serotypes	57	50

[a]Cases of bacterial diarrhea, inpatients and outpatients seen
during 1978 and 1979. (M.A. Karmali and P.C. Fleming, unpublished data.)

CHARACTERISTIC FEATURES OF CAMPYLOBACTERS

The Genus Campylobacter

The organisms in the genus Campylobacter are oxidase-positive,
microaerophilic, gram-negative bacilli. They are divided into two
groups based on their ability to produce catalase[1]. Three species,
Campylobacter jejuni, C. fetus subsp. fetus, and C. fetus subsp.
venerealis belong to the catalase-positive group. Two other species,
C. sputorum and C. bubulus, are catalase-negative[1]. Studies of plasmids are limited to work on strains of C. jejuni, although one strain
of C. fetus subsp. fetus (ATCC 27374) has been used as a recipient
in interspecies matings. The catalase-negative campylobacters are
not pathogenic for humans, and since nothing is known of their
plasmid content, they will not be discussed further. Campylobacter
fetus subsp. fetus causes abortion in cattle and sheep, but it is
occasionally implicated in some human infections. In contrast, C.
fetus subsp. venerealis is associated with sterility in cattle but
is not thought to be pathogenic for humans.

Campylobacters because of their morphology were once included
in the genus Vibrio, however studies of the guanine plus cytosine
(G + C) content of DNA from members of the two genera indicate that
they are unrelated[10]. DNA from strains of Campylobacter fetus subsp.
fetus and C. fetus subsp. venerealis has a G + C content of 34.4%;
DNA from strains of C. jejuni has a G + C content of 32.7%. The
genus Vibrio, however, comprises bacteria which contain DNA with a
G + C content of 40 to 53%[10].

Morphology of Campylobacters

Campylobacters are spirally curved rods which have a single polar flagellum at one or sometimes both ends of the cell. When examined by phase-contrast microscopy, the organism is motile with a characteristic corkscrew-like motion. Karmali et al. have shown that catalase-positive campylobacters may be differentiated morphologically[11]. Campylobacter jejuni is a small rod with tightly coiled spirals, which have a wave-length of 1.12 μm and an amplitude of 0.48 μm. The spirals of Campylobacter fetus subsp. fetus are intermediate in size with a mean wave-length of 1.8 μm and an amplitude of 0.55 μm. Of the three species, C. fetus subsp. venerealis form the largest spirals, with a mean wave-length of 2.43 μm and an amplitude of 0.73 μm.

Growth Conditions

The catalase-positive campylobacters are microaerophilic, growing best in an atmosphere in which the oxygen tension is reduced to 5-7%. Such an atmosphere may be achieved by evacuating two thirds of the air from an anaerobic jar (without catalyst) and replacing the evacuated air with carbon dioxide or a mixture of carbon dioxide and nitrogen[1,2,11]. Commercial gas generating systems (BBL, Oxoid) are also available.

Differential Features of Campylobacters

Table 2 shows characteristic features of C. jejuni and C. fetus subsp. fetus. These characteristics are important in the choice of temperatures for plasmid transfer, in the choice of antibiotic for counter-selection, and to allow differentiation of C. jejuni donors and C. fetus subsp. fetus recipients after plasmid transfer.

Table 2. Characteristics for the Differentiation of Campylobacter jejuni and Campylobacter fetus subspecies fetus

	Growth at			Resistance to nalidixic acid[a]	Resistance to cephalothin[a]
	25°C	37°C	42°C		
C. jejuni	-	+	++	S	R
C. fetus subsp. fetus	+	+	-	R	S

[a]S, susceptible: zone of inhibition surrounding disc containing 30 μg of nalidixic acid or cephalothin; R, resistant: no zone of inhibition.

EPIDEMIOLOGY AND PATHOGENESIS OF C. JEJUNI

The epidemiology of campylobacter enteritis is not well understood. The organism is a pathogen or commensal in a wide range of
animal species, including cattle, sheep, pigs, poultry, dogs, cats
and wild birds[2,6], consequently there is a large natural reservoir.
Ingestion of contaminated water[12] and unpasteurized milk[6,13,14]
has been implicated in some human infections. Serotyping schemes
are currently being developed[3,13,14,16] as one approach to understanding the epidemiology of campylobacter enteritis.

Little is known about the pathogenesis of C. jejuni. Studies
by Butzler and Skirrow using chick embryos and 8-day-old chicks indicate that pathogenesis depends on the direct invasive ability of
the organism although a few strains also produced a thermostable
enterotoxin[1]. The presence of blood in the stools from patients with
campylobacter enteritis also suggests an invasive process. Pathogenicity studies have been hampered by the lack of a suitable experimental model. Recently, however, Ruiz-Palacios et al.[17] reported
that the three-day-old chick may constitute a suitable animal model
for campylobacter enteritis.

ANTIBIOTIC RESISTANCE IN C. JEJUNI

Although campylobacter enteritis is usually self-limiting, antibiotics may be indicated for treatment of the more severe cases.
Erythromycin, tetracycline, and the nitrofuran derivative, furazoli-
done, have been recommended[18]. Approximately 1% of C. jejuni strains
isolated at The Hospital for Sick Children, Toronto, in 1978 and
1979 were resistant to erythromycin[19]. This result is similar to
the report of 0.5% erythromycin-resistant strains in the United
Kingdom[20]. Higher levels of erythromycin resistance were observed
in Belgium[18] and Sweden[21] where 9% of C. jejuni strains were erythromycin-resistant. In Toronto, studies are in progress to determine
if erythromicin resistance in C. jejuni is plasmid-mediated.

In the Toronto study[19], all C. jejuni isolates were susceptible
to nitrofurantoin with a minimal inhibitory concentration (MIC) of
$2 \mu g/ml$. About 20% of strains were resistant to $4 \mu g/ml$ of tetracycline; 12% showed high level resistance to tetracycline
(MIC $\geq 64 \mu g/ml$). The significant number of tetracycline-resistant
strains of C. jejuni in Toronto contrasts with the lower percentage
of European isolates resistant to this antibiotic. In Belgium,
Vanhoof et al.[18,22] showed that about 5 to 8% of clinical isolates
were tetracycline-resistant. In Sweden, however, Walder[23] found that
all clinical isolates of C. jejuni were susceptible to tetracycline.
In North America, owing to the high incidence of tetracycline-resistant C. jejuni, tetracycline may be of limited use in the treatment
of campylobacter enteritis.

ANTIBIOTIC RESISTANCE TRANSFER AND PLASMIDS IN C. JEJUNI

The relatively recent recognition of C. jejuni as a pathogen and the special conditions required for growth of the organism have delayed the study of plasmids in this genus. The first report of plasmids in C. jejuni was that of Austin and Trust[24], who found that approximately 19% of strains from various geographic locations contained plasmids. The molecular weights of these plasmids varied from 5.0 to 77×10^6. Only one isolate harboured more than one plasmid. Some of the strains of C. jejuni studied were resistant to antibiotics, but no direct correlation was made between antibiotic resistance and plasmid carriage[24].

Intraspecies Transfer of Tetracycline Resistance

At the Hospital for Sick Children, Toronto, clinical isolates of C. jejuni with MIC of tetracycline $\geq 64 \mu$gm/ml were studied. Tetracycline resistance was shown to be plasmid-mediated and transmissible within the genus Campylobacter[9]. A clinical isolate of C. jejuni, MK22, which had a tetracycline MIC of 128μg/ml, was used as the donor strain. The recipient strain, SD2, was a spontaneous nalidixic acid-resistant mutant of C. jejuni (MIC of tetracycline $\leq 4\mu$g/ml and of nalidixic acid = 256μg/ml). Tetracycline resistance transfer was performed using broth and filter mating methods. For both procedures, the strains were grown in a special medium devoid of blood (M.A. Karmali and P.C. Fleming, unpublished data). It contained per litre: Tryptone soya broth (Oxoid) 10g, special peptone (Oxoid) 5g, yeast extract (Oxoid) 5g, hemin 0.01g, TRIS (BDH) 0.75g, and sodium pyruvate 10g. Dithiothreitol (0.15g per litre) was added to the broth as a reducing agent and the pH adjusted to 7.2 by addition of hydrochloric acid. All solid media contained 3% agar to prevent swarming, which is a characteristic feature of C. jejuni[11].

Liquid matings were prepared by adding 0.5 ml of the donor culture to 1.0 ml of recipient culture and 1.0 ml of fresh broth. The mating mixtures were incubated at 42°C for 48 hours, then aliquots from the mating mixtures were diluted in 0.05M sodium phosphate buffer pH7.2. The C. jejuni transconjugants were selected on Diagnostic Sensitivity Testing agar (DST, Oxoid) containing 5% lysed horse blood, 50μg/ml nalidixic acid and 16μg/ml tetracyline. Filter matings were prepared by adding 0.5 ml of the donor culture to 1.0 ml of the recipient culture. The mating mixtures were collected on nitrocellulose filters (Millipore HA type, pore size 0.22 μm). The filters were placed on agar plates, containing the special medium plus 3% agar and incubated under reduced oxygen tension (7%) at 42°C for 48 hours. The filters were removed from plates, placed in tubes containing 1.0 ml of sterile phsphate buffer, and cells were separated from the filter by vortexing the tubes. Dilutions were made of the cell suspensions and the transconjugants were selected as described above.

The tetracycline resistance determinant was transferred from
C. jejuni strain MK22 to strain SD2. In broth matings, the frequency
of transfer was 2.4×10^{-6} transconjugants per recipient in a 48 hour
mating period at 42°C. For filter matings, the frequency of transfer was 5.0×10^{-4}; an increase in the transfer frequency of about
two hundred-fold. No significant difference in the transfer frequency of tetracycline resistance was noted when the temperature of
the mating mixtures was reduced from 42°C to 37°C.

Interspecies Transfer of Tetracycline Resistance

The higher transfer frequency observed for the filter-mating
procedure indicated that a solid surface facilitates intraspecies
transfer of the C. jejuni tetracycline resistance determinant.
As the filter-mating method is somewhat tedious, we used a plate-
mating procedure for the interspecies transfer studies.

Interspecies transfer was demonstrated with two donor strains
of C. jejuni, MK22, described above, and MK175, a clinical isolate
resistant to both tetracycline (MIC = 64µg/ml) and ampicillin
(MIC = 128µg/ml). The recipient strain was C. fetus subsp. fetus
ATCC 27374 (CIP 5396)[10], which is naturally resistant to nalidixic
acid (MIC = 256µg/ml). The strains were grown on Columbia base
agar (Gibco) containing 7% defibrinated horse blood (BA) and incubated for 48 hours, at 42°C for C. jejuni and at 37°C for C.
fetus subsp. fetus. The cells from the plates were suspended in
0.05M sodium phosphate buffer at 1×10^9 cells/ml. Aliquots of
0.15 ml of donor and recipient cell suspensions were mixed together
and spread over BA plates. The plates were incubated at 37°C for
48 hours. To select for C. fetus subsp. fetus transconjugants,
cells were washed off the plates, diluted and spread on DST agar
containing 5% lysed horse blood, 75µg/ml nalidixic acid and 16µg/ml
tetracycline.

Interspecies transfer of tetracycline resistance from clinical
isolates of C. jejuni to C. fetus subsp. fetus ATCC 27374 is shown
in Table 3. The tetracycline resistance determinant transferred
equally well to both the C. fetus subsp. fetus and C. jejuni recipients. Attempts were also made to transfer tetracycline resistance
to Escherichia coli. Three strains were used: E. coli K12, J53-1
(pro met gyrA), NM148 (Kr⁻Km⁺gyrA), a restriction deficient mutant
of E. coli K12, and the E. coli C strain RG176[25] which does not
possess the K restriction system. None of the three E. coli strains
was able to act as a recipient.

Mechanism of Transfer of C. jejuni Tetracycline Resistance Deter-
minants

Cell-free filtrates of the donor strains of C. jejuni MK22 and
MK175 could not promote the transfer of tetracycline resistance

Table 3. Interspecies Transfer of Tetracycline Resistance
from C. jejuni to C. fetus subsp. fetus[a]

Resistance pattern of C. jejuni isolate	Resistance determinant transferred[b]	Plasmid	Transfer frequency[c]
Tc	Tc	pMAK22	2.7×10^{-4}
ApTc	Tc	pMAK175	9.1×10^{-6}

[a]Tetracycline resistance determinants were transferred from
C. jejuni clinical isolates to C. fetus subsp. fetus ATCC 27374
in a 48 hour mating at 37°C.

[b]Ap, Ampicillin; Tc, tetracycline.

[c]Calculated as transconjugants per recipient.

determinants to strains of C. jejuni SD2 or C. fetus subsp. fetus
ATCC 27374 ($< 1 \times 10^{-8}$ transconjugants per recipient after a 48 hour
mating period). These results indicate that the transfer process
was not mediated by bacteriophage transduction. The addition of
DNase, at 100µg/ml, to the agar used in the plate-mating experiments,
also did not affect plasmid transfer frequencies. DNA transformation
therefore would not appear to be involved in the transfer process.
It appears most likely that transfer of C. jejuni tetracycline R determinants involves a plasmid-mediated conjugative process.

Isolation of C. jejuni Plasmid DNA

Physical isolation of plasmid DNA was performed using a modification of the method of Meyers et al.[26]. The DNA samples were
analyzed immediately after isolation by agarose gel electrophoresis
as described by Taylor and Levine[27]. Plasmid-enriched DNA fractions
were prepared from a total of four tetracycline-resistant clinical
isolates of C. jejuni isolated in Toronto. Tetracycline resistance
determinants could be transferred from all these strains to
C. jejuni SD2 and to C. fetus subsp. fetus ATCC 27374. Similar
extracts made from the recipient strains C. jejuni SD2 and C. fetus
subsp. fetus ATCC 27374 were plasmid-free. In contrast, all of
the above tetacycline-resistant campylobacters harboured a plasmid
with a molecular weight of approximately 38×10^{6}. A plasmid of the
same molecular weight was observed in tetracycline-resistant transconjugants of C. jejuni and C. fetus subsp. fetus.

Other Reports of Plasmids in Tetracycline Resistant C. jejuni

Goldstein and Acar have observed transfer of tetracycline resistance between strains of C. jejuni, although transfer to E. coli

was not achieved (F.W. Goldstein and J.F. Acar, personal communication). Cohen and Falkow noted the presence of a plasmid with a molecular weight of about 38×10^6 in a tetracycline resistant clinical isolate of C. jejuni (M.L.Cohen and S.Falkow, personal communication).

Ampicillin Resistance in C. jejuni

Recent studies in Toronto have indicated that ampicillin resistance, observed in approximately 15% of clinical isolates of C. jejuni, is associated with β-lactamase production by these strains (Karmali, D'Amico and Fleming, in preparation). MK175 is one such strain. Transfer of tetracycline resistance and the concomitant transfer of a 38×10^6 plasmid were observed in this strain (Table 3), however, ampicillin resistance was not cotransferred with tetracycline resistance, and is presumably not located on the same plasmid. As no other plasmid was visualized in DNA prepared from MK175, it is likely that ampicillin resistance in this strain is of chromosomal origin.

CONCLUSIONS

Transmissible plasmids encoding tetracycline resistance were identified in four clinical isolates of C. jejuni. The plasmids had molecular weights of 38×10^6. All four clinical isolates originated in Toronto, and it is possible that the plasmids are related and may have had a common source.

Transfer of plasmids in Campylobacter was facilitated on solid surfaces. A similar preference for a solid surface for mating has been noted for plasmids of some incompatibility groups in Enterobacteriaceae[28]. Our experiments indicate that DNA transformation and bacteriophage-mediated transduction are not involved in transfer of tetracycline resistance from C. jejuni. The process probably involves conjugation, via cell to cell contact.

Intraspecies transfer in C. jejuni was demonstrated, as well as interspecies transfer from C. jejuni to C. fetus subsp. fetus. The ability of C. fetus subsp. venerealis to act as a recipient, is currently being tested. Attempts to transfer campylobacter plasmids to E. coli were unsuccessful. Analogous host range limitations have been reported for other gram-negative organisms. Plasmids of the P2 incompatibility group from Pseudomonas aeruginosa could not be transferred to E. coli[29]. Apparently it is also difficult to transfer plasmids from Bacteroides fragilis to E. coli[30]. The reason for the failure of plasmids from one species to transfer to and/or replicate in a different species is, as yet, undetermined.

The studies reported here demonstrate that antibiotic-resistant campylobacters, like many pathogenic bacteria, may harbour resistance plasmids. Further work is required to determine both the source of these plasmids and the origin of their resistance determinants.

ACKNOWLEDGEMENTS

I thank my colleagues in the Department of Bacteriology, The Hospital for Sick Children, and the Department of Medical Microbiology, The University of Toronto, especially P.C.Fleming, M.A. Karmali, S.A. De Grandis, J.G. Levine, A.K. Allen and J.L. Penner.

This work was supported by a grant from The Medical Research Council of Canada. The author was also in receipt of a Medical Research Council Scholarship.

REFERENCES

1. Butzler, J.P. and M.B. Skirrow. Clinics in Gastroenterol. 8: 737-765 (1979).
2. Karmali, M.A. and P.C. Fleming. Can.Med. Assoc. J. 23: 1525-1532 (1979).
3. Butzler, J.P. in: "Modern Topics in Infection". J.D.Williams ed., pp.214-239. Heinmann, London. (1978).
4. Dekeyser, P., M. Gossuin, M. Detrain, J.P. Butzler and J. Sternon. J. Infect. Dis. 125: 390-392 (1972).
5. Skirrow, M.B. British Med. J. ii: 9-11 (1979).
6. Blaser, M.J., I.D. Berkowitz, F.M. LaForce, J. Cravens, L.B. Reller and W.L.L. Wang. Ann. Intern. Med. 91: 179-185 (1979).
7. Sack, R.B., R.C.Tilton, and A.S. Weissfeld. in "Cumulative Techniques and Procedures in Clinical Microbiology" 12, S.J. Rubin ed. pp. 1-13. ASM, Washington, D.C. (1980).
8. Smibert, R.M. Ann. Rev. Microbiol. 32: 673-709 (1978).
9 Taylor, D.E., S.A. De Grandis, M.A. Karmali and P.C. Fleming. Lancet ii: 797 (1980).
10. Veron, M. and R. Chatelain. Int. J. Syst. Bacteriol. 23: 122-134 (1973).
11. Karmali, M.A., A.K. Allen and P.C. Fleming. Int. J. Syst. Bacteriol. (in press-1981).
12. Tiehan, W. and R.L. Vogt. Morbidity Mortality Weekly Rep. 27: 207 (1978).
13. Abbott, J.D., B.A.S. Dale, J. Eldridge, D.M. Jones and E.M. Sutcliffe. J. Clin. Path.33: 762-766 (1980).
14. Robinson, D.A., W.J. Edgar, G.L. Gibson, A.A. Matcheff and L. Robertson. British Med. J. 1: 1171-1173 (1979).
15. Kosunen, T.U., D. Danielsson and J. Kjellander. Acta Path. Microbiol. Scand. Sect. B. 88:207-218 (1980).

16. Penner, J.L. and J.N. Hennessy. J. Clin. Microbiol. (in press-1980).
17. Ruiz-Palacios, G.M., E. Escamilla and N. Torres. 20th. Interscience Conference on Antimicrobial Agents and Chemotherapy, Abstract 697, ASM,Washington, D.C. (1980).
18. Vanhoof, R., M.P. Vanderlinden, R. Dierickx, S. Lauwers, E. Yourassowsky and J.P. Butzler. Antimicrob. Agents Chemother. 14: 553-556 (1978).
19. Karmali, M.A., S. De Grandis and P.C. Fleming. Antimicrob. Agents Chemother. (in press-1981).
20. Brunton, W.A.T., A.M.M. Wilson and R.M. Macrae. Lancet ii: 1385 (1978).
21. Walder, M. and A. Forsgren. Lancet ii: 1201 (1978).
22. Vanhoof, R., B. Gordts, R. Dierickx, H. Coigrau, and J.P. Butzler. Antimicrob. Agents Chemother. 18: 118-121 (1980).
23. Walder, M. Antimicrob. Agents Chemother. 16: 37-39 (1979).
24. Austen, R.A., and Trust, T.J. FEMS Microbiological Letters 8: 201-204 (1980).
25. Taylor, D.E., and R.B. Grant. Molec. Gen. Genet. 153: 5-10 (1977).
26. Meyers, J.A., D. Sanchez, L.P. Elwell and S. Falkow. J. Bacteriol. 127: 1529-1537 (1976).
27. Taylor, D.E. and J.G. Levine. J. Gen. Microbiol. 116: 475-484 (1980).
28. Bradley, D.E., D.E.Taylor and D.R. Cohen. J. Bacteriol. 143: 1466-1470 (1980).
29. Shahrabadi, M.S., L.E. Bryan and H.M. Van Den Elzen. Can. J. Microbiol. 21: 592-605 (1975).
30. Welch, R.A., K.R. Jones and F.L. Macrina. Plasmid 2: 261-268 (1979).

STUDIES ON DRUG RESISTANCE TRANSPOSONS IN HAEMOPHILUS INFLUENZAE R PLASMIDS

R. Laufs, R. Fock and P.-M. Kaulfers

Institut für Medizinische Mikrobiologie
und Immunologie der Universität Hamburg
Martinistr. 52, 2000 Hamburg 20
W-Germany

INTRODUCTION

The emergence of R plasmids in H. influenzae is of great clinical concern, since H. influenzae causes serious infections including meningitis, epiglottitis, pneumonia, and otitis media. Resistance to ampicillin (Ap), as well as to tetracycline (Tc) was shown to be plasmid linked (1, 2). The conjugative Haemophilus R plasmids that have been described are closely related to each other and have most of their base sequences in common independent of their geographical origins and their antibiotic resistance markers (3, 4). This paper examines whether these R factors arose as a result of the transposition of different resistance genes on to closely related indigenous H. influenzae plasmids or whether closely related R factors from the same incompatibility group with different resistance genes have now infected H. influenzae strains throughout the world.

MATERIALS AND METHODS

Bacterial strains, media, isolation of plasmid DNA, conjugation, DNA-DNA duplex studies and electron microscope DNA heteroduplex and homoduplex analysis have been recently described (5).

71

RESULTS

Relationship between the H. influenzae R plasmids

The H. influenzae R plasmids which were shown to be
self-transmissible have similar molecular properties.
The molecular weights of these R plasmids are between
30 to 40 Mdal and they have most of their base sequences in common as was shown by the analysis of plasmid
DNA homo- and heteroduplexes using the single-strand
specific endonuclease S1 (Table 1).

Table 1: Relationship between H. influenzae R plasmids

R plasmid	Resistance marker	Molecular weight (Mdal)	% DNA sequence homology with pKRE5367 (Ap^r)
pKRE5367	Ap^r	30	100
pFR16017	Tc^r	33	71
pHK539	Tc^r, Ap^r	36	80
pR1234	Tc^r, Cm^r	35	63
pHI706	Tc^r, Cm^r, Ap^r	38	81

Characterization of the resistance genes by molecular DNA-DNA hybridization using plasmids with known transposons as molecular probes

The presence of the ampicillin transposon Tn3 in the
ampicillin resistance specifying plasmids was demonstrated by molecular hybridization studies using the
5.5 Mdal plasmid RSF1030 (6) as a molecular probe. The
DNA-DNA duplexes between the ^{3}H-labeled RSF1030 DNA and
the ampicillin resistance specifying plasmids were
analysed using the single-strand-specific endonuclease,
S1, of Aspergillus oryzae (7). Plasmid RSF1030, which
contains the whole Tn3 representing 58 % of its total
DNA, had 49 % to 53 % of its base sequence in common
with the ampicillin resistance specifying H. influenzae
plasmids (Table 2).

As a molecular probe for the detection of the tetracycline resistance genes pKT007 (8) and a lambda phage
containing Tn10 (9) were used, which contains the whole
DNA sequence of Tn10. The homology ranged between 12 %

and 17 % indicating, that the tetracycline resistance inducing H. influenzae R plasmids contain the transposable element Tn10 (Table 2).

Table 2: Hybridization between ^{3}H-labeled RSF1030 (Tn3), pKTO07 (Tn10) and phage λ::Tn10 DNA and whole cell DNA from H. influenzae strains

Source of unlabeled DNA	DNA sequence homology with ^{3}H-labeled plasmid or phage DNA (%)		
	RSF1030 (Ap^r)	pKTO07 (Tc^r)	λ::Tn10 (Tc^r)
pKRE5367 (Ap^r)	51	0	0
pFR16017 (Tc^r)	0	28	17
pHK539 (Tc^r, Ap^r)	53	21	12

The presence of Tn9 in the R plasmids coding for combined tetracycline and chloramphenicol resistance could not be demonstrated as clear as the presence of Tn10 since only a small part of the lambda phage used as a molecular probe represented the DNA sequence of Tn9 (10). The presence of Tn9 was mainly indicated by analysis of homo- and heteroduplexes in the electron microscope.

Characterization of DNA sequences in the electron microscope specifying tetracycline, ampicillin and chloramphenicol resistance

Heteroduplex molecules between the different H. influenzae R plasmids were studied in the electron microscope. The plasmids specifying for ampicillin resistance were heteroduplexed with those specifying for tetracycline resistance. The heteroduplex molecules showed an insertion loop with the characteristics of Tn3 (6) and an insertion of a structure characteristic for Tn10 (9).

The H. influenzae R plasmids coding for combined resistances, however, showed unexpected insertions.

The plasmids coding for combined ampicillin and tetracycline resistance had the Tn3 integrated in one of the
inverted repeats of Tn10 close to its end toward the
Tc resistance specifying genes. The plasmid coding for
combined tetracycline and chloramphenicol resistance
carried a translocatable DNA segment composed of Tn10

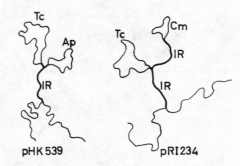

Fig. 1.   Diagram of self-annealed pHK539 (Tc^r, Ap^r)
          molecule shows the Tn3 (Ap^r) inserted in one
          of the inverted repeats (IR) of Tn10 (Tc^r) and
          the self-annealed pRI234 (Tc^r, Cm^r) shows the
          Tn9 (Cm^r) on long inverted repeats inserted in
          one of the inverted repeats of Tn10. Electron
          micrographs of formamide-spread single stran-
          ded plasmid DNA.

containing an insertion of the chloramphenicol resistance transposon Tn9 (11). Tn9 was found to be inserted into one of the components of the Tn10 inverted
repetitions and is itself flanked on both sides by long
inverted repetitions. The localisation of the integration site of Tn9 in one of the inverted repeats of
Tn10 was similar to that of Tn3 in Tn10 (Fig. 1).

The R plasmids coding for tripleresistance against tetracycline, chloramphenicol and ampicillin showed the same combined structure out of Tn10 and Tn9 as was found in the doubly resistant R plasmids (Tc^r, Cm^r). In addition the Tn3 integrated independently of the combined transposon at a different site of the plasmid core.

Transposition of Tn3

A 3.2 $\pm$ 0.2 Mdal DNA sequence of pKRE5367 as well as of pHK539 was transposed into the 5.5 Mdal plasmid RSF1010 (Su^r, Sm^r) (6) by conjugative transfer of the H. influenzae R plasmids to E. coli C600 carrying RSF1010 and selecting for ampicillin resistant clones. The resulting 8.7 $\pm$ 0.2 Mdal hybrid plasmid was shown to be RSF1010::Tn3 by analysis with restriction enzyme EcoR1 and electron microscope heteroduplex studies.

Multiple integration of drug resistance transposons

The H. influenzae R plasmids with the transposon Tn10 showed after prolonged growth in medium containing tetracycline one, two, three, four or even five copies of Tn10 integrated in the same plasmid. The minimum inhibitory concentration against tetracycline increased from 20 µg to 30 µg of tetracycline ml^{-1}. The molecular size of the DNA sequence between the integration sites was found to be similar in all molecules studied (Fig. 2).

The H. influenzae R plasmids with the tetracycline-chloramphenicol resistance transposon was integrated two or three times in the plasmids after their growth in medium containing tetracycline. The presence of multiple copies of the transposon correlated with higher minimum inhibitory concentrations against tetracycline as well as against chloramphenicol. The MICs had risen from 10 to 30 µg of tetracycline ml^{-1} and from 10 to 40 µg of chloramphenicol ml^{-1}. The intervening DNA segments between the integration sites had the same length as those found between the Tn10 copies found in the monoresistant strains (Fig. 2).

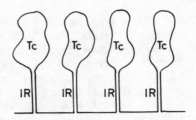

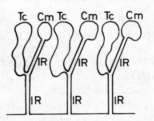

Fig. 2.   Schematic drawing of the multiple integration
           of Tn10 (Tc^r) in pFR16017 (Tc^r); 1 to 5 copies
           of Tn10 were found to be integrated in the
           same plasmid core in self-annealed molecules
           (top); one, two or three copies of the Tn10-
           Tn9 (Tc^r, Cm^r) transposons were found to be
           integrated in pRI234 (bottom). The intervening
           DNA sequences between the integration sites
           had the same molecular size in pFR16017 as
           well as in pRI234; IR: inverted repeats.

In vitro creation of multiresistant H. influenzae R plasmids

Doubly resistant H. influenzae strains were obtained by conjugational transfer of H. influenzae R plasmids carrying Tn3 and H. influenzae R plasmids carrying Tn10 within the H. influenzae isolates. R plasmids were obtained which contained Tn3 and Tn10 integrated at different sites in the same plasmid core and only in one out of ten molecules examined in the electron microscope the Tn3 was integrated in one of the inverted repeats of Tn10 as it was found in the doubly resistant natural isolates.

The Tn10 of pFR16017 as well as Tn3 of pKRE5367 was found to be integrated in the same plasmid core with the combined Tn10 - Tn9 transposon of pHK539 after conjugation of the different strains. However, Tn3 was never found linked to the combined Tn10 - Tn9 transposon.

Isolation of an indigenous H. influenzae plasmid

Fresh isolates of H. influenzae and H. parainfluenzae were examined by agarose gel electrophoresis for the presence of extrachromosomal DNA. Among 699 isolates only one H. influenzae type B isolate was found with the expected indigenous plasmid (pW266). Its molecular size was 27 Mdal and it had 82 % base homology with pKRE5367. This plasmid, which does not carry any detectable drug resistance markers, could not be regularely demonstrated by agarose gel electrophoresis and it seems possible that the chromosomal integration of pW266 is a frequent event (12).

DISCUSSION

The H. influenzae R plasmids examined are not replicate isolates of one plasmid clone. They not only have different molecular weights and different resistance markers, but also differ slightly in the base sequences of their plasmid cores. The presence of Tn3 in the ampicillin resistance specifying H. influenzae R plasmids was indicated by base sequence homology with the plasmid RSF1030 containing the Tn3 and the ampicillin resistance specifying DNA sequence was transposed from the H. influenzae plasmid pKRE5367 and pHK539 on to the E. coli plasmid RSF 1010. The genes for tetra-

cycline resistance were shown to be Tn10 by molecular
hybridization studies with a lambda phage containing
Tn10.

It was shown by electron microscopy that the H. influenzae P plasmids coding for combined tetracycline
and ampicillin resistance or combined tetracycline and
chloramphenicol resistance carried Tn3 or Tn9 integrated in one of the inverted repeats of Tn10. The passage
of the Tc plasmids in medium containing tetracycline
regularely resulted in the multiple integration of the
Tn10 or of the combined Tc-Cm transposon into the same
plasmid core. The multiple integration of the transposable elements was paralleled by an increase of the
resistance against Tc in the case of pFR16017 and
against Tc and Cm simultaneously in the case of pHK539.

The similarity between the cores of the H. influenzae R plasmids examined and the identity of the drug
resistance transposons with those found in the enterobacteriaceae is compatible with the hypothesis that the
H. influenzae R plasmids arose as a result of the transposition of different drug resistance transposons on
to closely related indigenous H. influenzae plasmids.
This idea is further supported by the isolation of an
indigenous plasmid which had the expected molecular
size and had almost all of its base sequences in common
with the H. influenzae R plasmids. Furthermore, the in
vitro creation of multiresistant H. influenzae plasmids
by conjugation of monoresistant and doubly resistant
strains revealed plasmids which were indistinguishable
from the multiresistant clinical isolates. An alternative hypothesis is that closely related R factors from
the same incompatibility group have now infected H. influenzae strains throughout the world. Such an incompatibility group, however, has not been detected yet.

ACKNOWLEDGMENTS

    This work was supported by the Deutsche Forschungs-
gemeinschaft, Bonn-Bad Godesberg, W. Germany. We thank
A. Koppe for excellent technical assistance.

LITERATURE

1. De Graaff, J., L.P. Elwell, and S. Falkow. 1976.
    Molecular nature of two beta-lactamase-speci-
    fying plasmids isolated from Haemophilus in-
    fluenzae type b. J. Bacteriol. 126: 439-446.

2. Elwell, L.P., J.R. Saunders, M.H. Richmond, and S.
    Falkow. 1977. Relationships between some R-
    plasmids found in Haemophilus influenzae. J.
    Bacteriol. 131: 356-362.

3. Laufs, R., and P.-M. Kaulfers. 1977. Molecular
    characterization of a plasmid specifying ampi-
    cillin resistance and its relationship to
    other R factors from Haemophilus influenzae.
    J. Gen. Microbiol. 103: 277-286.

4. Kaulfers, P.-M., R. Laufs, and G. Jahn.1978. Mole-
    cular properties of transmissible R factors of
    Haemophilus influenzae determining tetracy-
    cline resistance. J. Gen. Microbiol. 105:
    243-252.

5. Jahn, G., R. Laufs, P.-M. Kaulfers, and H. Kolenda.
    1979. Molecular nature of two Haemophilus in-
    fluenzae R factors containing resistances and
    the multiple integration of drug resistance
    transposons. J. Bacteriol. 138: 584-597.

6. Heffron, F., C. Rubens, and S. Falkow. 1977. Trans-
    position of a plasmid deoxyribonucleic acid
    sequence that mediates ampicillin resistance:
    identity of laboratory-constructed plasmids
    and clinical isolates. J. Bacteriol. 129:
    530-533.

7. Crosa, J.H., J. Brenner, and S. Falkow. 1973. Use
    of a single-strand specific nuclease for ana-
    lysis of bacterial and plasmid deoxyribonucleic
    acid homo- and heteroduplexes. J. Bacteriol.
    115: 904-911.

8. Timmis, K.N., F. Cabello, and S.N. Cohen. 1978.
    Cloning and characterization of EcoRI and
    HindIII restriction endonuclease-generated
    fragments of antibiotic resistance plasmids
    R6-5 and R6. Mol. Gen. Genet. 162: 121-137.

9. Kleckner, N., J.A. Swan, and M. Zabeau. 1978. Pro-
    perties of the translocatable tetracycline re-
    sistance element Tn10 in Escherichia coli and
    bacteriophage lambda. Genetics 90: 427-461.

10.   Alton, N.K., and D. Vapnek. 1979. Nucleotide se-
       quence analysis of the chloramphenicol re-
       sistance transposon Tn9. Nature 282: 1-6.

11.   Rosner, J.L., and M.M. Gottesman. 1977. Transposi-
       tion and deletion of Tn9: a transferable
       element carrying the gene for chlorampheni-
       col resistance, p. 213-218. In: A.I. Bukhari,
       J.A. Shapiro, and S.L. Adhya (ed.), DNA in-
       sertion elements, plasmids, and episomes.
       Cold Spring Harbor Laboratory, Cold Spring
       Harbor, N.Y.

12.   Stuy, J.H. 1980. Chromosomally integrated conju-
       gative plasmids are common in antibiotic-
       resistant Haemophilus influenzae. J. Bacte-
       riol. 142: 925-930.

PLASMIDS IN STREPTOCOCCI: A REVIEW

Donald J. LeBlanc

National Institute of Allergy and Infectious Diseases
National Institutes of Health
Bethesda, MD. 20205

INTRODUCTION

The genus Streptococcus contains several clinically, industri-
ally and ecologically important species, and many relevant properties resemble, phenotypically, similar traits known to be associated with plasmids among members of other bacterial genera. Studies
on the contributions of plasmids to the virulence and metabolic
versatility of the streptococci have, however, only recently begun.
The purpose of this review is two-fold: 1) to highlight some of the
major developments in the field of streptococcal plasmid biology
over the past eight years, and 2) to present data relevant to areas
of current activity in the field.

HISTORY OF STREPTOCOCCAL PLASMID BIOLOGY

The first report of plasmids in streptococci appeared in 1972
with the demonstration by Courvalin et al.[1] of plasmid-linked tetracycline and erythromycin resistance in a strain of Streptococcus
faecalis. In 1974, Jacob and Hobbs[2] provided the first conclusive
evidence for conjugal transfer of plasmid-borne multiple antibiotic
resistance in S. faecalis, and in 1975 Jacob et al.[3] described a
transmissible hemolysin plasmid in the same strain. These reports
stimulated several groups to become actively engaged in streptococcal plasmid research, but, with few exceptions[4,5,6,7], work
prior to 1976 was done with strains of S. faecalis. This was primarily due to difficulties in lysing other streptococcal species,
especially those obtained from natural sources. In 1976 Chassy[8]
reported that growth of streptococci in a rich medium supplemented
with threonine, which inhibits cell-wall cross linking, yielded
cells which could be rendered susceptible to detergent lysis fol-

lowing treatment with lysozyme. Using this approach, and adapting
existing plasmid enrichment techniques originally used for the isolation of plasmids from gram-negative bacteria, we[9], as well as others[10], were able to isolate and visualize directly on agarose gels,
plasmids from virtually any species of Streptococcus, and quite often from less than 10 ml of culture.

Another initial obstacle to the study of plasmids among the
streptococci was the unavailability of plasmid transfer systems in
this genus. All three of the major bacterial genetic transfer
systems, transduction, transformation and conjugation are now
available. Plasmids have been transferred by transduction among
Lancefield groups A and G[11], and between strains of group N[12] streptococci. Two strains have been used extensively for interspecies
transfer of plasmids by transformation, the group H Challis strain
of S. sanguis[13,14,15,16,17] and a group F isolate[18]. More recently
pneumococci have also been used for this purpose[19]. All three of
these strains exhibit physiological competence. So far, all
attempts to render other streptococcal species competent for transformation by artificial means have failed. Two types of "conjugation" systems have been described in the streptococci. The CIA,
or pheromone-enhanced mating system, which appears to be confined
to group D streptococci, is discussed in the paper by Clewell (this
volume). The second type of plasmid transfer requiring cell-to-cell
contact is facilitated by bringing donor and recipient cells together on a membrane filter. This system has been used for intra-
and interspecies transfer of a number of transmissible plasmids[15,
16,17,20,21,22,23].

With the development of plasmid transfer systems, and improved
plasmid isolation techniques, the role of extrachromosomal elements
in a variety of streptococcal functions has now been established.
Plasmid-mediated single and multiple antibiotic resistance has been
reported in most species of streptococci which are isolated from
human or animal sources[1,2,7,14,15,16,17,20,22,24,25]. Efstathiou
and McKay[26] have described a role of plasmids in the resistance of
S. lactis strains to inorganic ions such as silver, copper, chromate, arsenite and arsenate. Many clinical isolates of S. faecalis
are β-hemolytic on horse and human blood, but not sheep blood[27].
These hemolysins are often linked, if not identical, to bacteriocins
on plasmids which are usually transmissible[3,27,28]. Two transposons,
one carrying resistance to erythromycin[29] and the other tetracycline[30], have been identified in a strain of S. faecalis. We have
recently obtained preliminary results suggesting the presence of a
kanamycin-streptomycin resistance transposable element in a different
strain of S. faecalis (D. J. LeBlanc and L. N. Lee, unpublished observations). Plasmids may also play an important role in the
metabolism of the group N streptococci, as discussed below.

PLASMID—MEDIATED METABOLIC ACTIVITIES AMONG THE GROUP N STREPTOCOCCI

The ability of the group N, or dairy, streptococci to catabolize or produce a variety of organic compounds appears to be
plasmid-mediated. Plasmids have been implicated in the fermentation
of lactose[31,32], galactose[33], or sucrose[34], glucose-mannose[34] and
D-xylose[34]; in the utilization of citrate[35] and uric acid (J. A.
Breznac, personal communication); and in the production of pro-
teinases[31] and the small peptide antibiotic, nisin[34], in at least
some strains of the Lancefield group N streptococci. With the
exception of a few lactose plasmids, which have been shown to be
transmissible[36,37,38], and some lactose and proteinase plasmids
which have been transferred by transduction[12,39], all plasmid-
associated traits in this group of streptococci have been identified
by curing experiments.

We are currently using a new approach to learn more about the
group N metabolic plasmids. We have chosen the lactose pathway,
which is quite different from the corresponding pathway in enteric
bacteria, for our initial studies. Among streptococci lactose
enters the cell as a phosphorylated molecule by the activity of a
phosphoenolpyruvate-dependent phosphotransferase system[40], or PTS.
The lactose phosphate is then cleaved, by a phospho-β-galactosidase[41],
or P-β-gal, to glucose and galactose-6-phosphate, which are further
catabolized by glucose- and galactose-specific pathways. In collaboration with E. J. St. Martin we have recently employed the
Challis transformation system to obtain preliminary evidence suggesting that the structural genes for the two specific lactose pathway enzymes are carried by the lactose plasmid in a strain of S.
lactis. These results are summarized in Table 1. When S. lactis
strain DL11 was grown at the expense of lactose it possessed PTS
activity for both galactose and lactose in a ratio of 0.3 to 1[33].
Using an activity stain for P-β-gal (E. J. St. Martin, L. N. Lee
and D. J. LeBlanc, manuscript in preparation), on a polyacrylamide
gel containing total cell protein from strain DL11, we obtained a
molecular weight estimate for P-β-gal of 40,000. In contrast, a
lactose-grown wild-type culture of the Challis strain had a galactose to lactose PTS ratio of only 0.05 to 1, and its P-β-gal had
a molecular weight of 52,000. We isolated a lac-negative mutant of
the Challis strain, lac-8, which was missing P-β-gal activity, but
retained lactose PTS. This mutant was transformed by plasmid DNA
from the S. lactis strain, and selected for ability to grow on
lactose. These transformants exhibited the same galactose to lactose PTS ratios as the Challis strain, but now possessed a P-β-gal
activity with the same molecular weight as that of the donor strain.
A second mutant, lac-83, missing both lactose PTS and P-β-gal, was
isolated from the lac-8 mutant of Challis. When this strain was
transformed by plasmid DNA from strain DL11, it had PTS and P-β-gal
activities with the properties of the donor S. lactis strain.

Plasmid DNA could not be isolated from the Challis transformants, nor were they curable for lactose fermentation. We tentatively interpret this to mean that structural genes on the lactose plasmid from S. lactis have integrated into the Challis chromosome to re-store functions required for lactose metabolism. We are currently preparing labeled probes of whole lactose plasmid DNA, as well as restriction fragments, to locate the appropriate sequences on the plasmid, and to determine if, in fact, these sequences are inte-grated into the Challis chromosome. Similar approaches are also being used to examine other plasmid-mediated metabolic functions of the group N streptococci.

ANTIBIOTIC RESISTANCE

The streptococci, as with all other bacterial genera inhabiting human and animal niches, have become increasingly resistant to anti-biotics. Several of these resistance traits have.been shown to be plasmid-mediated in at least some streptococcal isolates. Plasmid-associated resistance to aminoglycosides and to chloramphenicol is mediated by antibiotic modifying enzymes which resemble in activity, but are clearly different from, their counterparts in gram-negative bacteria[24,25,42].

The vast majority of studies on antibiotic resistance plasmids in the streptococci have centered on resistance to erythromycin[7,13,14,15,16,18,20,21,22,23,29]. Streptococcal and staphylococcal plas-mids mediating resistance to this antibiotic are referred to as MLS plasmids because the mechanism of resistance, N^6-dimethylation of

Table 1.   Characterization of lactose[+] transformants of
S. sanguis by plasmid DNA from S. lactis

Strain	Gal/Lac PTS[a] Activity Ratio	P-β-Gal[b]
S. lactis DL11	0.30	40,000
S. sanguis (Challis)	0.05	52,000
S. sanguis lac-8	+	-
pDL1 X S. sanguis lac-8	0.07	40,000
S. sanguis lac-83	-	-
pDL1 X S. sanguis lac-83	0.29	40,000

[a]See reference 33 for assay procedure
[b]Assay procedure in (E. J. St. Martin, L. N. Lee, and
     D.J. LeBlanc, manuscript in preparation).

adenine in 23S ribosomal RNA, also results in resistance to other
macrolides, to lincosamides and to streptogramin B type antibiotics[43],
[44]. This mechanism is common among streptococci[44], Staphylococcus
aureus[43] and the producer of erythromycin, Streptomyces erythreus[45].
MLS plasmids isolated from several streptococci[16,44,46,47], as well as
staphylococci[44], all share at least some common sequences with each
other. With the exception of a few large MLS plasmids in strains of
S. faecalis[2,20], with transmissibility apparently limited to this
species, and one small non-transmissible plasmid isolated from a
strain of S. sanguis[14], the vast majority of MLS plasmids in streptococci have a very narrow molecular weight range, between 15 and
20 million, and a very broad range of hosts to which they may be
transferred by filter matings[15,16,20,21,22,23]. Not only can these
plasmids be conjugally transferred among virtually all species of
streptococci, but at least three intergeneric crosses have been
successfully attempted[48,49] (O. E. Landman et al., Abstracts of the
Annual Meeting of the American Society for Microbiology, p. 114,
1980). One of these MLS plasmids, pAMB1[50], often becomes partially
deleted following transfer to a new host. These deletions, which
range from approximately 2.3 to 18.8 kilobases, from a molecule
originally 25.7 kilobases in size, often result in the loss of
transmissibility. We have collected several of these deleted
molecules and are attempting to locate on a restriction map of the
original plasmid, and enumerate, plasmid functions required for
conjugation.

UNUSUAL PROPERTIES OF TETRACYCLINE RESISTANCE DETERMINANTS

Among gram-negative bacteria of clinical origin, tetracycline
resistance has almost always been associated with a plasmid[51]. However, Burdett[17] has reported that among 30 tetracycline resistant
group B streptococcal isolates, 27 could not be shown to harbor
tetracycline resistance plasmids. Similarly, in a recent study of
tetracycline resistant streptococci obtained from the human oral
cavity, we were able to isolate plasmid DNA from only 23 of 121
strains examined[52]. Yet, we have observed transfer, on membrane
filters, of resistance from 14 out of 50 of these isolates to a
strain of S. faecalis. Only 4 of the strains with transmissible
tetracycline resistance had detectable plasmids (D. J. LeBlanc and
L. N. Lee, unpublished observations).

Recent reports from two different laboratories appear to offer
possible explanations for these results. Guild and associates[19] have
demonstrated chromosomal linkage, by transformation, of a chloramphenicol and a tetracycline resistance determinant in a strain of
S. pneumoniae. These investigators subsequently observed conjugal
transfer of these determinants by filter matings to a recipient
strain of the same species[53]. No plasmid DNA could be isolated from
the donor or from transconjugant isolates. Franke and Clewell[30]

recently reported the conjugal transfer of a tetracycline resistance determinant located on a transposon between strains of S. faecalis, in the absence of a plasmid DNA. The authors suggest that the transposon may be a plasmid-like (or phage-like) element that lacks replicative autonomy while retaining specific information for transfer. We, in collaboration with J. A. Donkersloot, have been studying a transmissible tetracycline resistance determinant in a porcine isolate of S. mutans, which exhibits a somewhat different type of apparent plasmid-less transfer. S. mutans strain DL5 is resistant to high levels of streptomycin, MLS antibiotics and tetracycline. Extensive searches for plasmids in this strain, using several different methods, have all proven negative. Although MLS and streptomycin resistance could not be transferred by this strain, tetracycline resistance was, as shown in Table 2. When the JH2-2 strain of S. faecalis[2] was used as the recipient transfer occurred almost equally as well in broth matings as on filters. A recombination-deficient strain of S. faecalis, UV202[54], was also a good recipient. However, with a S. mutans strain, DR0001/1[21], as the recipient the transfer frequency was almost two orders of magnitude lower and occurred only on filters. One of these transconjugants, strain DL43, transferred tetracycline resistance to strain JH2-2, but at a low frequency and only on filters. Resistance was not transmissible from any of the S. faecalis transconjugants. As shown in Table 3, we have observed plasmid DNA in some transconjugant isolates. The S. mutans transconjugant, strain DL43, which can transfer tetracycline resistance, occasionally yielded a band in agarose gels with a migration rate consistent with a molecular weight of approximately 19 million. The S. faecalis transconjugants, which do not appear to transfer the resistance determinant, consistently yielded a plasmid with a molec-

Table 2. Transmissibility of a Streptococcus mutans tetracycline resistance determinant

Donor Strain	Recipient Strain	Conjugation[a] Frequency
S. mutans DL5	S. faecalis JH2-2	2×10^{-6} (F)[b]
		5×10^{-7} (B)
	S. faecalis UV202	1×10^{-6} (F)
	S. mutans DR0001/1	1×10^{-8} (F)
S. mutans DL43	S. faecalis JH2-2	1×10^{-8} (F)

[a] per input donor colony forming units
[b] (F) or (B) refer to filter or broth matings

Table 3. Properties of transconjugant isolates receiving
          tetracycline resistance from S. mutans DL5

Strain	Derivation	Plasmid (Mdal)	Curing Frequency[a]
DL5	S. mutans donor	–	≺ 0.3%
DL43	DL5 X S. mutans DR0001/1	19?	< 0.3
DL40	DL5 X S. faecalis JH2-2	8	4.5
DL178	DL5 X S. faecalis UV202	8	13.5

[a]Curing frequencies were determined after 40 to 50 generations
in the absence of tetracycline.

ular weight of 8 million. The covalently closed circular nature of
this latter plasmid species has been confirmed by dye buoyant density
gradient centrifugation. We have also examined these isolates for
spontaneous curing of tetracycline resistance following 40 to 50
generations in the absence of antibiotic. We could not detect curing
in either of the S. mutans strains, but the curing frequencies in a
JH2-2 transconjugant, strain DL40, and a rec⁻ transconjugant, DL178,
were relatively high. All cured strains examined had lost the 8
megadalton plasmid. We cannot yet explain all of these results, but
the system resembles, in some respects, those chromosomally integrated conjugative plasmids which appear to be common among antibiotic
resistant strains of Haemophilus influenzae[55,56]. We are currently
trying to isolate sufficient plasmid DNA from the transconjugants
to prepare labeled probes to investigate the possibility of chromosomal integration in the S. mutans strains.

We have recently observed yet another unusual property associated with tetracycline resistance in the streptococci. The JH1
strain of S. faecalis[2,3] harbors two transmissible plasmids, a 50
megadalton species, pJH1, mediating resistance to kanamycin, streptomycin, erythromycin and tetracycline, and a 35 megadalton species,
pJH2, coding for hemolysin and bacteriocin production. Each of
these plasmids can be transferred to the JH2-2 strain of S. faecalis
during broth matings. After conducting such a mating experiment we
recently obtained one transconjugant isolate with the properties
shown in Table 4. This isolate, strain DL172, was resistant to
tetracycline, but did not possess the other resistance traits associated with plasmid pJH1. Whereas the donor strain, JH1, was hemolytic
in the presence or absence of tetracycline, strain DL172 was hemolytic only in the presence of tetracycline, and contained a plasmid
intermediate in size between pJH1 and pJH2. Initially, we suspected

Table 4. Properties of S. faecalis strain JH1, JH2-2 and DL172

Property	JH1	JH2-2	DL172
Resistance to (μg/ml):			
Tetracycline	256	1	128
Kanamycin	10,000	500	500
Streptomycin	10,000	250	250
Erythromycin	1,000	1	1
Lincomycin	500	25	25
Hemolysis on Horse Blood:			
with tetracycline	+	no growth	+
without tetracycline	+	-	-
Plasmids present (Mdal)	50 & 35	none	43

that the tetracycline resistance determinant from plasmid pJH1 had
integrated into pJH2. However, when the 43 megadalton plasmid from
strain DL172 was purified, labeled with ^{32}P by nicked translation,
denatured and incubated with a blot containing pJH1 and pJH2, plus
chromosomal DNA from strain JH1, this plasmid hybridized with DNA
in the chromosome region and with plasmid pJH2, but not with pJH1.
We interpret these results to mean that a second tetracycline resistance determinant, from the chromosome of strain JH1, became integrated
into pJH2 and was transferred into strain JH2-2. Regardless of the
source of the tetracycline resistance determinant, it would appear
that the plasmid-mediated hemolytic activity was affected by the
presence of this DNA sequence, probably as a result of the location
and orientation of insertion. In support of this conclusion, Clewell
and associates[30] have recently described hyper- and non-hemolytic
isolates of S. faecalis strain DS16, resulting from site-specific
insertion of the tetracycline resistance transposon, Tn916, into the
hemolysin plasmid, pAD1.

CONCLUSIONS

     Although the existence of plasmids in the streptococci was only
demonstrated eight years ago, a great deal has been accomplished in
the area of streptococcal plasmid biology since then. Plasmids obviously play a significant role in the metabolism of the group N
streptococci and in antibiotic resistance and its dissemination among
several streptococcal species. Furthermore, the streptococci may be
an important link in the dissemination of antibiotic resistance among
gram-positive bacteria in general, particularly with regard to MLS
resistance. Our ability to answer many existing questions are
certainly now enhanced by the development of streptococcal recombinant DNA host-vestor systems recently described by Macrina et al.[57]
and by Behnke and Ferretti[58].

LITERATURE CITED

1. P. M. Courvalin, C. Carlier, and Y. A. Chabbert, Ann. Inst.
    Pasteur, 123:755 (1972).
2. A. E. Jacob and S. J. Hobbs, J. Bacteriol., 117:360 (1974).
3. A. E. Jacob, G. M. Douglas, and S. J. Hobbs, J. Bacteriol.,
    121:863 (1975).
4. L. L. McKay and K. A. Baldwin, Appl. Microbiol., 29:546 (1975).
5. B. R. Cords, L. L. McKay, and P. Guerry, J. Bacteriol.,
    117:1149 (1974).
6. G. M. Dunny, N. Birch, G. Hascall, and D. B. Clewell, J.
    Bacteriol., 114:1362 (1973).
7. D. B. Clewell and A. E. Franke, Antimicrob. Ag. Chemother.
    5:534 (1974).
8. B. M. Chassy, Biochem. Biophys. Res. Commun., 68:603 (1976).
9. D. J. LeBlanc and L. N. Lee, J. Bacteriol., 140:1112 (1979).
10. T. R. Klaenhammer, L. L. McKay, and K. A. Baldwin, Appl.
    Environ. Microbiol., 35:592 (1978).
11. S. A. Skjold, H. Malke, and L. W. Wannamaker, in: "Pathogenic
    Streptococci," M. T. Parker, ed., Reedbooks, Ltd., Windsor
    (1978).
12. L. L. McKay, K. A. Baldwin, and J. D. Efstathiou, Appl. Environ.
    Microbiol., 32:45 (1976).
13. D. J. LeBlanc and F. P. Hassell, J. Bacteriol., 128:347 (1976).
14. Y. Yagi, T. S. McLellan, W. A. Frez, and D. B. Clewell,
    Antimicrob. Ag. Chemother., 13:884 (1978).
15. H. Malke, FEMS Microbiol. Letters, 5:335 (1979).
16. V. Hershfield, Plasmid, 2:137 (1979).
17. V. Burdett, Antimicrob. Ag. Chemother., 18:753 (1980).
18. D. J. LeBlanc, L. Cohen, and L. Jensen, J. Gen. Microbiol.
    106:49 (1978).
19. N. B. Shoemaker, M. D. Smith, and W. R. Guild, J. Bacteriol.
    139:432 (1979).
20. J. D. A. vanEmbden, H. W. B. Engel, and B. vanKlingeren,
    Antimicrob. Ag. Chemother., 11:925 (1977).
21. D. J. LeBlanc, R. J. Hawley, L. N. Lee, and E. J. St. Martin,
    Proc. Natl. Acad. Sci. USA, 75:3484 (1978).
22. T. Horodniceanu, L. Bougueleret, N. El-Sohl, D. Bouanchaud,
    and Y. A. Chabbert, Plasmid, 2:197 (1979).
23. M. D. Smith, N. B. Shoemaker, V. Burdett, and W. R. Guild,
    Plasmid, 3:70 (1980).
24. T. Horodniceanu, L. Bougueleret, N. El-Sohl, G. Bieth, and
    F. Delbos, Antimicrob. Ag. Chemother., 16:686 (1979).
25. P. Courvalin, C. Carlier, and E. Collatz, J. Bacteriol., 143:
    541 (1980).
26. J. D. Efstathiou and L. L. McKay, J. Bacteriol., 130:257 (1977).
27. G. M. Dunny and D. B. Clewell, J. Bacteriol., 124:784 (1975).
28. D. R. Oliver, B. L. Brown, and D. B. Clewell, J. Bacteriol.
    130:948 (1977).

29. P. Tomich, F. An, and D. B. Clewell, J. Bacteriol., 141:1366 (1980).

30. A. E. Franke and D. B. Clewell, Cold Spring Harbor Symp. Quant. Biol. (In Press).

31. J. D. Efstathiou and L. L. McKay, Appl. Environ. Microbiol. 32:38 (1976).

32. D. G. Anderson and L. L. McKay, J. Bacteriol., 129:367 (1977).

33. D. J. LeBlanc, V. L. Crow, L. N. Lee, and C. F. Garon, J. Bacteriol., 137:878 (1979).

34. D. J. LeBlanc, V. L. Crow, and L. N. Lee, in: "Plasmids and Transposons: Environmental Effects and Maintenance Mechanisms" C. Stuttard and K. R. Rozee, eds. Academic Press, N. Y. (1980).

35. G. M. Kempler and L. L. McKay, Appl. Environ. Microbiol. 37: 316 (1979).

36. G. M. Kempler and L. L. McKay, Appl. Environ. Microbiol. 37: 1041 (1979).

37. L. L. McKay, K. A. Baldwin, and P. M. Walsh, Appl. Environ. Microbiol. 40:84 (1980).

38. M. J. Gasson and F. L. Davies, J. Bacteriol., 143:1260 (1980).

39. L. L. McKay and K. A. Baldwin, Appl. Microbiol., 28:342 (1974).

40. L. L. McKay, A. Miller III, W. E. Sandine, and P. R. Elliker, J. Bacteriol., 102:804 (1970).

41. T. A. Molskness, D. R. Lee, W. E. Sandine, and P. R. Elliker, Appl. Microbiol. 25:373 (1973).

42. P. M. Courvalin, W. V. Shaw, and A. E. Jacob, Antimicrob. Ag. Chemother., 13:716 (1978).

43. B. Wisblum, in: "Microbiology-1974," D. Schlessinger, ed. American Society for Microbiology, Washington, D.C. (1975).

44. B. Weisblum, S. B. Holder, and S. M. Halling, J. Bacteriol. 138:990 (1979).

45. M. Y. Graham and B. Weisblum, J. Bacteriol., 137:1464 (1979).

46. N. El-Sohl, D. H. Bouanchaud, T. Horodniceanu, A. Roussel, and Y. A. Chabbert, Antimicrob. Ag. Chemother., 14:19 (1978).

47. Y. Yagi, A. E. Franke, and D. B. Clewell, Antimicrob. Ag. Chemother., 7:871 (1975).

48. E. M. Gibson, N. M. Chace, S. B. London, and J. London., J. Bacteriol., 137:614 (1979).

49. H. W. B. Engel, N. Soedirman, J. A. Rost, W. J. van Leeuwen, and J. D. A. van Embden., J. Bacteriol., 142:407 (1980).

50. D. B. Clewell, Y. Yagi, G. M. Dunny, and S. K. Schultz, J. Bacteriol., 117:283 (1974).

51. S. Falkow, "Infectious Multiple Drug Resistance," Pion, Ltd.,

52. R.J. Hawley, L.N. Lee, D.J.LeBlanc, Ant.Ag.Chem.,17:372(1980).

53. N.B. Shoemaker, M.D. Smith, W.J. Guild, Plasmid,3:80 (1980).

54. Y. Yagi and D.B. Clewell, J. Bacteriol., 143:966 (1980).

55. J.H. Stuy, J. Bacteriol. 142:925 (1980).

56. M.C. Roberts and A.L. Smith, J.Bacteriol., 144:476 (1980).

57. F.L. Macrina, E.R. Jones, P.H. Wood,J.Bacteriol.143:1425(1980).

58. D.Behnke and J.J. Ferretti, J. Bacteriol., 144:806 (1980).

BACTERIAL PATHOGENICITY, AN OVERVIEW

Stanley Falkow

Department of Medical Microbiology
Stanford, University
Stanford, CA   94305

INTRODUCTION:

The majority of infectious diseases had begun to decline at the turn of the century with the understanding that potentially dangerous microbes could be transmitted by water, food and insects and by the application of sanitation and antisepsis. Since the birth of the modern antibiotic era some 45 years ago the incidence of bacterial disease has declined further and, despite the marvels of R plasmids we heard earlier today, most bacterial infections can be controlled, though usually not prevented, by chemotherapy. Some bacterial infections can be prevented by immunization although except for certain toxins, immunization is generally based on hit or miss whole organism vacccines. The fact is that if we understood more about how particular microorganisms caused infection it might be possible to devise rational means to prevent them.

Moreover, there is still the surprise of 'new' pathogens. The last decade alone has seen the emergence of the toxic shock syndrome (TSS) caused by certain strains of Staphylococcus aureus[1] and pneumonitis caused by Legionella pneumophila[2]. These organisms are, it seems to me, the responses of microorganisms to "civilization". Legionella seems to like water-cooling towers used for air-conditioning and are subsequently spread by aerosols while TSS staphylococci are associated primarily with increased tampon usage by women over the past decade. We might understand something of the selective pressures that have brought these organisms to the fore, we still don't understand why or even how they can cause disease.

In many parts of the world, in fact not far from this meeting hall, microbial diseases considered trivial by wealthy nations exact a heavy toll of mortality and morbidity. Diarrheal disease, leprosy, protozooan diseases, and infection with large parasites are the central problems. Widespread preventive measures are required. It would be easier to formulate these measures if we understand the mechanisms of infection.

In the following sections it is my intent to review general aspects of microbial pathogenicity. I shall not attempt to dwell on bacterial plasmids since the speakers that follow will do that and there have been several excellent reviews of the subject of plasmids and pathogenicity[3,4]. Rather I shall just summarize information that any interested individual might find in a textbook of medical microbiology or infectious disease text[5,6,7,8]. The references are few, the speculations are many. But it is in this way I hope to provide a perspective for the papers to come.

INFECTION AND DISEASE.

Thus far I have used the terms infection and disease inter-changeably. It is useful to distinguish between the two terms. Infection is the persistent presence of a microorganism on the sur-faces or within the tissue of the human body. The mere presence of the organism in the body however does not lead invariably to clinical illness, disease. In fact the production of disease in humans by most microorganisms is the exception rather than rule. It seems to me that disease occurs more as an abnormal event, an accident if you will, rather than an invariant outcome of infec-tion. Generally speaking most of the time something goes awry with normal host defence mechanisms and tips the host-parasite relation-ship from a relatively innocuous compromise to a potentially dangerous event.

Hence all of us at one time or another carry pneumococci, meningococci and streptococci without misfortune. But let there be some new factor thrown into the equation, trauma or a toxic insult like alcohol and we may not escape so lightly. Not unexpectedly the disease caused by a particular microorganism depends upon its properties, its pathogenicity. Pathogenicity is a relative term. Virutally any microorganism can cause disease when host defenses are suppressed or compromised. One can visit any burn unit or can-cer ward to see the devastation caused by 'ordinary micro-organisms'. However the term pathogen is generally employed to refer to an organism that causes disease in 'normal' hosts. Viru-lence properly refers to the degree of pathogenicity among strains within a given species. It should come as no surprise to the par-ticipants of this meeting that the genetic potential for patho-genicity may vary greatly between species of microorganisms. For example only about a dozen of the myriad of E. coli serotypes are regularly found as the causative agents of diarrheal disease.

The Pathogenesis of Infection

a. The initial events.

The inital encounter between a pathogenic microorganism and host involves a variety of factors. As a first step it is clear that sufficient numbers of the organism must be taken in by the human host before infection takes place. The numbers of organisms required to establish infection and disease varies dramatically. Some microbial species (for example Shigella flexneri) are so virulent that only a few hundred viable cells are required to establish clinical disease in a significant number of susceptible persons. In other instances, enteropathogenic E. coli for example, millions of viable cells are required. Since E. coli and Shigella flexneri are so closely related genetically, these differences will be presumably understood in the not too distant future - indeed Dr. Kopecko will speak to this question later on in the proceedings. In any event the offending microorganism must possess the genetic capacity to proliferate within the potential host; obviously the capacity to spread from host-to-host is of equal importance.

After an organism gains entry into a human host, a certain period of time (incubation period) elapses before clinical illness is apparent. It should be apparent also that the incubation period will be dependent upon the multiplication rate of an invading organism. Few microorganisms multiply as well in vivo as they do artificial culture media. Obviously a microorganism which has a doubling time measured in days (for example the tubercle bacillus) will tend to cause a more slowly evolving infection and disease than a microorganism which has a doubling time within a host of a few hours (for example, Salmonella typhimurium). In addition, just as in the laboratory the in vivo pH and oxygen tension must be satisfactory for growth.

We are still pretty much ignorant of the properties of cells after they have grown in vivo; most investigators grow their cultures on plates or in broth. In vivo growth can have an enormous affect on infectivity. It seems clear, as Professor Harry Smith[10] has suggested for many years now, that microbiologists should devise clever techniques to examine the properties of in vivo - grown cells as well as the more conveniently prepared laboratory grown cells of pathogens.

Finally, in analysing the initial encounter between the human and a pathogen it is worthwhile to see that despite differences in the required inoculum size, the capacity of proliferate in vivo etc. virtually all infections can be divided into a relatively few categories:

1.   Those in which the organisms have specific mechanisms for attaching to and sometimes penetrating the body surfaces of the human host.

2.   Microorganisms introduced into the body of the normal host by a biting arthropod.

3.   Organisms which are dependent upon previous tissue damage on severe impairment of host defense mechanisms for invasion to take place.

4.   Organisms capable of causing disease through the secretion of toxic substances. Such organisms may not even need to penetrate body surfaces to cause disease.

Few pathogens fall snugly into just one of these categories but, in the simplest possible terms, bacteria cause disease either because they invade tissue, or elaborate toxins.

Bacterial Attributes of Virulence

1.   The capacity to attach to the host cellular surface.

May microorganisms have the capacity of specifically adhere to host cells[11].   Indeed this adherence is highly evolved and is often quite specific for a certain host cell type.   In the oropharynx, for example, Streptococcus pyogenes synthesizes a specific surface protein, the M protein, that permits it to tightly adhere to pharyngeal cells but not to teeth or the epithelial cells of the cheek.   Similarly gonococci adhere to microvilli of columnar epithelial cells of the urogenital tract via pili and Bordetella pertussis specifically adhere to cilia on epithelial cells of the trachea.   We shall hear later on from Jan van Embden concering properties of plasmid-mediated pili of toxigenic E. coli that permit adherence to epithelial cells of the small bowel.   Thus many successful pathogens possess the capacity to 'stick' to the epithelial cell surface and the spread of the organism is very rapid on epithelial surfaces covered with liquid.   These adherence mechanisms point out one fundamental microbial strategy to circumvent host defense mechanisms and to increase their likelihood of establishing a host-parasite relationship.

2.   Spread of microorganisms in tissue.

Many infections stay pretty much confined to the epithelial cell surface and the organisms remain as extracellular parasites.

Such organisms may spread through the tissues effectively by mechanical means such as ciliary action, gravity, coughing, sneezing etc. Some degree of subepithelial spread will occur because of the death of host cells from microbial by-products. However, direct spread in the sub-epithelial tissue is often limited because of the connective tissue matrix. Some bacteria are known to elaborate specific enzymes including hyaluronidase that degrades the hayaluronic acid component of the connective tissue matrix and collagenase that breaks down the collagen of connective tissue. Other known bacterial enzymes and other extracellular factors thought to facilitate pathogenicity include coagulase (leading to the clotting of plasma), DNAse (thought to reduce the viscosity of exudates) as well as lecithinase and hemolysins both of which attack cell membranes). Whether one can asign specific roles in pathogenesis to any of these extracellular factors is not clear. Bacteria in general produce a variety of proteases and lipases that would theoretically play a role in bacterial pathogenesis. It is just as likely, however, that these enzymes play a role in bacterial nutrition and metabolism as they do in the infectious process. Certainly they can be considered as accessory determinants of pathogenesis at least in providing for the ease of mechanical spread of microorganisms throughout the tissue.

Most recently, a variety of pathogens that are largely restricted to the mucosal surface including Streptococcus mitis, S. pneumoniae, N. meningitidis, H. influenzae and N. gonorrheae have been found to elaborate a protease specific for human IgA12. This specificity coupled with the known antibacterial and anti-adhesive properties of IgA suggests that this enzyme may play an important role in pathogenesis although this has yet to be proved. Since the enzyme is found within microorganisms readily amenable to genetic study one can expect that it will be possible to assess the importance of this unusual class of enzymes. By the same token some bacteria, notably Streptococci and Staphylococci, actively bind the Fc portion of IgM, IgA and IgG. This property and antibody-specific proteases may all act to circumvent both specific and non-specific immune mechanisms.

3.   Invasion of epithelial cells.

Some bacteria regularly penetrate epithelial cells during the course of infection. Precisely how the microorganisms accomplish this is not known. For example, members of the Shigella and Yersinia group adhere to the host cell surface and enter the cytoplasm often causing a local breakdown in the host cell plasma membrane. This invasive process may be ultimately lethal to the cell. In other cases, for example in Salmonellosis, the penetration of the organism may not be fatal to the cell; it is almost as if the microbial cell is "passing through" to deeper tissue layers. This is not simply a passive phenomenon. One can easily isolate mutants of Salmonella, or plasmidless derivatives of Yersinia and Shigella which fail to invade tissue. Yet the precise biochemical mechanisms at play remain the subject to study. Plasmid-mediated determinants that confer invasiveness in Shigella and Yersinia will be discussed later on in this session.

4.   Subepithelial invasion.

Once an invading microorganism penetrates the basement membrane barrier it is exposed to important host defense mechanisms. The most important of these is the inflammatory response. The inflammatory response is a subject of considerable complexity. Suffice it to say that the host responds to a microbial insult by a prompt and vigorous change in its microcirculation. The reaction is the same for any part of the body - there is a dilatation of vessels and their permeability increases allowing the influx of serum, immunoglobulins and other proteins. Fibrinogen may be converted to fibrin so that a diffuse network is laid down to retard invading organisms. This is followed by active passage (diapedesis) of leucocytes and other cellular fractions into the insulted tissue. The lymphatics draining the affected area also become dilated, take up the inflammatory fluid and carry it to local lymph nodes where the macrophages lining the node act as filter agents.

It is at the subepithelial level that the battleground between the invading organism and the host take place. The outcome of the infection depends on the capacity of the inflammatory responses, particularly the phagocytes, to handle the invading microorganism and the microorganisms capacity to overcome normal host defense mechanisms. Two microbial factors that will be discussed in some detail at these meetings may come into play here. One of these, serum resistance, will be discussed by Ken Timmis. The other which is a more subtle but highly significant factor is the capacity of infecting microorganisms to sequester the free iron they require from growth from the host which in turn goes to great lengths to bind the iron in an unavailable form. Peter Williams' will describe to us the marvelous way that the Col V plasmid brings this capacity to certain E. coli strains.

a.   Anti-phagocytic factors of extracellular parasites.

A number of microorganisms have ways of interfering with phagocytic activity. The best known example is the bacterial capsule although there are other antiphagocytic surface components. For example, the pathogenic success of the pneumococcus and Streptococcus pyogenes are due to their capacity to avoid phagocytosis. Similarly the M protein of Streptococci and the pili of gonococci that provide specific adherence to certain target host cells also appear to be associated with their relative resistance to phago-

cytosis. In any event, encapsulation or the presence of an antiphagocytic surface is quite common in both gram positive and gram
negative microorganism. For most extracellular, parasites (those
that cannot survive within phagocytes) the antiphagocytic cell surface is the critical determinant of virulence. If one isolates
non-encapsulated mutants of pneumococci or cells that have lost
their antiphagocytic surface, the mutant cells are avirulent. If
one then isolates reversions or transfers genes conferring encapsulation virulence is regained. I am not aware there have been extensive genetic studies on most antiphagocytic determinants and
their specificity, however.

Some microorganisms, like Streptococcus pyogenes, not only
resist phagocytosis through the nature of its cell surface but also
because it elaborates a phagocytic poison, leukocidan. Similarly
some Staphylococci elaborate a substance that induces the granules
of white cells to discharge into its own cell cytoplasm; the white
cell is thus duped into killing itself rather than the microorganism. Such microbial tactics imply a long-standing evolutionary relationship between host and parasite that would be amenable
to genetic study.

b.   Antiphagocytic factors of intracellular bacteria.

Some bacteria like the tubercle bacillus, the leprosy bacillus
and the cause of undulant fever, Brucella sp. grow in macrophages
that phagocytose them. Their success as infectious agents depends
on this. It is not clear if these bacteria have specific receptors
that interact with the phagocytic surface or not. Clearly if a
phagocytosed microorganism is not exposed to the killing and diges-
tive processes of the phagocyte, it can survive and even multiply.
This indeed seems to be a factor leading to the survival of the
tubercle bacillus within macrophges.

The ways in which microorganisms survive within phagocytes is
not clearly understood. In this regard it is survival within
macrophages that is crucial. Polymorphs have a short lifespan but
macrophages live for comparatively long periods of time. Of
course, bacteria in a macrophage are protected against many antibiotics as well as antibody that cannot penetrate the macrophage
surface.

6.   Bacterial Toxins.

In my mind, bacterial toxins provide one of the more clear cut
examples of the polygenic nature of microbial pathogenesis. The
bacterial toxins are broadly divided into exotoxins, those that are
liberated in the environment from multiplying bacteria and endo-
toxins, those that are associated with the gram negative cell wall
and are released, in large part, upon death of the microorganism.

In some microorganisms the capacity to elaborate an exotoxin is the primary determinant of pathogenicity and the clinical symptoms in a patient can be accounted for by the action of the toxin alone. This is certainly true of botulism, staphylococcal food poisoning, tetanus, diphtheria, cholera and E. coli enterotoxins.

It is important, however, to make a distinction between the pharmocological action of pure exotoxin and the reality of its role in microbial pathogenesis. Undoubtedly in the case of botulism and staphylococcal food poisoning, the ingestion of preformed toxin in food will lead to clear-cut clinical disease; the microorganism need not multiply the host. One can duplicate diphtheria and tetanus, by parenteral toxin infection, and cholera and E. coli diarrhea by directly injecting toxin into ligated loops of bowel. Yet, many animals and man regularly carry toxigenic diphtheria bacilli and Clostridium tetani without apparent harm. Microbial cells which synthesize even large quantities of E. coli enterotoxin but lack the ability to effectively colonize the small intestine are innocuous to animals. Hence the important point to me is not that a purified toxin can cause injury when injected into an animal or a human but rather it is the sum total of toxigenicity coupled with the other determinants of the microorganism that is essential. C. tetani is innocuous if not introduced into tissue with a low redox potential; C. diphtheriae must be able to establish itself in the oropharynx (or a skin lesion), and multiply before the effects of intoxication can be appreciated. The delivery system is as important as the toxin. We still understand very little about the acessory determinants of pathogenicity in "purely" toxigenic pathogens.

At the end of this discussion of the general attributes of bacterial pathogenicity it is useful perhaps to note that rarely are invasiveness and toxigenicity completely separable. Invasive organisms often utilize factors of short-lived or local toxigenicity (a leukocidan, for example) while as noted above, toxigenic bacteria must possess at least some degree of bacterial multiplication and persistance in the tissues.

Plasmids and Pathogenicity

There has been a growing appreciation over the last decade that determinants carried by bacterial plasmids may directly contribute to bacterial pathogenicity. In the papers that follow we shall hear some of the details involving plasmid-mediated determinants of toxigenicity, adherence, serum resistance, invasiveness and iron scavanging. Many of us are fascinated by the fact that most bacterial toxins are associated with plasmids and bacteriophage. Why this should be I have no idea. It can not be accidental that this is so. Is this associated with the transmissibility of the genetic elements or their dispensability? Presumably the tactic that a plasmid-mediated determinant can be lost without affecting viability could be the most important factor. Under many circumstances we can imagine that a determinant of pathogenicity is a deterrent to microbial success. If it can be lost and later regained, it seems the best of both worlds.

Plasmid-mediated determinants of pathogenicity encompass a tantalizing array of elements and I believe we have yet but touched the tip of the iceberg. On the other hand, given the complexity of the steps in the pathogenesis of infection, the many genes that must be at play, the very dispensability of plasmids and the fact that only one or a few genes of pathogenicity are plasmid-mediated makes me a bit cautious in over interpreting their significance. For example we have shown that the heat labile enterotoxin of <u>E. coli</u> seems always to be plasmid-mediated while the closely related gene in <u>V. cholerae</u> is chromosomal[13]. Similarly there are chromosomal iron sequestering systems, determinants of serum resistance, hemolysins and invasive factors. This does not detract from the importance of plasmid-mediated determinants of virulence. Indeed because they can be so readily studied at the genetic and molecular level, they are of considerable importance to better understand pathogenicity. However, my guess is that the importance of plasmids to the pathogenicity of any particular organism lies more in the genetic flexability rather than the precise nature of the pathogenic determinant carried by plasmids.

REFERENCES

1. J. Todd, M. Fiskant, F. Kapral, and T. Welch. Toxic-shock syndrome associated with phage-group-1-staphylococci, Lancet ii, 1116 (1978).
2. Center for Disease Control, Legionnaires' Disease: Diagnosis and Management. Ann. Intern. Med. 88, 363 (1978).
3. K.N. Timmis and A. Puhler (ed), Plasmids of Medical, Environmental and Commercial Importance. Elsevier/North Holland Biomedical Press, Amsterdam (1979).
4. L.P. Elwell and P.L. Shipley, Plasmid-mediated factors associated with virulence of bacteria to animals, Ann. Rev. Microbiol. 34, 496 (1980).
5. C.A. Mims, The Pathogenesis of Infectious Disease, Academic Press, London (1976).
6. P.D. Hoeprich (ed) Infectious Diseses, Harper and Row, Hagerstown, MD (1977).
7. G.P. Youmans, P.Y. Paterson and H.M. Sommers, The Biologic and Clinical Basis of Infectious Diseases, W.B. Saunders, Philadelphia, PA (1979).
8. G.L. Mandell, R.G. Douglas, Jr., and J.E. Bennett, Principles and Practice of Infectious Diseases, John Wiley and Sons, New York, N.Y. (1979).

9. I. Orskov, F. Orskov, B. Jann, and K. Jann, Serology, Chemistry and Genetics of O and K antigens of Escherichia coli. Bacteriol. Rev. 41, 667 (1977).

10. H. Smith, Biochemical challenge of microbial pathogenicity, Bacteriol. Rev. 32, 164 (1968).

11. G.W. Jones, The attachment of bacteria to the surfaces of animal cells, in J.L. Reissig (ed) Receptors and Recognition, Sec. B, Vol. 3, Microbial Interactions, John Wiley and Sons, New York, N.Y. (1978).

12. J. Mestecky, J.R. McGhee, S.S. Crago, S. Jackson, M. Kilian, H. Kiyono, J.Ll Babb and S.M. Michalek. J. Reticuloend. Soc. 28, 450 (1980).

13. S.L. Moseley and S. Falkow, Nucleotide sequence homology between the heat-labile enterotoxin gene of Escherichia coli and Vibrio cholerae deoxyribonucleic acid, J. Bacterol. 144, 444 (1980).

CLONING AND EXPRESSION OF THE GENES ENCODING FOR THE ADHESIVE

ANTIGENS K88 AND K99

J.D.A.van Embden[1], F.K.de Graaf[2], F.R.Mooi[2],
W.Gaastra[2] and I.G.W.Bijlsma[3]

1) Rijksinstituut voor de Volksgezondheid, Bilthoven
2) Vrije Universiteit, Dept.of Microbiology, Biological
   Laboratory, Amsterdam
3) Rijks Universiteit Utrecht, Veterinary Faculty, Utrecht

INTRODUCTION

More than a decade ago, enterotoxigenic E.coli strains were
found to be associated with acute diarrhoea in young animals and
later such strains were also found to be involved in cases of human
diarrhoea. Enterotoxigenic E.coli strains release a heat labile toxin
and/or a heat stable toxin which effects the fluid and electrolyte
secretion in the intestine by activation of the mucosal enzymes
adenyl cyclase and guanyl cyclase, respectively[1,2]. A number of
proteinaceous surface antigens of enterotoxigenic E.coli have been
identified, that are involved in the colonization of the gut by
facilitating the adherence of the microorganism to the intestinal
mucosa. Enterotoxins and several of these colonization factors are
encoded by plasmids. The significance of organisms that possess
plasmid-mediated pathogenic characteristics is that they constitute
a genetic pool from which new lines of pathogenic organisms may
arise. To the research worker, they represent genetic material that
can be added or removed from organisms, thus permitting the construction of new lines which differ only from the parent microorganism by
the presence or the absence of one character. Smith and coworkers
exploited this idea to elucidate the pathogenesis of E. coli diarrhoea in animals. They showed in an elegant series of experiments
that the antigens K88 and K99 promote colonization of the intestine
by implanting K88 and K99 plasmids into non-pathogenic strains of
E. coli or alternatively by removal of these plasmids from pathogenic strains and subsequently feeding such modified strains to neonates[3,4,5]. The adhesion of K88 to the intestinal mucosa was demonstrated by Jones and Rutter[6]. Vaccination with K88 antigen results

in protection of neonatal animals by the antibodies induced in the colostrum[7],[8]. The K88 antigen is found on the surface of the E.coli cell as a thin filament of protein. Such filaments, also called pili or fimbriae, have been found among a great variety of bacteria. Among enterotoxigenic E.coli strains, 5 serologically unrelated pili have been found to be associated with adhesion and colonization of the intestine: K88, 987P, K99, CFA I and CFA II[9],[10],[11]. Each of these adhesive antigens is found among a characteristic set of serotypes of E.coli. E.coli strains producing the antigens K88 and P987 are found in diseased piglets, K99 mainly in calves and lambs and to a lesser extend in pigs. CFA I and CFA II have been associated with human strains. All five adhesive antigens share the following properties: The antigens are high molecular weight structures, composed of identical non-covalently linked polypeptides having molecular weights between 14,000 and 26,000. Each antigen can adhere to a specific set of animal cells, including erythrocytes and epithelial mucosa cells of the intestine; at temperatures of 18-20°C no or very little of the antigen is produced. Furthermore, the capability to produce pili is usually an unstable genetic trait. Although in certain cases this instability is due to the loss of plasmids which encode for the pili, this is not always the case. The protein of the adhesive antigens analysed are rich in hydrophobic amino-acids. Some of the properties of various pili are depicted in table 1. It is presumed that the pili recognize particular receptor structures on the surface of the animal cell. Until now no such receptors for any of the 5 adhesive antigens have been isolated and characterized in biochemical terms, although several attempts have been made[12],[13],[14]. In order to study the genetic organization and the expression of adhesive antigens we have cloned the genes encoding for K88 and K99.

Table 1. Properties of adhesive antigens of enterotoxigenic E.coli

Antigen	Diameter (nm)	Mol.weight sub unit	Genetic location	Origin
K88	2	25,000	plasmid	piglet
K99	3	18,500	plasmid	calf, lamb, piglet
987P	7	22,000	?	piglet
CFA I	6-9	14,000	plasmid	human
CFA II	7-8	?	plasmid	human

EXPRESSION AND CLONING OF THE K99 GENES

The K99 antigen is of particular interest with regard to its peculiar regulation of expression. Certain serotypes, like 08, 09, and 020, produce considerably less K99 than wild type strains of the serotypes 0101[15]. This regulation seems to be a host dependant trait because no difference in the level of K99 expression is observed when K99 plasmids of high and low producing serotypes are transferred to E.coli K12. Furthermore, K99 production is highly dependent on the composition of the growth medium. Because the K99 antigen is usually difficult to detect by agglutination with antiserum after growth on common media, Guinée et al.[16,17] developed a supplemented minimal medium. Isaacson showed that the amount of K99 on the surface of the cell is subject to catabolite repression: glucose repression could be overcome by addition of 0.5 mM cyclic AMP to the medium[18]. More dramatically, however, is the effect of the presence of alanine. When alanine is added to minimal medium at concentrations above 1 mM, the K99 production is less than 3% compared to that after growth in the absence of alanine[19]. By cloning of the K99 genes and introduction of mutations in these genes we hope to get more insight in this regulatory system. Plasmid pRI9901 was used for cloning of the K99 determinant and it originated from E.coli 0101:K99 strain B41. The K99 plasmid was transferred conjugally to E.coli K12 in order to separate it from the other 3 plasmids that are also present in B41. The K99 genes were cloned into the Hind III site of pBR322 and subcloned into the Bam HI site of pBR325. Four subclones were obtained which all contained a 4.5 Md BamHI fragment. Three of them expressed K99 and one clone produced very little K99 although the 4.5 Md was undistinguishable from the fragment of the other 3 subclones as analysed by multiply cutting enzymes on agarose gels[20]. Morris et al.[21] found spontaneous K99-negative mutants of B41 and analysis of plasmid DNA of this strain showed no difference with its K99-positive parental strain. Therefore, it seems likely that the expression of the K99 genes can be switched off, without loss of K99 DNA, perhaps by a mechanism analogous to the flagellar phages variation in Salmonella typhimurium[22]. Although the K99 genes were cloned on a multicopy vector, expression of K99 in E.coli K12 was low compared to the production of wild type strains. However, by introduction of the K99 recombinant plasmids into a wild 0101 strain, we obtained a strain that produced K99 more than 4-fold, compared to the best wild type producers. This again reinforces the idea that properties of the host play a major role in the expression of K99. By deletion of various regions in the cloned 4.5 Md K99 fragment the approximate location of the structural gene of the K99 subunit could be inferred between the coordinates 4.1 Kb and 5.8 Kb at the physical map as shown in figure 1. It is interesting a region about 1 Md distal from the K99 structural gene is required for K99 expression (as in pRI9915-11), whereas the more proximal region between 3-4 Kb can be deleted without much effect on the level of K99 expression.

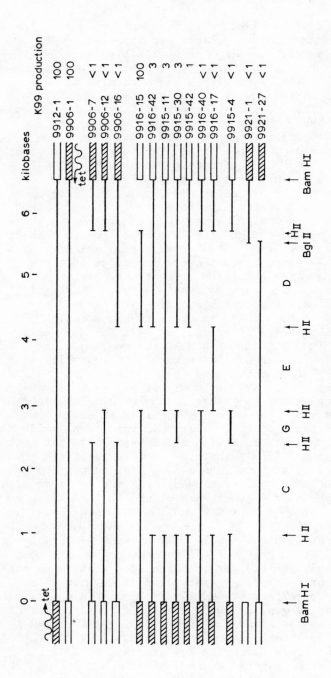

Figure 1. Expression of the K99 antigen by the recombinant plasmids pRI9912-1, pRI9906-1 and various deletion mutants. pRI9906-1 and pRI9912-1 contain the same K99 BamHI DNA fragment, but in different orientation. The direction of transcription of the tetracycline resistance gene of the vector pBR325 is indicated. Deletion mutants were obtained by partial digestion with Hind II (HII) or BamHI plus BglII. The production of K99 in E.coli K12 is measured by an enzyme-linked immunosorbent assay and it is expressed relative to that of pRI9912-1.

CLONING AND EXPRESSION OF THE K88 GENES

Much more is known of the K88 antigen. At least three different antigenic variants exist: K88ab, K88ac and K88ad[23]. Virtually all E.coli isolates that are K88+ have also the ability to ferment the trisaccharide raffinose[24]. Both characters are located on a single plasmid and therefore K88 can easily be transferred conjugally by selection of recipients on raf+. Shipley et al.[25] found that K88 is generally encoded by plasmids of a molecular weight of about 50 Md and these plasmids showed at least 97% polynucleotide homology. No or only slight differences are observed in the restriction enzyme digest patterns of K88ab, K88ac or K88ad plasmids and the plasmids of all 3 K88 variants contain a 7.7 Md <u>Hind</u> III fragment that encodes for the K88 determinant (25, Meyerink, unpublished). The presence of 2 copies of the IS1 sequence in direct orientation separated by a stretch of about 10 Md of DNA[26] explains the early observations of Let Bak et al.[27] on the dissociation of a 50 Md K88 plasmid into a 40 Md and a 10 Md component. The amino-acid sequence of about 90% of the K88ab subunit is established[28] and no differences between K88ab and K88ac in the sequenced part of the K88 subunit have been found. In contrast, the K88ad polypeptide differs from K88ab at least in 4 amino-acids.

Previously, we reported the cloning of the K88ab determinant. The smallest plasmid obtained that still expressed K88 was pFM205, which is composed of pBR322 and a 4.3 Md piece of K88 DNA[29]. We constructed derivatives of pFM205, having deletions in various regions of pFM205 and the expression was studied in minicells (see figure 2). pFM205 directs the synthesis of 6 non-vector encoded polypeptides in mini-cells. One of these (26 Kd) is identical to the K88ab subunit, because specific K88 antiserum precipitates this polypeptide as the only one. The K88 surface protein is translocated across the cyto-plasmic membrane and therefore one might expect that the mature K88 subunit is a product of proteolytic processing. By inhibition of the processing system with 9.5% ethanol, a 28 Kd K88 polypeptide was found in minicells, which indeed indicates the existence of a signal sequence about 20 amino-acids. This is consistent with preliminary DNA sequence data of the K88 coding region, which indicate that the K88 structural gene has a signal sequence of 22 amino-acids. Deletion of the genes encoding for the 17 Kd and the 81 Kd polypeptides (as in plasmids pFM222 and pFM77, respectively) affects the expression of K88 as an antigen. Extracts of cells carrying pFM222 or pFM77 bind only small amounts of anti-K88 antibodies, although the synthe-sis of the K88 subunit in minicells does not differ significantly from that in minicells carrying the parentel plasmid pFM205 (figure 2). Furthermore, the antigenic material of these mutants is much more thermolabile compared to wild type K88. Presumably, the 17 Kd and the 81 Kd polypeptides are involved in the assembly of the 26 Kd subunits to complete pili. The function of the other 3 polypeptides (27 Kd, 29 Kd and 30 Kd) which are also synthesized in minicells is present-ly unknown.

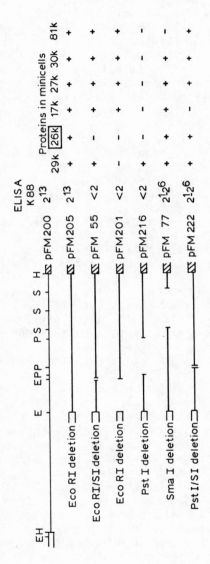

Figure 2. Polypeptide synthesis of the K88 recombinant plasmid pFM205 and deletion mutants in minicells. pFM205 is a deletion mutant of pFM200 obtained by EcoRI treatment and ligation. The level of K88 production was measured in E.coli K12 maxicells. The order of the 6 proteins as written in this figure corresponds to the gene order as derived from these data, except for the 30 K and the 27 K proteins. The mutual gene order of latter proteins is not yet known.

Jones and Rutter[6] found brush borders of pigs from certain litters that were not adhesive for K88+ E. coli. This "non-adhesive" phenotype was inherited as an autosomal recessive characteristic and the experiments showed the "non-adhesive" pigs conferred relative resistance to developing diarrhoea after challenge with K88+ entero-toxigenic E.coli. Recently, Bijlsma (unpublished) extended the study of Jones and Rutter and tested all 3 K88 variants in adhesion tests with brush borders from 42 pigs and piglets obtained from the slaughterhouse. He also found a "non-adhesive" phenotype, type E, to which none of the 3 K88 variants adhered. The brush borders of "adhesive phenotype", however, could be divided into 4 groups: phenotype A was adhesive for all 3 K88 variants, B for K88ab and K88ac, C for K88ab and K88ad and phenotype D only for K88ad (table 2). Preincubation of type A brush borders with an excess of purified K88ad antigen did not interfere with the adhesion of K88ab or K88ac bacteria, whereas K88ab completely blocked the adhesion of bacteria producing K88ac and vice versa.

Table 2. Adhesion of K88ab, K88ac and K88ad E.coli to brush borders of pigs

Brush border phenotype	Adhesion by K88ab	K88ac	K88ad	Number of pigs tested
A	+	+	+	11
B	+	+	−	6
C	+	−	+	11
D	−	−	+	3
E	−	−	−	11
			total	42

These experiments indicate that the antigenic variation of K88 is associated with differences in adhesive properties.

REFERENCES

1. D.J.Evans Jr., L.C.Chen, G.T.Curlin and D.G.Evans, Stimulation of adenyl cyclase by Escherichia coli enterotoxin, Nature New Biology 236: 137 (1972).
2. M.Field, L.H.Graf, W.J.Laird and P.L.Smith, Heat-stable entero-toxin of Escherichia coli: In vitro effects on guanylate cylase activity, cyclic GMP concentration, and ion transport in small intestine, Proc.Natl.Acad.Sci., USA 75:2800 (1978).
3. H.W.Smith and M.A.Linggood, Observations on the pathogenic properties of the K88, Hly and ENT plasmids of Escherichia coli with particular reference to porcine diarrhoea, J.Med. Microbiol. 4: 467 (1971).

4. H.W.Smith and M.A.Linggood, Further observations on Escherichia coli enterotoxins with particular regard to those produced by atypical piglet strains and by calf and lamb strains. The transmissible nature of these enterotoxins and of a K antigen possessed by calf and lamb strains, J.Med.Microbiol. 5: 243 (1972).

5. H.W.Smith and M.B.Huggins, The influence of plasmid and other characteristics of enteropathogenic E.coli on their ability to proliferate on the alumentory tracts of piglets, calves and lambs. J.Med.Microbiol. 11: 471 (1978).

6. G.W.Jones and J.M.Rutter, Role of K88 antigen in the pathogenesi of neonatal diarrhea caused by Escherichia coli in piglets, Infect.Immun. 6: 918 (1972).

7. S.D.Acres, R.E.Isaacson, L.A.Babiuk and R.A.Kapitany, Immunization of calves against enterotoxigenic colibacillosis by vaccinating dams with purified K99 antigen and whole cell bacterins, Infect.Immun. 25: 121 (1979).

8. J.M.Rutter and G.W.Jones, Protection against enteric disease caused by Escherichia coli - a model for vaccination with a virulence determinant? Nature 242: 531 (1973).

9. D.G.Evans, R.P.Silver, D.J.Evans Jr., D.G.Chase and S.L.Gorbach, Plasmid-controlled colonization factor associated with virulence in Escherichia coli enterotoxigenic for humans, Infect.Immun. 12: 656 (1975).

10. D.G.Evans and D.J.Evans Jr., New surface-associated heat-labile colonization factor antigen (CFA/II) produced by enterotoxigenic Escherichia coli of serogroups 06 and 08, Infect. Immun. 21: 638 (1978).

11. R.E.Isaacson, B.Nagy and H.W.Moon, Colonization of porcine small intestine by Escherichia coli: colonization and adhesion factors of pig enteropathogens that lack K88, J.Inf.Dis. 135: 531 (1977).

12. A.Faris, M.Lindahl and T.Wadström, GM_2-like glycoconjugate as possible erythrocyte receptor for the CFA/I and K99 haemagglutinins of enterotoxigenic Escherichia coli, FEMS Microbiology Letters 7: 265 (1980).

13. R.A.Gibbons, G.W.Jones and R.Sellwood, An attempt to identify the intestinal receptor for the K88 adhesin by means of a haemagglutination inhibition test using glycoproteins and fractions from sow colostrum, J.Gen.Microbiol. 86:228 (1975)

14. G.E.Jones, The attachment of bacteria to the surfaces of animal cells. In Microbial Interactions, Receptors and recognition, Series B, Vol. 3 (J.L.Riessig, Ed.). Chapman and Hall, London, pp. 139-176 (1977).

15. F.K.de Graaf, F.B.Wientjes and P.Klaasen-Boor, Production of K99 antigen by enterotoxigenic Escherichia coli strains of antigen groups 08, 09, 020 and 0101 grown at different conditions, Infect.Immun. 27: 216 (1980).

16. P.A.M.Guinée, W.H.Jansen and C.M.Agterberg, Detection of the
    K99 antigen by means of agglutination and immunoelectropho-
    resis in Escherichia coli isolates from calves and its
    correlation with enterotoxigenicity, Infect.Immun. 13:
    1369 (1976).
17. P.A.M.Guinée, J.Veldkamp and W.H.Jansen, Improved Minca medium
    for the detection of K99 antigen in calf enterotoxigenic
    strains of Escherichia coli, Infec.Immun. 15: 676 (1977).
18. R.E.Isaacson, Factors affecting expression of the Escherichia
    coli pilus K99, Infect.Immun. 28: 190 (1980).
19. F.K.de Graaf, P.Klaasen-Boor and J.E.van Hees, Biosynthesis
    of the K99 surface antigen is repressed by alanine, Infect.
    Immun. 30: 125 (1980).
20. J.D.A.van Embden, F.K.de Graaf, L.M.Schouls and J.S.Teppema,
    Cloning and expression of a deoxyribonucleic acid fragment
    that encodes for the adhesive antigen K99, Infect.Immun.
    29: 1125 (1980).
21. J.A.Morris, C.J.Thorns and W.J.Sojka, Evidence for two adhesive
    antigens on the K99 reference strain Escherichia coli B41,
    J.Gen.Microbiol. 118: 107 (1980).
22. J.Zieg, M.Hilmen and M.Simon, Regulation of gene expression by
    site-specitic inversion, Cell 15: 237 (1978).
23. P.A.M.Guinée and W.H.Jansen, Behavior of Escherichia coli K
    antigens K88ab, K88ac and K88ad in immunoelectrophoresis,
    double diffusion and hemagglution, Infect.Immun. 23,
    700 (1979).
24. H.W.Smith and Z.Parsell, Transmissible substrate-utilizing
    ability in Enterobacteria, J.Gen.Microbiol. 87: 129 (1975).
25. P.L.Shipley, C.L.Gyles and S.Falkow, Characterization of plas-
    mids that encode for the K88 colonization antigen, Infect.
    Immun. 20: 559 (1978).
26. R.Schmitt, R.Mattes, K.Schmid and J.Altenburger, Raf plasmids in
    strains of Escherichia coli and their possible role in entero-
    pathogenicity. In: Plasmids of Medical, environmental and
    commercial importance (K.N.Timmis and A.Pühler, Eds.)
    Elsevier Amsterdam, pp. 199-210 (1979).
27. A.Leth Bak, G.Christiansen, C.Christiansen and A.Stenderup,
    Circular DNA molecules controlling synthesis and transfer
    of the surface antigen (K88) in Escherichia coli, J.Gen.
    Microbiol. 73: 373 (1972).
28. W.Gaastra, P.Klemm, J.M.Walker and F.K.de Graaf, K88 fimbrial
    proteins: amino- and carboxyl terminal sequences of intact
    proteins and cyanogen bromide fragments, FEMS Microbiology
    Letters 6: 15 (1979).
29. F.R.Mooi, F.K.de Graaf and J.D.A.van Embden, Cloning, mapping
    and expression of the genetic determinant that encodes for
    the K88ab antigen, Nucleic Acids Research 6: 849 (1979).

INVASIVE BACTERIAL PATHOGENS OF THE INTESTINE: SHIGELLA VIRULENCE PLASMIDS AND POTENTIAL VACCINE APPROACHES

Dennis J. Kopecko, Philippe J. Sansonetti, Louis S. Baron, and Samuel B. Formal
Division of Communicable Diseases and Immunology
Walter Reed Army Institute of Research
Washington, D.C.   20012

INTRODUCTION

Bacterial diseases of the gastrointestinal tract usually occur by one of three overall mechanisms. The first mechanism, termed "intoxication," occurs by bacterial secretion of an exotoxin that oftentimes is preformed in food prior to ingestion by the host. This process is exemplified by staphylococcal or clostridial food poisoning. In contrast, the remaining two processes require living and multiplying disease agents. In the "enterotoxigenic" mechanism, as discussed elsewhere in this volume, bacteria colonize the small intestine, usually in the jejunum or duodenum. These bacteria multiply on the intestinal surface and elaborate an enterotoxin that stimulates excessive fluid and electrolyte efflux resulting in a watery diarrhea. Enteropathogenic Escherichia coli and Vibrio cholera serve as typical examples. Finally, a third group of organisms, termed "invasive," actually penetrate the epithelial mucosa of the large intestine. Subsequently, these organisms multiply intracellularly and disseminate within or through the mucosa. This latter mechanism, classically typified by Shigella and Salmonella, is now thought to be used by invasive strains of E. coli, Yersinia, and, possibly, Campylobacter. In contrast to other invasive bacterial diseases like salmonellosis in which the invading bacteria are disseminated throughout the host, shigellosis is a disease normally confined to the intestinal lining. Whereas toxigenic organisms generally require a large dose of organisms to cause disease, previous studies have shown that as few as ten virulent cells of Shigella can cause disease in humans. Thus, these features distinquish the toxigenic from the invasive mechanism of intestinal disease (see reviews[1,2]).

Two common and essential features of invasive bacteria are their ability to penetrate and to multiply within the epithelial cells of the colon[1,2]. Mutants of Shigella strains that fail to penetrate or that penetrate but cannot multiply intracellularly have been isolated. Both types of mutants are avirulent. The process of invasio has thus far been characterized in microscopic, but not biochemical detail. The first visible alteration in the host intestinal epithelium is a localized destruction of the microvilli, the outermost structure of the intestinal lining. The invading bacteria are then engulfed by means of an invagination of the intestinal cell membrane and are contained intracellularly within vaculoes. Subsequently, th microvilli are reestablished and intracellular bacterial multiplication occurs. These bacteria then destroy the vacuole and disseminate to adjacent cells, causing necrosis and resulting in acute inflammation and focal ulceration of the epithelium. The resulting dysentery is characterized by a painful, bloody and mucous diarrhea normally of relatively small volume.

Genetic studies of Shigella flexneri have previously resulted in the conclusion that virulence is multideterminant, with at least two widely separated bacterial chromosomal regions being required for invasion[1,2]. Furthermore, these studies have shown that not only is a smooth lipopolysaccharide bacterial cell surface necessary for intestinal invasion, but also that only certain O-repeat unit polymers are effective in this process; this is true for both shigellae and invasive E. coli. Until recently, plasmids did not appea to play a role in the invasion process or in the virulence of Shigella. Recent evidence amassed over the past three years, however, demonstrates that plasmids of Shigella are involved in the invasion process[3,4,5].

RESULTS

Colonial morphology transition of S. sonnei. Shigellosis is still an important disease worldwide, with approximately 15,000 case reported in the U.S. during 1980. Of the 4 species of Shigella, S. sonnei is currently responsible for greater than two-thirds of all shigellosis cases in the U.S. and Europe. Because of its importance this species was chosen as the initial focus of our studies. Unlike the other Shigella species, all S. sonnei strains fall into a single serotype. This serotype is due to a somatic antigen, termed form I, that is required for epithelial cell invasion. Chemical studies have revealed that the from I antigen is the O-side chain[6].

Upon restreaking on agar medium, smooth even-edged form I colonies generate at a relatively high frequency rough uneven-edged colonies, termed form II. Form II colonies appear in different strains at frequencies varying from 1 to 50%. Further study has shown that these rough colonies have irreversibly lost the form I antigen and are always avirulent due to the inability to invade epithelial cells[3,4]. The ability to penetrate epithelial cells can

easily be monitored using the guinea pig eye as an assay system[7].
Bacterial strains that can penetrate epithelial cells will elicit a
keratoconjunctivitis within 72 hours following inoculation of the
guinea pig eye with a bacterial suspension. This assay was used
exclusively throughout these studies.

   Plasmid analyses of form I and II strains. The high frequency
and irreversible nature of the form I to II transition, which always
resulted in the loss of virulence, suggested the involvement of a
plasmid in this phenomenon. Thus, the plasmid DNA's of various S.
sonnei strains, obtained from different parts of the world, were
examined[3]. Plasmid DNA's of 4 representative isogenic sets of form

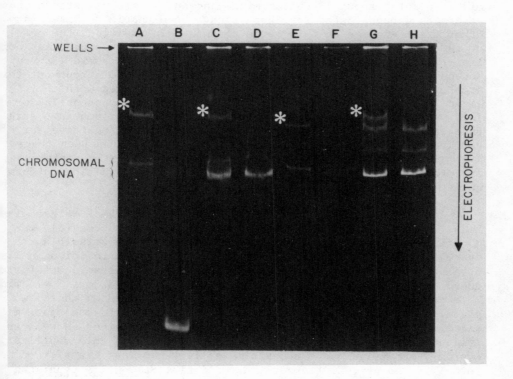

Fig. 1. Agarose gel electrophoretic profiles of circular plasmid
         DNA obtained from sets of isogenic form I and II S. sonnei
         strains. Plasmid profile of: (A) strain 53G form I; (B)
         53G form II; (C) 50E form I; (D) 50E form II; (E) 9774 form
         I; (F) 9774 form II; (G) MBI form I; and (H) MBI form II.
         The asterisks mark the large plasmids in the form I strains
         that are lost in form II derivatives. The gel position
         expected for fragmented chromosomal DNA is indicated. DNA
         isolation and gel electrophoresis procedures are described
         elsewhere[3].

I and form II S. sonnei strains are shown in Fig. 1. Each of the
DNA's from the form I strains contained a large plasmid which is es
timated, for most strains, to be 120 Mdal in size (Fig. 1A, C, E, G
This large plasmid is missing in all form II derivatives (Fig. 1B,
F, H). This observation has been independently confirmed[4].

Conjugal transfer studies. Direct proof that this large plasm
is involved in form I antigen synthesis and virulence can only be o
tained by reintroduction of this plasmid into a form II recipient c
with concomitant reestablishment of these properties. However, nei
ther the form I antigen nor virulence phenotypes are useful as sele
tive markers to monitor plasmid transfer. Therefore, we attempted
identify any marker of selective value expressed by the form I plas
mid. To date, about 175 biochemical and antibiotic resistance char
acters have been tested for, but we have been unable to detect any
other trait encoded on this large plasmid. In addition, the result
of further studies indicate that neither bacteriocin production nor
iron-chelating systems are encoded by this form I plasmid (Sansonet
Kopecko, and Formal; submitted for publication). To circumvent thi
problem, the form I plasmid was phenotypically tagged with the
ampicillin resistance transposon, Tn3, or with transposons Tn5 or
Tn10. These transposons were introduced into the appropriate strai
on a carrier F'_{ts} lac replicon that is temperature sensitive for
replication[3]. Strains in which the form I plasmid had been tagged
expressed the appropriate transposon-encoded antibiotic resistance;
and, this resistance was always lost during the transition to form
cells.

Attempts to detect conjugal self-transfer of these tagged plas
mids, using antibiotic selective pressure, were unsuccessful, indicating that these large plasmids are not self-transmissible. How
ever, two systems to mobilize the form I plasmid to recipient cells
have been developed. Initially, an F'_{ts} lac::Tn3 plasmid was intro
duced into an S. sonnei strain carrying a Tn3-tagged form I plasmid
We reasoned that recombination between the Tn3 units on these two
plasmids would result in the formation of a composite conjugative
plasmid. In fact, form I plasmid transfer was obtained as well as
evidence for the composite plasmid species[3]. Using this mobilizati
system, form I antigen synthesizing ability has been transferred to
form II S. sonnei, S. flexneri, E. coli K12, Salmonella typhi and
Serratia. These data strongly suggest that this S. sonnei plasmid
carries the structural genes for synthesizing the form I antigen.

Although F' lac-mediated transfer of the form I plasmid was
achieved, none of these form I transconjugants had reacquired virulence. Further studies, discussed later, have revealed that FI incompatibility (inc) group plasmids inhibit invasiveness. Thus, fur
ther attempts were made to mobilize the form I plasmid using variou
conjugative plasmids of ten different incompatibility groups. Oddl

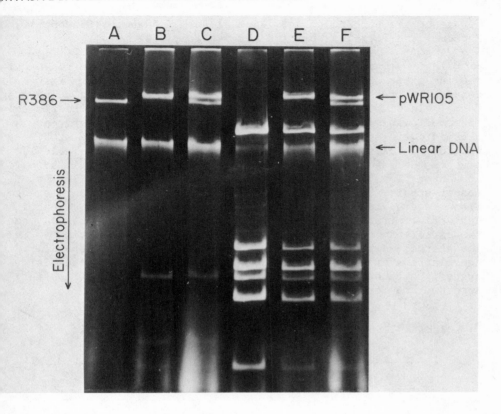

Fig. 2.   Mobilization of the form I plasmid by R386. The agarose
          gel electrophoretic profiles of circular plasmid DNA obtain-
          ed from donor, recipient, and transconjugant strains: (A)
          E. coli J53 carrying R386; (B) S. sonnei 482-79 carrying
          pWR105, a Tn5-tagged form I plasmid; (C) donor 482-79 with
          pWR105 and R386; (D) recipient form II S. sonnei Rudy; (E)
          Rudy transconjugant carrying pWR105; (F) Rudy transconjugant
          carrying pWR105 and R386. Experimental details are describ-
          ed elsewhere (Sansonetti, Kopecko, and Formal, submitted for
          publication)[3,12].

enough, only the R386 plasmid, of FI inc, was found capable of mobilizing the form-I plasmid. The plasmid DNA profiles of donor, recipient, and transconjugant strains from this mobilizing system are
shown in Fig. 2. Some transconjugants received only the form I
plasmid (Fig. 2E), while others also inherited the R386 plasmid
(Fig. 2F). Only transconjugants that did not contain the R386
plasmid were virulent, again verifying the virulence-inhibiting
nature of FI inc group plasmids. This mobilizing system has allowed
us to establish that form I antigen synthesizing ability and

virulence are encoded by the 120 Mdal form I plasmid (Sansonetti, Kopecko, and Formal; submitted for publication).

Incompatibility testing. Next, an attempt was made to identif the inc group of the form I plasmid. Various reference plasmids we conjugally transferred to an S. sonnei strain containing a Tn5-tagg form I plasmid. The resulting strains, purified on antibiotic sele tive media and each carrying the form I plasmid and a reference plasmid, were streaked onto MacConkey lactose agar. The stability the form I colony type was then monitored. As shown in Table 1, none of the reference plasmids, except R386, significantly affected the normal form I to II transition as compared to the wild-type S. sonnei strain. Control studies showed that all of these reference plasmids are stably maintained in the isogenic form II S. sonnei derivative strain. Virtually identical results were obtained when two different form I plasmids were tested for incompatibility. Although these experiments are hampered by the natural instability an nonselftransferability of the form I plasmid, these limited data suggest that the form I plasmid is of the FI inc group (Sansonetti, Kopecko, and Formal; submitted for publication).

Table 1. Incompatibility Between The Form I Plasmid
Of S. Sonnei 482-79 And Other Plasmids

Secondary Plasmid	Incompatibility Group	Colony Phenotype		
		I	I-II	II
		(% of 400 colonies)		
none	–	90.5	8.5	1
R386	FI	52.5	38	9.5
R1	FII	86.5	9.75	3.75
R124	FIV	84	13.5	2.5
R64-11	Iα	92.75	6.25	1
N3	N	91.5	7.5	1
R16	O	81.75	15.5	2.75
RP1	P	89.5	8.0	2.5
S-a	W	96	3	1
RA1	A	82.75	16.5	2.75

Virulence inhibition. As mentioned previously, the F'$_{ts}$ lac plasmid inhibited the virulence of form I-expressing S. sonnei strains. To examine this phenomenon in more detail, plasmids of various incompatibility groups were transferred to several invasive bacteria including S. sonnei, S. flexneri, S. dysenteriae and E. coli. Only a few representative plasmids and the virulence responses of two invasive strains are shown in Table 2, but all invasive strains responded similarly. Only the FI inc group plasmids and plasmid pED830 were observed to inhibit virulence. pED830, constructed in N. Willetts' lab, is a colicin E$_1$ derivative containing Tn3 and which has inserted into the Tn3 BamHl site a 45 kilobase (kb) BamHl fragment containing all of the F plasmid conjugal transfer genes[8]. These data indicate that plasmids of the FI inc group inhibit the ability of invasive organisms to penetrate epithelial cells. Furthermore, the gene(s) responsible for this inhibition is located on the 45 kb BamHl fragment that carries the conjugal transfer genes of the F plasmid (Sansonetti, Kopecko, and Formal; submitted for publication).

S. flexneri virulence plasmids. S. flexneri is a leading cause

Table 2. Effect Of Different Incompatibility Group
          Plasmids On The Virulence of Shigella Strains

Plasmid	Incompatibility Group	Virulence	
		S. sonnei 482-79 I	S. flexneri M4243
none	-	+	+
F'$_{114ts}$lac::Tn3	FI	-	-
F'$_{114ts}$lac	FI	-	-
pED830	(F tra genes)	-	-
R1	FII	+	+
222	FII	+	+
R124	FIV	+	+
R64	Iα	+	+
N3	N	+	+
R16	O	+	+

Virulence assessed by guinea pig keratoconjunctivitis assay.

of shigellosis in many parts of the world.   Initially, representative strains of the six serotypes of S. flexneri were examined for
plasmids.   Regardless of serotype, all strains were found to contain
multiple plasmid species and always contained at least one large
plasmid species of approximately 140 Mdal in size (unpublished data)
Upon restreaking virulent, smooth S. flexneri colonies on agar medium, granular colonial variants have recently been detected at a
frequency of about 0.1% in 4 of the 6 serotypes.   No reversion toward the original colonial morphology was observed when these variants were repurified on different media.   More importantly, all of
these granular derivatives proved to be avirulent.   Plasmid DNA
profiles of these avirulent granular derivatives were then compared
to those of the respective parental strains (Fig. 3).   Three of the
4 granular variants have lost the large 140 Mdal plasmid (Fig. 3B,
D, H), while in the fourth avirulent variant this plasmid appears to

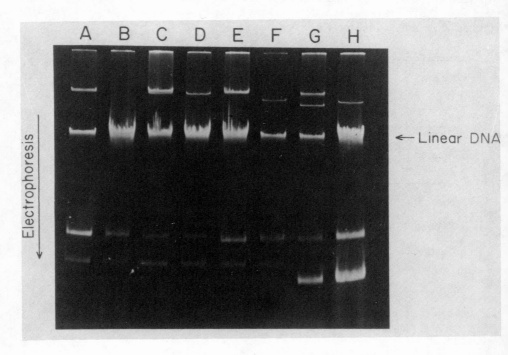

Fig. 3.   Agarose gel profiles of plasmid DNA obtained from virulent
S. flexneri (wells A,C,E,G) and their respective avirulent
derivatives (wells B,D,F,H).   (A,B) strain Z, serotype 1b;
(C,D) M4243, serotype 2a; (E,F) M90T, serotype 5; (G,H)
CCH060, serotype 6.   DNA isolation[12] and gel electrophores
procedures[3] are described elsewhere.   The DNA bands in (H)
migrated slightly behind the corresponding bands in (G),
because the DNA was overloaded in (H) to verify loss of the
largest plasmid.

have undergone a deletion (Sansonetti, Kopecko, Washington, and
Formal; manuscript in preparation). Although this evidence is not
conclusive, these data strongly suggest that plasmid-borne genes are
involved in the virulence of S. flexneri. To date, we have been
unable to obtain self-transfer of or detect selectable phenotypic
properties on these 140 Mdal plasmids. Thus, although these plasmids
appear to affect the ability of the bacterial host to penetrate
epithelial cells, the exact plasmid-mediated functions involved are
undetermined.

Vaccine strain construction. Parenterally administered Shigella
vaccines have not been successful, probably because shigellosis is an
infection limited to the superficial layer of the colonic mucosa.
Therefore, circulatory antibodies do not appear to be protective
against shigellosis. On the other hand, attenuated shigellae vaccines administered orally have been effective in protecting against
this disease, suggesting that the local intestinal immune response
is induced by the living oral vaccine[9]. However, attenuated Shigella
vaccines have not been widely used because of difficulties in isolating safe (i.e., nonreverting) and effective strains. Recently,
Germanier and Furer[10] have reported on the isolation and characterization of a galactose-epimeraseless (galE) mutant of Salmonella
typhi, the typhoid bacillus. This attenuated strain has been tested
in more than 15,000 volunteers and has been shown to be a safe and
highly effective oral vaccine[11]. We considered the possibility that
this strain might be modified so as to be protective also against
shigellosis due to S. sonnei. Therefore, the plasmid responsible
for S. sonnei form I antigen synthesis was mobilized, as described
earlier, into the galE S. typhi strain. The resulting derivative S.
typhi was shown to contain the form I plasmid. Furthermore, serological studies demonstrated that this derivative strain expresses
not only the somatic antigens of the S. typhi parent, but also the
S. sonnei form I antigen. It appeared that this derivative strain
would be a good vaccine candidate[5].

Mouse protection tests. To test the effectiveness of this vaccine, preliminary animal tests were conducted. Groups of mice were
inoculated with one of several vaccines or with a saline control.
Four weeks post-immunization, all mice were challenged with virulent
strains of S. typhi or S. sonnei and deaths were recorded 72 hours
after challenge (Table 3). Note that the living S. typhi galE
typhoid vaccine protected against the homologous challenge strain,
but not against the heterologous (i.e., S. sonnei) challenge. Similarly, the living S. sonnei vaccine protected against challenge by
S. sonnei, but not by S. typhi. However, the form I galE S. typhi
derivative vaccine protected against both challenge organisms[5].
These preliminary studies indicate that the form I-expressing galE
S. typhi strain is an effective immunizing agent in mice for protection against S. typhi and S. sonnei. Volunteer studies are
currently underway.

Table 3. Protection Of Mice Against S. typhi And S. sonnei Challenge With S. typhi And S. Sonnei Vaccines

Vaccine	Route of Immunization	Challenge Strain*	
		S. typhi Ty2	S. sonnei 53G?
Living S. typhi Ty21a	IP	0/12**	15/15
	SC	4/15	15/15
Living S. typhi-form I 5076-1C	IP	0/13	1/14
	SC	1/16	0/16
Living S. sonnei-53GI	IP	14/16	1/16
	SC	16/16	0/16
AKD*** S. typhi Ty2	IP	2/16	15/16
	SC	1/16	16/16
Saline	IP	10/10	10/10

* Challenges, suspended in 0.5 percent hog gastric mucin, were administered IP.

** Deaths recorded 72 hrs after challenge.
Total

*** Standard acetone-killed and dried typhoid vaccine.

SUMMARY

1. Shigella sonnei contain a 120 Mdal nonconjugative plasmid which appears to be in the FI inc. group. This plasmid codes for the structural determinants of the form I antigen which is thought to be essential for invasiveness. Other virulence properties, excluding iron-chelation, may reside on this plasmid.[3,4] (Sansonetti, Kopecko, Formal; submitted for publication).

2. All six serotypes of S. flexneri contain a large plasmid of approximately 140 Mdal, which also appears to be necessary for epithelial cell penetration. (Sansonetti, Kopecko, Washington, Formal; ms. in prep.).

3. A form I-expressing galE S. typhi vaccine strain has been constructed and has proven to be protective in mice against challenges with both virulent S. sonnei and S. typhi strains.[5]

4. This S. typhi galE strain Ty21a, which has been shown to be a safe and highly effective oral vaccine, should serve as a useful carrier strain for other antigens (e.g., colonization antigens or toxoids) to protect against a variety of different intestinal infections.[5]

REFERENCES

1. Formal, S.B., P. Gemski, R.A. Giannella, and A. Takeuchi. 1976.
Studies on the pathogenesis of enteric infections caused by invasive
bacteria, pp. 27-43. In: Acute Diarrhoea in Childhood - Ciba
Symposium, Vol. 42. Elsevier/North Holland.

2. Gemski, P. and S.B. Formal. 1975. Shigellosis: an invasive
infection of the gastrointestinal tract, pp. 165-169. In: Micro-
biology-1975, D. Schlessinger, ed., American Society for Microbiology, Washington, D.C.

3. Kopecko, D.J., O. Washington, and S.B. Formal. 1980. Genetic
and physical evidence for plasmid control of Shigella sonnei form I
cell surface antigen. Infect. Immun. 29:207-214.

4. Sansonetti, P., M. David, and M. Toucas. 1980. Correlation
entre la perte d'ADN plasmidique et le passage de la phase I
virulente a la phase II avirulente chez Shigella sonnei. C.R.
Acad. Sci. 290(D): 879-882.

5. Formal, S.B., L.S. Baron, D.J. Kopecko, O. Washington, C. Powell,
and C.A. Life. 1981. Construction of a potential bivalent vaccine
strain: introduction of Shigella sonnei form I antigen genes into
the galE Salmonella typhi Ty21a typhoid vaccine strain. Infect.
Immun. 31: (in press).

6. Kenne, L., B. Lindberg, K. Petersson, E. Katzenellenbogen, and
E. Romanowaska. 1980. Structural studies of the O-specific side-
chains of the Shigella sonnei phase I lipopolysaccharide. Carbo-
hydrate Res. 78: 119-126.

7. Sereny, B. 1955. Experimental Shigella conjunctivitis. Acta.
Microbiol. Acad. Aci. Hung. 2:293-296.

8. Johnson, D.A. and N.S. Willetts. 1980. Tn2301, a transposon
construct carrying the entire transfer region of the F plasmid. J.
Bacteriol. 143:1171-1178.

9. Mel, D.M., A.L. Terzin, and L. Vuksic. 1965. Studies on vaccination against bacillary dysentery. 3. Effective oral immunization against Shigella flexneri 2a in a field trial. Bull. Wld.
Hlth. Org. 32:647-655.

10. Germanier, R. and E. Furer. 1975. Isolation and characterization of galE mutant Ty21a of Salmonella typhi: a candidate strain
for a live, oral, typhoid vaccine. J. Infect. Dis. 131:553-558.

11. Wahdan, M.H., C. Serie, R. Germanier, A. Lackany, Y. Cerisier,
N. Guerin, S. Sallam, P. Geoffroy, A. Sadek El Tantaivi, and P.
Guesry. 1980. A controlled field trial of live oral typhoid
vaccine Ty21a. Bul WHO 58:469-474.

12. Casse, F., C. Boucher, J.S. Julliot, M. Michel, and J. Denaire.
1979. Identification and characterization of large plasmids in
Rhizobium meliloti using agarose gel electrophoresis. J. Gen.
Microbiol. 113:229-242.

PLASMID-SPECIFIED IRON UPTAKE BY BACTERAEMIC STRAINS

OF *ESCHERICHIA COLI*

Peter H. Williams and Philip J. Warner

Department of Genetics
University of Leicester
Leicester LE1 7RH, England

INTRODUCTION

Although *Escherichia coli* is a normally harmless major aerobic component of the gut flora of a healthy individual, some strains are invasive, and able to produce extraintestinal infections. *E. coli* has been isolated from urinary tract infections and from cases of neonatal meningitis and bacteraemia. Smith[1] reported that a significant proportion of *E. coli* strains associated with bacteraemia of humans and domestic animals harboured plasmids (ColV) specifying the narrow spectrum antibacterial protein colicin V. Furthermore, Cabello[2] found that many *E. coli* strains isolated from patients with meningitis carried such ColV plasmids. It has been unequivocally shown that possession of a ColV plasmid markedly enhances the virulence of *E. coli* strains in comparison with plasmid-free strains in experimental infections of a number of laboratory animals[1,2,3].

Investigations of the correlation between colicinogenicity and virulence have led to the identification of several ColV plasmid-associated characteristics which may be implicated in pathogenicity. Bacteria carrying a ColV plasmid show an enhanced ability to adhere to intestinal epithelium *in vitro*[4], while colicin V itself, detected in the laboratory by its ability to kill sensitive *E. coli* strains, may act synergistically with endotoxin to increase vascular permeability in the skin[5], and to depress macrophage activity in the peritoneal cavity of infected animals[6]. These may be crucial factors in the initiation of the invasive process. Binns et al[7] have cloned restriction fragments of the prototype plasmid ColV,I-K94 which specify increased resistance of bacteria to the bactericidal effects of antibody and complement in serum. It is difficult to assess the

123

importance of this, however, since the serum resistance of *E.coli*
isolates from meningitis was found to be unaffected by elimination
of ColV plasmids although lethality in experimental infections was
significantly reduced by curing[2].

Another characteristic controlled by ColV plasmids from bacteraemic strains of *E.coli* is the capacity to grow in conditions of iron
deprivation. It is this aspect that is considered in detail in this
communication.

There is now considerable evidence in the literature that the
concentration of free ferric cations in the tissues and fluids of the
body is critical to the outcome of the conflict between establishmen
of a bacterial infection and its suppression by the host animal[8].
Although present in body fluids, iron is predominantly unavailable
for microbial growth because it is strongly associated with iron
binding proteins (transferrin in serum, lactoferrin in secretions).
Inclusion of excess iron in the inoculum in experimental infections
enhances bacterial virulence[9]. Moreover, clinical conditions, such
as hepatitis, haemolytic anaemia, or haemorrhage due to severe viral
infection, which lead naturally to increased levels of free iron in
the body fluids are frequently associated with increased susceptibility to, and severity of, bacterial infections[8]. On the other
hand, an otherwise healthy body responds to infection in a number of
ways to reduce still further the level of free iron, and so deprive
invading bacteria of an essential growth requirement[8]. There may be
specific reduction of intestinal absorption of exogenous iron, and
increased iron flux from body fluids to hepatic storage sites; there
may also be increased synthesis of iron binding proteins and their
localisation at potential sites of infection. Thus, a bacterial
strain which is capable of overcoming such "nutritional immunity"[8]
by competing efficiently for iron with the iron binding proteins of
the host will be better able to proliferate rapidly after infection
and therefore elicit severe disease symptoms.

ColV PLASMIDS AND IRON STRESS

Since iron availability is crucial to the progress of a
bacterial infection, the possible involvement of ColV plasmids of
bacteraemic *E.coli* strains in iron uptake was investigated (table
1). Iron is normally present in low concentration in defined
minimal media as an impurity of the component chemicals. However,
addition of purified iron-free human transferrin to minimal medium
decreased the growth rate of plasmidless *E.coli* K-12 strain W3110
due to conversion of free iron to a relatively unavailable complexed
form. Saturation of iron binding sites of transferrin by excess
ferric ions reversed the inhibitory effect. On the other hand,
the same concentration of transferrin had no effect on the growth

Table 1. Effect of Transferrin on Bacterial Growth in
          Defined Minimal Medium

Bacterial strain		Mean generation time (min)	
Designation	Characteristics	−transferrin	+transferrin[a]
W3110	K-12, plasmidless	46	72 (47[b])
LG1327	W3110/ColV-H247	45	45
H247	bacteraemic *E. coli*	34	34
H247V⁻	cured derivative	34	55

[a]Transferrin was added at 250 µg/ml.

[b]$FeCl_3$ at 100 µM was added to growth medium.

rate of the colicinogenic human bacteraemic strain H247. Two
observations indicate that the ColV-H247 plasmid has a role in
acquiring sufficient iron for growth from the transferrin-complexed
state; transferrin significantly inhibited the growth of a cured
derivative of strain H247, while conversely a derivative of W3110
to which plasmid ColV-H247 had been transferred by conjugation was
unaffected by the presence of transferrin in the growth medium.
Identical results were obtained with ColV plasmids from bacteraemic
strains of calf (B188), pig (P72) and chicken (F70) origin and with
one of the prototype ColV plasmids ColV-K30[10,11].

Growth rate differences of this magnitude account for the
observed changes in constitution of mixed cultures of colicinogenic
and plasmid free bacteria during growth in conditions of iron
deprivation in immunoglobulin-free calf serum[10]. Furthermore, in
mixed infections of mice, the minority colicinogenic component of
the inoculum was reisolated as the predominant organism from dead
animals (table 2). When excess iron was included in the inoculum,
however, the relative proportions of the two strains recovered from
infected mice were similar to that of the inoculation mixture. Thus,
it is clear that ColV plasmids contribute to the ability of the cells
that harbour them to sequester iron under conditions of iron stress
both *in vivo* and *in vitro*. When iron is freely available the
selective advantage of colicinogenicity is abolished.

Table 2.   Effect of Iron on the Course of Mixed
Infections of Mice

% colicinogenic bacteria in inoculum[a]	Addition of Fe^{3+} [b]	% colicinogenic bacteria recovered[c]
1	-	87
1	+	2
11	-	100
11	+	16

[a]Mixtures of strains H247 and H247V$^-$ in the proportions
indicated were inoculated I/P into groups of 3 adult
white mice.

[b]Ferric ammonium citrate (20 mM).

[c]Peritoneal wash of dead mice.

ColV PLASMID SPECIFIED IRON UPTAKE

A number of routes of entry of iron into cells of enteric
bacteria have been described[12]. When the element is present at a
high concentration in the growth medium it enters in a passive,
non-specific fashion[13]. However, in conditions of iron deficit, the
synthesis and excretion of the catechol siderophore enterochelin are
induced[14], and the ferric-enterochelin complexes formed in the mediu
are subsequently actively transported into cells[15]. Alternatively,
compounds present in natural environments may be utilised for iron
uptake; an example is the fungal siderophore ferrichrome[16].

Mutants of *E.coli* K-12 defective in the synthesis of enterochelin are able to grow either if a high concentration of iron is
provided to allow passive entry (as in growth in nutrient medium),
or by addition to defined medium of an iron solubilising compound
such as sodium citrate which can be actively transported across the
cell membrane. The presence of plasmids ColV-H247, ColV-P72,
ColV-F70 or ColV-K30 in an enterochelin defective mutant, however,
abolishes the growth requirement for citrate[13], indicating the
activity of an efficient alternative iron uptake mechanism. This
has been demonstrated indirectly by observation of a plasmid-
specific sparing of the induction of synthesis of bacterial outer
membrane proteins that characteristically occurs when intracellular
iron concentrations are reduced[10,11]. Direct confirmation of the
operation of the plasmid-specified system comes from measurement of

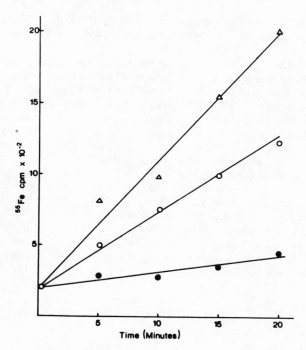

Figure 1.   Effect of the presence of a ColV plasmid on bacterial iron
uptake.   Strains LG1013 (plasmidless, enterochelin producing, O);
AN1937 (plasmidless, enterochelin deficient, ●); and LG1315 (AN1937
carrying ColV-K30, △) were grown in low iron medium, and the uptake
of $^{55}FeCl_3$ into washed, non-growing cells was determined[10],[11]

radioactive iron uptake into bacterial strains (fig.1). While the
enterochelin deficient mutant AN1937 did not actively take up ^{55}Fe
from the medium, a derivative carrying ColV-K30 (strain LG1315, Iu[+])
showed more efficient uptake of label than the plasmidless enterochelin producing control strain LG1013.

MECHANISM OF IRON UPTAKE

        Like the enterochelin-, citrate- and ferrichrome--mediated routes
for the uptake of iron, the ColV plasmid specified system is an
active process requiring the *tonB* gene product[10],[11]. It involves
iron chelation by an inducible hydroxamate siderophore[17].   The
observation that plasmid-free strains are not cross-fed by colicinogenic strains in mixed culture and infection suggests either
that the plasmid-coded iron chelator is cell bound, or that plasmid-
specified products act to transport an extracellular siderophore
into the cell.   Stuart et al[17] favour the former model on the basis

of their finding that hydroxamate compounds were chemically detectable[18] in cell pellets of ColV plasmid-carrying bacteria.

Genetic data, on the other hand, suggest that the plasmid
specified siderophore is a cell-free diffusible product[19]. Followin
mutagenesis and penicillin enrichment of strains LG1315 (enterocheli
deficient, carrying ColV-K30), mutants defective in plasmid promoted
iron uptake were isolated. All showed reduced virulence in experimental infections of mice. Moreover, they fell into two classes on
the basis of cross-feeding tests (table 3), defining two plasmid-
specified functions for the uptake of iron. One class (*iuc*) was
cross-fed by a strain carrying a wild type plasmid, and is therefore
postulated to lack an extracellular diffusible product for which the
cross-feeding strain compensates. The other mutant class (*iut*) was
not cross-fed by a strain producing extracellular chelator, but
was itself able to cross-feed mutants of the *iuc* class; thus it
produces normal siderophore, but is defective in some aspect of the
transport of siderophore into the cell. The behaviour of these
mutants cannot easily be reconciled with a cell-bound mode of action

Table 3. Cross-Feeding Tests[a]

Patch inoculum	Bacterial lawn		
Strain; Characteristics	LG1439[b] *entA*	LG1418 *entA*/ColV-K30*iuc*	LG1419 *entA*/ColV-K30*iut*
LG1315 *entA*/ColV-K30Iu[+]	−	+	−
LG1418[c] *entA*/ColV-K30*iuc*	−	−	−
LG1419[d] *entA*/ColV-K30*iut*	−	+	−

[a]Lawns of bacteria (10^7 cells/plate) on minimal agar containing
α α´-dipyridyl (160 µM) were patch inoculated as indicated.
Cross-feeding (+) was observed as a zone of growth of the
bacterial lawn around a particular patch; (−) indicates no
cross-feeding.

[b]Strain LG1439 is a colicin V insensitive derivative of strain
AN1937.

[c]No growth of patch inocula except on the LG1419 lawn.

[d]Poor growth of patch inocula.

of the plasmid-specified system. The general nature of the phenomenon is suggested by the finding that AN1937 derivatives carrying
plasmids ColV-H247 or ColV-P72 (from human and porcine bacteraemic
strains respectively) were also able to cross-feed *iuc* mutant strain
LG1418.

This type of test provides a sensitive quantifiable biological
assay for iron chelating activity. There is complete coincidence
of elution of biologically determined iron binding activity and
chemically determined hydroxamate material of strain LG1315 from
both Dowex-1 and Sephadex G-50 columns (fig. 2) indicating that
both tests measure the same plasmid characteristic. Furthermore
the *iuc* mutant LG1418, deduced from cross-feeding tests to be
deficient in chelator synthesis, was found to produce no detectable
hydroxamate material, while LG1419, the *iut* mutant defective in
transport of iron, produced 10-100 times more chelator (depending
on growth phase) than parental strain LG1315 on the basis of both
biological and chemical assays.

Furthermore, biological assays have confirmed the previous
observation[17] that cell pellets of exponentially growing cultures
of strains carrying wild-type ColV plasmids contain iron chelating
activity. Cell pellets were washed extensively, sonicated and
assayed for ability to promote the growth of *iuc* mutant LG1418 in
conditions of iron limitation. Approximately 10% of the total
biologically measurable activity produced by strain LG1315 was
associated with the cell pellet. Cell-associated activity in
sonicates and cell-free activity in culture supernatants eluted
identically from Sephadex G-50 columns.

Strain LG1418 is defective in plasmid specified siderophore
synthesis but it can grow in conditions of iron deficit if cell-
free siderophore is supplied exogenously. In this case also, biological activity was recovered from extensively washed, sonicated
cell pellets. These data suggest that the iron chelating material
associated with cell pellets was actively involved in iron uptake
into growing cells at the time of sampling. That is, it represents
the transient association of a diffusible chelator with a membrane
receptor rather than the more permanent involvement of siderophore
molecules as components of the bacterial membrane as suggested by
Stuart et al[17].

SELECTIVE ADVANTAGE OF COLICINOGENICITY

The siderophore elaborated by plasmid ColV-K30 has been identified by field desorption mass spectrometry as aerobactin (A.
Bindereif and J.B. Neilands, personal communication). This compound
was first purified from a strain of *Aerobacter aerogenes*[20], but has
subsequently been found to be synthesised by strains of *Shigella*[21]

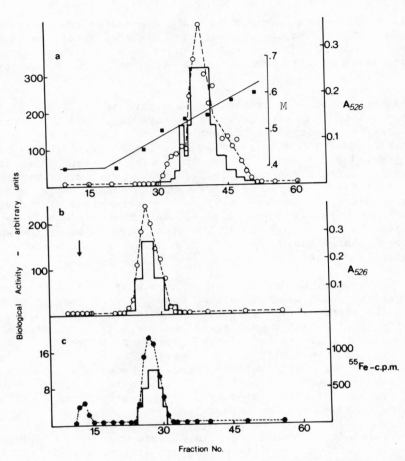

Figure 2.   Column chromatography of ColV plasmid specified siderophore.   In (a) culture supernatant of strain LG1315 was applied to
Dowex-1 and eluted with an ammonium chloride gradient (-■——■-);
eluant was tested for biological activity (histogram) and hydroxamate (O---O).   In (b) LG1315 culture supernatant material
concentrated approximately tenfold by Dowex-1 chromatography was
applied to a Sephadex G-50 column (25 cm x 1 cm); eluant was tested
for biological activity (histogram) and hydroxamate (O---O). The
void volume is marked by the arrow.   In (c) the sample was LG1315
culture supernatant to which were added 1 µC ^{55}FeCl$_3$ and then
excess transferrin to solubilise any non-complexed iron; the mixture
was applied to Sephadex G-50 and the column eluant was tested for
biological activity (histogram) and ^{55}Fe radioactivity (●----●).
Ferric-transferrin eluted in the void volume.   Biological activity
is defined as the reciprocal of the highest dilution of a sample
which allowed growth of LG1418 in conditions of iron limitation.
Hydroxamate compounds were determined colorimetrically (A$_{526}$) by
the method of Csaky[18].

and *Salmonella* (A. Bindereif and J.B. Neilands, personal communication) also. It is not known if aerobactin synthesis in these genera is plasmid mediated, but the observation raises interesting questions about the evolutionary origin of ColV plasmids carried by bacteraemic strains of *E.coli*. Of more immediate interest is the question of why aerobactin, a relatively low affinity iron chelator, should provide a selective advantage to bacterial strains that can also synthesise the high affinity siderophore enterochelin. It should be noted, however, that the synthesis of enterochelin, and its breakdown to release iron within a cell are expensive of metabolic energy[12]. We may speculate, therefore, that in conditions of extreme iron stress the operation of an iron uptake system which requires little energy, albeit a low affinity system, may be crucial to the survival of a bacterial cell.

ACKNOWLEDGEMENTS

We are grateful to R.H. Pritchard, I.B. Holland and G.S. Plastow for advice, helpful discussions and encouragement and to A. Bindereif and J.B. Neilands for communicating data before publication. This work was supported by project grant G979/461/C from the Medical Research Council and by funds from the University of Leicester.

LITERATURE CITED

1. H. W. Smith, *J.Gen.Microbiol.* 83:95-111 (1974)
2. F. Cabello, *in* "Plasmids of Medical, Environmental and Commercial Importance" K. N. Timmis and A. Pühler, eds., Elsevier-North Holland Biomedical Press, Amsterdam, pp155-160 (1979).
3. H. W. Smith and M. B. Huggins, *J. Gen. Microbiol.* 92:355-350 (1976).
4. J. Clancy and D. C. Savage, *Infect. Immun.* in the press (1981).
5. G. Ozanne, L.G. Mathieu and J.P. Baril, *Infect. Immun.* 17: 497-503 (1977).
6. G. Ozanne, L.G. Mathieu and J. P. Baril, *Rev. Can. Biol.* 36: 307-316 (1977).
7. M. M. Binns, D. L. Davies and K. G. Hardy, *Nature* 279:778-781 (1979).
8. E. D. Weinberg, *Microbiol. Rev.* 42:45-66 (1978).
9. J. J. Bullen, H. J. Rogers and E. Griffiths, *in* "Microbial Iron Metabolism", J. B. Neilands, ed., Academic Press, New York pp518-552 (1974).
10. P.H. Williams and H.K. George, *in* "Plasmids of Medical, Environmental and Commercial Importance", K. N. Timmis and A. Pühler, eds. Elsevier-North Holland Biomedical Press, Amsterdam pp161-172 (1979).
11. P.H. Williams, *Infect. Immun.* 26:925-932 (1979).

12.   H. Rosenberg and I. G. Young, *in* "Microbial Iron Metabolism",
      J.B. Neilands, ed., Academic Press, New York pp67-82 (1974).

13.   G. E. Frost and H. Rosenberg, *Biochim. Biophys. Acta* 330:90-101
      (1973).

14.   I. G. O'Brien and F. Gibson, *Biochim. Biophys. Acta* 215:309-402
      (1970).

15.   R. E. W. Hancock, K. Hantke and V. Braun, *J. Bacteriol.* 127:
      1370-1375 (1976).

16.   M. Luckey, J. R. Pollack, R. Wayne, B. N. Ames and J. B.
      Neilands, *J. Bacteriol.* 111:731-738 (1972).

17.   S. J. Stuart, K. T. Greenwood and R. K. J. Luke, *J. Bacteriol.*
      143: 35-42 (1980).

18.   T. Z. Csaky, *Acta Chem. Scand.* 2:450-454 (1948).

19.   P. H. Williams and P. J. Warner, *Infect. Immun.* 29:411-416
      (1980).

20.   F. Gibson, and D. I. Magrath, *Biochim. Biophys. Acta* 192:175-184
      (1969).

21.   S. M. Payne, *J. Bacteriol.* 143:1420-1424 (1980).

SERUM RESISTANCE IN E.COLI

Kenneth N. Timmis, Paul A. Manning, Christine Echarti,
Joan K. Timmis and Albrecht Moll
Max-Planck-Institute for Molecular Genetics
Berlin-Dahlem, West Germany

INTRODUCTION

Pathogenic bacteria that cause generalized infections or
meningitis invade the blood stream and are thereby distributed
throughout the body. Blood, or serum, contains a number of non-
specific (complement, lysozyme, phagocytes, iron-binding proteins,
etc.) and specific (antibodies, lymphocytes) agents that alone or
in combination lyse, kill or prevent the growth of the majority of
bacteria with which they make contact. Abilities to resist, evade
or inactivate these host defences constitute major components of
the virulence of invasive bacteria. At present little is known
about these bacterial properties or their molecular interactions
with host defences.

The role of resistance to serum/complement in the virulence
of invasive Gram-negative bacteria is indicated, on one hand, by
a substantial volume of epidemiological data[1-3] and, on the other,
by results obtained with experimental invasive bacterial infections, such as endocarditis, in laboratory animals[4,5]. We have
studied resistance to serum in E.coli and have found that two cellular components, an outer membrane protein and a polysaccharide
capsular antigen, are able to provide bacteria with substantial
resistance to serum.

RESULTS

The Plasmid R6-5 Surface Exclusion Gene traT Mediates Serum Resistance

Several groups have reported that certain plasmids of Gram-

133

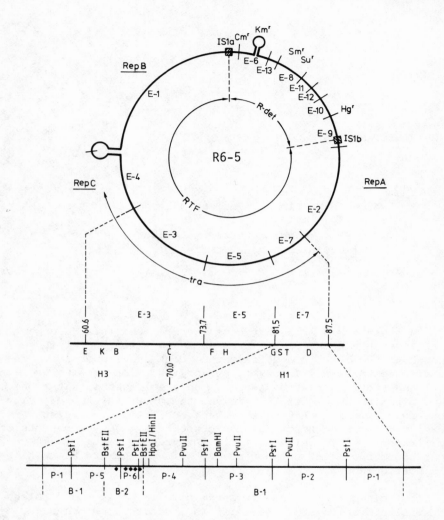

Fig. 1.   Physical and genetic map of plasmid R6-5. The R6-5 map
(top) is that of Timmis et al.[10]; cross bars indicate
EcoRI cleavage sites. The genetic map of the R6-5 tra
region (expansion, center) is that of Achtman et al.[11];
the bars above the map indicate EcoRI cleavage sites
whereas bars below the map indicate HindIII cleavage
sites. The detailed restriction map of the R6-5 EcoRI
fragment E-7 (bottom) is that of Moll et al.[12]. E, H, P,
and B numbers indicate restriction endonuclease fragments
generated by EcoRI, HindIII, PstI, and BstEII, respectively. The PstI and BstEII fragments of the E-7 fragment
are numbered according to size as they exist in the
pKT107 hybrid plasmid, and not according to size as they

exist in R6-5. The diamond symbols indicate the sites of insertion of Tn3 elements within the B-2 fragment in serum resistant-defective insertion mutant derivatives of the pKT107 plasmid. Abbreviations: Cm^r, Km^r, Sm^r, Su^r, and Hg^r, resistance to chloramphenicol, kanamycin, streptomycin, sulfonamide, and mercury salts, respectively; Rep and IS1, replication functions and insertion sequence 1; RTF, R-det, and tra, resistance transfer factor, resistance determinant, and transfer functions, respectively.

negative bacteria increase the resistance of E.coli strains to serum[6-8]. Plasmid R6-5[9] is a large (100kb), conjugative, multiple antibiotic resistance plasmid (Fig.1) that we have studied extensively and that is closely related to R100, one of the plasmids shown to specify serum resistance[6,8]. Table 1 shows that R6-5 provides a smooth strain of E.coli, E.coli 59rif, with almost complete resistance to serum and significantly elevates the resistance of a highly-sensitive rough strain, E.coli K-12, to low concentrations of serum.

In order to determine the approximate location of the serum resistance determinant on the R6-5 genome, we examined the ability of ColE1 hybrid plasmids carrying EcoRI fragments of R6-5[10] to confer upon E.coli K-12 host bacteria resistance to 3% rabbit serum. Only one type of hybrid plasmid was found to specify a serum resistance function, namely that which carries EcoRI fragment E-7[12]. A detailed restriction endonuclease cleavage map of the E-7 fragment is shown in Figure 1. For ease of subsequent genetic manipulations this fragment was cloned into the pACYC184 vector to form hybrid plasmid pKT107. This hybrid also confers resistance to serum upon E.coli K-12 (Table 1). Three genes, traS, traT and traD, that function in plasmid conjugation are known to be coded by fragment E-7[11]. The traS and traT genes encode proteins that are responsible for surface exclusion, the reduction in ability of bacteria carrying a conjugative plasmid to act as recipients when mated with donors carrying a closely related plasmid, whereas traD specifies a function involved in conjugal DNA transfer from donor to recipient bacteria[13].

Precise localization of the serum resistance gene was accomplished by transposon mutagenesis of the pKT107 plasmid[12]. Transposon Tn3 was introduced into pKT107 by standard procedures and insertion mutant derivatives that no longer specified serum resistance were identified using a recently-developed, colorimetric, rapid screening procedure[14]. Restriction endonuclease cleavage analysis of these mutant plasmids revealed that all Tn3 elements that had inactivated the serum resistance gene of pKT107 were located within a 600 bp BstEII fragment, B-2, although on different

Table 1.   Serum resistance levels of bacteria carrying plasmids that encode the traT protein or the K1 biosynthesis genes

Percent serum	P e r c e n t S u r v i v a l [a]						
	C600rif[b]	C600rif (R6-5) traT+	C600rif (pKT107) traT+	59rif[c]	59rif (R6-5) traT+	LE392[d]	LE392 (pKT172) K1+
0	100	100	100	100	100	100	100
1	97	315	286	—	—	107	246
2	12.5	245	263	—	—	0.18	731
3	0.62	192	182	—	—	0.05	1013
6	<0.001	6.7	9.1	139	333	<0.001	100.2
10	—	0.03	0.02	5.4	205	—	0.35
20	—	—	—	0.07	124	—	—
50	—	—	—	0.005	74.5	—	—
75	—	—	—	0.005	77.1	—	—

[a] Log phase bacteria were washed with phosphate-buffered saline (PBS), resuspended in PBS, diluted to a concentration of 2×10^7/ml and 0.5 ml of the cell suspension added to 2 ml of PBS containing serum at the indicated concentrations. The cell/serum mixtures were incubated at 37°C for 3 hr before dilution and plating for survivors[14];

[b] a rifampicin-resistant derivative of E.coli K-12 C600;

[c] a rifampicin-resistant derivative of E.coli 59, a smooth E.coli isolated from the feces of a healthy child[12];

[d] E.coli K-12 strain used as recipient for λ-packaged cosmid constructions, obtained from J. Collins.

PstI fragments, P-4, P-5 and P-6, that lie within or overlap with
the B-2 fragment (Fig.1). These insertion mutations localize the
serum resistance gene to a region thought to contain the traT surface exclusion gene.

Definitive identification of the serum resistance gene product was obtained by comparing plasmid-encoded proteins synthesized in minicells containing pKT107 or its serum resistance-nega-
tive Tn3 insertion derivatives. As can be seen in Figure 2, the
traS, traT and traD gene products were readily detected by polyacrylamide gel electrophoresis of radioactive proteins made by
minicells containing the pKT107 serum resistance-positive plasmid,
whereas the traT gene product could not be identified among the
proteins made by minicells containing the serum resistance-nega-
tive insertion mutant plasmids[12]. The traT gene product, a 25,000
dalton protein, is thus responsible for plasmid R6-5-specified
serum resistance.

The traT Protein is Located on the Outer Surface of the Outer Membrane

Complement is activated by cell surface structures and it is
the cell surface which is the site of action of the membrane attack unit of activated complement. It was therefore anticipated
that the traT protein, which mediates resistance to complement
killing, would either be localized on the cell surface or excreted
into the medium. We have compared the amounts of traT protein in
whole cells and in outer membrane preparations of these cells
(Triton X-100 insoluble component of the cell envelopes) and have
found that the majority of cellular traT protein is localized in
the outer membrane (Fig.2). It could be calculated from densito-
meter tracings of stained polyacrylamide gels of outer membrane
proteins that bacteria carrying the pKT107 plasmid contain about
20,000 copies of the traT protein per cell[12].

Outer membrane proteins may be located on the inner or outer
surface of the membrane, or may traverse it. In order to determine
whether the traT protein is exposed on the outer surface of the
outer membrane, we coupled ^{125}I to the surfaces of whole cells
using lactoperoxidase and analysed the labeled proteins by polyacrylamide gel electrophoresis, followed by autoradiography[15]. As
can be seen in Figure 2, the traT protein is labeled more heavily
than outer membrane proteins I and II*, which are larger and present in numbers of copies 5-fold greater than that of the traT
protein. This indicates that the traT protein is highly exposed on
the outer surface of the outer membrane. Similar findings have
been made on the F[15] and R100[16] traT proteins.

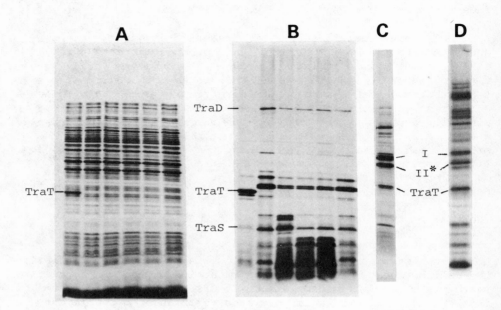

Fig. 2.   R6-5-specified serum resistance is mediated by the traT
          protein which is located on the outer surface of the cell
          outer membrane. Identification of the serum resistance
          gene product as the traT protein. (A,B) Analysis of plas-
          mid-encoded proteins synthesized in minicells. Minicells
          containing pKT107 (a) or its serum sensitive Tn3 inser-
          tion derivatives (b-f) were purified, radioactively la-
          beled with [35S]methionine, and analyzed by SDS-poly-
          acrylamide gel electrophoresis[12]. The gel was subsequent-
          ly stained (A) and autoradiographed (B). (b) pKT116;
          (c) pKT117; (d) pKT118; (e) pKT119; (f) pKT120. (C) Ana-
          lysis of outer membrane proteins of plasmid-carrying bac-
          teria. The outer membranes (Triton X-100-insoluble com-
          ponent of the cell envelope) of cells harboring pKT107
          were analyzed by SDS-polyacrylamide gel electrophoresis
          followed by staining[15]. (D) Analysis of proteins exposed
          on the cell surface. Cells harboring pKT107 were iodinat-
          ed with 125I in the presence of lactoperoxidase[15] and the
          total proteins analyzed by SDS-polyacrylamide gel elec-
          trophoresis, followed by autoradiography.

Table 2.   Serum resistant bacteria fail to cross protect
            sensitive bacteria

Bacterial strain	Percent Survival in 3% Serum[a]	
	After 60 min	After 180 min
A. CR34nal[b]	0.67	< 0.001
B. C600rif (pKT107)[c]	282	319
C. CR34nal +	2.33	< 0.001
C600rif (pKT107)[c]	237	320

[a]Bacteria were prepared as described in Table 1. At -30 min,
C600rif(pKT107) bacteria were added to serum solutions (B and C);
at 0 min, CR34nal bacteria were also added (A and C); at + 60 min
and + 180 min the bacterial suspensions were diluted and plated on
agar containing either nalidixic acid (50 μg/ml, for A and C) and
rifampicin (100 μg/ml; B and C);
[b]a nalidixic acid resistant mutant of E.coli K-12 CR34;
[c]present at 3 x the concentration of that of CR34nal.

Functional Aspects of the traT Protein

       Although we found no evidence of release of significant
amounts of traT protein from bacteria carrying the pKT107 plasmid,
the release of small quantities would not have been detected.
There are three possibilities regarding the mode of action of the
traT protein in serum resistance: (a) inactivation of one or more
components of complement in the fluid phase by released traT protein, (b) inactivation by cell-bound traT protein, or (c) prevention of the activation of complement by cell surface structures,
or inhibition of the lytic activity of activated complement on the
cell surface, due to a traT protein-mediated structural modification of the cell envelope. If the principal mechanism of serum resistance is inactivation of complement in the fluid phase, it
should be possible to protect serum sensitive bacteria by preincu-
bating the serum to be used with serum resistant cells. Table 2
shows that this is not the case: preincubation of 3% rabbit serum
with serum resistant bacteria (final concentration 6x10[6]/ml) for
30 min did not significantly increase the survival of serum sensitive bacteria (final concentration 2x10[6]/ml) that were subsequently added. This means that the traT protein does not inactivate complement components present in the fluid phase and that it
must mediate resistance as an integral component of the bacterial
outer membrane (see also ref.17).

As indicated above, the traT protein is responsible in part
for plasmid surface exclusion. In order to examine the functional
relationship between serum resistance and surface exclusion, we
have begun to isolate and analyse serum resistance-defective,
hydroxylamine-induced point mutant derivatives of the pKT107 plasmid. Twenty-two putative mutant plasmids of this type were initially identified by the rapid screening procedure, which measures
bacterial growth in the presence of serum, but only three were
subsequently confirmed as serum resistance-defective. The remaining seventeen mutant derivatives all caused substantial over-pro-
duction of the traT protein (up to 200,000 copies per cell)[18] and
all resulted in poor growth characteristics of host bacteria (the
rapid screening procedure is therefore a useful method for identifying bacterial mutants that exhibit altered regulation of the
synthesis of the traT protein, and also for mutants with altered
regulation of other structural components of the cell and that exhibit poor growth). Two of the three serum resistance-defective
plasmid derivatives have been examined: one of them, pKT147, specified normal surface exclusion (exclusion index of pKT107 with
R100drd:51) whereas the other, pKT145, exhibited greatly increased
surface exclusion (indices with R100drd of 45 and 1032, respectively). This suggests that surface exclusion and serum resistance
are independent activities of the traT protein, although a change
in the activity of traS in pKT145 cannot at this time be ruled out.

Outer membranes prepared from bacteria carrying the pKT145
and pKT147 plasmids did not exhibit detectable amounts of a 25,000
dalton protein and we conclude that these mutant plasmids no longer direct the synthesis of the traT protein, or that they direct
the synthesis of (a) traT protein in severely reduced amounts,
(b) a protein of altered molecular weight, or (c) a protein that
is no longer transported to the outer membrane. In view of the
fact that neither mutant plasmid specifies less than the normal
level of surface exclusion, alternatives (a) or (b) appear the
most plausible, although the isolation and analysis of more mutant
plasmids will be required before a firm conclusion can be drawn.

The K1 Capsular Antigen Mediates Bacterial Resistance to Serum

The K1 polysaccharide capsular antigen is an important virulence factor of E.coli strains that produce meningitis and septicaemia in neonates[19-21]. Its precise role in bacterial pathogenicity has not thus far been elucidated but it is known to reduce
the sensitivity of bacteria to phagocytosis[22] and some epidemiological data indicate that the K1 antigen also provides bacteria
with resistance to serum[23], although this latter conclusion has
recently been challenged[3,24,25].

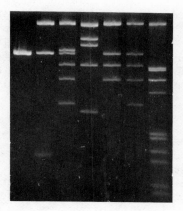

Fig. 3.   Cleavage of hybrid plasmids that specify K1 antigen biosynthesis with BamHI endonuclease. Plasmid DNA preparations were obtained, digested with BamHI restriction
endonuclease, and the fragments thereby generated analysed
by electrophoresis through a 0.8% agarose gel, as previously described[10]. From left to right: pHC79 (cosmid
vector), pKT168 (K1⁻), pKT169 (K1⁺), pKT170 (K1⁺), pKT171
(K1⁺), pKT172 (K1⁺), λ DNA cleaved with EcoRI and HindIII.
pKT170 is from the PstI gene bank; the remaining hybrid
plasmids are from the BamHI gene bank.

In order to be able to examine the serum resistance properties of essentially isogenic strains that differ only in their
ability to synthesize the K1 capsule, we have cloned the K1 biosynthesis genes in E.coli K-12 strain LE392. This was carried out
with the cosmid cloning — λ packaging system[26] using the pHC79
vector[26] and E.coli Bi 7509/41 (O7:K1:H⁻) DNA that had been partially cleaved with BamHI or PstI, to produce two gene banks. A
number of the clones in these banks were subsequently shown to produce precipitin haloes of specific antigen-antibody complexes,
when grown on agar plates containing meningococcus B antiserum
(the meningococcus B polysaccharide is identical to the K1 polysaccharide[17]), and hence to synthesize K1 antigen. Plasmid DNA was
prepared from four representative K1⁺ clones, three from the BamHI
gene bank and one from the PstI gene bank, and from one K1⁻ clone
and analysed by BamHI endonuclease cleavage (Fig.3). Comparison of
the digest patterns of the three hybrid plasmids from the BamHI
gene bank indicated that they possess three common BamHI fragments,
having sizes of approximately 20, 5.3 and 4.3 kb, which is consistent with the fact that they all specify biosynthesis of the K1
antigen.

Comparison of the serum resistance properties of the LE392 strain of E.coli K-12 and its K1[+] derivatives LE392 (pKT172) provided unequivocal evidence that the K1 capsular antigen provides bacteria with substantial protection against serum killing (Table 1). A similar conclusion has been arrived at by comparison of the serum resistance of K1[+] wild strains of E.coli and K1[-] mutant derivatives thereof[21,27].

DISCUSSION

At least two bacterial components, the R6-5 plasmid-determined traT outer membrane protein and the K1 polysaccharide capsular antigen, mediate resistance to complement killing; as anticipated, both are components of the cell surface.

The R6-5 traT protein is a 25,000 dalton polypeptide that is present in about 20,000 copies in plasmid pKT107-containing bacteria and that is highly exposed on the outer surface of the outer membrane. It provides resistance to complement not by inactivating complement components in the fluid phase but by modifying cell surface structure to prevent one or more steps in complement activation or action. It has been suggested that the traT proteins of the F and R100 plasmids, which are similar to that of R6-5 and which also mediate serum resistance (A. Moll, unpublished data), exist as multimeric aggregates in the outer membrane[15,16]. If this is also the case for the R6-5 traT protein, it is unlikely that it can be randomly distributed in the membrane and at the same time block all of the approximately 30,000 complement binding sites on the cell surface. Indeed, recent data show that there is little difference in the binding of complement components up to C8 to serum resistant and serum sensitive bacteria (ref. 17; Binns et al, this volume; D. Bitter-Suermann, personal communication). Taken together, these results suggest that the traT protein is localized at specific sites in the outer membrane, presumably sites of complement attack (adhesion zones between inner and outer membrane[28] ?), and that it functions either by inhibiting the binding of the terminal complement component C9 to form the membrane attack unit or, more likely, by inhibiting the action of the membrane attack unit.

The R6-5-type of serum resistance does not appear to be uncommon. ColV, a plasmid that is found in a high proportion of invasive strains of E.coli[21,29,30], has been shown to increase bacterial virulence[29,31] and to provide resistance to serum[31] via an outer membrane protein (Binns et al, this volume). Moreover, there appears to be a high degree of correlation between virulence, serum resistance, and the presence of an outer membrane protein in gonococcus[32].

On the other hand, capsules are also common attributes of invasive bacteria and these would appear to provide resistance to serum by a distinct, almost certainly less specific, mechanism that probably involves the shielding of cell surface structures which are ordinarily responsible for activating complement[33]. The fact that invasive strains of E.coli, Haemophilus, etc. frequently contain plasmids of the ColV and R6-5 type and synthesize capsules suggests that both types of serum resistance factor, outer membrane protein and capsule, may be important for bacterial virulence.

ACKNOWLEDGEMENTS

We thank D. Vogt and B. Kusecek for valued technical assistance, M. Binns, D. Bitter-Suermann, F. Cabello and R.P. Levine for stimulating discussions and for sharing their unpublished data, and J.B. Robbins and Bayer-Leverkusen for generous gifts of meningococcus B antiserum and ampicillin, respectively.

REFERENCES

1. G.K. Schoolnik, T.M. Buchanan, and K.K. Holmes, J. Clin. Invest. 58:1163-1173 (1976).
2. M.S. Simberkoff, I. Ricupero, and J.J. Rahal, Jr., J. Lab. Clin. Med. 87:206-217 (1976).
3. B. Björksten and B. Kaijser, Infect. Immun. 22:308-311 (1978).
4. G. Archer and F.R. Fekety, J. Infect. Dis. 134:1-7 (1976).
5. D.T. Durack and P.B. Beeson, Infect. Immun. 16:213-217 (1977).
6. A.M. Reynard and M.E. Beck, Infect. Immun. 14:848-850 (1976).
7. A. Fietta, E. Romero, and A.G. Siccardi, Infect. Immun. 18: 278-282 (1977).
8. P.W. Taylor and C. Hughes, Infect. Immun. 22:10-17 (1978).
9. R.P. Silver and S.N. Cohen, J. Bacteriol. 110:1082-1088 (1972).
10. K.N. Timmis, F. Cabello, and S.N. Cohen, Molec. Gen. Genet. 162:121-137 (1978).
11. M. Achtman, B. Kusecek, and K.N. Timmis, Molec. Gen. Genet. 163:169-179 (1978).
12. A. Moll, P.A. Manning, and K.N. Timmis, Infect. Immun. 28: 359-367 (1980).
13. P.A. Manning and M. Achtman, in: "Bacterial Outer Membranes: Biogenesis and Functions", M. Inouye, ed., Wiley, New York pp. 409-447 (1979).
14. A. Moll, F. Cabello, and K.N. Timmis, FEMS Lett. 6:273-276 (1979).
15. P.A. Manning, L. Beutin, and M. Achtman, J. Bacteriol. 142: 285-294 (1980).
16. D. Ferrazza and S.B. Levy, J. Bacteriol. 144:149-158 (1980).
17. R.T. Ogata and R.P. Levine, J. Immunol. 125:1494-1498 (1980).
18. P.A. Manning, C. Echarti, and K.N. Timmis, to be submitted.

19. J.B. Robbins, G.H. McCracken, E.C. Gotschlich, F. Orskov,
    I. Orskov, and L.A. Hanson, New Eng. J. Med. 290:1216-1220
    (1974).

20. M. Glode, A. Sutton, R. Moxon, and J.B. Robbins, Infect.
    Immun. 16:75-80 (1977).

21. F. Cabello in: "Plasmids of Medical, Environmental and Com-
    mercial Importance, K.N. Timmis and A. Pühler, eds.,
    Elsevier/North Holland, Amsterdam, pp. 155-160 (1979).

22. R. Bortolussi, P. Ferrieri, B. Bjorksten, and P.G. Cline,
    Infect. Immun. 25:293-298 (1979).

23. A.A. Glynn and C.J. Howard, Immunol. 18:331-346 (1970).

24. W.R. McCabe, B. Kaijser, S. Olling, M. Uwaydah, and L.A. Han-
    son, J. Infect. Dis. 138:33-40 (1978).

25. J. Pitt, Infect. Immun. 22:219-224 (1978).

26. B. Hohn and Hinnen, in: "Genetic Engineering, Principles and
    Methods, Vol 2, J.K. Setlow and A. Hollaender, eds.,
    Plenum, New York, pp. 169-183 (1980).

27. P. Gemski, A.S. Cross, and J.C. Sadoff, FEMS Lett. 9:193-197
    (1980).

28. M.E. Bayer, J. Gen. Microbiol. 53:395-404 (1968).

29. H.W. Smith, J. Gen. Microbiol. 83:95-111 (1974).

30. H.W. Smith and M.B. Huggins, J. Gen. Microbiol. 92:335-350
    (1976).

31. M.M. Binns, D.L. Davies, and K.G. Hardy, Nature 279:778-781
    (1979).

32. J.F. Hildebrandt, L.W. Mayer, S.P. Wang, and T.M. Buchanan,
    Infect. Immun. 20:267-273 (1978).

33. J.B. Robbins, R. Schneerson, W.B. Egan, W. Vann, and D.T. Liu,
    in: "The Molecular Basis of Microbial Pathogenicity,
    H. Smith, J.J. Skehel, and M.J. Turner, eds., Verlag Chemie,
    Weinheim, pp. 115-132 (1980).

ANTIBIOTIC RESISTANCE - A SURVEY

Julian E. Davies

Biogen S.A.
rte de Troinex 3
1227 Carouge/Geneva, Switzerland

The study of antibiotic resistance determinants is an active area of investigation that covers many aspects of plasmid biology. Thus, there is interest in, not only the biochemical mechanism by which the determinants express their resistance, but also in the distribution, origins and dissemination of resistance mechanisms. The problem of dissemination is particularly interesting since antibiotic resistance provides a convenient marker for the investigation of transposable elements. Parenthically, it should be added that plasmid-encoded resistance determinants are key components of all cloning vectors used in recombinant-DNA experimentation and "amp" and "tet" have become almost bywords in the field!

Although this brief review will focus on resistance to clinically useful antimicrobial agents, it should be remembered that R-plasmids may encode resistance to a wide variety of agents that are toxic to bacteria such as bacteriophages, bacteriocins, heavy metals, ionising radiation, serum components, detergents and other environmental poisons ; determinants exist (probably) that protect bacteria against toxic agents which have not yet been recognised. R-plasmids are the ultimate prophylactic agents (1).

In the past few years, studies of R-plasmid encoded antibiotic resistances have identified four distinct biochemical mechanisms that may be involved. These are listed in Table 1 together with some representative examples ; there are still some forms of antibiotic resistance that remain incompletely characterized in biochemical terms (for example, tetracycline, and certain forms of aminocyclitol and chloramphenicol resistance). In addition, resis-

Table I

Mechanisms of R-plasmid encoded antibiotic resistance*

Mechanism	Examples
Enɀymatic detoxification	β-lactams, chloramphenicol, aminocyclitols, pristinamicin
Alteration of target site	erythromycin-lincosamide
Altered uptake or retention by cell	tetracycline
By-pass sensitive step with drug-insensitive enzyme	sulphonamides, trimethoprim

* There are other resistance mechanisms known that are due to
  mutation and are not R-plasmid determined. In addition, there
  are classes of R-plasmid resistance (to chloramphenicol, aminocyclitols) that are uncharacterized biochemically.

tance to some antibiotics may involve a combination of biochemical mechanisms as exemplified by the aminocyclitols ; these agents
are detoxified inside the resistant organism which has the effect
of preventing strong binding to their target site (the ribosome)
necessary for uptake and maintenance of the drug inside the cell.
The overall result is that uptake of aminocyclitols into R^+ cells
is drastically reduced (2).

It is well-nigh redundant to discuss the appearance of new
forms (allomers) of resistance mechanisms that appear almost routinely with the continued selective pressure of antibiotic use in
human health and agricultural applications. The appearance of
β-lactamases with different substrate ranges and their spread to
different species and genera of bacteria is well-known and is

cause for concern now that penicillin-type resistance has been characterized in Neisseria, Hemophilus (3), and other important pathogenic genera. The presence of multiple-drug resistance in these organisms will certainly complicate therapy and in some instances the efficacy of the more advanced cephalosporins is threatened. Although penicillin-resistance in Streptococcus is not of the β-lactamase type its emergence has been a portent of other natural mechanisms of resistance to the β-lactams (4). A similar situation has been encountered in the case of the aminocyclitols and many mechanisms of resistance have (and continue to be) identified in Gram-negative and Gram-positive pathogens. The situation vis a vis aminocyclitols is more complex than that of resistance to β-lactams and other antibiotics since a variety of different aminocyclitol modifying enzymes exist in multiple allomeric forms with different substrate ranges (see Table II). More than one form of enzyme has been identified with respect to modification of the 6', 3', 2', 3 and 2" positions of aminocyclitols. For example in the case of modification at the 2"-OH group an allomeric form of adenylyltransferase has been reported recently, with a substrate range that includes the third-generation aminocyclitol amikacin (5) ; this drug was thought to be inert to resistance modification of this type (Fig. 1). The dissemination of such a resistance mechanism into other genera of Gram-negative bacteria could have serious consequences for aminocyclitol therapy of nosocomial infections. It is relevant at this point to voice some concern over the likelihood that large quantities of antibiotics may be used soon in industrial fermentations employing recombinant plasmids ; if "amp" or "tet" are used to maintain the plasmids involved it will be necessary to take steps to remove these agents before disposal of spent medium. As alternatives, the maintenance of plasmids in their hosts during industrial fermentations by other selective or genetically conditional methods should be investigated.

The mechanics of dissemination of R-plasmids and drug resistance is a complex problem ; many R-plasmids are non-conjugative (especially in Pseudomonas and Gram-positive organisms) and the mechanism of resistance spread in such genera in nature is not understood ; clearly transduction and transformation are mechanisms that could operate. However, it is apparent that even extremely rare events such as Staphylococcal-Streptococcal (6) conjugal exchange could lead to the establishment of a new group of resistance mechanisms in a hitherto "virgin" organism. Detailed nucleic acid and protein homology studies should throw some light on this question and positive support for Staphylococcal-Streptococcal exchange comes from the demonstration that the

Table II

Aminocyclitol-modifying enzymes

Enzyme	Typical substrates[+]
6'-acetyltransferase (AAC-6')	Kanamycin, tobramycin, amikacin, sisomicin, neomycin.
2'-acetyltransferase (AAC-2')	gentamicins
3-acetyltransferase (AAC-3)	gentamicins, tobramycin, kanamycin, neomycin, fortimicin
4'-adenylyltransferase (AAD-4')	tobramycin, amikacin, kanamycin, neomycin
2"-adenylyltransferase (AAD-2")	gentamicin, tobramycin, kanamycin
3"-adenylyltransferase (AAD-3")	streptomycin, spectinomycin
6-adenylyltransferase (AAD-6)	streptomycin
3'-phosphotransferase (APH-3')	neomycin, kanamycin
3"-phosphotransferase (APH-3")	streptomycin
2"-phosphotransferase (APH-2")	gentamicins, kanamycin
5"-phosphotransferase (APH-5")	ribostamycin, lividomycin
6-phosphotransferase (APH-6)	streptomycin

[+]These vary with the isozymic form of the enzyme.

macrolide-lincosamide resistance determinants in Staphylococcus and Streptococcus are homologous both in biochemical function and sequence (7).

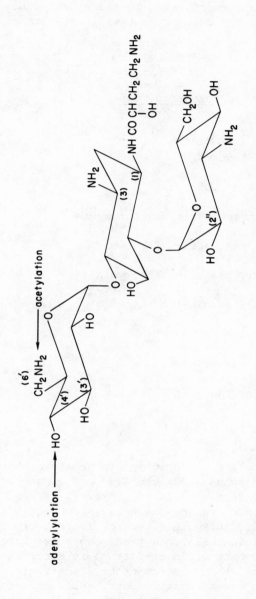

AMIKACIN

Figure I

With regard to the dissemination of resistance between replicons, transposable drug resistance provides a satisfactory mechanism for this exchange (8) and at present most, if not all drug
resistance genes can be demonstrated to transpose either singly or
in groups (Table III). The case of gentamicin resistance is inte-

Table III

Transposable drug resistances

β-lactams

chloramphenicol

streptomycin-spectinomycin

trimethoprim

erythromycin-lincomycin

gentamicin-tobramycin

sulphonamide

tetracycline

fosfonomycin

resting ; until recently transposition of these resistance genes,
in spite of the widespread use of the drug and occurence of resistant strains, had not been recognized. However, several examples
of gentamicin resistance transposition have now been identified
and the reason for difficulty in detection is probably due to the
fact that the gentamicin resistance transposons are large elements
in which the gene for gentamicin resistance is associated with at
least 3 or 4 other resistance determinants ; their size > 10 Md
prevented detection by transposition onto bacteriophage lambda
which could not accomodate such a large insert, even though λ is
normally a convenient receptor in transposition assays (9). Studies

of gentamicin resistance transposition from plasmid to plasmid
(by the use of incompatibility) have demonstrated the widespread
nature of transposable elements encoding gentamicin resistance
(10, 11). More recently in studies with a number of clinical isolates using bacteriophage P1 as a receptor for transposons, it has
been demonstrated that a large proportion of gentamicin resistance
determinants is capable of transduction either by transposition or
cointegration (12). To date most of the transposable resistance
elements that have been studied are from Gram-negative organisms,
and substantial information has been obtained with respect to their
structure and function. Only one Gram-positive transposable element
has been relatively well characterized, an erythromycin resistance
element (Tn551) that, interestingly, has short inverted repeat
sequences that share some homology with Tn3, the β-lactamase transposon of Gram-negative bacteria (13). In addition, there is strong
circumstantial evidence that the aminocyclitol resistance genes of
Staphylococci are transposable since the genes are associated with
invertible DNA structures of wide distribution and similar structure (14). However, definite proof of transposition is lacking.
It is worth noting that, with respect to the intrageneric exchange
of resistance mechanisms, most if not all Gram-positive resistance
genes have been found to be expressed in Gram-negative hosts, although the reverse has not been demonstrated.

No survey of R-plasmid encoded resistance can be complete
without some mention of recent studies on the sequences of the
resistance genes and their regulatory elements. The complete DNA
sequences of a β-lactamase (15), chloramphenicol acetytransferase
(16, 17) two aminocyclitol phosphotransferases (18, 19) and erythromycin ribosomal RNA methylase (20, 21), as well as partial
sequences for other genes are available. Of particular interest
is the regulatory region of the erythromycin resistance gene ;
sequence studies have led to the proposal that induction of the
expression of this gene (erythromycin resistance) can be explained
by antibiotic inhibition or slowing of ribosome movement over the
leader sequence to allow the formation of a new mRNA conformation
that exposes the initiator sequence to start translation. This
attentuation mechanism bears a strong resemblance to those proposed for the regulation of tryptophan, histidine, and threonine
biosynthesis. Sequences of the regulatory regions of point mutants
to constitutivity support the model since the single base changes
of the mutants are in sites that expose the initiator and allow
continuous translation (20, 22). It will be of interest to see
if the same situation obtains in Streptomyces erythreus, the erythromycin producing strain.

With regard to the regulation of other resistance determinants, much less is known. The Gram-negative chloramphenicol acetyltransferase (23) is a constitutive enzyme and is (apparently) regulated by catabolite repression only. The Gram-positive chloramphenicol acetyltransferase is inducible and it will be of interest to see how this gene is regulated - will it be like the attenuator-controlled erythromycin resistance of Staph aureus, or will it involve classical repressor-operator interactions ? In what way will chloramphenicol act as inducer ? There has been much nice work on the regulation of tetracycline resistance which functions through a typical repressor-operator interaction (24). It will be intriguing to know how the tetracycline actually interacts with the repressor ; will the same inducible mechanism obtain for the tetracycline resistance of Gram-positive R-plasmids ? The sequence of the aminocyclitol phosphotransferase 3'-I of Tn903 presents several interesting features, the gene is expressed in several eukaryotic organisms and the probable regulatory region has certain "eukaryotic" features (e.g. a Hogness box) that may well be associated with its capacity to be expressed well in a eukaryotic cytoplasm (25). Studies of the regulation of other resistance genes are eagerly awaited, since they may offer additional surprises concerning regulatory mechanisms.

To conclude this brief review, mention must be made of the ubiquity of antibiotic resistance mechanism in the microbial population of nature. In a variety of microorganisms other than clinical isolates, antibiotic resistance mechanisms have been characterized that are biochemically identical to those found in R-plasmid harboring organisms. In addition resistance mechanisms to new or rarely used antibiotics have been found in antibiotic producing organisms (Table IV). The detection of these mechanisms may be of predictive value in the design and modification of antibiotics in the future ; biochemical mechanisms of resistance to a given antibiotic may be very limited. The strong biochemical homology between resistance of clinical isolates and producers has been used as the basis of a hypothesis that R-plasmid-encoded resistance mechanisms may have evolved from antibiotic-producing organisms in nature. The failure to detect any nucleic acid homologies between the various determinants rules out the possibility of any direct (and recent) gene transfer between the different types of organisms (26). However, it will be interesting to see if DNA or protein sequence studies indicate any active site homologies. In the one case where two members of an allozymic group have been compared directly at the sequence level there is no evidence of any similarity in DNA or protein sequence (except that they contain the same bases and amino acids !) (Table V).

Table IV

Naturally-occurring (non R-plasmid) antibiotic resistance mechanisms

Resistance mechanism	Source
β-lactamase	Actinomycetes, Bacillus
chloramphenicol acetyltransferase	Actinomyces
erythromycin ribosome methylase	Actinomycetes, Bacillus
aminocyclitol acetyltransferases	Actinomycetes
aminocyclitol phosphotransferases	Actinomycetes, Bacillus
aminocyclitol adenylyltransfera- ses	Bacillus
thiostrepton ribosome methylase	Actinomyces
viomycin phosphotransferase	Actinomycetes
hygromycin phosphotransferase	Actinomycetes

Table V

Comparison of	APH(3')-I	APH(3')-II
M.W.	27k	23-25k
Amino acid residues	~ 280	~ 200 (sequence incomplete)
Base composition	44 % GC	63 % GC
K_m neomycin	2 uM	4 uM
Amino acid composition	high in asp arg~lys	asp~glu arg>lys

This would tend to indicate that, at least in the case of these two aminoglycoside-3'-phosphotransferases, evolution occurred independently from two different and entirely unrelated sources. Will we be able to find the sources, or possible replicons on the evolutionary route to these genes (enzymes) as they now exist ? Since some R-plasmid resistance determinants are (unlike Gram-negative chromosomal genes) expressed in Gram-positive cytoplasm, one might argue that the determinants are not typical Gram-negative genes even though they reside in such hosts.

ACKNOWLEDGEMENTS

I wish to thank N.I.H. and N.S.F. for their generous support of this work over the past 12 years. In addition I owe my gratitude to W. Piepersberg, S.A. Kagan, S. Harford, J. Leboul and K. Komatsu for their recent contributions to these studies. Drs. A. Oka, N. Grindley, H. Schaller, and B. Weisblum kindly provided much useful, and unpublished sequence information.

REFERENCES

1. J. Davies and D.I. Smith, Plasmid-determined resistance
        to antimicrobial agents, Ann. Rev. Biochem. 32:469 (1978).
2. L.E. Bryan and H.M. Van den Elzen, Effects of membrane-
        energy mutations and cations on streptomycin and genta-
        micin accumulation by bacteria : a model for entry of
        streptomycin and gentamicin in susceptible and resistant
        bacteria, Antimicrob. Ag. Chemother. 12:163 (1977).
3. S. Falkow, L.P. Elwell, M. Roberts, F. Heffron and R. Gill,
        The transcription of ampicillin resistance : nature of
        ampicillin resistant Hemophilus influenzae and Neisseria
        gonorrhea, in "R-factors, their properties and possible
        control", Berlin, Springer-Verlag, New York 1977 p. 115.
4. A. Tomasz, From penicillin-binding proteins to the lysis
        and death of bacteria : a 1979 view, Rev. Infect. Dis.
        1:434-467 (1979).
5. R.G. Coombe and A.M. George, A new plasmid-mediated amino-
        glycoside adenylyltransferase of broad substrate range
        that adenylylates amikacin, (submitted for publication).
6. D.B. Clewell, (pers. commun.) see this volume.

7. B. Weisblum, S.B. Holder and S.M. Halling, Deoxyribonucleic acid sequence common to staphylococcal and streptococcal plasmids which specify erythromicin resistance, J. Bacteriol. 138: 990-998 (1979).

8. S.N. Cohen. Transposable genetic elements and plasmid evolution. Nature 263:731 (1976).

9. D.E. Berg. Detection of transposable antibiotic resistance determinants with bacteriophage lambda, in "DNA insertion elements, plasmids and episomes". Cold Spring Harbor Laboratory, 1977 p 555.

10. M.E. Nugent, D.H. Bone and N. Datta. A transposon Tn732 encoding gentamicin/tobramycin resistance. Nature 282:422 (1980).

11. C.E. Rubens, W.F. McNeill, W.E. Farrar. Evolution of multiple antibiotic resistance plasmids mediated by transposable deoxyribonucleic acid sequences. J. Bacteriology 140:713 (1979).

12. W. Piepersberg and J. Davies (unpublished observations).

13. S.A. Khan and R.P. Novick. Terminal nucleotide sequences of Tn551, a transposon specifying erythromycin resistance in Staphylococcus aureus : homology with Tn3. Plasmid, 4:148 (1980).

14. G.S. Gray and T-S.R. Huang. Characterization of aminoglycoside-resistance plasmids in Staphylococcus aureus, Plasmid, in press.

15. J.G. Sutcliffe. Nucleotide sequence of the ampicillin resistance gene of Escherchia coli plasmid pBR322. Proc. Natl. Acad. Sci. U.S. 75:3737 (1978).

16. N.K. Alton and D. Vapnek. Nucleotide sequence analysis of the chloramphenicol resistance transposon Tn9. Nature, Vol. 282:864 (1979).

17. R. Marcoli, S. Iida, T.A. Bickle, Sequence of chloramphenicol transacetylase of transposon TnCam-204, Febs Lett. 110:11 (1980).

18. A. Oka, personal communication

19. H. Schaller, personal communication

20. S. Horinuchi and B. Weisblum. Posttranscriptional modification of mRNA conformation: a novel mechanism that regulates erythromycin-induced resistance. Proc. Natl. Scad. Sci. U.S. in press.

21. T. Gryczan, G. Grandi, J. Hahn, R. Grandi and D. Dubnau. Conformational alteration of mRNA structure and the posttranscriptional regulation of erythromycin-induced resistance. Nucl. Acids Res. in press.

22. S. Horinuchi and B. Weisblum. The control region for erythromycin resistance: free energy changes related to induction and mutation to constitutive expression. (Submitted for publication).

23. B. de Crombrugge, I. Pastan, W.V. Shaw and J.W. Rosner. Stimulation by cyclic AMP and ppGpp of chloramphenicol acetyltransferase synthesis. Nature 241:237 (1973).

24. H-L. Yang, G. Zubay and S.B. Levy. Synthesis of an R-plasmid protein associated with tetracycline resistance is negatively regulated. Proc. Nat. Acad. Sci (US) 73:1509 (1976).

25. A. Jimenez and J. Davies. Expression of a transposable antibiotic resistance element in Saccharomyces. Nature 287:869 (1980).

26. P. Courvalin, M. Fiandt and J. Davies. DNA relationships between genes coding for aminoglycoside-modifying enzymes from antibiotic-producing bacteria and R-plasmids. Microbiology, p 262 (1978).

REGULATION OF PLASMID SPECIFIED MLS-RESISTANCE IN BACILLUS

SUBTILIS BY CONFORMATIONAL ALTERATION OF RNA STRUCTURE

D. Dubnau, G. Grandi, R. Grandi, T.J. Gryczan
J. Hahn, Y. Kozloff and A.G. Shivakumar

Department of Microbiology
The Public Health Research Institute of the City
of New York, Inc.
New York, N.Y. 10016

INTRODUCTION

Resistance to the macrolide-lincosamide-streptogramin B (MLS) group of antibiotics, often mediated by plasmids, is widespread among clinically isolated strains of Staphylococcus and Streptococcus (1-5). The mechanism of resistance to these inhibitors of protein synthesis has been elucidated by B. Weisblum and his colleagues (6-8). MLS-resistance is associated with the presence of additional methyl groups (as N^6, N^6-dimethyl adenine) on 23S rRNA. This modification reduces the ribosomal affinity for the MLS antibiotics. In many cases exposure to a subinhibitory concentration of erythromycin (Em), results in induction of resistance to elevated levels of antibiotic. Although only Em and a few closely related macrolides like oleandomycin (Om) act as inducers, cultures exposed to these drugs acquire resistance to the entire range of MLS antibiotics. We will deal in this report with the MLS resistance specified by the 3.5 kb plasmid pE194. This entity was isolated from Staphylococcus aureus (9) and then transferred to Bacillus subtilis (10). All of our work has been carried out in the latter organism.

Certain features of induced resistance deserve emphasis. The regulatory system must possess some means of avoiding what appears to be an intrinsic dilemma: how to induce increased synthesis of a protein (ribosomal methylase - see below), by exposure to an inhibitor of protein synthesis (Em). This contradiction might be resolved kinetically or spatially. For instance, the Em-sensing

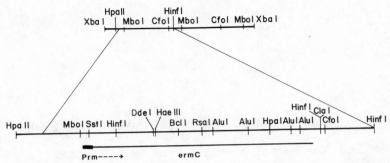

Fig. 1. Restriction endonuclease cleavage site map of pE194. The
plasmid is shown linearized at its single XbaI site. The
segment containing the ermC gene is shown in expanded form
and the position of the ermC determinant is indicated by a
horizontal bar. The location of the ermC promoter (Prm) and
the direction of transcription are also shown.

sites for induction may be separated physically from the ribosomes
which must translate the ribosomal methylase. Also, since resistance
is dependent on the specific methylation of rRNA, we can predict that
an economic regulatory system might sense both the intracellular concentration of Em and the existing extent of rRNA methylation. Such a
dual requirement for Em and unmethylated ribosomes as positive effec-
tors for methylase induction would generate a feedback loop, since
induced methylase will decrease the concentration of unmethylated
ribosomes. Such a system would be capable of maintaining a steady
state level of enzyme just sufficient to methylate newly synthesized
ribosomes.

The ermC gene and its product.

The inducible MLS-resistance specified by pE194 is encoded by
the ermC gene. This determinant specifies a 29,000 dalton polypeptide, the synthesis of which has been shown to be induced by Em
(11). Cloning of restriction fragments and deletion analysis have
defined the location of the ermC gene on the pE194 physical map
(12,13). The gene is located between the single SstI and ClaI sites
(Fig. 1). These studies have also served to confirm the essential
role of the 29 K protein in MLS resistance. The direction of transcription and the location of the ermC promoter have been established
by RNA polymerase binding studies, deletion analysis, transcription
mapping and by DNA sequencing (12,13). The promoter is near the
single SstI site and transcription of ermC proceeds from left to
right on the map (Fig. 1). Recently, we have purified to homogeneity
an inducible ribosomal methylase specified by pE194 (unpublished).

This enzyme co-electrophoreses with the 29 K protein on SDS-poly-acrylamide gels. The methylase requires S-adenosyl methionine and methylates only "free" 50S ribosomes in vitro.

Induction is Posttranscriptional.

Using the B. subtilis minicell system (11,14), we have estab-lished that induction of the ermC gene product is mediated post-transcriptionally (15). Enhanced synthesis of the 29 K protein occurs in response to an inducing (27nM) concentration of Em, even after transcription is arrested by the addition of either rifampicin or streptolydigin. This enhancement is specific; synthesis of the other four known pE194 polypeptides is unaffected by this concen-tration of Em. Tylosin (Ty), a non-inducing macrolide antibiotic, does not stimulate synthesis of the 29 K protein. These experiments also reveal that Em (and not Ty) specifically lengthens the func-tional half-life of the 29 K protein transcript, since the synthetic capacity of the minicells for this protein decays very slowly in the presence of both rifampicin and Em. Although we suspect that stabi-lization of ermC mRNA by Em is a secondary consequence of enhanced translation, it may very well be an important factor contributing to the all-over induction of ribosomal methylase.

Induction Requires a Ribosomal Em-Binding Site.

Minicells pre-incubated in the presence of Em cannot be induced when the drug is washed away and then added back (15). Instead, methylase synthesis continues at the basal (uninduced) rate. This is easily explained in terms of the feedback loop postulated above, since pre-induced cells contain methylated ribosomes. The non-inducibility of pre-induced cells is consistent with the notion that a ribosomal Em-binding site is required for induction. In support we cite two more observations. First, all Em-sensitive ermC mutants studied to date, are hyper-inducible for the mutant protein (15). This strongly indicates that a feedback mechanism is operative during induction of the normal methylase and is consistent with the hypothesis that an unmethylated ribosomal site is required for in-duction. Second, we can perturb the Em-binding site by introducing ole-1, a chromosomal mutation which alters ribosomal protein L17 and results in a low-level resistance to Em (G. Williams and I. Smith, pers. commun.; 16). Ribosomes isolated from ole-1 cultures bind Em poorly in vitro (15). Minicells from an ole-1 strain carrying pE194 cannot be induced to synthesize the ribosomal methylase at an ele-vated rate by the usual inducing concentrations of Em. Once again we are led to the conclusion that a ribosomal Em binding site is required for induction. If an Em-ribosome complex must form in order for induction to occur, then the system has an effective way to meter the intracellular concentrations of both Em and unmethylated

(Em-sensitive) ribosomes as postulated above. These properties of
the system seem eminently consistent with our conclusion that induction is regulated posttranscriptionally.

Regulatory Mutants.

     Selection of colonies capable of growth on Ty in the absence
of Em, permits ready isolation of constitutive (tyc) mutants (10).
These plasmid mutations result in elevated levels of methylase in
the absence of induction (11; unpublished). The map location and
the nature of the tyc mutations strongly support the posttranscriptional model of methylase regulation. Out of 21 spontaneous
tyc mutants which we have studied, 12 contained plasmids of larger
molecular weight than the pE194 parent. Restriction endonuclease
mapping of the "extra" DNA present in these molecules revealed that
this material (ranging in size from about 100 to 600 base pairs)
was inserted between the single SstI and HaeIII sites of pE194
(Fig. 1). Several other tyc mutations which do not appear to result
in larger plasmids, were mapped by marker rescue (17) and found to
be located near the HaeIII site (unpublished). Thus, the tyc
mutations are located at the promoter proximal end of ermC. If
these mutations exert their effects posttranscriptionally, as does
Em-induction, we would expect that the mutations might be located
within the transcribed portion of ermC. In this respect they would
be unlike operator-promoter mutants which are themselves usually
not transcribed. This expectation was confirmed for two mutants,
tyc-16 and tyc-9 which result from insertions of about 100 and 600
base pairs respectively. The sizes of the tyc-16, tyc-9 and wild
type ermC transcripts were measured in a blotting-hybridization
experiment. The ermC transcript, normally about 0.97 kb in size,
was enlarged by about 0.1 and 0.6 kb in the mutants (13). Thus the
tyc mutations most likely act posttranscriptionally as does Em-
induction. Two tyc mutants have been sequenced and will be
described below.

Structure of the ermC Gene.

     The ermC gene has been entirely sequenced (13). A portion of
the sequence, corresponding to the promoter proximal region is re-
produced in Fig. 2. Transcription-mapping has confirmed that transcription initiates near the tandem A residues at positions 196-197
(13). Centered about 10 bases upstream from this position is a
TATAAT sequence which is a typical prokaryotic consensus "-10
sequence" (18). The sequence contains a single open reading extending from an ATG codon at 337 to a TAA termination codon at position
1069 (not shown). This is sufficient to encode a protein of 244
amino acids with molecular weight 28,947, in agreement with the
known molecular weight of the ribosomal methylase. Thus the sequenc

TCGTAATTAAGTCGTTAAACCGTGTGCTCTACGACCAAAACTATAAAACCTTTAAGAACTTTCTTTTTTTACAAGAAAAAAGAAATTAGATAAATCTCT 99

CATATCTTTTATTCAATAATCGCATCCGATTGCAGTATAAATTTAACGATCACTCATCATGTTCATATTTATCAGAGCTCGTGCTATAATTATACTAAT 198
                                                  MboI   -35   SstI   -10

                    MetGlyIluPheSerIluPheValIluSerThrValHisTyrGlnProAsnLysLys
TTTATAAGGAGGAAAAAATATGGGCATTTTTAGTATTTTTGTAATCAGCACAGTTCATTATCAACCAAACAAAAAATAAGTGGTTATAATGAATCGTTA 297
     S.D.1   HinfI

                              MetAsnGluLysAsnIluLysHisSerGlnAsnPheIluThrSerLysHisAsnIluAsp
ATAAGCAAAATTCATATAACCAAATTAAAGAGGGTTATAATGAACGAGAAAAATATAAAACACAGTCAAAACTTTATTACTTCAAAACATAATATAGAT 396
                              S.D.2

LysIluMetThrAsnIluArgLeuAsnGluHisAspAsnIluPheGluIluGlySerGlyLysGlyHisPheThrLeuGluLeuValLysArgCysAsn
AAAATAATGACAAATATAAGATTAAATGAACATGATAATATCTTTGAAATCGGCTCAGGAAAAGGCCATTTTACCCTTGAATTAGTAAAGAGGTGTAAT 495
                              DdeI   HaeIII

Fig. 2.   The promoter proximal portion of the ermC sequence (13) is
           presented. The coding strand is shown. The promoter is
           located near the SstI cleavage site and the inferrred RNA
           polymerase binding and recognition elements are denoted as
           "-10" and "-35." The probable transcriptional initiation
           point at 196-197 and the direction of transcription are
           marked by an arrow. The inferred ribosomal binding sites
           are indicated as "S.D.1 and S.D.2" and probable trans-
           lational start codons are shown by wavy underlining. The
           stop codon for the 19 amino acid peptide is denoted by
           double underlining.

defines a 141 base leader sequence, between positions 197 and 337.
Within this leader are several noteworth features summarized in
Fig. 2 and 3. SD1 and SD2 (Shine-Dalgarno sequences (19) represent
probable ribosomal binding sites, possessing 7 and 9 base comple-
mentarities with the terminal 3' sequences of bacillus 16S rRNA
(20-22). Correctly situated downstream from SD1 and SD2 are ATG
codons. The first potentially initiates translation of a 19 amino
acid polypeptide. The second almost certainly initiates methylase
synthesis. In addition to these features, the leader region contains
6 complementary segments (I-VI) which permit folding into several
possible stem-loop structures (Fig. 3). Within two of these potential structures (A & B), the ATG codon for methylase synthesis and
part of SD2 are buried within a base-paired region. In structure C,
SD2 and its associated ATG codon are unpaired. In all of these
possible structures, SD1 and its ATG codon are exposed and therefore
available for interaction with a ribosome.

       Fig. 3 also indicates the locations of the tyc-1 and tyc-16
mutations (13). tyc-1 substitutes A for C at position 317. tyc-16
inserts an extra 109 base pairs between positions 321-322. The

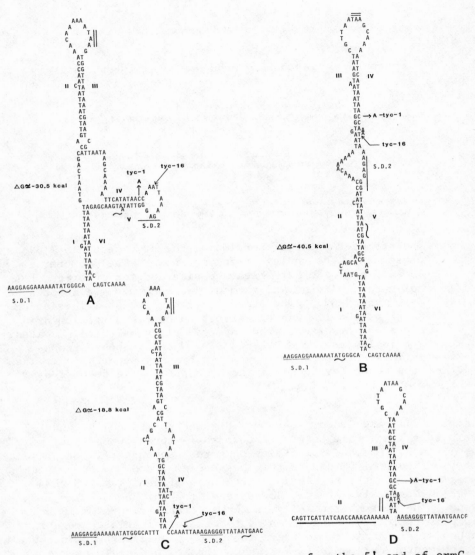

Fig. 3.   Hypothetical hairpin structures for the 5' end of ermC
mRNA.   The sequences are written with thymine residues to
facilitate comparison with Fig. 2.   The locations of the
tyc-1 base change and the tyc-16 insertions are indicated.
Calculated energies of structures A and B (inactive) and C
(active) are given (31,32).   The inferred ribosomal binding
sites and start and stop codons are denoted as in Fig. 2.
The heavy bar on structure D is meant to suggest the
approximate location of a ribosome, stalled in the presenc
of Em.

inserted DNA is a direct tandem duplication of the 109 residues
immediately downstream from the point of insertion.

We will now suggest a model for the regulation of ribosomal
methylase synthesis, which is based on the features of the ermC
system described above.

Translational Attenuation.

Several of the features of the ermC system are reminiscent of
the attenuation mechanisms proposed for regulation of a number of
amino acid biosynthetic operons (23-28). These features include
the presence of a leader with extensive potential secondary structure, the possible translation of a short polypeptide within the
leader sequence and a requirement for a ribosome as a positive
effector. We propose that ribosomal methylase synthesis is regulated by an attenuation-like mechanism, but entirely on the translational level. Other, less attractive alternatives have been
discussed (13). The present model suggest that mRNA folding determines the rate of methylase synthesis and that this folding can be
influenced by tyc mutations as well as by Em-induction. The transcriptional attenuation models (23-28) hold that depletion of an
amino acyl tRNA species causes stalling of a ribosome at a sensitive
site during leader-peptide translation. This in turn induces isomerization of the nascent mRNA, which removes a structural feature
required for the termination of transcription. Consequently, transcription of the structural genes can occur. Our model of translational attenuation suggests that Em causes ribosome stalling
during translation of the 19 amino acid peptide which results in
refolding of the already completed transcript into an active configuration for methylase synthesis. This mechanism is consistent with
a large body of work which points to the importance of mRNA secondary
structure in regulating translation by masking or exposing initiation
sequences (29,30).

Some Specific Features of ermC Regulation.

In minicells and in whole cells a basal level of methylase is
produced without induction (11 and unpublished). The basal synthesis corresponds to about 5% of the induced level. This can be
explained by the spontaneous refolding of inactive structures (A
and B) into an active form e.g. C. (Fig. 3). The calculated energies of these structures (31,32) suggest that they are stable enough
to exist in the cell. Considerable uncertainties are associated
with these calculations however, making quantitative assertions
about the equilibrium ratios of active and inactive forms very
dangerous. Nevertheless, A, B and C should be in equilibrium with
one another, with the concentrations of A and B being higher than

that of C.   The tyc-1 mutation elevates the basal level 2-4 fold
(unpublished).   This mutation increases the calculated energy of A
from -30.5 to -22.5 Kcal/mol and that of B from -40.5 to -31.6.   On
the other hand, by permitting the formation of several additional
base pairs, the stability of the tyc-1 mutant form of C is, if
anything, slightly increased (from -18.8 to -19.4 Kcal/mol).   Thus
an increase in the concentration of C would be expected to occur,
leading to an increased basal synthesis, as observed.   tyc-16 permits an entirely new structure to form, since complementary segments
V and VI are duplicated.   The inserted DNA should form structures
identical to A and B, but with the "original" V and VI segments
located downstream, in an exposed configuration and contiguous with
the remaining protion of the ermC coding sequence.   This arrangement
should result in enhanced basal synthesis as observed.

The translational attenuation model of induction presupposes
that a ribosome can bind at SD1 and initiate translation of the 19
amino acid peptide.   Inhibition of this ribosome by a bound molecule
of Em, will result in stalling within segments I or II.   Ribosomal
stalling, we suggest, induces isomerization of structure A or B to
generate D, exposing SD2 and the methylase start codon.   We will
first consider this model in the light of what is known about the
mode of Em action.   This antibiotic appears to slow the movement of
ribosomes on mRNA (33).   Em binds to "free" ribosomes and to polysomes, from which peptidyl tRNA has been removed.   It binds poorly
to native polysomes (33,34).   Em (and Om) inhibit neither initiation
complex formation, nor formation of the first peptide bond (35,36).
These macrolides seem to inhibit translocation or transpeptidization
only when the nascent peptidyl tRNA has grown to some (unknown)
chain length (37).   In addition to size, the chemical nature of the
polymerized amino acid residues is an important determinant of Em
sensitivity, with bulky and hydrophillic amino acids contributing to
enhanced susceptibility (38).   Other MLS antibiotics, such as Ty,
can inhibit formation of the first peptide bond following initiation
(36).   We would expect then, that Em will bind to a 50S ribosome
before or immediately following initiation of 19 amino acid peptide
synthesis.   When the peptidyl tRNA reaches a critical length and
when the appropriate amino acid substituents are polymerized, the
ribosome will stall.   In Escherichia coli, initiating ribosomes protect 30-35 bases in mRNA from the action of RNAse A (39).   Thus it
is plausible to suggest that ribosome stalling within segments I or
II will sequester segment II leading to the freeing of segment III
(Fig. 3).   This will result in formation of structure D directly
from B.   Freeing of III within structure A will also increase the
concentration of D, since the III-IV structure is more stable
(-15.0 Kcal/mol) than IV-V (-11.7 Kcal/mol).   This model can also
accomodate the failure of Ty and other MLS antibiotics to act as
inducers of ermC expression.   Em and Om may induce because they permit the nascent peptidyl tRNA to elongate somewhat before ribosome
stalling occurs.   Ty would be expected to prevent formation of the

first peptide bond (fmet-gly) thus possibly stalling the ribosome in a position which does not induce isomerization to an active structure. Whether a given MLS antibiotic acts as an inducer should therefore depend on the details of molecular structure in a given system. A dramatic feature of the transcriptional attenuation system is the presence of several tandem repeat amino acid codons which comprise a site of extraordinary sensitivity to depletion of a specific amino acyl tRNA (23-28). It is tempting to speculate that the 19 amino acid peptide is likewise a specialized sensor of Em. In fact, polylysine synthesis seems particularly sensitive to the action of Em (40). Perhaps the HisTyrGlnProAsnLysLys sequence at the C-terminus of the peptide comprises a string of bulky hydro- phillic residues for sensing the presence of Em (38).

The translational attenuation model surmounts the dilemma posed initially, since it separates the Em-sensing device from the ribo- somes which translate the methylase structural sequence. Since induction can occur at low (∿20nM) Em levels and since ribosomes are half-saturated in vitro by Em at about 1μM (15) most of the ribosomes which bind and initiate at the newly exposed SD2 sequence will be uninhibited. Once translation of methylase begins, increased Em concentrations will have no effect, since Em does not bind to poly- somes (33,34). Slow colony formation can occur when uninduced cells carrying pE194 are seeded on plates containing as much as 8mM Em (unpublished). Since a basal level of methylase exists in this sys- tem, some methylated ribosomes presumably are also present prior to induction. Em will cause non-methylated ribosomes to stall within the coding sequence for the 19 amino acid peptide, thus exposing SD2 by isomerization of the mRNA. If a rare methylated ribosome then attaches and initiates, methylase will be synthesized. Thus, the ingridients are present for a slow exponential escape from inhibi- tion by high concentrations of Em, a bacteriostatic agent.

Some Features of Posttranscriptional Regulation.

RNA polymerase (41-43), gene 32 protein of T4 (44), ribosomal proteins (41,42,45-48) and proteins of RNA bacteriophage (30) all seem to be regulated on the level of translation and all are pro- teins capable of interaction with nucleic acid. The ribosomal methylase of pE194 clearly fits into this category. The former systems also seem to be regulated autogenously, by direct binding of each protein to specialized secondary structures at the 5' end of mRNA. Methylase induction is at least formally autogenous, although the feedback loop is probably mediated via rRNA methylation. Direct autogenous regulation of methylase synthesis by binding of the protein to mRNA has not been excluded and it is tempting to speculate by analogy, that such direct autorepression operates.

We gratefully acknowledge discussions with I. Smith, E. Dubnau, R.P. Novick, L. Mindich and R. Losick. We thank L. Kohl for expert secretarial assistance. This work was supported by NIH Grant AI1031 and ACS Grant VC-300. G.G. was partially supported by funds from Farmitalia C. Erba S.p.A., Milan, Italy.

REFERENCES

1. Clewell, D.B. and Franke, A.E. (1974) Antimicrob. Ag. Chemother 5, 534-537.
2. Courvalin, P.M., Carlier, C. and Chabbert, Y.A. (1972) Ann. Inst. Pasteur (Paris) 123, 755-759.
3. Horodniceanu, T., Bouanchaud, D.H., Bieth, G. and Chabbert, Y.A (1976) Antimicrob. Ag. Chemother. 10, 795-801.
4. Jacobs, M.R., Koornhof, H.J., Robins, Browne, R.M., Stevenson, C.M., Vermaak, Z.A., Freiman, I., Miller, G.B., Witcomb, M.A., Isaacson, M., Ward, J.I. and Austrian, R. (1978) New Engl. J. Med. 299, 735-740.
5. Otaya, H. (1971) In Drug Action and Drug Resistance in Bacteria (S. Mitsuhashi, ed.) University Park Press, Baltimore.
6. Lai, C.-J. and Weisblum, B. (1971) Proc. Nat. Acad. Sci. USA 68, 856-860.
7. Lai, C.-J., Dahlberg, J.E. and Weisblum, B. (1973) Biochemistry 12, 457-460.
8. Lai, C.-J., Weisblum, B., Fahnestock, S.R. and Nomura, M. (1973 J. Mol. Biol. 74, 67-72.
9. Iordanescu, S. (1976) Arch. Roum. Path. Exp. Microbiol. 35, 111 118.
10. Weisblum, B., Graham, M.Y., Gryczan, T. and Dubnau, D. (1979) J. Bacteriol. 137, 635-643.
11. Shivakumar, A.G., Hahn, J. and Dubnau, D. (1979) Plasmid 2, 279-289.
12. Shivakumar, A.G., Gryczan, T.J., Kozlov, Y.I. and Dubnau, D. (1980a) Molec. gen. Genet. 179, 241-252.
13. Gryczan, T.J., Grandi, G., Hahn, J., Grandi, R. and Dubnau, D. (1980) Nucl. Acids Res. 8, 6081-6097.
14. Reeve, J.N., Mendelson, N.H., Coyne, S.I., Hallock, L.L. and Cole, R.M. (1973) J. Bacteriol. 114, 860-873.
15. Shivakumar, A.G., Hahn, J., Grandi, G., Kozlov, Y. and Dubnau, D. (1980b) Proc. Nat. Acad. Sci. USA 77, 3903-3907.
16. Tipper, D.J., Johnson, C.W., Ginther, C.L., Leighton, T. and Wittman, H.G. (1977) Molec. gen. Genet. 150, 147-159.
17. Contente, S. and Dubnau, D. (1979b) Plasmid 2, 555-571.
18. Rosenberg, M. and Court, D. (1979) Ann. Rev. Genet. 13, 319-353
19. Shine, J. and Dalgarno, L. (1974) Proc. Nat. Acad. Sci. USA 71, 1342-1346.
20. Shine, J. and Dalgaron, L. (1975) Nature 254, 34.
21. Sprague, K.U., Steitz, J.A., Grenley, R.M. and Stocking, C.E. (1977) Nature 267, 462.

22. Woese, C., Sogin, M., Stahl, D., Lewis, B.J. and Bowen, L. (1976) J. Mol. Evol. 7, 197.
23. Barnes, W.M. (1978) Proc. Nat. Acad. Sci. USA 75, 4281-4285.
24. Di Nocera, P.P., Blasi, F., Di Lauro, R., Frunzio, R. and Bruni, C.B. (1978) Proc. Nat. Acad. Sci. USA 75, 4276-4280.
25. Gardner, J.F. (1979) Proc. Nat. Acad. Sci. USA 76, 1706-1710.
26. Gemmill, R.M., Wessler, S.R., Keller, E.B. and Calvo, J.M. (1979) Proc. Nat. Acad. Sci. USA 76, 4941-4945.
27. Zurawski, G., Brown, K., Killingly, D. and Yanofsky, C. (1978) Proc. Nat. Acad. Sci. USA 75, 4271-4275.
28. Zurawski, G., Elseviers, D., Stauffer, G.V. and Yanofsky, C. (1978) Proc. Nat. Acad. Sci. USA 75, 5988-5992.
29. Miller, J.H. (1974) Cell 1, 73-76.
30. Steitz, J.A. (1979) In Biological Regulation and Development, Vol. 1. Gene Expression. (R.F. Goldberger, ed.) pp. 349-399. Plenum Press, New York.
31. Borer, P.N., Dengler, B. and Tinoco, Jr., I., Uhlenbeck, O.C. (1974) J. Mol. Biol. 86, 843-853.
32. Tinoco, Jr., I., Borer, P.N., Dengler, B., Levine, M.D., Uhlenbeck, O.C., Crothers, D.M. and Gralla, J. (1973) Nature New Biology 246, 40-41.
33. Tai, P.-C., Wallace, B.J. and Davis, B.D. (1974) Biochemistry 13, 4653-4659.
34. Pestka, S. (1974) Antimicrob. Ag. Chemother. 5, 255-267.
35. Kubota, K., Okuyama, A. and Tanaka, N. (1972) BBRC 47, 1196-1202.
36. Mao, J.C.-H. and Robishaw, E.E. (1971) Biochemistry 10, 2054-2061.
37. Pestka, S. (1977) In Molecular Mechanisms of Protein Biosynthesis (H. Weissbach and S. Pestka, eds.) pp. 467-553, Academic Press, New York.
38. Mao, J.C.-H. and Robishaw, E.E. (1972) Biochemistry 11, 4864-4872.
39. Steitz, J.A. (1975) In RNA Phages (N.D. Zinder, ed.) pp. 319-352. Cold Spring Harbor Laboratory, Cold Spring Harbor, N.Y.
40. Cerná, J., Jonák, J. and Rychlík, I. (1971) Biochem. Biophys. Acta 240, 109-121.
41. Dennis, P.P. and Fiil, N.P. (1979) J. Biol. Chem. 254, 7540-7547.
42. Fiil, N.P., Friesen, J.D., Downing, W.L., Dennis, P.P. (1980) Cell 19, 837-844.
43. Ishihama, A., Fukuda, R., Kajitani, M. (1980) Molec. Gen. Genet. 179, 489-496.
44. Lemaire, G., Gold, L. and Yarus, M. (1978) J. Mol. Biol. 126, 73-90.
45. Fallon, A.M., Jinks, C.S., Strycharz, G.D. and Nomura, M. (1979) Proc. Nat. Acad. Sci. USA 76, 3411-3415.
46. Dean, D. and Nomura, M. (1980) Proc. Nat. Acad. Sci. USA 77, 3590-3594.
47. Yates, J.L. and Nomura, M. (1980) Cell 21, 517-522.
48. Yates, J.L., Arfsten, A.E. and Nomura, M. (1980) Proc. Nat. Acad. Sci. USA 77, 1837-1841.

CONTROL AND DNA STRUCTURE OF THE ampC β-LACTAMASE GENE OF

ESCHERICHIA COLI

Bengtåke Jaurin, Thomas Grundström, Sven Bergström and
Staffan Normark
Department of Microbiology
University of Umeå
S-901 87 Umeå, Sweden

INTRODUCTION

Escherichia coli K-12 is coding for a β-lactamase which
hydrolyzes the β-lactam ring of both cephalosporins and penicillins including ampicillin. Its structural gene, ampC, has been
mapped to 93.8 min on the E. coli chromosome (Burman et al., 1973;
Grundström et al., 1980). The level of ampC β-lactamase is stric -
ly proportional to the gene dosage, and to the ampicillin resistance (Normark et al., 1977). These features enabled us to directly select for ColE1 ampC hybrid clones within the collection of
ColE1 hybrids prepared by Clarke and Carbon (Clarke and Carbon,
1976; Edlund et al., 1979). One ColE1 ampC hybrid plasmid was
physically mapped and the location of ampC within this plasmid was
deduced by subcloning (Grundström et al., 1980). We could thereby
demonstrate that the ampC gene was present on a 1,370 bp DNA segment. By selecting for various degrees of ampicillin resistance
a number of E. coli mutants have been isolated that hyperproduce
the ampC β-lactamase due to mutations in ampA, a control sequence
region for ampC (Grundström et al., 1980).

In this paper we report the complete nucleotide sequence for the
ampC operon. We also show that ampA contains both a promotor and
an attenuator. Mutations in both types of control sequences may
cause elevated production of ampC β-lactamase. The relative
synthesis of ampC β-lactamase increases with growth rate (Jaurin
and Normark, 1979). We present data suggesting that the growth
rate dependent regulation of ampC is due to antitermination of
transcription at the ampC attenuator.

RESULTS AND DISCUSSION

Nucleotide sequence of the ampC gene

The entire ampC gene with flanking sequences was DNA sequenced using the procedure of Maxam and Gilbert (Fig. 1). To localize the beginning of the coding region for ampC, the order of the twelve N-terminal amino acids of purified ampC β-lactamase was determined by Edman degradation. A complete correspondence was found with the codons stretching from base +117 to base +152. The nearest translation start sequence appeared nineteen codons before the N-terminal amino acid, alanine, of the purified enzyme. This means that the primary translational product of ampC carries a nineteen amino acid long N-terminal extension. This extension has all the structural features of a signal peptide.

The ampC β-lactamase consists of 358 amino acids and has a molecular weight of 39,600. It is therefore considerably larger than previously sequenced β-lactamases (Ambler, 1979). The four previously sequenced β-lactamases all show a preference for substrates of the penicillin group and are therefore penicillinases, whereas the ampC β-lactamase is a cephalosporinase. The four sequenced penicillinases all show extensive sequence homologies with each other (Ambler, 1979). Short blocks of amino acid residues that show homology between the ampC β-lactamase and the consensus sequence of the four sequenced penicillinases are shown in Fig. 2. Outside the homologous amino acid blocks very little, if any, amino acid sequence homology is found between the ampC β-lactamase and the penicillinases. Only one β-lactamase apart from ampC has been sequenced on DNA level, namely the bla gene of pBR322 (Sutcliffe, 1978). Upon comparing the DNA sequence of these two genes, small sequence homologies were found even in regions outside the blocks coding for homologous amino acid residues. This may indicate that the bla and the ampC genes have evolved from a common ancester gene. An active site peptide fragment of the chromosomally encoded β-lactamase of Pseudomonas aeruginosa has recently been sequenced (S. G. Waley, personal communication). The deduced amino acid sequence showed a significant degree of homology with the region around serine 80 in the ampC β-lactamase. Clearly this suggests that serine 80 is the reactive residue at the active site. The ampC β-lactamase like all four sequenced penicillinases exhibit regions of amino acid sequence homology with some sequenced D-alanine carboxypeptidases (Fig. 2). As these latter groups of enzymes also contain a reactive serine in the active site (Yocum et al., 1979) we speculate that cephalosporinases, penicillinase, and D-alanine carboxypeptidases may have a common evolutionary origin.

The DNA sequences at positions -13 to -8 (-T-A-C-A-A-T-) and -35 to -30 (-T-T-G-T-C-A-) (Fig. 1) show a five out of six base-pair homology with the conserved -10 and -35 regions of promotors,

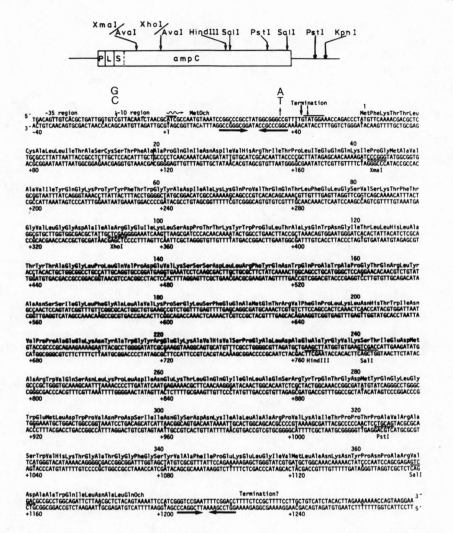

Figure 1. Upper part: Restriction enzyme map for enzymes that cut at most twice in the ampC region. The box displays the location of the ampC gene. P, L, and S indicate promotor region, leader region, and signal peptide, respectively. Lower part: DNA sequence of the ampC gene from Escherichia coli K-12. The three letter abbreviations for the amino acids of the ampC β-lactamase appear directly over their three-base codons and they are numbered (every 20th amino acid) starting from the first methionine. The positions of restriction enzyme sites are marked with a horizontal line between the strands, and the names of the enzymes are written below the strands. The start of transcription is marked by +1 and the wavy arrow. The major and minor termination points of the attenuator are (Continuation next page)

respectively (Siebenlist et al., 1980). By RNA sequencing it was possible to demonstrate that the adenine at position +1 is the first base of the β-lactamase mRNA. The β-lactamase leader-DNA is 59 basepair long. In this leader we find a nine basepair long, exclusively G-C containing, dyad symmetry at nucleotide positions

ampC β-lactamase	NH2 211 - AlaLeuAsp - 17 - GlnSerAsnLeuLysProLeu - 6 - LeuGlnGln - 36 - SerAspAsn - 41 - GluLysGluLeu - 27 COOH	
Penicillinases	17–22 - AlaLeuAsp (GluIle) - 17–18 - AlaSer* (Met) Thr-N-LysAlaLeu (ValIle) - 5 - LeuGlnGln (GluArg) (Ser) - 44–46 - SerAspAsn - 33 - GluProGluLeu (Ile) (Thr) - 109–124	
D-alanine carboxypeptidase	13 - LeuValAsp - 18 - AlaSer*MetThrLysMet - - -	

Figure 2: Regions showing amino acid sequence homologies between the ampC β-lactamase, four sequenced penicillinases (Ambler, 1979) and the sequenced N-terminal part of the D-alanine carboxypeptidase of *Bacillus stearothermophilus* (Yocum et al., 1979). The number of amino acids separating the blocks of homology and the termini of the proteins are given. Where the four penicillinases differ from each other, the stretches are indicated as intervals. Within the parenthesis are given the amino acid residues in the case where one of the penicillinases differ from the others. -N- means that four different amino acids are found at that position. Underlined amino acids represent homologous residues found in at least two of the three groups of proteins. The serine residues marked with stars have been shown to bind active site-directed substrate analogous for the D-alanine carboxypeptidase, and the β-lactamase I of *B. cereus*.

(Continuation Fig. 1)
indicated by vertical solid and dashed arrows, respectively. Solid horizontal lines designate possible ribosome binding sites. The regions of dyad symmetry in the attenuator and the possible operon terminator are marked by horizontal arrows. The boundary between the signal peptide and the mature β-lactamase is marked by a vertical dashed line. The -35 and -10 regions of the β-lactamase promotor are indicated. The ampP15G16 G-C insertion and the ampL35A A-T transversion are indicated.

+17 to +25 and +29 to +37. This symmetrical DNA sequence is followed by a stretch of four T residues on the non-coding strand. Thus,
this region has all the features of a terminator for transcription.
In vitro transcription studies have indeed revealed that about 94%
of all initiated transcripts are terminated with base +41 at their
3' end. Thus, the ampC gene was found to be controlled by attenuation of transcription.

The XhoI/KpnI DNA segment that carries most of the structural
gene ampC (Fig. 1) was ^{32}P-labelled by nick translation and used
as a DNA probe in Southern blotting experiments with restriction
endonuclease digests of chromosomal DNA from a number of enterobacterial genera (Fig. 3). The ampC probe hybridized to DNA fragments of the same size in strains of Escherichia coli, Shigella
sonnei, Shigella flexneri, Salmonella typhimurium, Serratia
marscesens and Klebsiella pneumoniae. Therefore, a region with
extensive sequence homologies to that of the ampC gene is present
in all tested members of the Enterobacteriacae. It therefore seems
likely that the chromosomal β-lactamases within these genera constitute a very related group of enzymes.

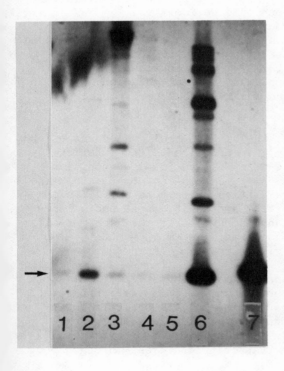

Figure 3: Hybridization of a
^{32}P-labelled XhoI/KpnI ampC
probe to XhoI/PvuII digests of
enteric DNAs. The XhoI/KpnI
ampC probe was 1060 bp large.
This fragment was 90 bp larger
than the XhoI/PvuII fragment.
Lane 1, S. typhimurium
lane 2, S. sonnei
lane 3, S. flexneri
lane 4, K. pneumoniae
lane 5, S. marscesens
lane 6, E. coli
lane 7, ampC probe.
The location of the ampC hybridization fragment is indicated
by the arrow.

Mutations leading to overproduction of the ampC β-lactamase

i) Promotor mutations
     The resistance of E. coli K-12 to ampicillin is 1 µg/ml. At
an incidence of about 10⁻¹⁰ mutants are found with a fifteenfold
increase in both resistance to β-lactam antibiotics and production of the ampC β-lactamase. One such mutant was isolated several
years ago and the mutated control sequence region was denoted ampA
(Eriksson-Grennberg, 1968). Plasmid derivatives carrying the mutation was isolated, and the ampA region was physically mapped, and
DNA sequenced. The mutation leading to a fifteenfold increase in
β-lactamase production was found to be a G-C insertion between
positions -16 and -15 in the ampC promotor (Fig. 1). This mutation
denoted ampP15G16 (previously ampA1), is an up-promotor mutation,
because in vitro transcription of an 1.5 kb SacII-XhoI DNA fragment carrying the mutation resulted in the increased synthesis of
both the short leader transcript and a long run off transcript.
The ampP15G16 mutation increases the distance between the conserved sequences of the ampC promotor. The mutation indicates that
the sterical arrangement between the two conserved regions is important for efficient initiation of transcription.

ii) Attenuator mutations
     From an E. coli K-12 strain carrying the up-promotor mutation
ampP15G16 spontaneous mutants with a further four to tenfold increase in β-lactamase production could be isolated.
These mutants fell into two groups with respect to genetic stability. The group of mutants unstable in a rec⁺ background was found
to carry multiple tandem repeats of the ampC region of the E.
coli chromosome (Edlund et al., 1979). The genetically stable mutants were each found to contain an additional mutation in the
same 370 bp DNA segment as where ampP15G16 had been mapped
(Grundström et al., 1980).

     The nucleotide sequence of the ampC control region was estab-
lished in one such double mutant. In addition to the mutation
ampP15G16 a transversion from C-G to A-T was found at position
+35. This amp leader mutation denoted ampL35A occurred within the
ampC attenuator. When a DNA fragment carrying both ampP15G16 and
ampL35A was transcribed in vitro no synthesis of the short leader
transcript was observed. Instead, the amount of the long run off
transcript was further increased. Thus, the ampL35A mutation abolishes the terminator located within the ampC leader.

     In a coupled in vitro transcription-translation system the
ampL35A mutation leads to a fourfold increase in the synthesis of
the ampC pre- β-lactamase. This corresponds to the fourfold increase in the steady state amount of β-lactamase found in vivo
at high growth rates. In the in vitro transcription system the
ampL35A mutation increased the transcriptional read-through about

sixteenfold (from about 6 per cent to virtually 100 per cent). This
suggests that in vivo, and in the coupled transcription-translation
system one or several factors decrease the degree of termination
at the wild type attenuator.

The relative amount of the ampC β-lactamase increases with
growth rate (Jaurin and Normark, 1979). The amount of a majority
of the more abundant E. coli proteins exhibit a similar positive
correlation with growth rate. This group of proteins includes ribosomal proteins, elongation factors, aminoacyl-tRNA-synthetases as
well as the subunits of the RNA polymerase (Pedersen et al., 1978).

The growth rate response of an E. coli strain carrying the
ampP15G16 promotor mutation was investigated. The specific amount
of ampC β-lactamase increased proportionally with growth rate as
in the wild type (Table 1). However, in an E. coli double mutant

Table 1. Relative amount of ampC β-lactamase produced in strains
LA51 and TE18 at different growth rates.

LA51[a]		TE18[a]	
k[b]	relative amount[c]	k[b]	relative amount[c]
0.33	1.00	0.26	8.90
0.47	1.25	0.33	8.83
0.95	1.87	0.50	8.65
1.39	2.47	0.97	8.73

[a] The E. coli K-12 strain LA51 carries the ampP15G16 up-promotor
mutation. Its derivative TE18 carries in addition the attenuator mutation ampL35A.

[b] Growth rates are expressed as k, the first-order constant,
in units of hour^{-1}, as calculated from the expression
$k = \ln2/\text{mass doubling time in hours}$.

[c] The relative amount of ampC β-lactamase produced is based on the
relative area obtained from rocket immunoelectrophoresis.

carrying both the ampP15G16 and the ampL35A mutations, the growth
rate dependent regulation was abolished. Thus, in this mutant, the
level of β-lactamase was constantly high. There was no change in
β-lactamase level within a threefold variation in growth rate
(Table 1). This suggested that a functional attenuator is required for growth rate dependent regulation. Attenuators have been
found within the leader DNA of a number of amino acid biosynthetic
operons, e.g. the trp operon (Crawford and Stauffer, 1980).

Unlike these operons, the 41 bases long ampC leader transcript has no coding region for a leader peptide. Moreover, the ampC leader RNA cannot form any alternative secondary structure that would preclude formation of the terminator stem. However, in the ampC leader RNA the first three bases are complementary to a sequence near the 3' end of 16S RNA. At bases 8 to 13 is an initiation codon (AUG) directly followed by an ochre stop codon (UAA). The amp leader RNA has therefore the potential to bind a ribosome

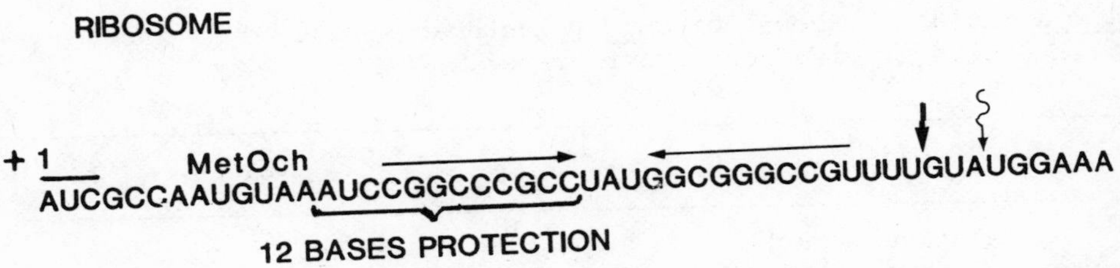

RIBOSOME

+1   MetOch

AUCGCCAAUGUAAAUCCGGCCCGCCUAUGGCGGGCCGUUUUGUAUGGAAA

12 BASES PROTECTION

Figure 4: A model for growth rate dependent attenuation of transcription. Hypothetical protection by the ribosome is thought to prevent formation of the termination stem, leading to read-through (see text for Discussion). The stippled area represents a ribosome. Start of transcription is marked by +1. The solid line designate a possible basepairing with the 3' end of 16S RNA. Met and Och stands for initiation codon (Methionine) and stop codon (Ochre), respectively. The termination stem is indicated by the horizontal arrows. The major and minor termination points of the attenuator are displayed by vertical solid and wavy arrows, respectively.

and form an initiation complex. If a ribosome binds to the nascent ampC leader it would preclude the formation of the terminator stem and loop structure and favour transcriptional read-through. The amount of ribosomes per cell mass increases with growth rate. Our current hypothesis is therefore that the concentration of ribosomes is the factor that regulates the degree of anti-termination at the ampC attenuator (Fig. 4).

We have studied the growth rate response of a number of clinical E. coli isolates that hyperproduces the ampC β-lactamase. The
response was abolished in one of the isolates but retained in the
remaining five isolates tested. This suggests that both promotor
and attenuator mutations may be selected for in the in vivo situation.

ACKNOWLEDGEMENTS

This work was supported by grants from the Swedish Natural
Science Research Council (Dnr 3373) and from the Swedish Medical
Research Council (Dnr 5428).

REFERENCES

Ambler, R. P. 1979. Amino acid sequences of β-lactamases, in:
     "Beta-Lactamase", J. M. T. Hamilton-Miller, J. T. Smith, eds.,
     Academic Press, London, pp. 99-125.
Burman, L. G., Park, J. T., Lindström, E. B., and Boman, H. G.
     1973. Resistance of Escherichia coli to penicillins. X. Iden-
     tification of the structural gene for the chromosomal peni-
     cillinase. J. Bacteriol. 116: 123-130.
Clarke, L., and Carbon, J. 1976. A colony bank containing synthe-
     tic ColEl hybrid plasmids representative of the entire E.
     coli genome. Cell 9: 91-99.
Crawford, J. P., and Stauffer, G. V. 1980. Regulation of trypto-
     phan biosynthesis. Ann. Rev. Biochem. 49: 163-195.
Edlund, T., Grundström, T., and Normark, S. 1979. Isolation and
     characterization of DNA repetitions carrying the chromosomal
     β-lactamase gene of Escherichia coli K-12. Molec. Gen. Genet.
     173: 115-125.
Eriksson-Grennberg, K. G. 1968. Resistance of Escherichia coli to
     penicillins. II. An improved mapping of the ampA gene. Genet.
     Res. 12: 147-156.
Grundström, T., Jaurin, B., Edlund, T., and Normark, S. 1980.
     Physical mapping and expression of hybrid plasmids carrying
     chromosomal β-lactamase genes of Escherichia coli K-12.
     J. Bacteriol. 143: 1127-1134.
Jaurin, B., and Normark, S. 1979. In vivo regulation of chromoso-
     mal β-lactamase in Escherichia coli. J. Bacteriol. 138: 896-
     902.
Normark, S., Edlund, T., Grundström, T., Bergström, S., and
     Wolf-Watz, H. 1977. Escherichia coli K-12 mutants hyperpro-
     ducing chromosomal β-lactamase by gene repetitions. J.
     Bacteriol. 132: 912-922.
Pedersen, S., Block, P. L., Reeh, S., and Neidhardt, F. C. 1978.
     Patterns of protein synthesis in E. coli: a catalog of the
     amount of 140 individual proteins at different growth rates.
     Cell 14: 179-190.

Siebenlist, U., Simpson, R. B., and Gilbert, W. 1980. E. coli RNA
    polymerase interacts homologously with two different promotors.
    Cell 20: 269-281.
Sutcliffe, J. G. 1978. Nucleotide sequence of the ampicillin re-
    sistance gene of Escherichia coli plasmid pBR322. Proc. Natl.
    Acad. Sci. USA 75: 3737-3741.
Yocum, R. R., Waxman, D. J., Rasmussen, J. R., and Strominger,
    J. L. 1979. Mechanism of penicillin action: Penicillin and
    substrate bind covalently to the same active site serine in
    two bacterial D-alanine carboxypeptidase. Proc. Natl. Acad.
    Sci. USA 76: 2730-2734.

MECHANISMS OF PLASMID-DETERMINED

HEAVY METAL RESISTANCES

Simon Silver

Department of Biology
Washington University
St. Louis, Missouri 63130 U.S.A.

INTRODUCTION

Many plasmids of both Gram negative and Gram positive bacteria have genes determining resistances to a wide range of toxic inorganic cations and anions, including ions of mercury (and organomercurials), cadmium (in Gram positives only), arsenic, antimony, bismuth, chromium, silver and tellurium. Three years ago, we reviewed the available information on the physiological and biochemical bases of these resistances, as well as the genetic structures that govern them (Summers and Silver, 1978). Here I will try to summarize both the overall picture and newer findings.

MERCURY AND ORGANOMERCURIAL RESISTANCES

Plasmid-determined resistance to Hg^{2+} and to organomercurials occurs in both Staphylococcus aureus (Novick and Roth, 1968) and Escherichia coli (Smith, 1967). The frequency of Hg(II) resistance determinants among clinical isolates can be well over 50% (e.g. Nakahara et al., 1977a and b) and among the collection of over 800 plasmids introduced into E. coli K-12 in Drs. Datta and Hedges' laboratory, about 25% conferred Hg(II) resistance (Schottel et al., 1974). There are differences in frequencies of these resistances. Although Cd(II)-resistance is found with high frequency in S. aureus of both human and animal origin, Hg(II)-resistance is common in human hospital staph but rare or absent in non-hospital human and animal S. aureus (Lacey, 1980; Witte et al., 1980).

We have found a small number of resistance patterns for organomercurials among strains with plasmids: (a) In E. coli over

90% of the mercury-resistance plasmids confer resistance to the
organomercurials merbromin and fluorescein mercuric acetate (FMA)
but to no other tested organomercurial (Fig. 1). We called these
"narrow spectrum" mercurial-resistance plasmids (Weiss et al.,
1978b), since the other 4% "broad spectrum" plasmids additionally
conferred resistances to phenylmercuric acetate (PMA) and thimerosal. The plasmids in Pseudomonas aeruginosa also divided into
"narrow" and "broad" spectrum with regard to resistance to organomercurials (Clark et al., 1977); however, about 50% of the plasmids
tested fell into each class. Furthermore, the "narrow spectrum"
Pseudomonas plasmids also conferred resistance to p-hydroxymercuri-
benzoate (pHMB) and the "broad spectrum" Pseudomonas plasmids
showed still additional resistance to methylmercuric and ethyl-
mercuric compounds (Clark et al., 1977; Weiss et al., 1978b).
Only a single pattern has been found with S. aureus plasmids
(Weiss et al., 1977,1978b), but this pattern is different yet in

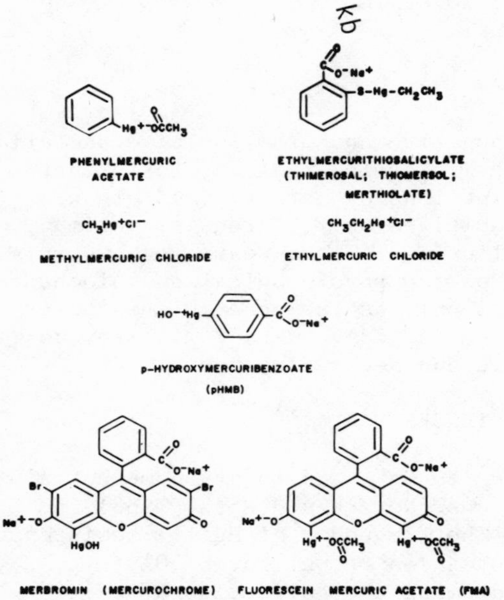

Fig. 1.   Structures of the
organomercurial compounds.

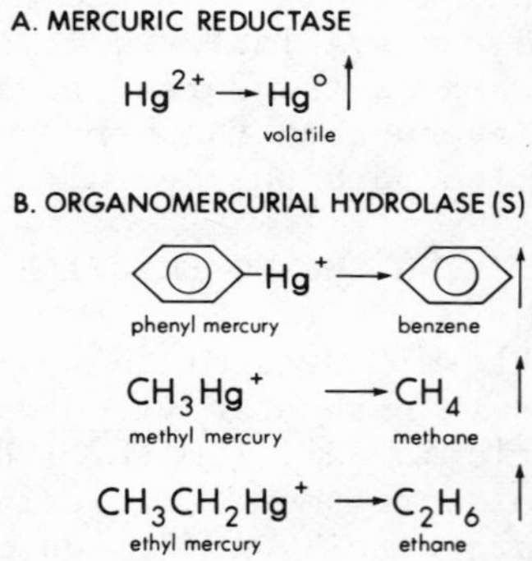

Fig. 2.   Enzymatic detoxification of Hg(II) and organomercurials.

that all the S. aureus plasmids conferred resistances to PMA,
pHMB and FMA but not to thimerosal or to merbromin. Recently,
Hg(II)-resistant plasmid-bearing Bacillus have become available
(Timoney et al., 1978; K. Izaki, in press; D. Reanney, personal
communication). These plasmids all conferred a pattern of resistance to Hg(II) and organomercurials identical to that in S.

aureus (T.G. Kinscherf, unpublished). Thus plasmids confer resistances to a range of organomercurials, and each type of organism
shows only a small number of resistance patterns. To a limited
extent these patterns can be correlated with plasmid incompatability groups (Schottel et al., 1974; Weiss et al., 1978b).

Enzymatic Mechanism of Mercury and Organomercurial Detoxification

Hg^{2+} resistance results from enzymatic detoxification leading
to the volatilization of mercury from the growing bacterial
culture. This was discovered independently in two laboratories
in Japan (Tonomura and Kanzaki, 1969; Furukawa and Tonomura,
1972; Komura et al., 1971; Izaki et al., 1974) and our own (Summers
and Silver, 1972). The volatile mercury was shown to be metallic
$Hg°$ in each case and the enzyme responsible is the mercuric
reductase enzyme.

Several organomercurials were also enzymatically detoxified
to volatile compounds. These include methylmercury, ethylmercury,
PMA, pHMB and thimerosal (Fig. 2); benzene is produced from PMA,
methane from methylmercury and ethane from ethylmercury, and
these have been identified by gas chromatography. The enzymes
responsible for cleaving the Hg-C bond are organomercurial lyases.
In a soil pseudomonad (for which a plasmid has never been demonstrated), Tezuka and Tonomura (1976,1978) were able to separate
two small soluble lyase enzymes. Both have molecular weights of
about 19,000 and require thiol reagents such as thioglycolate.
The two lyases were difficult to separate by chromatographic
methods, but when this was accomplished (Tezuka and Tonomura,
1978), it was found that one enzyme cleaved PMA, pHMB and methylmercury, while the other enzyme cleaved only PMA and pHMB. With
a plasmid-containing E. coli, there was no evidence for hydrolysis
of pHMB (Weiss et al., 1978b) and Schottel (1978) was unable to
separate the two lyases. Nevertheless, kinetic analysis indicated
that there were two enzymes active toward PMA but only one active
toward methyl-and ethylmercury. The E. coli organomercurial
lyases appeared to have a somewhat greater molecular weight, but
otherwise the general properties of the enzymes from the soil
pseudomonad and E. coli were rather similar.

Mercuric reductase has been studied in greater detail both
with plasmid-bearing E. coli (Izaki et al., 1974; Schottel, 1978)
and with the soil pseudomonad (Furukawa and Tonomura, 1972). The
intact enzyme has a molecular weight of about 180,000 and consists of three identical subunits (Schottel, 1978), each containing
an FAD molecule. The enzyme is strictly NADPH-dependent and one
NADPH is oxidized per Hg(II) reduced (Schottel, 1978).

Antibodies have been prepared against purified mercuric
reductases coded by two different plasmids in E. coli (Kinscherf,

in preparation). All reductases tested (obtained from different
Gram negative sources) reacted with these antibodies as shown by
inhibition of enzyme activity and formation of precipitin bands
on double-diffusion gels. The enzymes divided into two major
subclasses, based on only partial immunological identity. The
prototype enzyme of the first class is coded by transposon
Tn501, the first well-studied mercuric resistance transposon
(Bennett et al., 1978). This enzymological class also includes
mercuric reductases governed by a variety of plasmids found in
clinical isolates of enteric bacteria and P. aeruginosa, in
marine pseudomonads, and in Pseudomonas putida (the MER plasmid).
The MER plasmid harbors a transposon, Tn1861, which appears
indistinguishable (Friello and Chakrabarty, 1980) from Tn501
(Bennett et al., 1978) which originated in a clinical P. aeruginosa
isolate. That is one strong conclusion from studies of plasmid-
determined mercuric resistance: the same system appears widely
in clinical isolates and in bacteria from other environments.
The second immunological subgroup of the Gram negative mercuric
reductases has as its prototype the enzyme coded by plasmid R100,
one of the earliest and most thoroughly studied of the antibiotic
resistance plasmids. It is with this plasmid that the genetic
structure of the mercuric resistance operon was recently studied
(Foster et al., 1979; Nakahara et al., 1979). This subgroup also
includes enzymes from plasmids of a wide variety of incompatability
groups and also the enzyme determined by a second characterized
Pseudomonas mercury transposon, Tn502 (Kinscherf, in preparation;
Stanisich, in preparation). Although all of the mercuric reductases from Gram negative bacteria were immunologically related,
the antibodies prepared against the two classes of Gram negative
enzymes did not cross react with mercuric reductases from S.
aureus strains and marine and soil Bacilli. These enzymes from
Gram positive sources showed similar masses and functional requirements to those from E. coli (Weiss et al., 1977), but they are
immunologically distinct from the Gram negative enzymes.

     To summarize briefly the current understanding of plasmid-
determined mercuric and organomercurial resistances: (a) These
occur widely in both Gram positive and Gram negative species and
are the best understood of all plasmid-coded heavy metal resistances. (b) Resistance is due to enzymatic detoxification of the
mercurials to volatile compounds of lesser toxicity that escape
from the growth media. (c) The enzymes responsible (mercuric
reductases and organomercurial lyases) have been purified and
studied in vitro.

CADMIUM RESISTANCE IN S. AUREUS

     Plasmid-determined cadmium resistance has been found only in
S. aureus (Novick and Roth, 1968). In some clinical collections,
Cd(II) resistance is the most common of the S. aureus plasmid

resistances, exceeding in frequency both mercury and penicillin
resistances (Nakahara et al., 1977a). Gram negative cells without
plasmids are just as resistant to Cd(II) as are staph cells with
plasmids (Nakahara et al., 1977b), probably because of relatively
reduced Cd(II) uptake by the cells (Silver, unpublished).

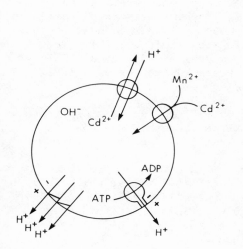

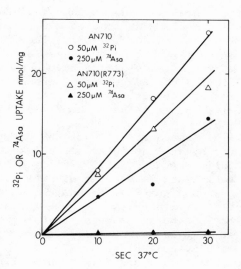

Fig. 3. Model for Cd^{2+} uptake
and efflux systems (from Tynecka
et al., 1981).

Fig. 4. Arsenate and phosphate
uptake by sensitive and resistant E. coli (from Silver et al.,
1981).

        The mechanism of Cd(II) resistance is a constitutive block
on the accumulation of Cd(II) by the resistant cells (Chopra,
1970, 1975; Tynecka et al., 1975). This was initially considered
a direct permeability block (Chopra, 1975), but it was later
found that Cd(II) enters S. aureus cells as an alternative substrate for the cellular Mn(II) transport system (Weiss et al.,
1978a; Silver, 1978). Resistance prevented Cd(II) accumulation
through this transport system. Most recently, it has been shown
that the lowered accumulation is due to a plasmid-coded efflux
system that rapidly excretes Cd(II) rather than a direct effect
on the uptake process itself (Tynecka et al., 1981). Fig. 3
shows the current model of Cd(II) resistance including the shared
Mn(II)/Cd(II) uptake system found in both sensitive and in resistant S. aureus cells and the Cd(II)/H$^+$ exchange system that
functions only in resistant cells (Tynecka et al., 1981). Studies
with membrane vesicles (R.D. Perry, in preparation) support this
picture by showing identical kinetic parameters for Cd(II) and
Mn(II) transport in right-side out vesicles from sensitive and
from resistant cells. Unfortunately, the type of inside-out

vesicle studies used by McMurry et al. (1980) to demonstrate a
similar efflux transport system for tetracycline in plasmid
containing E. coli have not succeeded in S. aureus.

ARSENATE, ARSENITE AND ANTIMONY(III) RESISTANCES

Arsenic and antimony resistances are governed by the same S.
aureus plasmids that code for other heavy metal resistances
(Novick and Roth, 1968). The first arsenic-resistance plasmid in
E. coli was found by Hedges and Baumberg (1973) and more recently
many similar plasmids have been isolated (Smith, 1978). The
first detailed report of arsenate, arsenite and antimony(III)
resistances is, however, still in press (Silver et al., 1981). I
will summarize here the basic findings of that paper.

Arsenate, arsenite and antimony(III) resistances are coded
for by an inducible operon-like system in both S. aureus and E.
coli (Silver et al., 1981). All three ions induce all three
resistances. Genetic studies with S. aureus plasmids demonstrate
that the gene for arsenate resistance is different from but
closely linked to the gene for arsenite resistance, which in turn
may not be the same as that for antimony(III) resistance (Novick
et al., 1979). Bi(III) is a gratuitous inducer of this system
with E. coli plasmid R773, which does not confer Bi(III) resistance (Leahy and Silver, unpublished).

The mechanism of arsenate resistance is a reduced accumulation
of arsenate by induced resistant cells. Arsenate is normally
accumulated via the cellular phosphate transport systems, of
which bacterial cells appear to have two (Silver, 1978). Phosphate
protects cells from arsenate toxicity, just as high Mn(II) protects
sensitive S. aureus from Cd(II) toxicity (R.D. Perry, unpublished).
The separateness of arsenate and arsenite resistances was shown
by the finding that phosphate did not protect against arsenite
(Silver et al., 1981). The presence of the resistance plasmid
does not alter the kinetic parameters of the cellular phosphate
transport systems, not even the K_i for arsenate as a competitive
inhibitor of phosphate transport. This finding, coupled with
direct evidence for plasmid-governed efflux of arsenate, suggests
that the arsenate resistance system will be an efflux transport
system (Silver et al., 1981), similar to that described above for
Cd(II).

We do not know the mechanism(s) of arsenite or of antimony
resistances. Arsenicals and antimonial compounds are toxic by
virtue of inhibiting thiol-containing enzymes (e.g. Albert,
1973). Some dithiol reagents such as BAL (British anti-Lewisite)
protect against arsenicals and antimonials. We have experimentally eliminated two possible hypotheses for arsenite and antimony
resistances proposed in our earlier review (Summers and Silver,

1978). Arsenite is <u>not</u> oxidized to the less toxic arsenate by
plasmid-bearing <u>E</u>. <u>coli</u> or <u>S</u>. <u>aureus</u> (Silver et al., 1981).
Growing resistant cells do <u>not</u> excrete soluble thiol compounds
into the medium to bind arsenite and antimony, since pre-growth
of resistant cells in medium containing these toxic ions does not
allow subsequent growth of sensitive or of uninduced resistant
cells (Silver et al., 1981). We are left only with untested
hypotheses of an alteration in uptake or a change in a key intracellular target.

SILVER RESISTANCE

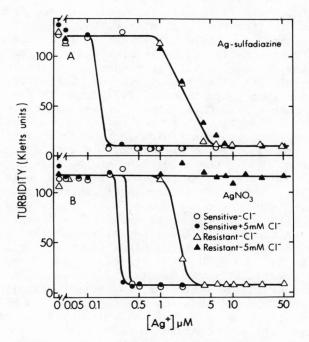

Fig. 5. Resistance of <u>E</u>. <u>coli</u> strains J62 (sensitive) or J62
(pSC35) (resistant) to Ag sulfadiazine and $AgNO_3$ in low and high
Cl^- (Silver and Leahy, unpublished).

Silver-resistance plasmids are among the more recent discov-
eries of the heavy metal resistance plasmids (McHugh et al.,
1975; Annear et al., 1976; Summers et al., 1978; Bridges et al.,
1979). These resistance plasmids have been found (not surprisingly) following the widespread use of silver salts as topical
treatments for extensive burns (e.g. Fox, 1968). Only one known
Ag^+ resistance plasmid was transferrable by conjugation (McHugh
et al., 1975). However, R.W. Hedges (personal communication)

produced a recombinant between plasmid R1 and a Ag^+ resistance
plasmid from <u>Citrobacter</u> (Hendry and Stewart, 1979) and introduced
it into an <u>E. coli</u> K-12 strain. We have been studying it for
much of the last year, since Hedges insisted that "Silver must
not ignore silver-resistance," and can report here some progress
and a somewhat supported hypothesis for the mechanism of Ag^+-
resistance. Silver resistance is constitutive in <u>E. coli</u>, like
Cd(II) resistance in <u>S. aureus</u>, but unlike Hg(II), arsenate-,
arsenite-, and antimony-resistances. The plasmid-determined
resistance is very great and the ratio of minimum-inhibitory
concentrations can be greater than 1000:1 (Fig. 5B). The level
of resistance is strongly dependent upon available halide ions;
and without Cl^-, there is relatively little difference between
the cells with or without a plasmid (Fig. 5B). Br^- and I^- at
concentrations far below those required for Cl^- confer resistances
on both plasmid-less cells and cells with the plasmid. These
results have led to our current hypothesis that both sensitive
and resistant cells bind Ag^+ tightly and are killed by effects on
cell respiration (Bragg and Rainnie, 1974) and other cell surface
functions (Rosenkranz and Carr, 1972; Fox and Modak, 1974). Once
bound extracellularly, Ag^+ enters the cells and is found in high
speed centrifugal supernatant fluids (unpublished data). Ag^+
precipitates with Cl^-, as the solubility product for AgCl is only
1.6×10^{-10} M at 25°C (and those for AgBr and AgI are significantly
lower yet). The hypothesis is that the sensitive cells bind Ag^+
so tightly that they extract it from AgCl, whereas the cells with
the resistance plasmid do not compete successfully with
Ag-halide precipitates for Ag^+. Because topically applied $AgNO_3$
ointments caused tissue chloride loss, silver sulfadiazine has
significantly replaced $AgNO_3$ in clinical practice (Fox, 1968).
As seen in Fig. 5A, the $AgNO_3$-resistance plasmid confers resistance as well towards silver sulfadiazine. However, added Cl^-
was without effect on the inhibitory concentrations of silver
sulfadiazine. This result was expected, since it is known that
adding NaCl to solutions of silver sulfadiazine does not cause
AgCl precipitates to form. Although many Ag^+-resistant clinical
isolates have determinants of sulfadiazine resistance as well,
these determinants can be on separate plasmids (Hedges, personal
communication). The function of sulfadiazine in topical preparations is not to inhibit bacterial growth directly (the concentrations released are too low; Fox, 1968), but rather to bind silver
in a form subject to slow release.

OTHER HEAVY METAL RESISTANCES

There are many other plasmid heavy metal resistances (Summers
et al., 1978; Summers and Silver, 1978). Yet, we know nothing
today about the mechanisms of resistances to bismuth, boron,
cobalt, nickel, tellurium or zinc ions. Chromate resistance in a
pseudomonad isolated from river sediment seems to be due to

reduction of toxic Cr(VI) to less toxic Cr(III) (Bopp and Ehrlich, Abstract Q111, 1980 A.S.M. Meetings) and this resistance appears to be plasmid determined (Chakrabarty, personal communication). However, caution on this point is needed, since bacteria capable of oxidizing toxic As(III) to less toxic As(V) are also known, but this turned out not to be the mechanism of plasmid-governed resistance (Silver et al., 1981). Hopefully, at future plasmid symposia our understanding of the mechanisms of these heavy metal resistances will be beyond the space limits of such a brief review. We need to start asking why these resistances occur at high frequencies in clinical isolates that have experienced no apparent selection with mercurials, arsenicals, antimonials etc.

ACKNOWLEDGMENTS

Recent work in our laboratory on these topics has been supported by grants from the National Science foundation PCM79-03986 and the National Institutes of Health AI15672.

REFERENCES

Albert, A. 1973. pp. 392-397, in: "Selective Toxicity, Fifth Edition," Chapman and Hall, London.

Annear, D.I., B.J. Mee, and M. Bailey. 1976. J. Clin. Path. 29: 441-443.

Bennett, P.M., J. Grinsted, C.L. Choi, and M.H. Richmond. 1978. Mol. Gen. Genet. 159: 101-106.

Bragg, P.D., and D.J. Rainnie. 1974. Canad. J. Microbiol. 20: 883-889.

Bridges, K., A. Kidson, E.J.L. Lowbury, and M.D. Wilkins. 1979. Brit. Med. J. 1: 446-449.

Chopra, I. 1970. J. Gen. Microbiol. 63: 265-267.

Chopra, I. 1975. Antimicrob. Agents Chemother. 7: 8-14.

Clark, D.L., A.A. Weiss, and S. Silver. 1977. J. Bacteriol. 132: 186-196.

Foster, T.J., H. Nakahara, A.A. Weiss, and S. Silver. 1979. J. Bacteriol. 140: 167-181.

Fox, C.L., Jr. 1968. Arch. Surg. 96: 184-188.

Fox, C.L., Jr., and S.M. Modak. 1974. Antimicrob. Agents Chemother. 5: 582-588.

Friello, D.A., and A.M. Chakrabarty. 1980. pp. 249-259, in: "Plasmids and Transposons: Environmental Effects and Maintenance Mechanisms," C. Suttard, and K.R. Rozee, eds., Academic Press, New York.

Furukawa, K., T. Suzuki, and K. Tonomura. 1969. Agric. Biol. Chem. 33: 128-130.

Furukawa, K., and K. Tonomura. 1971. Agric. Biol. Chem. 35: 604-610.

Furukawa, K., and K. Tonomura. 1972. Agric. Biol. Chem. 36: 217-226.

Hedges, R.W., and S. Baumberg. 1973. J. Bacteriol. 115: 459–460.

Hendry, A.T., and I.O. Stewart. 1979. Canad. J. Microbiol. 25: 915–921.

Izaki, K., Y. Tashiro, and T. Funaba. 1974. J. Biochem. 75: 591–599.

Komura, I., T. Funaba, and K. Izaki. 1971. J. Biochem. 70: 895–901.

Lacey, R.W. 1980. J. Gen. Microbiol. 119: 437–442.

McHugh, G.L., R.C. Moellering, C.C. Hopkins, and M.N. Swartz. 1975. Lancet 1: 235–240.

McMurry, L., R.E. Petrucci, Jr., and S.B. Levy. 1980. Proc. Natl. Acad. Sci. U.S.A. 77: 3974–3977.

Nakahara, H., T. Ishikawa, Y. Sarai, and I. Kondo. 1977a. Zentralbl. Bakteriol. Parasitenkd. Infektionkr. Hyg. 1 Abt. Orig. A. 237: 470–476.

Nakahara, H., T. Ishikawa, Y. Sarai, I. Kondo, H. Kozukue, and S. Silver. 1977b. Appl. Envir. Microbiol. 33: 975–976.

Nakahara, H., S. Silver, T. Miki, and R.H. Rownd. 1979. J. Bacteriol. 140: 161–166.

Novick, R.P., E. Murphy, T.J. Gryczan, E. Baron, and I. Edelman. 1979. Plasmid 2: 109–129.

Novick, R.P., and C. Roth. 1968. J. Bacteriol. 95: 1335–1342.

Rosenkranz, H.S., and H.S. Carr. Antimicrob. Agents Chemother. 2: 367–372.

Schottel, J.L. 1978. J. Biol. Chem. 253: 4341–4349.

Schottel, J., A. Mandal, D. Clark, S. Silver, and R.W. Hedges. 1974. Nature 251: 335–337.

Silver, S. 1978. p. 221–324, in: "Bacterial Transport," B.P. Rosen, ed., Marcel Dekker Inc., New York.

Silver, S., K. Budd, K.M. Leahy, W.V. Shaw, D. Hammond, R.P. Novick, G.R. Willsky, M.H. Malamy, and H. Rosenberg. 1981. J. Bacteriol., in press.

Smith, D.H. 1967. Science 156: 1114–1116.

Smith, H.W. 1978. J. Gen. Microbiol. 109: 49–56.

Summers, A.O., G.A. Jacoby, M.N. Swartz, G. McHugh, and L. Sutton. 1978. pp. 128–131, in: "Microbiology 1978," D. Schlessinger, ed., American Society for Microbiology, Washington, D.C.

Summers, A.O., and S. Silver. 1972. J. Bacteriol. 112: 1128–1236.

Summers, A.O., and S. Silver. 1978. Annu. Rev. Microbiol. 32: 637–672.

Tezuka, T., and K. Tonomura. 1976. J. Biochem. 80: 79–87.

Tezuka, T., and K. Tonomura. 1978. J. Bacteriol. 135: 138–143.

Timoney, J.F., J. Port, J. Giles, and J. Spanier. 1978. Appl. Environ. Microbiol. 36: 465–472.

Tonomura, K., and F. Kanzaki. 1969. Biochim. Biophys. Acta 184: 227–229.

Tynecka, Z., Z. Goś and J. Zajac. 1981. J. Bacteriol., in press.

Tynecka, Z., J. Zając, and Z. Goś. 1975. Acta Microbiol. Pol. 7: 11–20.

Weiss, A.A., S.D. Murphy, and S. Silver. 1977. J. Bacteriol. 132: 197-208.

Weiss, A.A., S. Silver, and T.G. Kinscherf. 1978a. Antimicrob. Agents Chemother. 14: 856-865.

Weiss, A.A., J.L. Schottel, D.L. Clark, R.G. Beller, and S. Silver. 1978b. p. 121-124, in: "Microbiology-1978," D. Schlessinger, ed., American Society for Microbiology, Washington, D.C.

Witte, W., N. Van Dip, and R. Hummel. 1980. Z. Allg. Mikrobiol. 20: 517-521.

CONJUGATION AND RESISTANCE TRANSFER IN STREPTOCOCCI
AND OTHER GRAM POSITIVE SPECIES: PLASMIDS, SEX PHEROMONES
AND "CONJUGATIVE TRANSPOSONS" (A REVIEW)

Don B. Clewell

Depts. of Oral Biology and Microbiology
Schools of Dentistry and Medicine
    and The Dental Research Institute
The University of Michigan
Ann Arbor, MI 48109

Until recently, information on the nature of conjugation and
related gene transfer in Gram positive bacteria has been relatively
scarce. Although conjugation among the actinomycetes has been known
for many years,[1,2] fertility plasmids have, so far, been recognized
in only a single strain of a single species in this group. Streptomyces coelicolor strain A3(2) harbors two conjugative plasmids, SCP1
and SCP2[3-5]; and whereas SCP2 has been isolated and characterized[5,6],
efforts to isolate SCP1 have been unsuccessful. The latter determines the synthesis of the antibiotic methylenomycin[7] and, when
integrated into the bacterial chromosome, will mobilize chromosomal
segments to SCP1$^-$ strains with almost 100 percent efficiency[8].

It has been only eight years since the phenomenon of plasmid
transfer in Gram positive eubacteria was first described[9], and conjugative plasmids have now been identified in a number of species of
streptococci, as well as in Clostridium perfringens (Table 1). A
report as early as 1964[10] had claimed a high frequency of transfer
(2.2 per donor) for a chloramphenicol resistance mutation (presumably
on the chromosome) in Streptococcus faecalis. There was no evidence
for plasmid involvement, and such a high frequency of chromosomal
transfer has not been confirmed. It was not until nine years later
that conjugal transfer was again reported--again in S. faecalis.
Tomura et al.[11] reported on the transfer of a hemolysin-bacteriocin
determinant at relatively high frequency (up to 5.8 x 10^{-2} per
donor). While direct evidence for a plasmid bearing this property
was not provided, it is likely that this was the case. [Hemolysin-
bacteriocin activity was subsequently shown to be plasmid-borne in a
number of other hemolytic (bacteriocinogenic) strains of S.

191

faecalis[12-16].. Interestingly, these two activities appear to represent one and the same protein[17,18].] About the same time, Jacob and Hobbs[9] presented evidence for conjugal transfer of multiple drug resistance from S. faecalis strain JH1 and were the first to show the direct involvement of plasmid DNA. Strain JH1 actually harbored two conjugative plasmids, a 50 Mdal R-plasmid pJH1, and a 38 Mdal hemolysin-bacteriocin plasmid pJH2[9,13]. In both of the above reports[9,11], transfer occurred in broth in a matter of hours; transfer was DNase resistant, and evidence against transduction was provided. Thus, cell to cell contact seemed a requirement for transfer.

Additional evidence for conjugative plasmids in S. faecalis[12-16, 19-27] as well as in other streptococci[28-37], and even Clostridium perfringens[38, 39], soon followed (see Table 1); and it was shown that, like the case in Gram negative bacteria, nonconjugative plasmids[12, 16, 40] and even chromosomal markers[41,42] could also be mobilized.

Table 1. Gram Positive Species with Naturally
Occurring Conjugative Plasmids

Bacteria	References
Actinomycetes	
Streptomyces coelicolor	3-5
Eubacteria	
Streptococcus faecalis (Group D)	9, 12-16, 19-27
Streptococcus pyogenes (Group A)	28-30
Streptococcus agalactiae (Group B)	31-34
Streptococcus lactis (Group N)	35,36
Streptococcus sp. (Group C)	37
Streptococcus sp. (Group G)	37
Clostridium perfringens	38,39

Some attention has been focused recently on pAMβ1, a 17 Mdal conjugative plasmid determining erythromycin resistance. This resistance is representative of the so-called MLS phenotype (i.e., resistance to macrolides, lincosamides and streptogramin B). Originally identified in S. faecalis strain DS5[43], pAMβ1 has been shown to have a broad host range. Its transfer into different species of streptococci was first shown by LeBlanc and co-workers[44], and it now has been shown to establish in nine different species of streptococci[28, 31, 44, 45, 46]. In addition, it has been observed to transfer into Lactobacillus casei[46], Staphylococcus aureus[26, 47] and Bacillus subtilis (O. Landman, personal communication). Interestingly, in S. faecalis, the transferability of pAMβ1 is dramatically inhibited if pAMγ1 or pAD1 is also present in the donor strain; the latter two plasmids remain highly transmissible (Brown and Clewell, unpublished). It is also noteworthy that pAMβ1 has been useful in the construction of streptococcal cloning vehicles[48].

MLS-resistance plasmids resembling pAMβ1 in size (15–20 Mdal) have been identified in S. faecalis[25, 49, 49a], S. pyogenes[29, 30, 50], and S. agalactiae[31-34], as well as in Lancefield groups C and G[37]. One S. pyogenes plasmid, pAC1[30] was found to be more than 90 percent homologous with pAMβ1[51]. [A report[52] showing homology of MLS-resistance determinants in streptococci (including pneumococci) and staphylococci suggests that this determinant has a common origin in Gram positive bacteria.] Malke[28] recently showed that pAC1 (called pDC10535 by him) could be transferred from S. pyogenes to several other species including S. faecalis. In the same report, a rather comprehensive study showed that several MLS-resistance plasmids from different sources transfer (on filter membranes) between strains of streptococcal groups A, B, D and H. Other recent studies demonstrated transfer of drug resistance between strains of groups A, B and D[20, 26, 32], and several MLS-resistance plasmids identified in group B streptococci were transferrable to group B, D, F and H recipients[31]. R-plasmid transfer between S. pneumoniae and streptococcal groups A, B and D[26,52a] and between Staphyloccus aureus and groups A, B and D[26,47] has also been reported.

Conjugative systems recently described in group N streptococci[35, 36] involve transfer of the ability to metabolize lactose. Interestingly, variants which donate at high frequency and exhibited an unusual cell-aggregation phenotype were readily generated[35] (L. McKay, personal communication).

SEX PHEROMONES IN STREPTOCOCCUS FAECALIS

In Streptococcus faecalis there appear to be two basic types of conjugative plasmids. There are those such as pAD1, pOB1, pPD1, pJH2, pAMγ1, pAMγ2 and pAMγ3, which transfer at relatively high frequency (10^{-3} to 10^{-1} per donor) in broth[13, 19, 53, 54] (Yagi, Brown, and Clewell, unpublished); and there are those such as pAMγ1, pAC1, pIP501, and pSM15346, which transfer poorly in broth (usually less than 10^{-4}, and in most cases, less than 10^{-6} per donor), but which transfer well (10^{-4} to 10^{-2}) when the matings are carried out on filter membranes[28, 31] (Brown and Clewell, unpublished). The reason for these differences is now becoming clear. Those systems which

transfer well in broth, make use of sex pheromones to generate cell
to cell contact, whereas those that transfer poorly in broth do not.
As illustrated in Fig. 1, recipient strains have been found to excrete soluble, protease-sensitive, heat-stable substances which
induce donor cells to become adherent[19, 53, 54]. This induction
facilitates the formation of mating aggregates arising from random
collisions of these non-motile cells. Since cell-free filtrates of

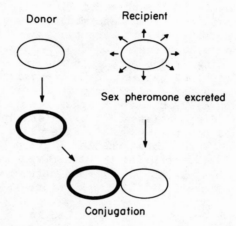

Fig. 1. Expression of sex pheromone by recipient and response by
         donor containing a conjugative plasmid (see text).

recipients also elicit an aggregation (clumping) response when mixed
with donors, this substance has been referred to as "clumping-inducir
agent" (CIA). When filtrates of recipients are mixed with donor
cells for 20-50 min prior to a short (10 min) mating with recipients,
the frequency of plasmid transfer is increased by several orders of
magnitude. CIA, therefore, can be viewed as a sex pheromone. The
response of donor cells to CIA requires both RNA and protein

synthesis, but not DNA synthesis[19]. The acquisition of a conjugative plasmid results in a "shutting off" of endogenous CIA production; and the cell with the newly acquired plasmid becomes responsive to exogenous CIA.

Interestingly, donors harboring different conjugative plasmids respond to different CIAs[53]. A given recipient actually produces multiple pheromones; and the acquisition of a given plasmid shuts off the production of only the related pheromone, while the cell continues to produce other pheromones which can induce other donors with different conjugative plasmids. The pheromones are now identified by relating them to the plasmid originally used to detect them. Thus, cPD1 refers to the CIA to which strains harboring pPD1 respond. Similarly, the other activities are identified as cAMγ1, cOB1, etc.

Studies have now shown that, in addition to an aggregation response, the pheromone induces a function(s) more directly related to plasmid transfer[55]. This was revealed by analyzing isogenic donor-donor matings using derivatives of pAD1 containing two distinguishable transposons (Tn916[42] and Tn917[56, 57]). It was reasoned that if the sole function of the pheromone (cAD1) was to induce aggregation, then once the cells aggregated, transfer should occur equally well in both directions--regardless of which donor was induced with cAD1 prior to mating. It was found, however, that when only one of the donors was induced, transfer occurred only in the direction from the induced to the uninduced strain. If both donors were induced, transfer occurred in both directions. Thus, the pheromone must also induce a "preparation" for plasmid transfer, the nature of which is not known. Conceivably, the pheromone induces a polycistronic operon [perhaps somewhat analogous to the Tra operon of certain conjugative plasmids in Gram negative bacteria (for reviews, see ref. 58, 59)] which, in addition to having determinants related to aggregation, also determines functions related to transfer.

Pheromone activity can be quantitated using a simple microtiter plate system[53]; the highest dilution of filtrate (using serial 2 fold dilutions) that still induces clumping in appropriate responder (donor) cells is taken to represent the pheromone titer. The titer for a given filtrate varies somewhat with the particular responder system; this depends on the conjugative plasmid as well as the host. (Titers typically range from 4-64.) In general, it would seem to be disadvantageous to produce "too much" sex pheromone, or for donors to be "too sensitive"; such behavior would result in donors becoming induced when they are "too far" away from recipients to make contact.

The production of pheromones by recipient cells was found to closely parallel cell growth[53]. In the case of certain plasmid-free strains such as JH2-2 or DR1, CIA activity in filtrates leveled

off as cells entered stationary phase. In the case of other strains
such as OG1 or ND539, both liquefaciens subspecies, activity in
filtrates rapidly disappeared as cells entered stationary phase. It
is likely that this decrease is due to degradation by the protease
("gelatinase") produced by these strains (i.e., the liquefaciens
subspecies). [A recently derived mutant of OG1, which fails to
degrade gelatin, produces CIA activity which does not decrease as
the cells enter stationary phase (Yagi, Craig and Clewell, unpublished).]

Recent data have shown that pheromone-induced donor cells have
a new antigen on their surface[60]. A highly specific rabbit antiserum prepared against induced pPD1-containing cells (the serum was
absorbed with uninduced cells) was found to readily cross-react with
different donors (induced) harboring several different conjugative
plasmids (pAD1, pOB1, pAMγ1, pAMγ2 and pAMγ3)[60]. The surface material has been referred to as aggregation substance (AS); and, being
sensitive to trypsin and pronase, it must be proteinaceous. When
submitted to specific immunological staining procedures involving
conjugated horse-radish peroxidase and analyzed by electron microscopy, an amorphous surface material (presumably representing AS)
could be visualized on the surface of induced, but not uninduced,
cells[60]. Pilus-like structures were not seen; however, the possibility that small, difficult to resolve microfimbriae may coat the
surface, remains.

AS probably binds to a specific substance, designated binding
substance (BS) located on the surface of both recipients and donors.
The interaction of AS and BS requires divalent cations and, interestingly, also phosphate ions[60].

Krogstad et al.[61] recently presented electron micrographs of
mating mixtures of S. faecalis, showing what appears to be inter-
cellular connections between chains of streptococci in the absence
of fimbriae or pili. (While the latter system represented a "high
frequency" transfer system, evidence for pheromone involvement was
lacking.) Similar "connections" have been observed in pheromone-
induced aggregates of cells harboring pPD1[62]; however, preparations
of uninduced cells also showed such connections. Thus, in this
case at least, it was not clear whether the observed "connections"
were an actual reflection of "conjugal contact", or an artifact of
the preparation.

The chemical nature of the pheromones is currently being
examined. Their sensitivity to proteases [including exopeptidases
(R. Craig, unpublished)], as well as heat stability and dialyz-
ability suggests that they are small peptides. [It was originally
reported that CIA was sensitive to trypsin[19]. However, subsequent
studies have shown that this was probably due to chymotrypsin

contamination. Purer preparations of trypsin fail to inactivate
cPD1, cAD1, cAMγ1, or cOB1, whereas chymotrypsin inactivates all of
these activities (Craig and Clewell, unpublished).] Analyses of
cPD1 on molecular sizing columns suggest a molecular weight of less
than 1000[54].

Examination of 100 clinical isolates of S. faecalis showed that
34 percent exhibit a CIA response to a filtrate of the plasmid-free
strain OG1-10, and 72 percent excreted cPD1[53]. Interestingly, the
ability to respond to, as well as produce CIA activities, was significantly more frequent among strains resistant to one or more
drugs as compared to drug sensitive strains[53]. Thus, pheromones
may contribute to the evolution of drug resistance in this species.
A recipient producing numerous sex pheromones would probably be a
prime "target" for R-plasmids which confer pheromone responses, or
which can be mobilized by such systems. [In the case of pAMγ1,
pAMγ2 and pAMγ3, it is worth noting that these plasmids, all having
nearly identical molecular weights and previously indistinguishable
from each other in their original host (S. faecalis strain
DS5[12, 43]), have each been shown to determine responses to different pheromones (Yagi, Brown, Craig and Clewell, unpublished).]

Whereas several of the above-mentioned pheromone-responding
plasmid systems (pAD1, pAMγ1, pOB1 and pJH2) determine hemolysin
(bacteriocin), this phenotype is not necessarily related to the
ability to respond. For example, pPD1, pAMγ2 and pAMγ3 do not determine hemolysin, but confer a pheromone response (Brown, Yagi and
Clewell, unpublished). [While it was believed earlier that pPD1
determined a hemolysin[53], this has recently been shown not to be
the case. We now know that in the original isolate (strain 39-5),
hemolysin is actually determined by a different conjugative plasmid,
pPD5, which has a similar molecular weight and which frequently
transfers together with pPD1 (Brown, Yagi and Clewell, unpublished).
pPD1, however, does determine a bacteriocin activity.] Also, of the
34 clinical isolates mentioned above which exhibited CIA responses,
only nine were hemolytic.

A model[53] has been proposed (Fig. 2) to explain the relationship between plasmids, pheromones, and the aggregation phenomenon.
The model schematically shows a plasmid-free recipient strain that
produces two different pheromones, cA and cB; two isogenic donor
strains harboring the conjugative plasmids pA or pB are also shown.
All three strains have the chromosomally determined binding substance (BS). Plasmid pA determines the ability to respond to cA;
and, at the same time, through an IcA (inhibitor of cA) gene, prevents production of endogenous cA. (Alternatively, an inactivation
of cA could be involved). Similarly, plasmid pB allows its host to
respond to cB and prevents the production of endogenous cB via gene
IcB. The response of the donor cell to the pheromone is depicted as

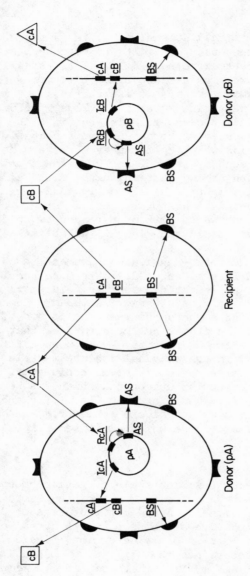

Fig. 2.   A model showing various donor and recipient relationships with respect to the synthesis of and response to sex pheromones.   cA and cB are the determinants of sex pheromones cA and cB. BS represents the determinant for binding substance (BS) which is located on the cell surface. IcA and IcB are determinants for substances which repress (or inactivate) endogenous cA or cB. RcA and RcB are determinants of regulatory proteins which respond respectively to cA or cB resulting in a "turning on" of the determinant AS which produces aggregation substance (AS) which locates itself on the cell surface. Once a donor has responded to a sex pheromone, AS can now bind to BS which is located on recipients and also donors. Taken from ref. 53.

an interaction (directly or indirectly) of the latter with "res-
ponding substance" (repressor or activator?) determined by gene
RcA or RcB, which in turn, activates AS synthesis. As, which could
be either plasmid (as shown in Fig. 2) or chromosonally determined,
locates itself on the cell surface where it can "recognize" BS.
(It is clear from the model how induced donors can self aggregate
as well as bind to recipients).

The fact that a single recipient strain of S. faecalis may
produce numerous sex pheromones specific for different donors seems
at first surprising, since it is possible that such cells have never
before encountered the "related" plasmids. Conceivably, the pheromones may have other functions in the recipient or represent degradation products of larger proteins. Plasmids might then have
evolved in such a way as to take advantage of such molecules to
facilitate their dissemination.

CONJUGAL TRANSFER IN THE ABSENCE OF PLASMIDS
(CONJUGATIVE TRANSPOSONS?)

When multiply resistant clinical isolates of S. pneumoniae
began to appear a few years ago[63, 64], efforts by several research
groups to reveal R-plasmids were unsuccessful[65-70] (Brown and
Clewell, unpublished). Recently, there have been reports showing
that resistance determinants in S. pneumoniae are capable of transfer to recipient strains on membrane filters by a DNase-resistant
process[69, 71]. Plasmid-free transfer has been observed in S.
faecalis[42, 72], in groups A, B F and G streptococci[73], and certain
oral streptococci[74] (D. LeBlanc, personal communication); and there
are indications that it may also occur in Clostridium difficile[75].

Shoemaker, Smith and Guild[71] reported that two plasmid-free
isolates of S. pneumoniae (BM6001 and N77) could transfer Tc- and
Cm-resistance determinants on membrane filters at a frequency of
10^{-6} per donor. Transfer was resistant to DNase; however, transfer
of an Em^r chromosomal mutation (ery-2) marker could be eliminated
by DNase. The two resistance markers cat and tet had earlier been
shown by transformation studies to be closely linked and were
shown both physically and genetically to represent insertions
(referred to as Ω cat tet) in the bacterial chromosome[67]. In
matings, about 90 percent co-transfer of cat and tet was observed;
however, while tet could transfer without cat, the reverse did not
occur[71]. Also, Cm^r, Tc^s derivatives could be generated by transformation, but they failed to donate cat by conjugation. It was
estimated that cat had a size of 4-6 kb, whereas tet was greater
than 30 kb[67].

Buu-hoi and Horodniceanu[69] reported that several plasmid-free

clinical isolates of S. pneumoniae could transfer resistance traits
not only into S. pneumoniae recipients (by filter mating), but also
to group B and group D strains. In some of these cases, transfer
occurred en bloc as: Tc^r and Cm^r; Tc^r and MLS^r; or Tc^r, Cm^r, MLS^r
and Km^r. Similar observations were made in clinical isolates of
Group A, B, F and G streptococci[73].

Franke and Clewell have reported that a transferrable Tc-
resistance determinant located on the chromosome of S. faecalis
strain DS16 is located on a 10 Mdal transposon[42, 72]. Designated
Tn916, this element was shown to insert at multiple sites into
several different conjugative plasmids at a frequency of about
10^{-6}. Transposition of Tn916 from the chromosome to the conjugative plasmid pAD1 is Rec-independent, as is its ability to transfer
in the absence of plasmid DNA (at a frequency of $\sim 10^{-8}$). (Transfer
of Tc-resistance was not reduced if either the donor or the recipient was Rec^-.) Transfer involved the entire transposon; after
introduction of a conjugative plasmid into transconjugants, typical
transposition to plasmid DNA could be detected. Transfer from a
plasmid-free donor required cell to cell contact; extensive efforts
to implicate transformation or transduction by a variety of means
were unsuccessful. [It is noteworthy that S. faecalis has never
been transformable (despite exhaustive efforts to obtain transformation), nor have transducing phages ever been reported in this
species.]

After transfer from the plasmid-free strain DS16C3, some
transconjugants have been found to retransfer Tn916 at an elevated
frequency ($\sim 10^{-6}$), about 100-fold higher than "normal"[76]. Interestingly, the transposition frequency from the chromosome to a
subsequently introduced pAD1 is also elevated about 100-fold in
such strains[76], suggesting a common step for both transfer and
transposition.

It has also been shown that after Tn916 transfer, insertion
can occur at different sites on the recipient chromosome[76]. This
was done in the following way. Insofar as Tn916 has a single
Hind III cleavage site, Hind III digests of chromosomal DNA containing Tn916 should give rise to two fragments, X and Y, which
constitute the transposon-host DNA junction fragments. With the
"Southern blot" hybridization technique, using an EcoR1 fragment
of pAD1::Tn916 (there are no EcoR1 sites in Tn916) as a probe,
hybridization with the two fragments (X and Y) readily occurs.
However, the size of the detectable X and Y fragments varies
greatly in chromosomal DNA preparations obtained from different
transconjugants (including those from secondary matings), a result
which would be expected if Tn916 were located at different sites
on the chromosome. (It is noteworthy that this result also is
strong evidence against the location of Tn916 on a plasmid which
had escaped physical detection.)

It is likely that Tn916 determines (at least in part), functions related to its own transfer; at a size of 10 Mdal there would seem to be room for such genetic information. Thus, transfer could simply represent an elaborate transposition event where the donor and recipient replicons are in different cells. A model generated from an earlier proposal[42, 72] is suggested in Fig. 3, where the transposon is shown to excise and then have the option to: i) re-insert onto the chromosome (perhaps at a different location); ii) insert onto a resident plasmid; or iii) transfer to another cell.

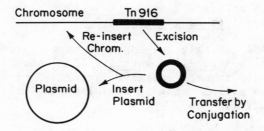

Fig. 3.   Model showing Tn916 as a "conjugative transposon" (see text).

After transfer into the recipient, insertion might be facilitated by "zygotic induction" of an "integrase" (the related transposase?). Since transfer probably occurs by a single strand (i.e., plasmid-like) process, a copy of the transposon would remain in the donor and might still be capable of reinserting into host DNA.

In view of the growing evidence in a number of species of streptococci for conjugal transfer in a plasmid-free environment, it will be interesting to see the extent to which these systems represent "conjugative transposons". In this regard, Guild's group (unpublished) has recently shown that Tn916 has homology with the transferrable tetracycline element that they have studied in S. pneumoniae[71].

CONCLUSIONS

While many aspects of conjugation in Gram positive bacteria appear similar to the more heavily studied Gram negatives, there are in certain cases characteristics which, so far, appear distinct. Clear evidence for sex pheromones in bacteria other than S. faecalis (Gram positive or Gram negative) has not yet been reported, although sex-related chemotactic factors in E. coli[77] and S. typhimurium[78] have been suggested. Pheromone-related behavior is well known, however, in yeast, fungi and higher organisms[79, 80]. "Conjugative transposons" are also yet to be reported in Gram negative bacteria; however, there are recent indications that such elements may indeed occur in Bacteroides fragilis[81, 82].

The use of recently developed cloning systems in Streptococcus sanguis[48, 83], and Bacillus subtilis[84, 85] should begin to simplify genetic analyses in Gram positive bacteria, and it is likely that rapid progress will be made in revealing the molecular bases of conjugal transfer.

REFERENCES

1. D. A. Hopwood, Ann. N.Y. Acad. Sci. 81:887 (1959).
2. D. A. Hopwood and M. J. Merrick, Bacteriol. Rev. 41:595 (1977).
3. A. Vivian, J. Gen. Microbiol. 69:353 (1971).
4. D. A. Hopwood, K. F. Chater, J. E. Dowding, and A. Vivian, Bacteriol. Rev. 37:371 (1973).
5. M. J. Bibb, R. F. Freeman, and D. A. Hopwood, Mol. Gen. Genet. 154:155 (1977).
6. H. Schrempf, H. Bujard, D. A. Hopwood, and W. Goebel, J. Bacteriol. 121:416 (1975).
7. L. F. Wright, and D. A. Hopwood, J. Gen. Microbiol. 95:96 (1976).
8. D. A. Hopwood, and H. M. Wright, in: "Second International Symposium on the Genetics of Industrial Microorganisms", K. D. MacDonald, ed., Academic Press, London, New York, and San Francisco (1976).
9. A. Jacob and S. J. Hobbs, J. Bacteriol. 117:360 (1974).
10. R. E. Raycroft and L. N. Zimmerman, J. Bacteriol. 87:799 (1964).
11. T. Tomura, T. Hirano, T. Ito, and M. Yoshioka, Jpn. J. Microbiol. 17:445 (1973).

12. G. Dunny and D. Clewell, J. Bacteriol. 124:784 (1975).
13. A. Jacob, G. I. Douglas and S. J. Hobbs, J. Bacteriol. 121: 863 (1975).
14. M. L. Frazier, and L. N. Zimmerman, J. Bacteriol. 130:1064 (1977).
15. D. Oliver, B. Brown and D. Clewell, J. Bacteriol. 130:948 (1977).
16. P. Tomich, F. An, S. Damle and D. Clewell, Antimicrob. Ag. Chemother. 15:828 (1979).
17. T. D. Brock, and J. M. Davie, J. Bacteriol. 86:708 (1963).
18. P. A. Granato and R. W. Jackson, J. Bacteriol. 100:865 (1969).
19. G. Dunny, B. Brown and D. Clewell, Proc. Nat. Acad. Sci. USA 75:3479 (1978).
20. J. van Embden, H. Engel, and B. van Klingeren, Antimicrob. Ag. Chemother. 11:925 (1977).
21. H. Marder and F. H. Kayser, Antimicrob. Ag. Chemother. 12:261 (1977).
22. P. Courvalin, C. Carlier and E. Collatz, J. Bacteriol. 143: 541 (1980).
23. D. Krogstad, T. R. Korfhagen, R. C. Moellering, Jr., C. Wennersten, and M. N. Swartz, J. Clin. Invest. 61:1645 (1978).
24. T. Horodniceanu, L. Bougueleret, N. El-Solh, G. Bieth, and F. Delbos, Antimicrob. Ag. Chemother. 16:686 (1979).
25. J. D. A. van Embden, N. Soedirman, and H. Engel, Lancet i: 655 (1978).
26. H. Engel, N. Soedirman, J. Rost, W. van Leeuwen and J. D. A. van Embden, J. Bacteriol. 142:407–413 (1980).
27. E. Romero, M. Perduca, and L. Pagani, Microbiologica 2:421 (1979).
28. H. Malke, FEMS Microbiol. Lett. 5:335 (1979).
29. D. Behnke, V. I. Golubkov, H. Malke, A. Boitsov, and A. Totolian, FEMS Microbiol. Lett. 6:5 (1979).
30. D. Clewell and A. Franke, Antimicrob. Ag. Chemother. 5:534 (1974).
31. V. Hershfield, Plasmid 2:137 (1979).
32. T. Horodniceanu, L. Boogueleret, N. El-Solh, D. Bouanchaud and Y. Chabbert, Plasmid 2:197 (1979).
33. T. Horodniceanu, D. Bouanchaud, G. Biet and Y. Chabbert, Antimicrob. Ag. Chemother 10:795 (1976).
34. N. El-Solh, D. H. Bouanchaud, T. Horodniceanu, A. F. Roussel, and Y. A. Chabbert, Antimicrob. Ag. Chemother. 14:19 (1978).
35. M. J. Gasson and F. L. Davies, J. Bacteriol. 143:1260 (1980).
36. L. L. McKay, K. A. Baldwin, and P. M. Walsh, Appl. Env. Microbiol. 40:84 (1980).
37. L. Bougueleret, G. Bieth, and T. Horodniceanu, J. Bacteriol., in press (1981).
38. G. Brefort, M. Magot, H. Ionesco, and M. Sebald, Plasmid 1:52 (1977).
39. J. I. Rood, V. N. Scott, and C. L. Duncan, Plasmid 1:563 (1978).

40. D. Oliver, B. Brown, and D. Clewell, J. Bacteriol. 130:759 (1977).

41. A. Franke, G. Dunny, B. Brown, F. An, D. Oliver, S. Damle, and D. Clewell, in: "Microbiology 1978", D. Schlessinger, ed., Am. Soc. Microbiol., Washington, D.C. (1978).

42. A. Franke and D. B. Clewell, J. Bacteriol. 145:494 (1981).

43. D. Clewell, Y. Yagi, G. Dunny and S. Schultz, J. Bacteriol. 117:283 (1974).

44. D. J. LeBlanc, R. J. Hawley, L. N. Lee, and E. J. St. Martin, Proc. Nat. Acad. Sci. USA 75:3484 (1978).

45. M. J. Gasson and F. L. Davies, FEMS Lett. 7:51 (1980).

46. E. M. Gibson, N. M. Chace, S. B. London, and J. London, J. Bacteriol. 137:614 (1979).

47. D. Schaberg, D. Clewell, L. Glatzer, This volume.

48. F. L. Macrina, K. R. Jones, and P. H. Wood, J. Bacteriol. 143: 1425 (1980).

49. P. M. Courvalin, C. Carlier, O. Croissant, and D. Blangy, Molec. Gen. Genet. 132:181 (1974).

49a. M. M. Corb and M. L. Murray, FEMS Microbiol. Lett. 1:351 (1977).

50. H. Malke, H. E. Jacob, and K. Storl, Molec. & Gen. Genetics 144:333 (1976).

51. Y. Yagi, A. Franke and D. Clewell, Antimicrob. Ag. Chemother. 7:871 (1975).

52. B. Weisblum, S. Holder and S. Halling, J. Bacteriol. 138:990 (1979).

52a. M. D. Smith, N. B. Shoemaker, V. Burdett, and W. R. Guild, Plasmid 3:70 (1980).

53. G. Dunny, R. Craig, R. Carron and D. Clewell, Plasmid 2:454 (1979).

54. D. Clewell, R. Craig, G. Dunny, R. Carron and B. Brown, in: "Plasmids and Transposons: Environmental Effects and Maintenance Mechanisms", C. Stuttard and K. R. Rozee, eds., Academic Press, Inc., N. Y. (1980).

55. D. Clewell and B. Brown, J. Bacteriol. 143:1063 (1980).

56. P. Tomich and D. Clewell, Cold Spr. Harb. Symp. Quant. Biol. 43:1217 (1978).

57. P. Tomich, F. An and D. Clewell, J. Bacteriol. 141:1366 (1980).

58. M. Achtman, and R. Skurray, in: "Microbial Interactions (Series B, Receptors and Recognition, Vol. 3)", J. L. Reissig, ed., Chapman and Hall, London (1977).

59. N. Willets and R. Skurray, Ann. Rev. Genet. 14:41 (1980).

60. Y. Yagi, R. Kessler, B. Brown, D. Lopatin and D. Clewell, This volume.

61. D. J. Krogstad, R. M. Smith, R. C. Moellering, Jr., and A. R. Parquette, J. Bacteriol. 141:963 (1980).

62. G. Dunny, Ph.D. Thesis, Univ. of Michigan (1978).

63. Center for Disease Control, Morbidity and Mortality Weekly Rep. 26:285 (1977).

64. M. Jacobs, H. Koornhof, R. Robins-Browne, C. Stevenson, I. Freiman, M. Miller, M. Witcomb, M. Isaacson, J. Ward and R. Austrian, N. Eng. J. Med. 299:735 (1978).

65. A. Dang-Van, G. Tiraby, J. Acar, W. Shaw, and D. Bouanchaud, Antimicrob. Ag. Chemother. 13:577 (1978).

66. R. M. Robins-Browne, M. Gaspar, J. Ward, I. Wachsmuth, H. Koornhof, M. Jacobs and C. Thornsberry, Antimicrob. Ag. Chemother. 15:470 (1979).

67. N. B. Shoemaker, M. D. Smith and W. R. Guild, J. Bacteriol. 139:432 (1979).

68. F. Young, and L. Mayer, Rev. of Infect. Dis. 1:55 (1979).

69. A. Buu-hoi, and T. Horodniceanu, J. Bacteriol. 143:313 (1980).

70. M. Smith and W. R. Guild, J. Bacteriol. 137:735 (1979).

71. N. Shoemaker, M. Smith and W. Guild, Plasmid 3:80 (1980).

72. A. Franke and D. Clewell, Cold Spr. Harb. Symp. Quant. Biol. 45: in press (1980).

73. T. Horodniceanu, L. Bougueleret, and G. Bieth, Plasmid, in press (1981).

74. D. LeBlanc, This volume.

75. C. J. Smith, S. M. Markowitz, and F. Macrina, submitted for publication.

76. C. Gawron-Burke, A. Franke and D. B. Clewell, This volume.

77. J. F. Collins and P. Broda, Nature 258:722 (1975).

78. M. Bezdek, and J. Soska, Folia Microbiol. 17:366 (1972).

79. T. R. Manney and J. H. Meade, in: "Microbial Interaction (Series B, Receptors and Recognition, Vol. 3)", J.L. Reissig, ed., Chapman and Hall, London (1977).

80. G. Kochert, Ann. Rev. Plant. Physiol. 29:461 (1978).

81. T. D. Mays, F. L. Macrina, R. A. Welch and C. J. Smith, This volume.

82. F. P. Tally, M. J. Shimell and M. H. Malamy, This volume.

83. D. Behnke and J. J. Ferretti, J. Bacteriol. 144:806 (1980).

84. P. S. Lovett and K. M. Keggins, Methods in Enzymology 68: 342 (1979).

85. D. Dubnau, T. Gryczan, S. Contente and A. G. Shivakumar, in: "Genetic Engineering", Vol. 2, J. K. Setlow and A. Hollander, eds., Plenum, New York (1980).

SITES AND SYSTEMS FOR CONJUGAL DNA TRANSFER IN BACTERIA

Neil Willetts

Department of Molecular Biology
University of Edinburgh
Edinburgh   EH9 3JR, Scotland

Plasmids isolated from Gram-negative bacteria can be divided into two major groups: large plasmids (>30 kb) that determine conjugation systems, and small plasmids (<10 kb) that do not. However, it was observed many years ago that a representative small non-conjugative plasmid, ColE1, was mobilised with high efficiency if the cell also contained an appropriate conjugative plasmid (Clowes, 1963), and more recent data for other non-conjugative plasmids suggests that this might generally be the case.   Indeed, ColE1 contributes not only an "origin of transfer" DNA sequence (oriT), but also mobilisation genes that are essential for its own transfer (Inselburg, 1977; Dougan and Sherratt, 1977). Interestingly, about one-third of the total plasmid DNA is devoted to conjugation, both for conjugative plasmids such as F, and for non-conjugative plasmids such as ColE1; this compares to the 5-10 fold smaller proportion required for autonomous replication.

The importance of conjugation to plasmids is underlined by the large percentage of them that encode conjugation systems, by the likelihood that even small non-conjugative plasmids frequently carry an oriT and perhaps mobilisation genes, and by the relatively large proportion of the plasmid DNA dedicated to this function. From an evolutionary point of view this importance is not surprising, since as a result plasmid genes are better able to survive.   Firstly, conjugation allows plasmids repeatedly to express their "phenotype" genes (which, as in the case of anti- biotic resistance, typically confer only a transient advantage) in different hosts in different environments.   Secondly, conjugation is essentially a replication process, and allows plasmid genes to replicate faster than host chromosomal genes.   This can give rise, for example, to "infectious spread" of a conjugative plasmid

through a bacterial population. ͺTransmissible non-conjugative
plasmids may have the additional advantages of exploiting several
types of conjugation systems (with the corollary of a wider host
range) and of their small size being compatible with a high copy
number.

    In this paper I shall discuss the requirements that must be
satisfied for a replicon to be transferred by conjugation, and
review the inter-relationships that have been observed between
different conjugation systems.

Conjugation systems determined by plasmids belonging to different incompatibility groups

    Most, if not all, conjugation systems so far studied are
physiologically similar, and two separate though connected
components can be recognised: mating pair formation with a
potential recipient cell, for which the plasmid-encoded extracellular pilus is essential, and conjugal DNA metabolism that
subsequently transfers and replicates the plasmid DNA from its oriT
site. For the purposes of this article, the first component will
be abbreviated to Mpf and the second to Dtr.

    Despite this overall similarity, numerous distinct and non-
interacting conjugation systems have been identified. The pilus
provides one important means of classifying conjugation systems,
since pili differ in their morphology and serology, in the
particular varieties of male-specific bacteriophages that they
adsorb, and in their abilities to allow conjugation in liquid,
as opposed to solid, medium (Table 1; Bradley, 1980; Bradley et al,
1980). A second method is to determine whether non-piliated
($Mpf^- Dtr^+ oriT^+$) mutants of one plasmid can be transferred by the
conjugation system of a second (Willetts, 1970 and unpublished
data). By these means, the conjugation systems of plasmids
falling into different incompatibility groups can be compared: the
data presently available suggest that plasmids with similar
conjugation systems belong either to a single incompatibility group

Table 1.   Pilus types

Plasmid group	Pilus morphology	Pilus diameter (nm)	Isometric RNA phage	Filamentous single-strand DNA phage	Lipid-cont. double-strand DNA phage
I	Flexible	6	–	If1	–
F	Flexible	9	f2, Qβ	f1	–
X	Flexible	9	–	–	–
P	Rigid	8	PRR1	Pf3	PR4
N	Rigid	9.5	–	Ike	PR4
W	Rigid	12	–	–	PR4

(as for IncN, P, W or X plasmids) or to one of a small collection of
incompatibility groups (as for the IncF or IncI "complexes"). Furthermore, the lack of complementation between different conjugation systems implies that recognition of a particular oriT sequence by a Dtr
system, and of a particular Dtr system by an Mpf system, are both
highly specific processes.

Because of the large proportion of plasmid DNA devoted to conjugation, plasmids with similar conjugation systems share a large proportion (40-80%) of DNA homology, while plasmids with different
systems do not (<10%). These percentages are for plasmids from the
six groups listed above (Falkow et al, 1974). The absence of DNA
homology itself provides an indication that the conjugation systems
determined by a particular pair of plasmids are likely to be dissimilar.

The F conjugation system

In the case of IncF plasmids, sufficient information is available to provide a substantial genetic and molecular basis for understanding the Mpf and Dtr components of the conjugation system. This
information has been reviewed recently by Willetts and Skurray (1980)
and will be briefly summarised here.

Approximately 33 kb of DNA is required to determine the F conjugation system, and about 20 conjugation genes have been identified
(Fig. 1). Those contributing to the Mpf system are traALEKBVWCUNFHG.
The pilin precursor protein is encoded by traA (Minkley et al, 1976),
and most of the other genes are required for the (unknown) pathway
whereby this is chemically modified and erected into the pilus structure. traG is needed not only for pilus synthesis, but also - together
with traN - for stabilisation of mating pairs. As might be expected,
the products of all these genes are located in the cell envelope.

Genes necessary for the Dtr system are traMYDIZ. Of these,
traYZ probably determine an endonuclease that reversibly nicks one
DNA strand at oriT - even in the absence of Mpf (Everett and
Willetts, 1980). In response to Mpf, the traMI products may
trigger Dtr by displacing the YZ endonuclease from the nicked

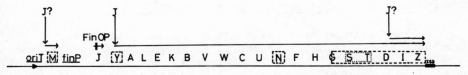

Fig. 1. A map of the F conjugation region. Letters above the line
indicate tra genes. Those not required for pilus formation are
boxed. The various tra operons and their regulatory systems are
indicated.

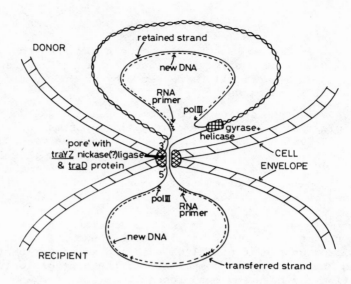

Fig. 2   A model for conjugation

form of the plasmid DNA and allowing the strand separation (to which
the traD product may contribute) required for initiation of DNA
transfer and synthesis from oriT.   Host proteins such as RNA polymerase, DNA polymerase III and gyrase play important roles in the
latter two processes.   The traZ and traI proteins, together with
the host proteins listed, are located in the cytoplasm, whereas the
traY and traM components of the nicking and triggering functions
and the traD protein are found in the cell envelope, where they
perhaps serve to connect the Mpf and Dtr systems, and to locate the
oriT sequence strategically at the inner cell surface.

A model for conjugation is illustrated in Fig. 2;   one
additional feature of this is that the 3' and 5' termini of the
transferred strand are both linked to a presumptive membrane-located
transfer complex.   This would account for the RNA primer requiremen
for donor conjugal DNA synthesis and for accurate and efficient
recA- and tra-independent recircularisation of the transferred stran
in the recipient cell.

Specificity of the Dtr systems of F-like plasmids

F-like plasmids synthesise morphologically and serologically
similar pili that adsorb (though with varying efficiencies) the
same male-specific phages, and their transfer regions are largely
homologous.   Indeed, all F-like plasmids tested (including R100-1,
R1-19, ColV2 and ColVBtrp) allow transfer (via complementation or
perhaps successful Mpf-Dtr interaction) of Mpf⁻ mutants of F.
However, F mutants in the Dtr genes traMYIZ are not always transferred by other F-like plasmids, indicating that there are differen

Table 2. Complementation of piliated Flac tra mutants

Flac mutation	Complementation (%) by	
	R1-19	R100-1
traM102	0.03	0.1
traY::EDλ4	0.60	1.5
traN548	82	48
traG42	50	61
traD38	73	76
traI41	58	1.0
traΔIZ337	41	3.0

Plasmids with complementation patterns similar to F itself
are ColV2, ColB2, ColVBtrp and R124; to R1-19 are R538-1
and ColB4; and to R100-1 are R6 and R136.

allelic forms of these genes.   Table 2 presents data to illustrate
this point, and lists the three groups into which F-like plasmids
can be arranged on this basis.   It is the paired traY and traM, and
traZ and traI, specificities that suggests that the traYZ endonuclease and the traMI triggering function both act at oriT, within
which there may be two domains.

An implication of these observations is that the oriT sequences
of the three groups of F-like plasmids differ from each other.   This
has been verified directly in one case, since pED806, a pBR322
derivative into which the F oriT (but no tra genes) has been cloned,
is efficiently transferred by Flac but not by an Ap^S R1-19 variant
or by R100-1.

Despite the differences between their Dtr systems, it should be
emphasized that the Mpf system of any F-like plasmid will serve to
transfer an Mpf⁻Dtr⁺ mutant of any other F-like plasmid, whereas this
is not the case for plasmids with unrelated conjugation systems.

Mobilisation of non-conjugative plasmids

Small naturally-occurring non-conjugative plasmids are often
transferred efficiently and specifically by one or more types of
conjugative plasmid (Table 3).   This may prove to be the general
rule for all non-conjugative plasmids once sufficient conjugation
systems have been tested to allow the appropriate one(s) to be
identified.   For example, although it has been known for some time
that IncI plasmids mobilise non-conjugative IncQ plasmids such as
RSF1010 with relatively low efficiency, we have recently found that
IncP plasmids mobilise RSF1010 with 100% efficiency in both E.coli
and P.aeruginosa (Willetts and Crowther, 1981).   Neither IncN nor
IncW plasmids, which like IncP plasmids determine rigid pili that
adsorb the male-specific phage PR4, mobilised RSF1010.   IncP

Table 3.   Mobilisation of non-conjugative plasmids

Conjugative plasmid	Group	Transfer (% of conjugative)				
		ColE1	CloDF13	ColE2	pSC101	RSF1010
R64-11	I	70		80	0.5	6
Flac	F	100	133	<0.01	10^{-5}	10^{-3}
R1-19	F	40	83	<0.01	10^{-3}	10^{-3}
R100-1	F	0.1	93			10^{-3}
R751	P	48			13	100
R388	W	1				10^{-2}

Data are taken from: Reeves and Willetts, 1974; Hardy, 1975; Warren et al, 1978, 1979; Willetts, 1980; and Willetts and Crowther, 1981.

plasmids were also fairly efficient at mobilising pSC101.

The efficiency, specificity and recA-independence of the mobilisation of non-conjugative plasmids indicate that these plasmids contain an oriT sequence from which conjugal transfer can be initiated. This sequence is probably similar to that at which the protein-DNA "relaxation complexes" of ColE1 and some (but not all) other small plasmids are nicked in response to ionic detergents or other stimuli (Clewell and Helinski, 1969). However, caution must be exercised in comparing conjugal DNA metabolism by F, which is relatively well understood, and by ColE1, which is not. Some of the fundamental questions that remain unanswered for ColE1 are whether a pre-existing unique DNA strand is transferred undirectionally, and in what orientation; whether donor conjugal DNA synthesis replaces this strand, and what primes this synthesis; and what the role(s) of the ColE1 mobilisation gene(s) are. Furthermore, despite extensive efforts, we have been unable to identify an F relaxation complex.

The oriT sequence of a non-conjugative plasmid is often, perhaps always, recognised by a Dtr system (which might function in a different way to that of a conjugative plasmid) determined by the plasmid's own "mobilisation" genes (Warren et al, 1978). These genes are essential for mobilisation, indicating that the Dtr system of the conjugative plasmid is of different specificity and therefore probably dispensable. This is indeed the case for mobilisation of ColE1 or CloDF13 by F, since the F traMIZ genes (and the traD gene, for CloDF13 - but not for ColE1) are not required (Table 4; Willetts, 1980). Complementation of Dtr⁻ mutants of ColE1 by ColK but not by ColE2 (Warren and Sherratt, 1977) shows that different non-conjugative plasmids encode different Dtr systems (and therefore have different oriT sequences), even when they are mobilised by the same conjugative plasmid (R64-11 in this case). Similar

Table 4.   Mobilisation by Flac tra mutants

Flac mutant	Function lost	Transfer (%)	
		ColE1	CloDF13
tra$^+$	-	27	36
traA	pilus synthesis	0.002	0.002
traG ⎫	stabilisation of	<0.001	<0.004
traN ⎭	mating pairs	0.016	0.014
traM ⎫	triggering	21	38
traI ⎭		10	32
traIZ	triggering and nicking	18	32
traD	strand separation?	<0.001	51

experiments show that even the 2.3 kb miniplasmid p15A is efficiently mobilised if ColE1 and F are present to provide the necessary Dtr and Mpf systems (Chang and Cohen, 1978), and therefore contains an oriT sequence.

It is clearly essential that the conjugative plasmid's Mpf system should specifically recognise the non-conjugative plasmid's Dtr system (or, possibly, a second DNA sequence other than oriT on the plasmid to be transferred).   In either case, the success or failure of this recognition process can account for the ability or otherwise of a non-conjugative plasmid to be mobilised by a particular conjugative plasmid.   Insufficient information is available for any clear understanding of the molecular requirements for successful Mpf-Dtr interaction;   the data in Table 3 emphasise the complexities of the patterns already observed.   In this connection the versatility of ColE1 is of particular note;   this plasmid can be efficiently mobilised by IncF (although excluding, curiously, R100-1), IncI and IncP plasmids.

Mobilisation of replicons without an oriT

Replicons that do not carry an oriT sequence, or carry one that is non-functional because of the absence of Dtr or Mpf systems of appropriate specificities, can be conjugally transferred only if they become covalently linked by recombination to a functional oriT sequence.   This type of mobilisation is of particular importance for the special case where the mobilised replicon is the bacterial chromosome, since the resultant interchange of genes may accelerate bacterial evolution (Reanney, 1976).

Mobilisation of the E.coli K12 chromosome by F is due mainly to inefficient host-encoded recombination between the short regions of homology provided by insertion sequences present in both replicons (Davidson, 1975).   Chromosome mobilisation by autonomous F and Hfr formation are both reduced about 100-fold if the cell is

Table 5. Transpositional mobilisation

Conjugative plasmid	Non-conjugative plasmid	Relevant transposon (source)	
R1-19ΔKm	pSC101	Tn3	(C)
Flac	chromosome::Mu cts	Mu cts	(NC)
Flac	mini-R1	Tn3	(NC)
R388	pMB8::Tn3Δ596	Tn3Δ596 (+RSF1010::Tn3Ap^s)	(NC)
F	pBR322	γδ	(C)
R1-19ΔKm	mini F-Km	Tn3	(C)
R68.45	pBR325ΔAp	IS21	(C)

References (in order) are: Lopecko and Cohen, 1975; Faelen
and Toussaint, 1976; Goebel et al, 1977; Gill et al, 1978;
Guyer, 1978; Crisona et al, 1980; Willetts et al, 1981.

recombination-deficient (Moody and Hayes, 1972; Cullum and Broda,
1979) or if all the insertion sequences are deleted from F by
in vitro means (Willetts and Johnson, unpublished data).

Where no such homology exists, mobilisation can be detected
as the result of cointegrate formation during transposition of a
transposable DNA sequence from the conjugative to the non-
conjugative replicon, or vice versa (Table 5). This mechanism
probably accounts for host chromosome mobilisation by the IncP
plasmid variant R68.45, since this contains the highly
transposable IS21 (Willetts et al, 1981).

Conclusions

The requirements that must be satisfied for a replicon to be
transferred by conjugation are that (a) it must contain (or be
covalently linked to) an oriT sequence; (b) the cell in which the
replicon exists must synthesise a DNA transfer and replication (Dtr)
system that specifically recognises this oriT; and (c) the cell
must also synthesise a system for stable mating pair formation with
recipient cells (Mpf) that specifically recognises this Dtr system
(or possibly a second specific DNA sequence near to oriT).   The
Dtr and Mpf systems, though often encoded by the replicon itself,
can be provided in trans by other replicons.

References

Bradley, D.E., 1980, Plasmid 4: 155-169
Bradley, D.E., Taylor, D.E. and Cohen, D.R., 1980, J.Bacteriol.
    143: 1466-1470
Chang, A.C.Y. and Cohen, S., 1978, J.Bacteriol. 134: 1141-1156
Clewell, D.B. and Helinski, D.R., 1969, Proc.Nat.Acad.Sci.USA
    62: 1159-1166

Clowes, R.C., 1963, Genet.Res. 4: 162-165

Crisona, N.J., Nowak, J.A., Nagaishi, H. and Clark, A.J., 1980,
    J.Bacteriol. 142: 701-713

Cullum, J. and Broda, P., 1979, Plasmid 2: 358-365

Davidson, N., Deonier, R.C., Hu, S. and Ohtsubo, E., 1975,
    Microbiology - 1974, 56-65

Dougan, G. and Sherratt, D.S., 1977, Molec.Gen.Genet. 151: 151-160

Everett, R. and Willetts, N., 1980, J.Mol.Biol. 136: 129-150

Faelen, M. and Toussaint, A., 1976, J.Mol.Biol. 104: 525-539

Falkow, S., Guerry, P., Hedges, R.W. and Datta, N., 1974,
    J.Gen.Microbiol. 85: 65-76

Gill, R., Heffron, F., Dougan, G. and Falkow, S., 1978,
    J.Bacteriol. 136: 742-756

Goebel, W., Lindennaier, W., Pfeifer, F., Schrempf, H. and
    Schelle, B., 1977, Molec.Gen.Genet. 157: 119-129

Guyer, M., 1978, J.Mol.Biol. 126: 347-365

Hardy, K., 1975, Bact.Rev. 39: 464-515

Inselburg, J. 1977, J.Bacteriol. 132: 332-340

Kopecko, D.J. and Cohen, S.N., 1975, Proc.Nat.Acad.Sci.USA
    72: 1373-1377

Minkley, E.G., Polen, S., Brinton, C.C. and Ippen-Ihler, K., 1976,
    J.Mol.Biol. 108: 111-121

Moody, E.E.M. and Hayes, W., 1972, J.Bacteriol. 111: 80-85

Reanney, D., 1976, Bact.Rev. 40: 552-590

Reeves, P. and Willetts, N.S., 1974, J.Bacteriol. 120: 125-130

Warren, G. and Sherratt, D.J., 1977, Molec.Gen.Genet. 151: 197-201

Warren, G.J., Twigg, A.J. and Sherratt, D.J., 1978, Nature
    274: 259-261

Warren, G.J., Saul, M.W. and Sherratt, D.J., 1979, Molec.Gen.Genet.
    170: 103-107

Willetts, N.S., 1970, Molec.Gen.Genet. 108: 365-373

Willetts, N.S., 1980, Molec.Gen.Genet. 180: 213-217

Willetts, N.S. and Skurray, R., 1980, Ann.Rev.Genet. 14: 41-76

Willetts, N.S. and Crowther, C.C., 1981, Genet.Res., in press.

Willetts, N.S., Crowther, C. and Holloway, B.W., 1981, Plasmid
    submitted.

CONJUGATIVE PILI OF PLASMIDS IN ESCHERICHIA COLI K-12

AND PSEUDOMONAS SPECIES

David E. Bradley

Faculty of Medicine
Memorial University of Newfoundland
St. John's, Newfoundland, Canada A1B 3V6

SUMMARY

There are three basic morphological forms of conjugative pili
for plasmids transferable to Escherichia coli K-12: thin flexible,
thick flexible, and rigid. Plasmids determining rigid pili transfer
at least 2000X more efficiently on a solid surface compared with in
a liquid. The majority of such plasmids are naturally derepressed
for transfer and pilus synthesis. The following Pseudomonas plasmids determine rigid pili: Rms148 (IncP-7), TOL (IncP-9), and R91.5
(IncP-10). Several new plasmid-specific bacteriophages have been
found to adsorb to the sides or tips of conjugative pili.

INTRODUCTION

F pili were the first conjugative pili to be identified,[1] and
were quickly implicated as organelles of plasmid transfer.[2,3] Conjugative pili have since been found for all incompatibility groups
in Escherichia coli K-12,[4] and for some in Pseudomonas (see below).
However, the requirement of pili for conjugation has only been
demonstrated in three cases: F pili,[2,3] I pili,[5] and W pili.[6] Conjugative pili are of direct value in plasmid identification and
classification when their morphological and serological characteristics are compared. The classification of plasmids by incompatibility (for review see reference 7) correlates well with pilus
serotyping on the basis that similar pili (serologically related)
are determined by plasmids within an incompatibility group. However,
while different incompatibility groups of plasmids usually have
unrelated pili, there are a few exceptions: C pili are related to
J pili for example.[8] A direct result of studying pilus morphology
has been the discovery that certain types of conjugative pili are

217

structurally fragile, and this is linked with poor transfer efficiency in liquids. However, when bacteria carrying these plasmids
are mated on a solid surface such as an agar plate, transfer efficiency is dramatically increased.[9] This paper reviews these aspects
and describes some new observations on Pseudomonas conjugative pili.

METHODS FOR STUDYING CONJUGATION AND CONJUGATIVE PILI

     The standard method for plasmid transfer in the past has been
mating in a liquid environment (broth), but the identification of
surface mating systems[9] suggests that in many cases a plate mating
method would be more appropriate as follows. A nalidixic acid-
sensitive donor and a nalidixic acid-resistant recipient are grown
in shake culture to an absorbance of 1.0 at 620 nm wavelength, and
equal volumes of the cultures are mixed. 0.3 ml of the mixture is
spread on a nutrient non-selective plate predried at 37°C for 20
minutes uncovered. The bacterial suspension is allowed to dry on
the plate at the appropriate incubation temperature for the plasmid
or host strain (5-10 minutes). The plate is then covered and incubated for 55 minutes for mating. The cells are washed off quantitatively with three washes of 1.0 ml of broth using a wire
spreader to resuspend them. After adjusting the suspension volume
to 3.0 ml, serial dilutions are spread on selective plates
(nalidixic acid counterselection to prevent further plate mating)
for incubation and the counting of transconjugant colonies. This
procedure allows the introduction of mating inhibitors such as
inactivated pilus-specific bacteriophages into the mixture on the
mating plate. A concurrent comparative liquid mating can be
carried out by adding 0.3 ml of the initial mating mixture to 1.0
ml of broth, incubating this for 1 hour, then making the volume up
to 3.0 ml and plating serial dilutions as above.

     Pili determined by derepressed plasmids can be prepared for
electron microscopy by mounting them on specimen grids from a very
thick bacterial suspension.[4] For repressed plasmids, the "temporary
derepression" method of growth often improves pilus yields. Loop-
fuls of 6 hour non-selective plate cultures of donor and recipient
(both "bald") are spread evenly on a transconjugant-selecting plate
after suspending them in a drop of broth. Overnight incubation
gives confluent growth which is used for electron microscopy.

MORPHOLOGICAL AND SEROLOGICAL RELATIONSHIPS AMONG CONJUGATIVE PILI

     The morphological and serological relationships of conjugative
pili correlate well with the existing plasmid classification based
on incompatibility.[8] Three basic morphological types of pilus have
been identified: thin flexible (Fig. 1), thick flexible (Fig. 2),
and rigid (Fig. 3). Thin flexible pili (thickness about 6 nm) are
determined by plasmids in the I complex of incompatibility groups,
and also IncB and IncK plasmids. Immune electron microscopy has

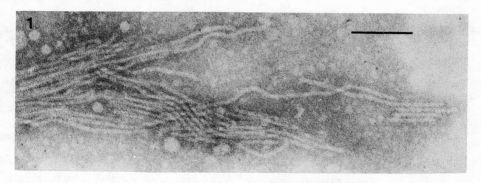

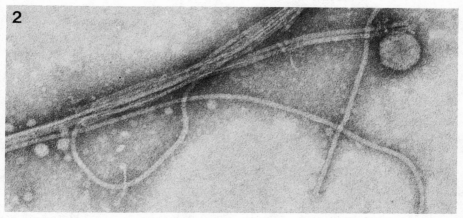

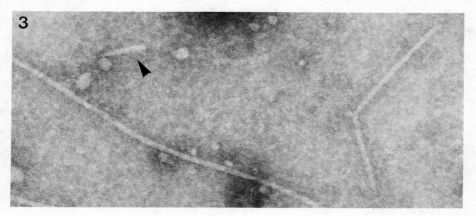

Fig. 1.   Thin flexible I_α pili from E. coli J53(R64drd11). Bar
          for Figs. 1-3, 100 nm.
Fig. 2.   Thick flexible H2 pili from E. coli JE2571(pIN32).
Fig. 3.   Rigid N pili determined by E. coli JE2571(N3). Arrow
          marks a very short pilus, which is common.

revealed two distinct serotypes, the I_α serotype for pili of $IncI_\alpha$, $IncI_\gamma$, IncB, and IncK plasmids, and the I_2 serotype for I_2 and I_δ pili. I_ζ pili reacted with antisera to both I_α and I_2 pili, the first reaction being the stronger. While a relationship between IncB and $IncI_\alpha$ plasmids has been established,[10] the possibility that IncK plasmids belong to the I complex is unexpected. Thick flexible pili (diameter about 9 nm) are determined by plasmids of incompatibility groups C, D, the F complex, H1, H2, J, T, V, X, com9, and the single plasmid (one which forms its own incompatibility "group") F_olac. Of these, C pili were found to be related to J pili, and com9 pili to F_olac pili, the remainder being unrelated. In a recent study (D. E. Bradley, unpublished), it was found that the pili of a transferable plasmid coding for the production of heat-stable entero-toxin (plasmid TP224; strain E7476 in reference 11) were serological-ly related to F_olac and com9 pili. TP224 was compatible with both F_olac and R71 (com9); it probably forms its own incompatibility "group" (M. McConnell, personal communication).

Rigid pili, which are fragile and easily broken, were deter-mined by plasmids of incompatibility groups M, N, P, U (a tentative new group as yet unpublished), and W, as well as the unclassified plasmid R775 (R. W. Hedges, unpublished). There was no relation-ship between the pili of any of these groups.

Tests on pili of plasmids within incompatibility groups showed serological identity with two exceptions. pHH1457 (V. Hughes, personal communication), while IncD, did not determine D pili. Its thick flexible pili were serologically unrelated to any others in the morphological group. pDT201 (D. E. Taylor et al., Plasmid, in press), while IncM, determined pili which were serologically related to those of plasmids in the F complex, most strongly to FII pili. It cannot therefore be stated that pili for all plasmids within a given incompatibility group are related, although exceptions are very rare.

The morphological classification of conjugative pili is neces-sarily somewhat subjective since it depends upon their appearance in the electron microscope, and some inaccuracies could arise. For example, X pili were obviously thick and flexible when obtained from overnight plates.[4] However, R6K, the naturally derepressed proto-type IncX plasmid, only determined large numbers of pili during the exponential phase of growth on plates (D. E. Bradley, unpublished), and these appeared much shorter (Fig. 4) and could easily be mis-taken for rigid pili.

Another IncX plasmid, R485, illustrates the usefulness of serological techniques for pilus identification. R485 determines very thin pili only 5 nm thick,[12] which are not typical X pili. This, together with its ill-defined incompatibility relationship with R6K, suggested that it might not be truly IncX. However, the

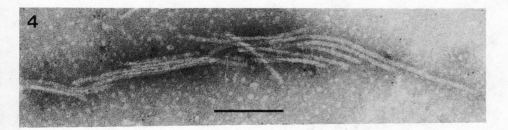

Fig. 4. Aggregate of short thick flexible X pili from a 6 hour
plate culture of E. coli JE2571(R6K). Bar marker 100 nm.

temporary derepression growth method revealed that, in addition to
the thin pili, thick filaments which labeled with antiserum to X
pili were produced (not illustrated). A possible function of the
thin pili may be to provide the host organism with the ability to
adhere to surfaces, since strains carrying the plasmid adhere very
much better to electron microscope specimen support films than those
without it.

RELATIONSHIP OF PILUS MORPHOLOGY WITH OPTIMUM MATING ENVIRONMENT

The use of plate mating allows a direct comparison to be made
between the transfer efficiencies of a plasmid on a solid surface
and in a liquid. By this means, Bradley et al.[9] compared the transfer frequencies on plates with those obtained in broth for representative plasmids from most incompatibility groups. Table 1 aligns
the plasmids according to optimum mating environment as indicated by
the ratio plate mating frequency/broth mating frequency. A ratio
near 1 shows that transfer frequencies were similar in both environments, with higher ratios demonstrating correspondingly greater surface mating efficiencies. It was expected that all plasmids determining thick flexible pili might transfer equally well in both
environments, but it can be seen that those in incompatibility groups
C, D, T, and X are considerably more efficient on a solid surface
than in a liquid. As was expected, all plasmids determining rigid
pili transferred very much more efficiently on plates, and in most
cases transfer frequencies were at derepressed levels. The broth
matings normally used to transfer these plasmids had erroneously
suggested that they were naturally repressed.

COMPARISON OF STATE OF PILUS SYNTHESIS (REPRESSED OR DEREPRESSED)
WITH PLASMID TRANSFERABILITY

It was possible to ascertain from the number of conjugative
pili found in the electron microscope whether or not they were determined constitutively (derepressed synthesis; see reference 8). This
could then be correlated with the transfer frequency obtained in the
plasmid's optimum mating environment. It might be thought that all

Table 1. Classification of Plasmid Mating Systems Based on
          Optimum Environment for Conjugal Transfer

Type of mating system[a]	Pilus morphology	Inc group[b]	Representative plasmid	Transfer frequency ratio plate/broth[c]
Universal	Thin flexible	I$_\alpha$	R64	0.9
		K	pTM559	0.51
	Thick flexible	FII	R100	0.73
		H1	R27	5.5
		J	R391	0.9
		V	R753	0.35
		com9	R71	1.55
Surface preferred	Thick flexible	C	RA1	45
		D	R711b	180
		T	Rts1	265
		X	R6K	250
Surface obligatory	Rigid	M	R446b	16,150
		N	N3	10,200
		P	RP1	2,100
		U	RA3	7,900
		W	Sa	36,450

[a]"Universal", transfer equally good in a liquid or on a solid surface; "surface preferred", transfer significantly better on a solid surface compared with in a liquid; "surface obligatory", transfer fairly low in a liquid and very high (derepressed) on a surface
[b]Single representatives only are included for incompatibility group complexes I, F, and H. IncU is tentative and unpublished (R. W. Hedges, personal communication).
[c]Transfer frequencies on plates divided by frequencies in broth.

plasmids determining conjugative pili constitutively would transfer at derepressed frequencies ($>10^{-1}$ transconjugants/donor/hour). However, representative plasmids from incompatibility groups D (R711b) and T (Rts1) determined pili constitutively but transferred at repressed frequencies. In summary, the following naturally occurring plasmids (as opposed to laboratory derepressed mutants) were repressed for both pilus synthesis and transfer: R64 (IncI$_\alpha$), TP114 (IncI2), and pTM559 (IncK), each of which determined thin flexible pili; RA1 (IncC), R100 (IncFII), R27 (IncH1), R478 (IncH2), R391 (IncJ), R753 (IncV), TP228 (IncX), and R71 (com9), which determined thick flexible pili. Plasmids which determined pili constitutively and were derepressed for transfer were as follows: R6K (IncX), which determined thick flexible pili; R831b (IncM), N3 (IncN), RP1 (IncP), RA3 (IncU), and Sa (IncW), which determined rigid pili. Notably, R6K is a naturally derepressed IncX plasmid, but other IncX plasmids appear to be repressed. Apart from the exceptions already indicated, the IncM plasmid R446b was repressed for pilus synthesis although it transferred at 1.4 X 10^{-1} transconjugants/donor/hour Possibly, like R6K, R446b only determines M pili in large numbers during the exponential phase of bacterial growth. It must be emphasized that, while a plasmid is derepressed in one bacterial species such as E. coli, it may well be repressed in another. Loss of derepression might also occur on transfer between different strains of the same species.

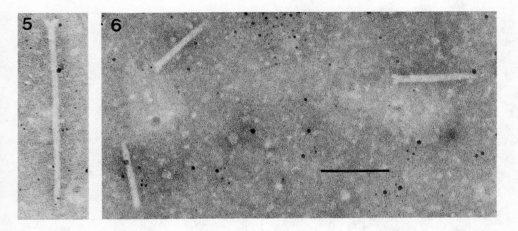

Figs. 5, 6.   P-7 pili (rigid) determined by Rms148 derepressed in
host P. aeruginosa PAO1150.1.   Bar 100nm.

DETERMINATION OF PILI BY SOME PLASMIDS OF PSEUDOMONAS SPECIES

Conjugative pili have been identified for Pseudomonas incompatibility group P-1 only with any degree of certainty.   They are
rigid and thinner than average.[13]   P-7, P-9, and P-10 pili can now
be added (D. E. Bradley, unpublished).   Pili determined by Rms148
(IncP-7) are short, rigid, and synthesized constitutively by PAO
strains of Pseudomonas aeruginosa carrying the plasmid (Figs. 5, 6).
TOL (IncP-9) appears to determine two kinds of pilus at a repressed
level, one thick and rigid (Fig. 7), and the other thinner and
flexible (Fig. 8).   However, the latter could be a metabolic product.   P-10 pili are determined by R91.5 (R91 derepressed),[14] and are
again rigid.   They are determined constitutively (Fig. 9).   Six of
the ten incompatibility groups of Pseudomonas species[14,15] remain to
be screened for pili, and all of them except IncP-1 for the surface
mating characteristics of their plasmids.

PLASMID-SPECIFIC BACTERIOPHAGES

Plasmid-specific bacteriophages such as fd[16] and R17[17] are
useful for identifying plasmids.   Also, if plaques are formed, conjugative pilus receptors are determined constitutively.   The isolation of five new phages by J. N. Coetzee and colleagues (see
F. A. Sirgel et al., J. Gen. Microbiol., in press, for phage C-1)
greatly extends their usefulness.   From Table 2 (single examples
only are included for F-specific phages), it can be seen that phages
have now been found for the majority of incompatibility groups,
although the host ranges of many are overlapping.   All the phages
tested adsorb to conjugative pili.   They can be divided into two

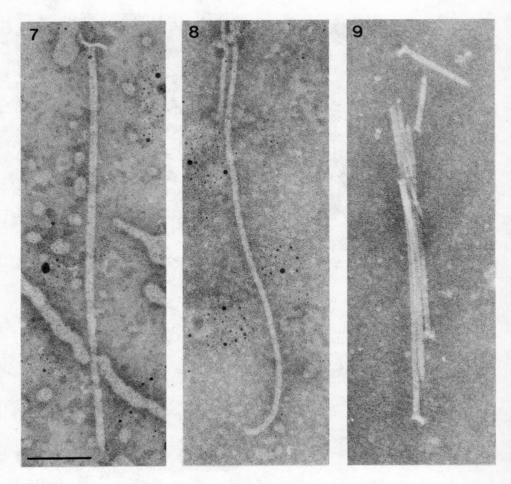

Fig. 7. Rigid TOL pilus from <u>P</u>. <u>putida</u> AC37(TOL). Bar marker for
         Figs. 7-9, 100 nm.
Fig. 8. Thick flexibile filaments associated with TOL.
Fig. 9. Rigid P-10 pili determined by R91.5.

general classes: RNA phages adsorbing to the sides of pili, and the
tip-adsorbing filamentous and tailed types. The first are highly
specific, while the tip-adsorbing phages are relatively non-specific

CONCLUSION

     Studies of conjugative pili must clearly be extended. For
example, it is desirable to demonstrate unequivocally that all
types are required for mating. A new experimental approach to this

Table 2.   Plasmid-Specific Bacteriophages

Bacteriophage designation	Type	Inc specificity[a]	Adsorption site (pilus type)
R17	RNA	FI-FIV	Thick flexible
fd	Filamentous	FI-FIV, D, $F_o lac$	Thick flexible
If1, If2, PR64FS	Filamentous	I complex,	Thin flexible
UA6[b], $F_o lac$[c]	RNA	$F_o lac$	Thick flexible
C-1[c]	RNA	C_o	Thick flexible
C-2[c]	Filamentous	C	Not yet tested
t[c]	RNA	T	Thick flexible
X[c]	Filamentous	X, M, N, U, (W), R775	Thick flexible (X only), rigid
IKe	Filamentous	N, (P),	Rigid
PRD1, PR4	Lipid	N, P, W	Rigid
PRR1	RNA	P	Rigid
Pf3	Filamentous	$(P)^d$	Not yet tested
J[c]	Short-tailed	C, D, J	Not yet tested

[a] Plaques formed with most derepressed plasmids. Plasmids in parentheses show multiplication with titer increase test only. <u>Pseudomonas</u> incompatibility groups not included.
[b] Isolated by G. D. Armstrong[19], serologically related to phage $F_o lac$.
[c] Isolated by J. N. Coetzee and colleagues (manuscripts in preparation).
[d] Does not plaque on <u>Escherichia coli</u> strains but forms hazy plaques on <u>Pseudomonas aeruginosa</u>.

is to block receptor sites on recipient cells by introducing purified pili into mating mixtures. Preliminary experiments with N and P pili have been successful using plate mating.[13] The functional role of pili in conjugation is still not fully understood, although the concept that they attach to recipient cells by their tips, and bring about cell-to-cell contact by retraction, is fairly well supported by experimental evidence.[18] How this model would apply to surface mating systems has not yet been considered. The chemical and physical structures of rigid pili remain to be examined; one would expect them to be different from flexible pili, of which only those of F and $F_o lac$ have been extensively studied.[19,20]

ACKNOWLEDGMENTS

I am grateful to all those who kindly supplied plasmids, to J. N. Coetzee for his new plasmid-specific phages, and to Doris Cohen for valuable technical assistance. The author's work was supported by the Medical Research Council of Canada (Grant No. MA5608).

REFERENCES

1. C. C. Brinton, <u>Trans</u>. <u>N</u>. <u>Y</u>. <u>Acad</u>. <u>Sci</u>., 27:1003 (1965).

2. K. A. Ippen and R. C. Valentine, Biochem. Biophys. Res. Commun.,
    27:674 (1967).
3. C. P. Novotny, W. S. Knight, and C. C. Brinton, J. Bacteriol.,
    95:314 (1968).
4. D. E. Bradley, J. Bacteriol., 141:828 (1980).
5. V. Harden and E. Meynell, J. Bacteriol., 109:1067 (1972).
6. D. E. Bradley, in "Pili," D. E. Bradley, E. Raizen, P. Fives-
    Taylor, J. Ou, ed., International Conferences on Pili,
    Washington, D. C. (1978).
7. N. Datta, in "Plasmids of Medical, Environmental and Commercial
    Importance," K. N. Timmis and A Pühler, ed., Elsevier/North-
    Holland, Amsterdam (1979).
8. D. E. Bradley, Plasmid, 4:155 (1980).
9. D. E. Bradley, D. E. Taylor, and D. R. Cohen, J. Bacteriol.,
    143:1466 (1980).
10. S. Falkow, P. Guerry, R. W. Hedges, and N. Datta, J. Gen.
    Microbiol., 85:65 (1974).
11. S. M. Scotland, R. J. Gross, T. Cheasty, and B. Rowe, J. Hyg.
    Camb., 83:531 (1979).
12. D. E. Bradley, Plasmid, 1:376 (1978).
13. D. E. Bradley and T. Chaudhuri, in "Plasmids and Transposons,"
    C. Stuttard and K. R. Rozee, ed., Academic Press, New York
    (1980).
14. G. A. Jacoby, R. Weiss, T. R. Korfhagen, V. Krishnapillai,
    A. E. Jacob, and R. W. Hedges, J. Bacteriol., 136:1159 (1978).
15. G. A. Jacoby, in "Microbiology-1977," D. Schlessinger, ed.,
    American Society for Microbiology, Washington, D. C. (1977).
16. D. A. Marvin and H. Hoffmann-Berling, Nature (London), 197:517
    (1963).
17. W. Paranchych and A. F. Graham, J. Cell. Comp. Physiol., 60:199
    (1962).
18. C. P. Novotny and P. Fives-Taylor, J. Bacteriol., 117:1306
    (1974).
19. G. D. Armstrong, L. S. Frost, P. A. Sastry, and W. Paranchych,
    J. Bacteriol., 141:333 (1980).
20. W. Folkhard, K. R. Leonard, S. Malsey, D. A. Marvin, J. Dubochet,
    A. Engel, M. Achtman, and R. Helmuth. J. Mol. Biol., 130:
    145 (1979).

THE PATHWAY OF PLASMID TRANSFORMATION IN PNEUMOCOCCUS

Walter R. Guild and Charles W. Saunders

Department of Biochemistry
Duke University
Durham, North Carolina   27710

SUMMARY

Plasmids transform Streptococcus pneumoniae by a process involving low efficiency assembly of replicons from fragments of single strands that have entered the cell separately. Transformation of preexisting replicons is much more efficient. We have cloned the erm gene of pIP501 into pMV158, which so far as we know is the first example of cloning in a pneumococcus host-vector system.

INTRODUCTION

Plasmids have not been found in drug resistant clinical isolates of Streptococcus pneumoniae, which instead carry R determinants inserted into their chromosomes (1, 2). However, a few laboratory strains carry the 2 Md cryptic pDP1 (3), and several R plasmids have been introduced into laboratory strains by conjugation (4, 5) or by transformation (1, 4, 6). We have examined the transformation of pneumococcus by the 3.5 Md tet plasmid pMV158, isolated from a group B streptococcus (7). The results appear useful in thinking about plasmid rearrangements and cloning strategies in streptococci. Here we review work described in three recent papers (8-10) and report the successful cloning of a gene in pneumococcus.

The normal entry pathway for donor DNA in naturally competent pneumococcus, and apparently in S. sanguis and B. subtilis, involves binding and nonspecific cutting of donor duplexes on the cell surface followed by entry of one of the strands of the donor fragments and degradation of the other (11-13). If this is also the major pathway used for plasmid transformation in these gram positive species, it

227

predicts that plasmid replicons have to be assembled inside the
recipient cell from fragments of the original donors, as has been
shown for transfection by phage DNA in pneumococcus (14).

RESULTS

We first established that transformation by pMV158 appears to
share binding and entry steps with chromosomal transformation, in
that both required the competent state of the cell surface and a
membrane endonuclease needed for the single strand entry pathway,
and that both were inhibited to comparable extents by competitor
DNA (although a larger plasmid was less inhibited) (8).

We then examined which forms of plasmid DNA were active and
characterized their relative contributions to the total transformants
observed. In doing so, we paid close attention to the results from
B. subtilis, where multimeric forms of very high specific activity
were shown to contaminate other fractions and could give misleading
results (15, 16). The problem was to know whether activity comigrating with a physically detectable DNA form was due to that form or to
another of high specific activity. In particular, in the size range
of pMV158, monomer open circles (OC) migrate in 0.5% - 1.0% agarose
gels very close to closed circular (CC) dimers (9), and in sucrose
gradients dimer OC cosediments with monomer CC (9, 10, 17). A single
separation by either method was not sufficient to allow conclusions
as to which form contributed the activity, particularly since it was
quickly evident that much of the activity was due to dimers or higher

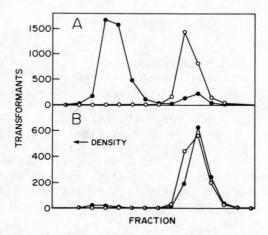

Fig. 1. Plasmid transforming activity in dye-buoyancy gradients
         before (A) and after (B) digestion of a cleared lysate with
         S1 nuclease. Filled symbols, pMV158; open, chromosomal
         reference marker. Twice as much DNA was put into B as into
         A (from ref. 10).

multimers which were often undetectable by fluorescence of gels
stained with ethidium bromide (EtBr). Later work showed that at most
5% of pMV158 DNA was in dimeric forms and that often only a fraction
of this was CC. We therefore used combinations of methods to separate and identify which plasmid form contributed a given transforming
activity, and then characterized these further with respect to
kinetics and relative activities.

Transformants arose from DNA in both the CC and non-CC regions
of EtBr-CsCl gradients, with the fraction in each region varying from
preparation to preparation (1, 8). On deliberately cutting a cleared
lysate by treatment with S1 nuclease, over 99% of the activity
disappeared from the CC region, and that in the non-CC region,
representing almost all the surviving activity, increased slightly
(Fig. 1). Therefore, non-CC forms clearly could transform but had
much lower activity per molecule than the CC forms (10).

The critical results came from analysis of the behavior of
transforming activity in fractions separated by preparative gel
electrophoresis, using automated collection of fractions from a large
agarose slab gel, the "Gene Machine" described by Polsky et al. (18).
Well resolved peaks of activity were found and the activities in a
number of them were examined by various combinations of sedimentation
velocity, dye-buoyancy, analytical gel electrophoresis, kinetic
response, and sensitivity to S1 nuclease. The profile of a preparation in which almost all activity was in CC forms is shown in Fig. 2.
Analytical gels showed that CC monomer coeluted with peak A and that
OC monomer was the only plasmid form visible in peak B. However,
98% of the activity in peak B banded as CC in an EtBr-CsCl gradient,

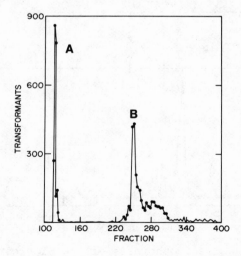

Fig. 2.   Preparative electrophoretic fractionation of pMV158
          transforming activity (from ref. 9).

and most of it had the sedimentation velocity expected for dimer CC;
that in peak A was 100% CC in EtBr-CsCl and had the velocity of
monomer CC. On examining kinetics, transformation varied with the
square of DNA concentration in peak A; the material in peak B gave
linear concentration response (9).

Fig. 3 shows the electrophoretic profile of activity in the
preparation of Fig. 1 that had been digested with S1 nuclease before running (10). Essentially all the activity banded as non-CC
in dye-buoyancy gradients. Beneath the R_f scale are shown the
positions expected for various forms from analytical gels run under
similar conditions and, for monomer forms, observed directly in
analytical gels of single fractions from this or similar runs (that
in Fig. 2 used different conditions and was not directly comparable
for R_f).

Fig. 4 shows the sedimentation velocity distributions in the
initial cleared lysate before (A) and after (B) S1 treatment and of
fractions 51, 68, and 152 from the run of Fig. 3. There was too
little activity in fraction 41 to confirm that it was due to monomer
linear DNA, but the strong presumption is that it was. The combined
results of these runs provided strong evidence that CC, OC, and
linear forms of both monomers and dimers were active, but that the
non-CC forms were much less active than the CC forms per molecule.
A small fraction of the total activity may have come from trimers or
higher multimers sedimenting rapidly (Fig. 4A, 4B) and eluting near
fractions 80-95 in Fig. 3.

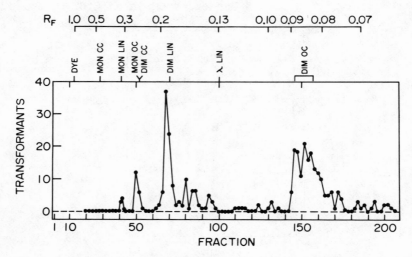

Fig. 3. Preparative electrophoresis of the S1 treated lysate in
         Fig. 1B (from ref. 10).

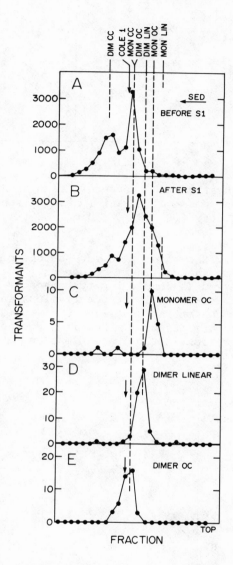

Fig. 4. Sedimentation velocity distributions of pMV158 transforming
activity (see text). Positions indicated at the top are
predicted from the relations of Clowes (17), relative to
the internal ^{3}H-ColE1 standard. Panels C, D, and E show
the activities in fractions 51, 68, and 152, respectively,
from Fig. 3 (from ref. 10).

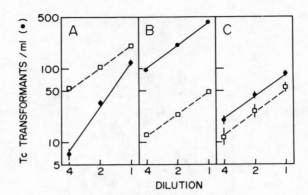

Fig. 5.   DNA concentration dependence of transformation for pMV158
          (●) and chromosomal marker (□). A, monomer OC (fr. 51);
          B, dimer linear (fr. 68); C, dimer OC (fr. 152) (ref. 10).

        As did CC forms, the monomer OC gave second order kinetics
while the dimer forms showed linear responses (Fig. 5). When a
cleared lysate was used as donor, the response curve was the sum
of a linear component seen at low concentrations and a multi-hit
component at higher concentrations (Fig. 6). That is, the fraction
of the transformants arising from monomers increased from undetectable at low concentration in the transformation tube to a majority
at higher concentrations.

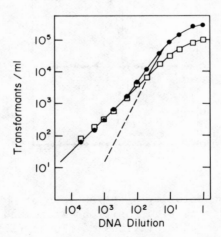

Fig. 6.   Dose-response curve for a cleared lysate containing pMV158
          (●) and a chromosomal marker (□). It was coincidence
          that the numbers were the same at high dilution. The dashed
          line indicates a slope of 2.0 (from ref. 8).

Unique linear products of digestion with either of two restriction enzymes that cut at single sites showed essentially no transforming activity ($\leqslant$ 0.1% of that of CC forms). However, a mixture of the two separate digests transformed at a level comparable to that of the mixture of linear monomers produced by S1 nuclease, near 1% of that of an equal weight of CC monomer. In another experiment, monomer CC, dimer CC, and dimer OC forms were first separated electrophoretically and then digested with S1. Surviving activities were 2.6, 2.8, and 72% respectively (10).

MODEL

Fig. 7 summarizes our interpretation of the pathway of plasmid transformation in pneumococcus. We believe that it will prove to be similar in S. sanguis and probably in B. subtilis, although it remains to be established why monomer plasmids are not active in the latter system (15, 16). Quantitative estimates of absolute efficiency imply that less than 1% of the cells that receive the minimum number of strand fragments are in fact transformed. We have suggested that this reflects intracellular degradation of the first strand while it awaits the entry of the second, and that this process may be more extensive in B. subtilis than in pneumococcus (10).

In S. sanguis, Macrina et al. have shown that multimeric forms of pVA736 contribute the majority of the transforming activity and that the monomer CC band cut from gels is active with second order kinetics (19). In contrast, data forcing one to invoke cooperation between donor strands is lacking in B. subtilis. However, based on the similarities of the chromosomal transformation pathways in these

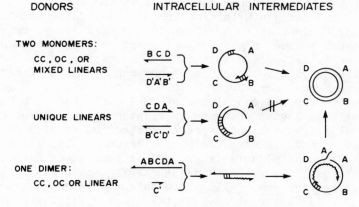

Fig. 7.   Intracellular assembly of plasmid replicons from single
           strand fragments in pneumococcus. See text (from ref. 10).

gram positive species, Dubnau et al. (24) have suggested a model
similar to ours for the processing of multimeric plasmid DNA in
B. subtilis.

A recent report on transformation of pneumococcus by other
plasmids reached some conclusions similar to ours (6). These authors
concluded from a single separation by gel electrophoresis that OC
monomer was active, whereas we found that activity comigrating with
monomer OC was almost entirely due to dimer CC, unless we had first
digested the preparation with S1. They found cooperation between
restriction digests, as did we. Although our results differ in some
quantitative respects, such as relative activities of the various
forms, the major qualitative difference is in the kinetics for monomer donors, where they did not recognize the second order response.

IMPLICATIONS

Assembly of replicons from fragments of single strands represents physical recombination, and the low efficiency suggests that
the rare successes result from minimal pairings just sufficient to
generate a circle carrying intact replication functions. In this
situation sequence rearrangements may be expected to occur wherever
partial homologies allow them, and those generating smaller replicons
should have a selective advantage. We have observed an extensive
deletion during transformation of the 20 Mdal pIP501 (4), and Behnke
et al. have seen several examples of deletion during transformation
of S. sanguis by a derivative of pSM19035 (20).

CLONING IN PNEUMOCOCCUS

The fragmentation on entry and the resulting low overall efficiency of establishing new replicons in the recipient implies that
recovering plasmids created by in vitro recombination will be more
difficult than if the donor molecule remained intact. However, the
efficiency of adding new information to a partially homologous replicon already present is much higher, as in chromosomal transformation
and in marker rescue in phage transformation (21). Dubnau's laboratory has explicitly demonstrated this for plasmid transformation in
B. subtilis (22, 23). Using this approach, we have cloned the erm
(MLS^r) gene from a derivative of pIP501 into pMV158. Digests of pDP
treated with Hind III and S1 and of pMV158 treated with S1 were
treated with T4 ligase and used to transform a recipient carrying
pMV158. MLS^r transformants were recovered and lysates of several of
these transformed the same recipients again at high efficiencies
while transforming plasmid-free cells at much lower efficiencies.
The transformants carry plasmids of varying sizes and some of these
carry both tet and erm, making them potentially useful for further
cloning. So far as we are aware, this is the first successful
cloning in a pneumococcus host vector system.

ACKNOWLEDGMENTS

     This work has been supported by grant GM21887 from the National
Institutes of Health and by contract DE-AS05-76EV03941 from the
Department of Energy to WRG. CWS is a genetics trainee under grant
1 T32 GM07754 from the N.I.H.

REFERENCES

1. Shoemaker, N.B., M.D. Smith, and W.R. Guild. 1979. J. Bacteriol.
         139:432-441.
2. Smith, M.D., S. Hazum, and W.R. Guild. 1981. (ms. in prep.).
3. Smith, M.D., and W.R. Guild. 1979. J. Bacteriol. 137:735-739.
4. Smith, M.D., N.B. Shoemaker, V. Burdett, and W.R. Guild. 1980.
         Plasmid 3:70-79.
5. Engel, H.W.B., N. Soedirman, J.A. Rost, W.J. van Leeuwen, and
         J.D.A. van Embden. 1980. J. Bacteriol. 142:407-413.
6. Barany, F., and A. Tomasz. 1980. J. Bacteriol. 144:698-709.
7. Burdett, V. 1980. Antimicrob. Agents Chemother. 18:753-760.
8. Saunders, C., and W.R. Guild. 1980. Mol. Gen. Genet.180:573-578.
9. Saunders, C., and W.R. Guild. 1981. Mol. Gen. Genet. 181: 57-62.
10. Saunders, C., and W.R. Guild. 1981. J. Bacteriol., in press.
11. Morrison, D.A. and W.R. Guild. 1973. Biochim. Biophys. Acta
         299:545-556.
12. Lacks, S. 1977. in J. Reissig (ed.), "Microbial Interactions."
         Chapman and Hall, London.
13. Lacks, S. 1979. J. Bacteriol. 138:404-409.
14. Porter, R.D., and W.R. Guild. 1978. J. Virol. 25:60-72.
15. Canosi, U., G. Morelli, V. Sgamarella, and T.A. Trautner. 1978.
         Mol. Gen. Genet. 166:259-267.
16. Mottes, M., G. Grandi, V. Sgamarella, U. Canosi, G. Morelli, and
         T.A. Trautner. 1979. Mol. Gen. Genet. 174:281-286.
17. Clowes, R.C. 1972. Bacteriol. Rev. 36:361-405.
18. Polsky, F., M.H. Edgell, J.G. Seidman, and P. Leder. 1978. Anal.
         Biochem. 87:397-410.
19. Macrina, F.L., K.R. Jones, and R.A. Welch. 1980. Pers. commun.
20. Behnke, D., H. Malke, M. Hartmann, and F. Walter. 1979. Plasmid
         2:605-616.
21. Green, D.M. 1966. J. Mol. Biol. 22:1-13.
22. Contente, S., and D. Dubnau. 1979. Plasmid. 2:555-571.
23. Gryczan, T., S. Contente, and D. Dubnau. 1980. Mol. Gen. Genet.
         177:459-467.
24. Dubnau, D., S. Contente, and T.J. Gryczan. 1980. in S. Zadrazil
         and J. Sponar (eds.), "DNA - Recombination Interactions
         and Repair." Pergamon Press, Oxford and New York.

PLASMIDS OF THE GONOCOCCUS

P. Frederick Sparling, Gour Biswas, James Graves, and
Eleanore Blackman

Departments of Medicine and Bacteriology
University of North Carolina School of Medicine
Chapel Hill, N. C.   27514

There are at least four naturally-occurring plasmids in the
gonococcus (Table 1).   This paper will review the structure,
origins and functions of these plasmids, insofar as known or can
be reasonably inferred.   Certain hybrid plasmids which have been
of particular interest in delineating early steps in entry of DNA
into competent gonococci are also discussed.

Table 1. Plasmids of <u>Neisseria gonorrhoeae</u>

Plasmid Size	Designation	Mol% G+C	Function	Ref.
2.7	pFA1, pLE2600	50	ND[a]	1-4
3.4	pFA7, pMR0200	41	Pc^r	4,5
4.7[b]	pFA3, pMR0360	41	Pc^r	4,5
7.5	pFA10	ND	Pc^r	5
24.5	pFA2, pLE2450	50	Tra$^+$	4,6,7
28.0[c]	pFA14	ND	Pc^r, Tra$^-$	5

[a] Not determined.
[b] Recombinant plasmid pFA3 Ω pFA1, resulting from entry of
pFA3 by transformation into a pFA1-containing recipient.
[c] Recombinant plasmid pFA3 Ω pFA2, resulting from entry of
pFA3 by transformation into a pFA2-containing recipient.

237

CRYPTIC PLASMIDS

Most gonococcal isolates contain an approximately 2.7 Mdal cryptic plasmid.[2,3,4,8] The structure of this plasmid is highly conserved, although small deletions or differences in restriction-endonuclease sites have been documented.[9,10] The function(s) of this plasmid have been elusive. There is no evidence that the 2.7 Mdal plasmid (or any other gonococcal plasmid) is involved in control of piliation, iron utilization, or resistance to serum. We have recently observed that strains lacking the 2.7 Mdal plasmid are apparently aberrant in several respects, including their propensity to be highly opaque in their colonial morphology. We have attempted to introduce the native 2.7 Mdal plasmid into plasmidless strains by transformation or conjugation, selecting for entry of a 4.7 Mdal Pc^r plasmid and scoring on agarose gels for coincident entry of the 2.7 Mdal plasmid. None of over 100 Pc^r transformants or transconjugants also acquired the 2.7 Mdal cryptic plasmid. Attempts to cure strains of their cryptic plasmid have also been unsuccessful. Failure to construct isogenic derivatives varying in presence of the 2.7 Mdal plasmid has prevented serious study of its function(s).

PENICILLINASE PLASMIDS

In 1976, strains of gonococci were isolated in the United Kingdom, U.S.A., and in South East Asia which produced a TEM-1 type β-lactamase.[11] The bla gene (penicillinase production) was carried on either a 3.4 or 4.7 Mdal plasmid.[5,11] (Earlier papers considered the sizes of these plasmids as 3.2 and 4.4 Mdal, but these estimates were probably slightly too low.) Isolates of Pc^r gonococci in the U.S.A. and Asia generally contained the 4.7 Mdal plasmid, whereas African and European isolates usually contained the 3.4 Mdal plasmid.[12] Strains of Pc^r gonococci from Asia and the U.S.A. also often contained a 24 Mdal conjugative plasmid, and were either prototrophic or proline-requiring; European-African isolates were frequently arginine-requiring, and rarely contained a 24 Mdal conjugative plasmid.[12] These observations suggested nearly simultaneous origin of two related but epidemiologically distinct clones of Pc^r gonococci in different geographic areas.

Roberts, Elwell, and Falkow showed by DNA-DNA hybridization that gonococcal Pc^r plasmids were closely related to each other and to previously characterized Ap^r plasmids of about 4 Mdal isolated in Haemophilus influenzae.[4] The 4.7 and 3.4 Mdal gonococcal Pc^r plasmids have a base content of about 41 mol.% G+C, which is similar to Haemophilus DNA but unlike the approximately 50% mol.% G+C in other gonococcal plasmids and chromosomal DNA.[1,4,6] These data suggested that the gonococcal Pc^r plasmids could have been transferred into gonococci from Haemophilus.

This speculation was strengthened by demonstration of a 4.7 Mdal Haemophilus Pc^r plasmid with HpaII, AluI and BamHI restriction-endonuclease fragment structure identical with the 4.7 Mdal gonococcal Pc^r plasmid. This strain of <u>Haemophilus</u>, which was isolated in 1974 (before the advent of Pc^r gonococci), could conjugally transfer its Pc^r plasmid into gonococci. The Haemophilus Pc^r plasmid was very unstable in a gonococcal host, even in the presence of penicillin or ampicillin.[13] It is also possible, of course, that the similar 4.7 Mdal Pc^r plasmids observed in gonococci and <u>Haemophilus</u> were transferred into each from another unknown source.

Introduction of the gonococcal 4.7 Mdal Pc^r plasmid into an isogenic Pc^s gonococcal recipient by transformation frequently resulted in formation of deleted plasmids, varying in size from 2.3 Mdal to 3.4 Mdal. The most common class of transformation-induced deleted Pc^r plasmid was 3.4 Mdal, which was identical in restriction-endonuclease fragment structure to the naturally-occurring 3.4 Mdal plasmids.[5] Deletions were observed with both 4.7 Mdal Pc^r plasmid transforming DNA prepared from cesium chloride-ethidium bromide density gradients, and with more highly purified preparations from subsequent sucrose gradients. Similar deletions were not observed during serial passage of strains carrying the 4.7 Mdal Pc^r plasmid in vitro, nor after transfer of the same plasmid into gonococci by conjugation or into <u>E. coli</u> by transformation.[5] Thus, it was proposed that entry of plasmids by transformation may produce linear fragments, and that recircularization may have resulted in formation of the 3.4 Mdal Pc^r plasmid from the 4.7 Mdal Pc^r plasmid. This event is perhaps more plausible if one considers the uniform competence for transformation of virtually all naturally-isolated gonococci,[14] and the propensity of gonococci to autolyze and thereby release transforming DNA.

The gonococcal Pc^r plasmids, like the small Haemophilus Pc^r plasmids, contain about 40% of the ampicillin-resistance transposon Tn2, including one of the two terminal inverted repeats.[11,15] This almost certainly means that the gonococcal <u>bla</u> gene cannot undergo transposition into new sites. Hybrid <u>bla</u> plasmids have been observed after transformation into certain recipients, but these are probably the result of classical recombinational events and not transposition (see below).

For several years the prevalence of Pc^r gonococci in the U.S.A. and Europe remained low, although in certain areas of the Far East up to 50% of all gonococci were Pc^r.[12] Very recently, there have been several outbreaks of Pc^r gonococcal infections in the U.S.A. and Europe, which may portend greater problems in the future. The prevalence of Pc^r gonococci in the U.S.A. is apparently still less than 1.0% of all isolates, however, and thus

currently recommended regimens for treatment in the U.S.A. have
not included routine use of drugs such as spectinomycin or cefoxitin, which are known to be effective for Pc[r] gonococcal infections.[16,17]

CONJUGATIVE PLASMIDS

    Shortly after the discovery in 1976 of Pc[r] gonococci, it was
shown that many gonococci could conjugally transfer their Pc[r]
plasmid to other gonococci, E. coli, or certain other Neisseria
such as N. flava.[18]   The ability to act as a conjugal donor
depended on presence of an approximately 24 Mdal plasmid, which
carried no detectable markers for drug, heavy metal, or ultraviolet resistance, but efficiently mobilized itself and also the
smaller non-self-transferable Pc[r] plasmids into suitable recipients.[6]   Transfer was mediated by an Anderson Class II system.[6]
Nearly 50% of Pc[r] gonococci isolated in the Far East carried a 24
Mdal conjugative plasmid,[12] whereas only 12 of 156 (8%) tested
Pc[s] gonococci carried a similar plasmid.[6] This suggested that
Pc[r] plasmids may be conjugally transferred between gonococci in
nature.

    The structure of a limited number of the 24 Mdal conjugative
plasmids has been studied. All had similar (but not identical)
restriction digest fragment structures.[6]   There were remarkable
differences in function, however, when different 24 Mdal plasmids
were introduced into a strain carrying the non-self-transferable
4.7 Mdal Pc[r] plasmid pFA3. Some 24 Mdal plasmids mobilized the
Pc[r] plasmid with a frequency of about 1×10^{-3} per donor cell,
whereas others did not mobilize it at detectable frequency.[6]   In
other strains, the same 24 Mdal plasmids were all capable of mobilizing the 4.7 Mdal Pc[r] plasmid.[6]   Certain deletions of the 4.7
Mdal Pc[r] plasmid completely prevented mobilization by the 24 Mdal
conjugative plasmid.[5]   Thus, efficiency of conjugation was dependent on both plasmid and host strain factors, many of which have
not been well characterized.

    Recent evidence showed that the gonococcal conjugal system
was naturally derepressed, with frequencies of Pc[r] plasmid transfer up to 10% per donor CFU in a 90 minute mating on membrane
filters.[19]   Efficiencies of transfer were often reduced, sometimes by orders of magnitude, in crosses between unrelated gonococcal strains, or between unrelated species (N. flava, E. coli).
Maximum frequencies of Pc[r] plasmid transfer were only detected
when low concentrations of penicillin (about 8-fold greater than
the MIC of the recipient strain) were used to select the transconjugants; this was necessary because of the low single-cell resistance of gonococci carrying a Pc[r] plasmid.[19]   Despite evidence
that gonococcal conjugation is derepressed, no sex pili have been
observed yet.

The interaction between conjugal donor and recipient cells is poorly understood. Addition of purified lipopolysaccharide isolated from the donor did not reduce frequencies of conjugal transfer of a 4.7 Mdal Pc^r plasmid (unpublished data). Outer membrane protein structure did influence conjugation, however. Gonococci are known to undergo relatively high-frequency bidirectional variation in expression of a series of closely related, heat-modifiable, outer membrane proteins of about 2800 daltons;[19] cells containing these proteins are termed opaque, whereas those without these proteins are transparent. In a series of experiments with isogenic donors and recipients varying in presence of the "opacity proteins", conjugation efficiencies were at least 10-fold higher in transparent x transparent than opaque x opaque crosses.[19] One might have expected the reverse result, since opaque gonococci are much more likely to clump and therefore each opaque CFU contains many more cells. Perhaps the heat-modifiable outer membrane opacity proteins reduce efficiency of mating pair formation. The 24 Mdal plasmid has no effect on outer membrane proteins, and no surface exclusion in conjugation has been observed.[19]

Many laboratories have attempted to demonstrate conjugal transfer of chromosomal genes. Initial results were promising, since recombinants for a variety of chromosomal markers were observed in prolonged filter matings, apparently due to a DNase-resistant transfer mechanism.[20] At least three laboratories have since shown, however, that the apparent initial successes were probably due to transformation which occurred despite initial addition of DNase. No differences in transfer frequencies were observed in isogenic donors which varied only in presence of the 24 Mdal conjugative plasmid.[19,21,22] Norlander et al[21] reported that 24 Mdal plasmids enhanced the transformation-competence of recipient cells, but we were unable to confirm their claim (unpublished data).

HYBRID Pc^r PLASMIDS

When the 4.7 Mdal Pc^r plasmid pFA3 was introduced by transformation into a recipient which contained the 2.7 Mdal cryptic plasmid pFA1 and the 24 Mdal conjugative plasmid pFA2, rare hybrid Pc^r plasmids were formed.[5] One of these, designated pFA10, was about 7.5 Mdal in mass, and has been shown to be a nearly complete cointegrate between pFA1 and pFA3 (unpublished data). Another, designated pFA14, was about 28 Mdal and has been shown to be a recombinant of pFA3 into the conjugative plasmid pFA2 (unpublished data). The insertion into pFA2 rendered it conjugation deficient (Tra$^-$). We have studied these hybrid plasmids in some detail, because of their markedly enhanced activity in transformation (Table 2).

Table 2. Transformation Frequencies With Native and Hybrid Pc^r
          Plasmids Into An Isogenic Pc^s Recipient[a]

Plasmid	Mass (Mdal)	Pc^r Transformants Per µg DNA per 10^8 Recipient Cells
pFA3	4.7	10
pFA10[b]	7.5	60,000
pFA14[c]	28.0	140,000

[a] The recipient contained pFA1 and pFA2.
[b] pFA10 is a pFA3 Ω pFA1 hybrid.
[c] pFA14 is a pFA3 Ω pFA2 hybrid.

We recently have completed experiments which provide a
rational basis for the markedly increased transformation efficiency of the hybrid Pc^r plasmids pFA10 and pFA14. Two mechanisms
are involved: marker rescue, and sequence specific uptake of
transforming DNA.

The evidence for marker rescue is straightforward. When the
hybrid Pc^r plasmid pFA14 (pFA2 Ω pFA3) was introduced by transformation into competent isogenic recipients which lacked any
plasmid, or which contained only the unrelated plasmid pFA1, Pc^r
transformants were rare ($\leq 10^{-7}$ per µg plasmid DNA). When Pc^r
plasmids were reisolated from the transformants, they were always
much smaller than the original 28 Mdal donor plasmid. In contrast, when the pFA2 pFA3 Pc^r hybrid (pFA14) was introduced into
the same isogenic recipient, excepting that it now contained the
homologous plasmid pFA2, Pc^r transformants were obtained at 1000-
fold increased frequency, and each of the tested transformant Pc^r
plasmids was of the same size (28 Mdal) and restriction-digest
fragment structure as the donor plasmid pFA14 (Table 3). We hypothesized that there probably were endonucleases which linearized
the incoming Pc^r plasmid, resulting in rare recircularized Pc^r
transformant plasmids of reduced size; however, when the recipient
contained a resident replicon homologous with much of the incoming
Pc^r plasmid, the linearized Pc^r plasmid was "rescued", possibly by
recombination with the resident plasmid. The putative endonucleases were presumably not restriction endonucleases, since the
experiments were done entirely with DNA isolated from the single
strain used as recipient. (These experiments will be presented in
detail elsewhere.)

Table 3. Marker Rescue During Transformation of the Gonococcus
          With the Hybrid 28 Mdal Pc^r Plasmid pFA14 (pFA3 Ω pFA2)

Recipient Plasmid Content[a]	Pc^r Transformants per μg DNA per 10^8 Recipient Cells	Deleted Plasmids in Transformants/ Total Tested
PFA1	18	13/13[b]
pFA1, pFA2	20,000	0/14

[a]The donor Pc^r plasmid is a stable recombinant between the Pc^r
plasmid pFA3 and the native gonococcal conjugative plasmid pFA2.
The donor DNA was isolated from the strain used in subsequent
transformations; the Pc^s recipients were identical excepting for
the addition to one of them (by conjugal transfer) of pFA2.
[b]Pc^r plasmids were isolated from individual transformants and were
compared on horizontal agarose gels to the size of the donor
plasmid pFA14.

There is a second reason for increased transformation efficiency of the hybrid Pc^r plasmids: acquisition of resident gonococcal DNA containing sequence(s) required for efficient uptake by
competent cells. It was shown earlier that non-homologous DNA did
not compete effectively against gonococcal DNA during transformation.[23] We have confirmed and extended this evidence for specificity of gonococcal DNA uptake, using the Pc^r hybrid plasmid
pFA10. The hybrid Pc^r pFA10 (pFA3 Ω pFA1) has been shown to be
10 to 30-fold more active in transformation of a plasmid-free
recipient strain than the naturally-occurring Pc^r plasmid pFA3.
Since there was no detectable plasmid DNA in the recipient,
marker rescue of the hybrid plasmid by a homologous resident
replicon seemed unlikely. (pFA10 is relatively more active in
transformation of recipients containing a 2.7 Mdal cryptic
plasmid, presumably because of homology with the pFA1 portion of
pFA10 - "marker rescue".) Since the experiments were done in a
completely isogenic background, differences due to restriction
modification also seemed implausible. There was no evidence for
increased formation of multimeric forms of the hybrid pFA10;
rather, monomeric DNA isolated on sucrose gradients seemed to
account for the great majority of transforming activity. Thus,
we reasoned that the hybrid pFA10 probably had sequences required
for uptake which were not present on the parent plasmid pFA3, and
that these sequences were probably on the pFA1 (2.7 Mdal cryptic
plasmid) component of pFA10.

The structure of pFA10 is known in considerable detail. It has seven major Msp1 fragments, or which one (M2, 3000 bp) is composed entirely of DNA from the native gonococcal 2.7 Mdal plasmid pFA1. Two other Msp1 fragments contain smaller amounts of pFA1 DNA, plus a majority of DNA from the original Pc^r plasmid pFA3. All other Msp1 fragments contain DNA entirely derived from pFA3. Competent gonococcal cells were briefly exposed to ^{32}P-end-labeled Msp1 fragments of pFA10, followed by digestion with DNase-1 to remove all fragments not taken up. The cells were then carefully washed. DNA extracted from the washed cells was separated on agarose gels, and autoradiography repeatedly demonstrated that the only fragment taken up was the 3000 bp M-2 fragment derived entirely from the native 2.7 Mdal cryptic plasmid pFA1. Thus gonococci, like Haemophilus,[24] recognize specific sequences during DNA uptake. The gonococcal sequences appear to be different from the 11 bp Haemophilus uptake sequence,[25] since Haemophilus DNA did not compete with gonococcal DNA during transformation. (These experiments will be presented in detail elsewhere.)

CONCLUSIONS

The hybrid Pc^r gonococcal plasmids have proven highly useful in better understanding early events in gonococcal transformation. Much remains to be learned however. What is the precise mechanism for marker rescue? What is the nature of the gonococcal DNA sequence required for uptake? What is the receptor for uptake? Why is this receptor apparently inactive in non-piliated non-competent gonococci? Can the hybrid pFA10, which contains nearly all of the ubiquitous 2.7 Mdal cryptic plasmid, be used to identify the functions of the cryptic plasmid? Can future hybrid plasmids be constructed which will effectively mobilize the chromosome in conjugation? Can these or similar plasmids be used as cloning vehicles, so as to understand the basis for many other unresolved problems concerning the biology and pathogenicity of the gonococcus? We believe the answer to many of these questions is affirmative.

ACKNOWLEDGEMENTS

Many of the preliminary experiments were performed by T. Sox. This work was supported by Public Health Service grant AI15036 from the National Institute of Allergy and Infectious Diseases.

REFERENCES

1. L. W. Mayer, K. K. Holmes, and S. Falkow, Characterization of plasmid deoxyribonucleic acid from Neisseria gonorrhoeae, Infect. Immun. 10:712 (1974).

2. P. W. Stiffler, S. A. Lerner, M. Bohnhoff, and J. A. Morello,
    Plasmid deoxyribonucleic acid in clinical isolates of
    Neisseria gonorrhoeae, J. Bacteriol. 122:1293 (1975).
3. G. Biswas, S. Comer, and P. F. Sparling, Chromosomal location
    of antibiotic resistance genes in Neisseria gonorrhoeae,
    J. Bacteriol. 125:1207 (1976).
4. M. Roberts, L. P. Elwell, and S. Falkow, Molecular character-
    ization of two beta-lactamase-specifying plasmids isolated
    from Neisseria gonorrhoeae, J. Bacteriol. 131:557 (1977).
5. T. E. Sox, W. Mohammed, and P. F. Sparling, Transformation-
    derived Neisseria gonorrhoeae plasmids with altered
    structure and function, J. Bacteriol. 138:510 (1979).
6. T. E. Sox, W. Mohammed, E. Blackman, G. Biswas, and P. F.
    Sparling, Conjugative plasmids in Neisseria gonorrhoeae,
    J. Bacteriol. 134:278 (1978).
7. F. C. Tenover, L. W. Mayer, and F. E. Young, Physical map of
    the conjugal plasmid of Neisseria gonorrhoeae, Infect.
    Immun. 29:181 (1980).
8. M. Roberts, P. Piot, and S. Falkow, The ecology of gonococcal
    plasmids, J. Gen. Microbiol. 114:491 (1979).
9. R. S. Foster and G. C. Foster, Electrophoretic comparison of
    endonuclease-digested plasmids from Neisseria gonorrhoeae,
    J. Bacteriol. 126:1297 (1976).
10. J. K. Davies and S. Normark, A relationship between plasmid
    structure, structural lability, and sensitivity to site-
    specific endonucleases in Neisseria gonorrhoeae, Molec.
    gen. Genet. 177:251 (1980).
11. L. P. Elwell, M. Roberts, L. W. Mayer, and S. Falkow,
    Plasmid-mediated beta-lactamase production in Neisseria
    gonorrhoeae, Antimicrob. Agents Chemother. 11:528 (1977).
12. P. L. Perine, C. Thornsberry, W. Schalla, J. Biddle, M. S.
    Siegel, K.-H. Wong, and S. E. Thompson, Evidence for two
    distinct types of penicillinase-producing Neisseria gonor-
    rhoeae, Lancet 2:993 (1977).
13. P. F. Sparling, T. E. Sox, W. Mohammed, and L. F. Guymon,
    Antibiotic resistance in the gonococcus: Diverse mecha-
    nisms of coping with a hostile environment, in "Immuno-
    biology of Neisseria gonorrhoeae," G. F. Brooks, E. C.
    Gotschlich, K. K. Holmes, W. D. Sawyer, and F. E. Young,
    eds., American Society for Microbiology, Washington, D.C.
    (1978).
14. P. F. Sparling, Genetic transformation of Neisseria gonor-
    rhoeae to streptomycin resistance, J. Bacteriol. 92:1364
    (1966).
15. R. Laufs, P.-M. Kaulfers, G. Jahn, and U. Teschner, Molecular
    characterization of a small Haemophilus influenzae plasmid
    specifying β-lactamase and its relationship to R factors
    from Neisseria gonorrhoeae, J. Gen. Microbiol. 111:223
    (1979).

16. A. Percival and C. A. Hart, Rationale for antimicrobial
     therapy of infections caused by multiply resistant
     Neisseria gonorrhoeae, in "Immunobiology of Neisseria
     gonorrhoeae," G. F. Brooks, E. C. Gotschlich, K. K.
     Holmes, W. D. Sawyer, and F. E. Young, eds., American
     Society for Microbiology, Washington, D.C. (1978).

17. C. Thornsberry, J. W. Biddle, P. L. Perine, and M. S. Siegel,
     Susceptibility of Neisseria gonorrhoeae from the United
     States and the Far East (β-lactamase negative and
     positive) to antimicrobial agents, in "Immunobiology of
     Neisseria gonorrhoeae," G. F. Brooks, E. C. Gotschlich, K.
     K. Holmes, W. D. Sawyer, and F. E. Young, eds., American
     Society for Microbiology, Washington, D.C. (1978).

18. B. I. Eisenstein, T. Sox, G. Biswas, E. Blackman, and P. F.
     Sparling, Conjugal transfer of the gonococcal penicil-
     linase plasmid, Science 195:998 (1977).

19. G. D. Biswas, E. Y. Blackman, and P. F. Sparling, High-
     frequency conjugal transfer of a gonococcal penicillinase
     plasmid, J. Bacteriol. 143:1318 (1980).

20. M. Roberts and S. Falkow, Plasmid-mediated chromosomal gene
     transfer in Neisseria gonorrhoeae, J. Bacteriol. 134:66
     (1978).

21. L. Norlander, J. Davies, and S. Normark, Genetic exchange
     mechanisms in Neisseria gonorrhoeae, J. Bacteriol. 138:756
     (1979).

22. V. I. Steinberg and I. D. Goldberg, On the question of
     chromosomal gene transfer via conjugation in Neisseria
     gonorrhoeae, J. Bacteriol. 142:350 (1980).

23. T. J. Dougherty, A. Asmus, and A. Tomasz, Specificity of DNA
     uptake in genetic transformation of gonococci, Biochem.
     Biophys. Res. Commun. 86:97 (1979).

24. K. L. Sisco and H. O. Smith, Sequence-specific DNA uptake in
     Haemophilus transformation, Proc. Natl. Acad. Sci. USA
     76:972 (1979).

25. D. B. Danner, R. A. Deich, K. L. Sisco, and H. O. Smith, An
     eleven base pair sequence determines the specificity of
     DNA uptake in Haemophilus transformation, Gene 11:311
     (1980).

GENETIC ORGANIZATION AND EXPRESSION

OF NON-CONJUGATIVE PLASMIDS

H. John J. Nijkamp and Eduard Veltkamp

Department of Genetics, Biological Laboratory

De Boelelaan 1087
Amsterdam, The Netherlands

INTRODUCTION

Non-conjugative plasmids are plasmids that are not able to
transfer themselves to other cells without the help of a conjugative system provided by the large, so-called conjugative plasmids.
Non-conjugative plasmids are small plasmids. Their M.W. generally
does not exceed 10 Megadaltons. Furthermore, they are multicopy
plasmids; that means that they are usually present to the extend
of 10-20 copies per chromosome. As all other small DNA molecules,
the non-conjugative plasmids are very attractive for basic research. Over the past ten years studies on plasmids were focused
on basic questions dealing with gene-function, gene-organisation,
gene-expression, mechanism and control of replication, and plasmid
mobilisation. And, ever since it became apparent that plasmids
are a very useful tool in genetic engineering also a lot of work
has been done on the construction of appropriate vector molecules.

The availability of mutants is of discisive importance in the
study on the genetic organisation and gene functions of plasmids.
Over the past five years new approaches became available for the
construction and isolation of plasmids mutants and for the study
of their behaviour. Construction and isolation of plasmid mutants
can, in addition to classical methods, be achieved by insertion
of transposable elements into plasmid DNA and plasmid deletions/
hybrids can be constructed in vitro by using appropriate restriction nucleases. Besides these methods of "site-directed" mutagenesis, new DNA sequencing procedures as well as techniques to
study gene expression in vivo (minicells and maxicells) and in
vitro (cell-free systems) have become available that allows
detailed characterisation of plasmid mutants.

247

This brief review on the genetic organisation and expression
of non-conjugative plasmids, will be focussed mainly on the small
bacteriocinogenic E. coli plasmids CloDF13 (originally from
E. cloacae DF13) and ColEl, because these plasmids have been
studied quite well.

GENETIC MAP OF BACTERIOCINOGENIC PLASMIDS

Glancing at a genetic map of a non-conjugative plasmid, e.g.
of CloDF13 (Fig. 1), one can observe, to a certain extend, a
clustering of those sites and genes that are functionally related.
In the region involved in replication the origin of replication
as well as the genetic information essential for the control of
replication is located. The adjacent region is involved in
bacteriocinogenicity; three genes are located in this region.
Another cluster is located at the lefthand side of the map. This
region is responsible for the mobilisation of the plasmid, a
mobilisation that is regular for the transfer of the non-
conjugative plasmid to other cells. In addition to these genes,
regions have been located that are involved in the maintenance of
the plasmid, the inhibition of the propagation of RNA phages and
the transfer of certain other plasmids and the inhibition of the
multiplication of DNA phages.

The ColEl and CloDF13 proteins that have been identified
both, in vivo (using E. coli minicells) and in vitro are listed
in Table 1. CloDF13 encodes at least for 10 polypeptides; the sum
of their M.W. comprises about 70% of the coding capacity of
CloDF13. In case of ColEl about 13 plasmid encoded polypeptides
have been identified. The sum of their M.W, amounts to about
400 KD., which is significantly more than the coding capacity of
ColEl. Some of these polypeptides may be breakdown products of
other proteins. The functions or presumptive functions of these
proteins are also listed in Table 1.

Fig. 2 shows the RNA species produced by CloDF13 in CloDF13
containing minicells. About 15 of these RNA bands are CloDF13
specific: four of them (indicated in Fig.2) have been mapped
precisely.

FUNCTIONS SPECIFIED BY CloDF13 AND ColEl

In this section the different plasmid regions as well as
their functions will be discussed in more detail. In Fig. 3, the
region to the left of gene H is the region involved in replication.
Although a description of the mechanisme of vegetative plasmid
replication is out of the focus of this paper, it is relevant to
mention that these small plasmids are fully dependent for their
replication on enzymes specified by the host. The CloDF13 replication starts at the origin (2,8%) and proceeds uniderectional.

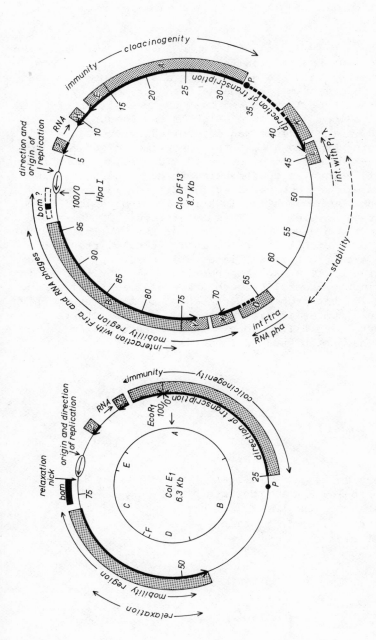

Figure 1. Comparison of the genetic and functional maps of the bacteriocinogenic plasmids ColE1 and CloDF13 32. The single Eco R1 site defines the zero point on the ColE1 map whereas the single HpaI site is used as reference point on the Clo DF13 map. Both maps have been orientated in such a way that they can easily be compared. bom indicates the basis of mobilization. For references see text. The inner circle on the ColE1 map represents the HaeII cleavage map.

The sequences upstream the replication origin are required for
autonomous replication and may reflect a regulatory role in the
initiation of plasmid replication.

What are the mean features of this region? (1) RNA primer for
the initiation of DNA replication is synthesized starting from
promoter P3. Actually this RNA molecule is a pre-primer, because
it is processed into a primer by RNAase H as was shown by Itoh
and Tomizawa for ColEl[1]. They showed that the pre-primer of ColEl
is 555 nucleotides long. In case of CloDF13 the length of this
pre-primer is 580 nucleotidesas was determined by Stuitje et al.[2]
(2) Codon analysis[3] has shown that the pre-primer might code for
a basic, arginin-rich protein of about 45 amino acids, both for
ColEl and CloDF13, since an open reading frame is present. However, such a protein has not yet been identified. (3) A small RNA
molecule of about 100 nucleotides (RNA-100) is synthesized from
the opposite strand of CloDF13[4]. This RNA molecule is therefore
complementary to the 5' end of the preprimer RNA. A similar situation exists in case of ColEl[5,6,7,8]. Interestingly, the transcription of the pre-primer is initiated at a position where the
RNA-100 is terminated. The crucial question is whether this region
has a function in the control of vegetative plasmid replication.
In order to tackle that problem, replication control mutants have
been isolated in a number of different ways. A few mutants in
replication control, so called copy mutants because of an increased copy number, have been studied in detail.

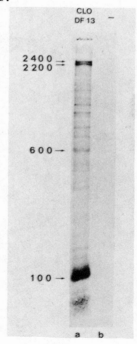

Figure 2.
SDS-urea polyacrylamide gel electrophoresis of ³H-labeled RNA synthesized
in minicells harboring the CloDF13
cop3 plasmid (track a) or in plasmidless minicells (track b)[4].

TABLE 1

PROTEINS ENCODED BY COL E1 AND CLO DF 13

Col E1		Clo DF13	
mw x 10^{-3}	Function	mw x 10^{-3}	Function
62	mobility[a]	64	cloacin DF 13[d]
58	colicin E1[b]	62	mobility, RNA phage int.[d]
44	unknown	21	unknown
41	unknown	18	unknown
36	unknown	17	RNA phage int.[d]
33	unknown	12.5	unknown
30	unknown	11	DNA phage int., stability? [d]
27	unknown	10	unknown
17	mobility[a]	8.5	immunity[d,e]
15	mobility[a]	6.5	transport of cloacin
14	immunity[c]		
10	mobility[a]		
6.5	unknown		

[a] The presumptive function of these proteins is based on the fact that the molecular weights of these proteins correspond to those isolated from relaxable DNA[31].

[b] Identification of colicin E1 protein is based on identical molecular weights of labeled and purified colicin protein[37,38,39] immunological crossreactivity[40], and the effect on polypeptide synthesis of mutations affecting colicin activity[37,39]. Possible breakdown products of colicin E1, based on their reaction with colicin E1 antiserum, are omitted from this table.

[c] Identification of this protein is based on effects on polypeptide synthesis of mutations affecting immunity activity[39].

[d] The identification of these proteins is based on the effects on protein synthesis of mutations affecting the activities described[41,27,35,25,26].

[e] The aminoacid sequence of purified immunity protein has been determined as well as the DNA base sequence of the immunity gene[18]. This table is taken from Veltkamp and Stuitje[32].

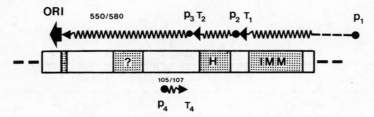

Figure 3. Transcriptional maps of the CloDF13 and ColEl DNA
          regions containing the origin of replication (ORI) as well
          as the genes coding for the bacteriocin and immunity (IMM)
          proteins. ●─▶: direction of transcription. The estimated
          length of the RNA molecules is given in nucleotides.
          [?] : CloDF13 and ColEl homologous sequences that
          might code for protein. P1 indicates the cloacin promotor;
          T1 and T2: termination site 1 and 2.

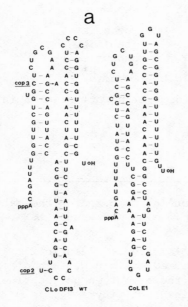

a

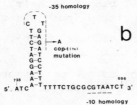

b

Figure 4A

Possible secondary structure for the
105 and 107 nucleotide RNAs.
The CloDF13 copy mutations cop3
(G→A) and cop1 (C→U) are indicated.

Figure 4B

Possible secondary structure of the
DNA region involved in the termination
as well as initiation of the downstream transcription[2,3].
The possible RNA polymerase recognition (-35 homology) and binding site
(-10 homology) involved in initiation
of primer precursor RNA synthesis are
indicated. Downstream transcription
proceeds from left to right. The cop1
ts (G→A) is indicated.

For instance two non-conditional CloDF13 copy mutants have been mapped by base sequence analysis[2]. Both mutations cop2, cop3 are located within the region encoding for the RNA-100 suggesting that this RNA molecule modulates the rate of initiation of DNA synthesis in a negative way. However, the situation is complex, because these mutations do alter, at the same time, also the pre-primer RNA. In our laboratory we have also located a conditional copy control mutation cop1-Ts[2], a mutation that causes both, an increase in plasmid copy number and cell death at increased temperature. This ts mutation has been located in the terminator, T2, of the bacteriocin operon[2]. Also, a Col E1 copy mutation has been located by Polisky et al.[10].

Fig. 4A shows the 100 n.RNA molecules of CloDF13 and ColE1. They can be folded in a similar way, although the sequences differ to about 30%[2]. Apparently the secondary structure is very important for the functionning of this RNA[9]. The sequence of the first loop at the 5' end (GCUCUC) of the RNA-100 of CloDF13 is identical to that of ColE1. The sequence of the second and the third loop of CloDF13 (UCCCCA) are identical. These loops sequences are also identical in ColE1 (GUUGGUAGC). However, the latter sequences of CloDF13 differ from those of ColE1. An interesting question is whether these differences might be the reason for the fact that CloDF13 and ColE1 are compatible.

As indicated earlier, the cop1-Ts mutation (G→A transition) is located in the terminator region (T2) of the bacteriocin operon. This terminator region overlaps with the promotor sequence for the synthesis of the pre-primer RNA (Fig. 4B). Therefore, the effect of the cop1-Ts mutation, a temperature inducible plasmid copy number, could be the result of read through of transcription. We postulate that the formation of the pre-primer RNA is regulated in different ways: (1) The synthesis of the pre-primer RNA is negatively controlled by the RNA-100, e.g. by the formation of a RNA-RNA or RNA-DNA hybrid, (2) The synthesis of the pre-primer RNA may be also controlled by transcriptional activities of the bacteriocin operon since promotor P3 overlaps the terminator T2 of the bacteriocin operon (Fig.3) the leftward transcription of this operon might influence the rate of pre-primer synthesis, (3) Additional controls might operate at or around the origin of replication by the formation of the primer and/or start of DNA synthesis.

Adjacent to the replication region, a DNA region is located that is involved in bacteriocinogenicity (Fig.5). This region code for the production of the antibiotic protein cloacine DF13 in case of CloDF13 and colicin E1 in case of ColE1. Both proteins have been purified and characterized.[11,12,13,14]. Cells carrying these plasmids are immune to the lethal effect of their homologous

bacteriocines. The genes responsible for this immunity have been
located both for ColE1[15,16] and for CloDF13[17,18]. The CloDF13
immunity substance has been purified and characterized in our
laboratory as a protein of 85 amino acids[18,19,20]. This protein
is able to inactivate the cloacin protein by the formation of an
immunity protein-cloacin complex[21]. The cloacin and immunity gene
can be induced by e.g. mitomycin C or UV. The mechanism of
regulation has not yet been elucidated.

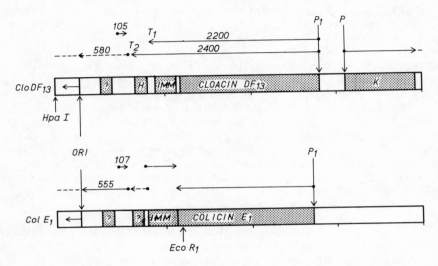

Figure 5. Regulatory sites involved in CloDF13 and ColEl
          replication. Presumed promotors and terminators are
          indicated by ● and ← respectively. The direction of
          transcription is indicated by an arrow. The estimated
          length of the RNA molecules is given in nucleotides.

Recent data show that this CloDF13 region encodes for two classes
of RNA molecules; the transcription of these RNA molecule is
initiated at the cloacin promotor, located at 32%[4]. The
transcription of the first class, consisting of 2200 nucleotides
RNA terminates at terminator T1, while the second class,
consisting of 2400 nucleotides RNA overlaps the first class and
terminates at T2[4]. This latter transcript does not only contain
the message for the cloacin and immunity proteins, but it also
codes for the third protein, protein H. This latter protein has
been identified as a 5800 daltons protein and is localized as
an innermembrane protein. The synthesis of this protein largely
depends on a functional cloacin promotor (P1). What is the function
of protein H? If we raise the level of protein H in the cell by
either induction with mitomycin C or by gene dosage effect using

a thermosensitive copy mutant, the cells will die and will lyse
as well. When gene H is missing e.g. by deletion, the bacterial
cells will still die in this experiment, but cells wil not lyse
anymore. Protein H is likely involved in the lysis of the cell
under these circumstances[23]. The natural function of protein H
could be the transport of the cloacin-immunity protein complex
through the cell envelope, because H⁻ cells accumulate this complex inside the cell[23].

With respect to ColE1 the situation seems to be different.
The direction of transcription of the immunity gene is the
opposite of that of CloDF13[6,24]. That means that in case of
ColE1 the genes for colicin, the immunity protein and the
hypothetical protein H (gene H is likely present also in ColE1
because of the presence of an open reading frame) are not part
of one transcriptional unit.

In Fig. 1, the CloDF13 region next to the bacteriocin operon,
two genes (K and L) have been identified[25]. In contrast to the
transcription of the bacteriocin operon, the transcription of
this region proceeds clockwise[4]. Gene L is involved in an interaction with the development of double standed DNA phages.
Although certain transposon insertions in gene K have the same
effect as insertions in gene L, it could be demonstrated that
this effect is due to a polar effect on gene L. The gene L
product inhibits the multiplication of phages like Pl, Tl, and λ,
leading to a reduced burstsize and an altered phage morphology[25].
It is important to note, that plasmids, even small plasmids, can
affect the propagation of phages and that, in general, one should
be aware of such phenomena in case of phage typing of bacteria.

The neighbouring area (Fig.1) plays a role in the stable
maintenance of the plasmid CloDF13. Deletion of this region in a
CloDF13 copy mutant gives rise to large multimeric plasmid
molecules and finally to loss of the plasmids from the cell[27].
Integration of an ampicillin transposon (Tn901) restores the
stability. Probably the Tn901 transposon, like Tn3[23], provides for
a system that resolves multimeric molecules into monomeric
molecules, a system that the CloDF13 deletion mutant is missing.
The stability region has, like the replication control region, a
function in incompatibility[23] (Stuitje, unpublished observations).

PLASMID MOBILIZATION

Genetic studies reveal that the transfer of CloDF13 and ColE1
does not entirely depend on the conjugative plasmid, but also on
genetic information present in case of non-conjugative
plasmids[22,27,28,29]. Three CloDF13 genes (B, X and Y) have been

identified that are involved in mobilization of CloDF13[22]. Mutations
in either of these genes can be complemented by the wild type
CloDF13, but not by the wild type ColE1. The gene products for
mobilization are not exchangeable between CloDF13 and ColE1[22]. One
type of mutant cannot be complemented at all[27]. The location of such
a cis-acting sequence, named bom[30] (basis of mobilization) is
interesting because it is very close or may be even identical to
the site where the three protein components of the ColE1 relaxation
complex[31] are bound and where upon relaxation a single strand nick
is produced bij one of these proteins. This nick is considered as
one of the steps in the initiation of transfer replication. At the
moment none of the three proteins present in the relaxation complex
have been identified as one of the gene products of the mobilization
genes.

     The bom site in CloDF13 and ColE1 is distanced only a few
hundred base pairs downstream the origin of regetative replication
and this might be significant for the transfer of these plasmids.
A model that includes a relationship between the vegetative plasmid
replication process and the plasmid mobilization process has been
discussed by Veltkamp and Stuitje[33]. A conjugative plasmid, like F.
is required for the transfer of non-conjugative plasmids. The
question is whether all transfer genes of F are required for the
transfer of non-conjugative plasmids. Obviously, the F tra genes,
involved in mating pair formation are required, but F tra genes
required for the replication and transfer of F itself, like tra
M, I, and Z are not required for the transfer of CloDfl3 and
ColE1[33,34,27]. A difference between these plasmids is that the
tra D gene product is required for ColE1 transfer[33], but not for
CloDF13 transfer[27]. Apparently, CloDFl3 produces its own tra D
like product.

     One of the mobilization genes, gene B and also gene D, located
next to the mobilization region, are responsible for a reduced
propagation of male specific RNA phages and for an inhibition of
the transfer of F and ColE1[35]. Likely their gene products inhibit
the function of the F tra D product[36].

     In Fig.1 most of the present knowledge about the genetic
constitution of ColE1 and CloDF13 have been summerized. If we
compare both bacteriocinogenic plasmids, it is evident that the
overall genetic organization is very similar. However, many
differences exist, not only at the level of base sequences and
transcription patterns but also at the level of the action of the
gene products. Probably, this is the reason that certain gene
products are not exchangeable between CloDF13 and ColE1. Although
during the past 10 years, a reasonable amount of progress have been
made with respect to the genetic organization and expression of
non-conjugative plasmids, like ColE1 and CloDF13, many questions
have still to be answered for a clear comprehension of the
molecular biology of non-conjugative plasmids.

REFERENCES

1. T. Itoh, and J. Tomizawa, Proc. Nat. Acad. Sci. U.S.A.
   77:2450 (1980).
2. A.R. Stuitje, C.E. Spelt, E. Veltkamp, and H.J.J. Nijkamp,
   Nature, in press.
3. A.R. Stuitje, E. Veltkamp, J. Maat, and H.L. Heyneker,
   Nucleic Acid Res., 8:1459 (1980).
4. P.J.M. van den Elzen, R.N.H. Konings, E. Veltkamp, and
   H.J.J. Nijkamp, J. Bacteriol., 144:579 (1980).
5. A.D. Levine, and W.D. Rupp, in:"Microbiology 1978", p.lbo,
   D. Schlessinger, ed., A.S.M., Washington D.C. (1979).
6. R.K. Patient, Nucleic Acid Res., 6:2647 (1979).
7. P.T. Chan, J. Lebowitz, and D. Bastia, Nucleic Acid Res.,
   5:1247 (1979).
8. M. Morita and A. Oka, Eur. J. Biochem., 97:425 (1979).
9. R.H. Pritchard, This book.
10. B. Polisky, M. Muesing, J. Tamm, and H.M. Shepard, This book.
11. F.K. de Graaf, L.E. Goedvolk-de Groot, and A.H. Stouthamer,
    Biochim. Biophys. Acta, 221:556 (1970).
12. F.K. de Graaf, H.G.D. Niekus, and J. Klootwijk, FEBS Lett.,
    35:161 (1973).
13. S.A. Schwarz, and D.R. Helinsky, J. Biol. Chem., 246:6318 (1971).
14. S. Farid-Sabet, J. Biol. Chem., 253:982 (1978).
15. F. Heffron, M. So and B.J. McCarthy, Proc. Nat. Acad. Sci.
    U.S.A., 75:6012 (1978).
16. D.J. Sherratt, G. Dougan, M. Saul, B. Sunar, A. Twigg, and
    G. Warren, Contrib. Microb. Imm., 6:180 (1979).
17. E. Veltkamp, H. van de Pol, A.R. Stuitje, P.J.M. van den Elzen,
    and H.J.J. Nijkamp, Contrib. Microb. Imm., 6:111 (1979).
18. P.J.M. van den Elzen, W. Gaastra, C.E. Spelt, F.K. de Graaf,
    E. Veltkamp, and H.J.J. Nijkamp, Nucleic Acid Res.,
    8:4349 (1980).
19. A.J. Kool, A.J. Borstlap, and H.J.J. Nijkamp, Antimicrob.
    Agents Chemo ther., 8:76-85 (1975).
20. A.J. Kool, C. Pols, and H.J.J. Nijkamp, Antimicrob. Agents
    Chemo ther., 8:67 (1975).
21. F.K. de Graaf and P. Klaassen-Boor, Eur. J. Biochem.,
    73:107 (1977).
22. H. van de Pol, Thesis, Free University, Amsterdam (1980).
23. M.J.J. Hakkaart, E. Veltkamp, and H.J.J. Nijkamp,
    unpublished results.
24. A. Oka, N. Nomura, M. Morita, H. Sugisaki, K. Sugimoto, and
    M. Takanami, Mol. Gen. Genet., 172:151 (1979).
25. H. van de Pol, E. Veltkamp, and H.J.J. Nijkamp, Mol. Gen. Genet.,
    178:535 (1980).
26. A.R. Stuitje, E. Veltkamp, P.J.M. van den Elzen, and
    H.J.J. Nijkamp, Nucleic Acid Res., 5:1801 (1978).

27. H. van de Pol, E. Veltkamp, and H.J.J. Nijkamp, Mol. Gen. Genet.
    160:139 (1978).
28. G. Dougan, M. Saul, G.J. Warren, and D. Sherratt, Mol. Gen.
    Genet., 158:325 (1978).
29. J. Inselburg, and P. Ware, J. Bacteriol., 132:321 (1977).
30. G.J. Warren, A.J. Twigg, and D.J. Sherratt, Nature, 274:259
    (1978).
31. M.A. Lovett, and D.R. Helinski, J. Biol. Chem., 250:8796 (1975).
32. E. Veltkamp and A.R. Stuitje, Plasmid, in press.
33. G. Alfaro, and N.S. Willetts, Genet. Res., 20:279 (1972).
34. N.S. Willetts, and J. Maule, Mol. Gen. Genet., 169:325 (1979).
35. H. van de Pol, E. Veltkamp, and H.J.J. Nijkamp, Mol. Gen.
    Genet., 168:309 (1979).
36. N. Willetts, Mol. Gen. Genet., 180:213 (1980).
37. R.B. Beagher, R.C. Tait, M. Betlach, and H.W. Boyer, Cell,
    10:521 (1977).
38. G. Dougan, and D.J. Sherratt, Mol. Gen. Genet., 151:151 (1977).
39. J. Inselburg, and B. Appelbaum, J. Bacteriol., 133:1444 (1978).
40. Y. Ebina, F. Kishi, T. Nakazawa, and A. Nakazawa,
    Nucleic Acid Res., 7: 639 (1979).
41. P.M. Andreoli, N. Overbeeke, E. Veltkamp, J.D.A. van Embden,
    and H.J.J. Nijkamp, Mol. Gen. Genet., 160:1 (1978).

STURCTURE-FUNCTION RELATIONSHIPS IN ESSENTIAL REGIONS FOR PLASMID REPLICATION

Avigdor Shafferman, David M. Stalker, Aslihan Tolun,
Roberto Kolter and Donald R. Helinski

Department of Biology
University of California at San Diego
La Jolla, CA   92093

INTRODUCTION

The development of recombinant DNA techniques has made possible
the isolation of segments of a plasmid DNA molecule that are essential for plasmid replication and stable maintenance in a bacterial
host. The discovery of rapid methods for the determination of the
nucleotide sequence of DNA fragments and the development of in vitro
systems for plasmid DNA replication permit a detailed analysis of
the structure-function relationships of these various DNA segments.
Such an analysis has been carried out on the essential region for
plasmid R6K DNA replication. In addition segments of the replication regions of plasmids R6K and F that are involved in plasmid
incompatibility have been isolated and analyzed. A striking feature
of the essential region of replication of plasmids R6K, F and the
broad host range plasmid RK2 [also studied in our laboratory[1-5]] is
the presence of direct repeats of nucleotide sequences. The important role of these direct repeats in both plasmid replication and
incompatibility and the major structural features of the essential
region for plasmid R6K replication will be considered in this article.

GENERAL PROPERTIES OF PLASMID R6K

The antibiotic resistance plasmid R6K is 38 kb in size and
specifies resistance to the antibiotics streptomycin and ampicillin[6].
This multi-copy plasmid (10-15 copies per chromosome equivalent) is
a member of incompatibility group X. The positions of three origins
of replication, designated α, β and γ, and a unique terminus of
replication have been determined on a restriction map of this

259

plasmid (Fig. 1)[7-10]. At least two of the origins, α and β, exhibit
in *Escherichia coli* sequential, bi-directional replication toward
an asymmetrically located terminus [11,12]. An *in vitro* system has
been developed from *E. coli* for the replication of plasmid R6K and
its derivatives[13,14]. The frequency of usage of the α, β and γ
origins *in vitro* (0.20:0.43:0.37, respectively) differs from that
observed *in vivo* where the α origin is used predominantly[9,10].

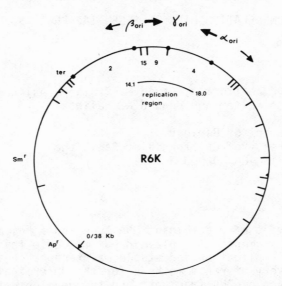

Figure 1. Physical and genetic map of R6K. The arrows indicate
the sequential bi-directional mode of replication of replication
origins α and β. 2, 15, 9 and 4 refer to specific Hind III fragments. The positions of other Hind III sites, the Bam H1 (↑)
site and EcoRI (▼) sites also are indicated. ■ter refers to the
terminus of replication.

CONSTRUCTION OF PLASMID R6K DERIVATIVES

A variety of restriction endonucleases have been used to delete
regions of R6K non-essential for replication[8,15]. The replication
region of plasmid R6K, encompassing all three replication origins,
is approximately 4 kb in length and includes Hind III fragments 2,
15, 9 and 4. A number of low molecular weight derivatives of R6K,
capable of autonomous replication, have been obtained. We have
found that Hind III fragments 15 and 9 and a portion of 4 are common to all of these fragments[15]. This minimal replication region,
depicted in Fig. 2, consists of two separate components: the γ
origin and a structural gene, designated *pir*, which acts *in trans*
to support the replication of the γ origin[16]. Interruption of the
junction between Hind III fragments 4 and 9 by insertion of DNA
fragments results in inactivation of the γ origin. Similar attempts

in our laboratory to derive minimal replicons for the α and β
origins have not been successful.

Studies with the *in vitro* R6K replication system identified
the π protein as the trans-acting product of the *pir* gene[14]. This
35,000 dalton protein is required for the initiation of R6K replication in a cell-free *E. coli* system[14].

NUCLEOTIDE SEQUENCE OF THE R6K γ-REPLICON

The nucleotide sequence of the entire π gene-γ origin replicon
(consisting of 1583 bp) has been determined[17,18]. The γ origin component of this replicon has been delineated by the insertion of the
Tn5 transposon into a number of sites in the γ origin region and
determination of the effect of the Tn5 insertions on γ origin
activity[19].

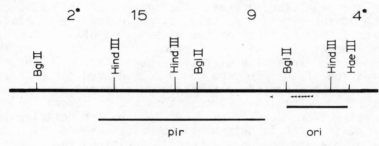

Figure 2.   Map of the R6K γ-replicon. The locations of the *pir* gene
and γ origin (ori) of replication are indicated. The arrow heads
represent the positions of the 22 bp nucleotide sequence repeats.

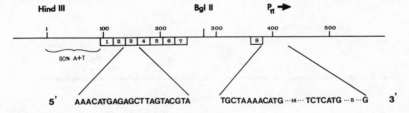

Figure 3.   Major features of the nucleotide sequence of the γ
origin region of R6K[17,18]. Nucleotide sequences of one of the
direct repeats and putative RNA polymerase recognition and binding
sites in the promoter region (P$_\pi$) of the π gene also are indicated.

The functional γ origin was found to consist of a 260 bp region
extending from a short distance to the left of the junction of
Hind III fragments 4 and 9 (Fig. 3) to just before the Bgl II site
in Hind III fragment 9. The γ origin includes seven tandem 22 bp
direct repeats. Removal of three or more of the direct repeats
results in loss of origin activity[19]. As indicated in Fig. 3, an

eighth direct repeat of 22 bp is located in the putative π gene
promoter region. The nucleotide sequence of the R6K γ-replicon
contains only one large open reading frame[18] for translation that
spans Hind III fragments 2, 15 and 9[18]. This sequence encodes for
a polypeptide of 35,000 molecular weight which is in good agreement
with the size estimate of the π protein.

ROLE OF THE π PROTEIN IN R6K REPLICATION

     Both *in vivo* and *in vitro* evidence have been obtained for the
essential role of the π protein in plasmid R6K replication[14,16].
In addition, studies with the *in vitro* system for R6K replication
have provided evidence for the requirement for the π protein in the
initiation of R6K replication. The analysis of Tn5 transposition
mutants and deletions of the γ origin region also has established
a role of the 22 bp direct repeats in γ origin activity[19]. If π
functions as a regulatory protein, the control of initiation of
replication at the γ origin conceivably could involve a relatively
simple circuit that consists of the interaction of π as a positive
regulatory element with the direct repeats within the γ origin and
the autoregulated expression of the *pir* gene (Fig. 4). Autoregulated expression of the *pir* gene would be mediated conceivably by
interaction of the π protein with the eighth direct repeat in the
putative π promoter region. To test this model several *in vitro*
plasmid constructions were carried out to vary the cellular level
of π protein, in order to determine the effect of π protein concentration on plasmid copy number[20]. In addition, the effect of
the presence of π protein on *pir* gene promoter activity *in vivo*
was determined[20].

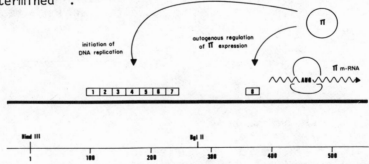

Figure 4. Model for the role of the π protein in the initiation
of R6K replication. The numbered boxes indicate the positions of
the eight 22 bp direct repeats.

AUTOGENOUS REGULATION OF EXPRESSION OF THE *pir* GENE

     If the expression of π is autogenously regulated, then a
change in the number of the *pir* genes per cell is not expected to
affect the concentration of π protein in that cell. To obtain

bacteria carrying different copies of the *pir* gene, isogenic strains of *E. coli* were either made lysogenic with a λ-*pir* hybrid phage[16] or transformed with a ColEI-*pir* recombinant plasmid (maintained at 20-40 copies per chromosome equivalent). The amount of π per cell was monitored by the *in vitro* R6K replication assay using extracts prepared from the λ-*pir* lysogens and the ColEI-*pir* transformants[20]. Similar amounts of π were recovered from both cell types. Thus at least a 20-fold increase in *pir* gene dosage has no significant effect on the concentration of π in the cell. These results are consistent with an autoregulated expression of the *pir* gene.

Nucleotide sequence analysis identified a putative promoter for the expression of the *pir* gene. That the *pir* gene contains its own transcriptional promoter was shown by fusing the putative *pir*-promoter to the *lac* Z gene[20]. Plasmids carrying the *pir*-*lac* fusion allowed expression of β-galactosidase (Fig. 5).

β-Galactosidase Activity in Cells Harboring Operon Fusions

Strain	Plasmids	β-Gal Units	%
MC1000	none	0	0
MC1000	pRK419	0	0
MC1000(λpir)	none	0	0
MC1000	pMC81	41	2
MC1000	pRK776	1364	81
MC1000	pRK776, pRK419	1443	85
MC1000	pRK775	1686	100
MC1000	pRK775, pRK419	763	45
MC1000(λpir)	pRK775	1118	66

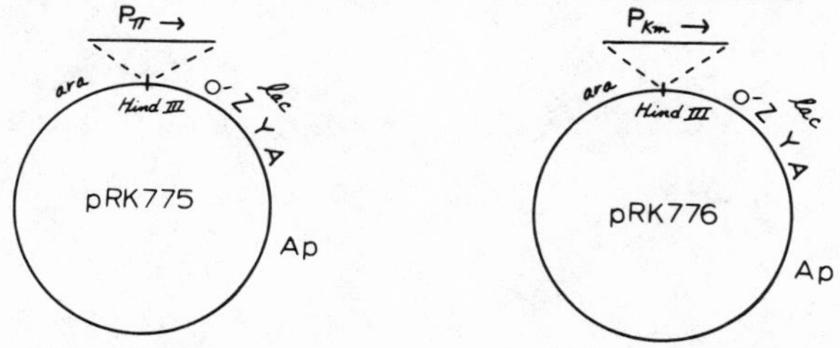

Figure 5. The construction of plasmid pCM81 was described[21]. Plasmids pRK775 and pRK776 are derivatives of pCM81. Plasmid pRK665[20] and pRK419[15] were the sources of the Hind III fragments containing the *pir* and the *kan* promoters, respectively.

When π protein is provided *in trans* by λ-*pir* or plasmid pRK419, a significant reduction in the levels of β-galactosidase expression from the *pir*-*lac* plasmid is observed (Fig. 5). The π protein has no effect on the expression of β-galactosidase from the kanamycin resistance promoter (Fig. 5). These results indicate that the π protein interacts with its own promoter region and thereby regulates its own expression.

π PROTEIN IS NOT THE REGULATORY ELEMENT FOR THE INITIATION OF
REPLICATION

A fundamental role assigned to π in the working model (Fig. 4)
is its ability to regulate positively the frequency of initiation
of R6K DNA replication. This regulatory role of π was tested by
placing the expression of π under different promoters and assaying
for the effects of different cellular levels of π on the copy number of derivative of the R6K plasmid. We were able to isolate an
R6K Hinf I fragment that contains the *pir* gene but is deleted for
the region containing the *pir* promoter sequence and the first five
nucleotides from its putative translational start signal. This
fragment was fused to a tryptophan promoter fragment containing
the first seven codons of the N-terminus of TrpE, which provides
a promoter sequence, a ribosomal binding site and a translational
start signal. The correct reading frame was provided by the introduction of EcoRI linkers between the *pir* and the *Trp* fragments.
Cells carrying either one of the four plasmids depicted in Fig. 6
were transformed subsequently with the R6K γ origin plasmid pRK526[16].
By varying conditions for tryptophan expression, the copy number of
pRK526 could be determined for varying cellular concentrations of
the π protein. Concentration of the π protein was assayed either
by following synthesis in minicells or by the *in vitro* R6K replication assay.

	Copy No. γ-ori	S-Met (minicells)	activity (in vitro rep.)
pRK665	18	1.0	1.0
pAS751 Repressed	18	1.3	0.057
Derepressed	17	7.0	N.D.
TrpR⁻	17	7.0	5.4
pAS752	18	0.1	0.85
pAS754	3	≤0.1	<0.01

Figure 6. The effect of variation of π concentration on the copy
number of a γ origin plasmid. All constructs are pBR322 derivatives
pRK665 contains the entire *pir* operon; pAS751, pAS752 and pAS754
carry the π sequences without the *pir* promoter. pAS752 and pAS756
differ in orientation of insertion of the π coding sequence in the
EcoRI site of pBR322. pAS754 and pAS751 differ in that the latter
also contains the tryptophan promoter fragment.

There is some discrepancy between the results obtained from minicells and the *in vitro* assay (Fig. 6). Nevertheless, regardless of the method for determining π concentration, the results show that varying the concentration of π in the cell over a 70-95 fold range has no effect on the copy number of the R6K γ origin plasmid. Recently this analysis was extended to the entire R6K replicon (includes all three origins of replication) with similar results. These observations argue against a positive regulatory role of π in replication. For the last construction (pAS754), shown in Fig. 6, the level of π was too low to be detected by the methods used and the copy number of pRK526 correspondingly is very low. In addition pRK526 is maintained unstably under non-selective conditions. This result is consistent with a minimal requirement of this essential initiation protein for stable maintenance of the plasmid.

π PROTEIN IS REQUIRED FOR ACTIVITY OF ALL THREE ORIGINS OF REPLICATION

The failure to isolate the most frequently used origins of replication *in vivo* (α and β) even when π is supplied *in trans*, raised the question of whether or not the requirement for π is limited to replication from the γ origin. To answer this question, *in vitro* site specific insertions were carried out, taking advantage of previous information that two Hind III recognition sites span the coding sequence for π. For the insertions a small Hind III fragment of 58 bp that was constructed by dimerization of a 29 bp segment located on pBR322 between the EcoRI and Hind III sites was employed. The EcoRI site provided an easy marker for the mapping of the site of insertion as well as a convenient tool for further genetic rearrangements. Figure 7 summarizes the data from these experiments. In the construction of pAS808 the 58 bp fragment is inserted in the junction of Hind III fragments 9 and 15 which corresponds to the N-terminus of the π protein. This plasmid was found to be unable to replicate in a *pol* A strain of *E. coli* unless a functional π protein is supplied *in trans*. It can be concluded therefore that replication of R6K from any one of the three origins requires the π protein.

Contrary to previous observations (Fig. 7, pRK693/Hin) insertion of this 58 bp fragment in the junction of Hind III fragments 9 and 4 (pAS865 and pAS807) did not abolish the γ origin activity. This unexpected finding may be due to the fact that the 58 bp insert is composed of two tandem inverted repeats and may therefore acquire a structure which would not adversely affect the structure of the γ origin.

THE γ ORIGIN REGION IS REQUIRED *in cis* FOR α AND β ORIGIN ACTIVITY

Plasmid pAS904, a deletion mutant of the R6K replicon that is missing the Hind III fragment 9, was constructed. Hind III fragment

9 contains a major part of the N-terminus of π together with the
essential seven 22 bp repeats of the γ origin (Fig. 2). Plasmid
pAS904, which contains both the α and the β origins of replication,
cannot be maintained in *E. coli* even when π is supplied *in trans*.
Thus, replication of R6K from the α or β origins requires the π
protein, which may be supplied *in trans*, and a *cis* interaction of
the γ origin region with α and β.

It is conceivable that the proposed interaction of the π
protein with the direct repeats of the γ origin region activates
also the α and β origins either via a transcriptional activation
event or by promoting the synthesis of RNA transcripts that subsequently are processed into a functional   initiation primer
specific for the α and β origins.

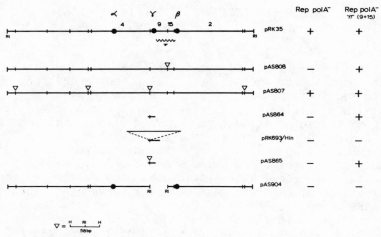

Figure 7. Ability of R6K derivatives to replicate in an *E. coli*
*pol*A strain. *Pol*A⁻ π (9+15) refers to a λ *pir* lysogen of the *pol*A
strain. Each triangle in the third line represents a different
plasmid carrying the 58 bp insert; pAS807 refers to an insert at
Hind III junction 9 and 4. Plasmids pAS807, pAS808 and pAS904 are
pSF2124 derivatives. pAS864, pAS865 and pRK693 are pBR322 derivatives. The pRK693/Hin represents a group of plasmids carrying
individual Hind III fragments from R6K (except Hind III-4) inserted
into the Hind III 9/4 junction.

DIRECT REPEATS OF NUCLEOTIDE SEQUENCES FUNCTION IN PLASMID
INCOMPATIBILITY

The region of R6K containing the seven 22 bp direct repeats,
which is required for replication from the α, β or γ origins, also
expresses R6K incompatibility. A segment of R6K containing the
seven 22 bp direct repeats, but non-functional as a replicon, was
cloned into the normally compatible plasmids pBR322 and pACYC184.

When these two hybrid plasmids were introduced into the same cell,
they behaved as an incompatible pair. Moreover, when hybrid plasmids were constructed that carried fewer copies of the 22 bp repeats.
the level of incompatibility correspondingly decreased (S. Yang, unpublished observations).

Direct repeats also have been identified in an incompatibility
region of the plasmid mini-F, a low molecular weight derivative of
the F plasmid[22,23]. The mini-F *incC* region of about 600 bp (45.8
- 46.4 Kb on F plasmid map) had been cloned on a ColEI replicon and
the resulting plasmid pRF7 was shown to express incompatibility with
mini-F derivatives (M. Kahn, unpublished results). Mutations[24] have
been obtained in the region 45.1 - 46.4 Kb [i.e. *incB* (45.1 - 45.8
Kb) plus *incC*], that result in a higher copy number and a loss of
incompatibility. The nucleotide sequence of the *incC* region was
analyzed to determine whether this region has the capacity to encode for a repressor protein. The nucleotide sequence[25] revealed
a very limited coding capacity; the largest putative polypeptides
with an ATG translational start signal are only 4.1 K and 3.4 K.
A striking feature of this region, however, is the presence of five
22 bp direct repeats within a 251 bp segment. Fig. 8 summarizes
the prominent features of this 453 bp region. To determine whether
it is a polypeptide or the direct repeat region that is required
for incompatibility, deletions were made in plasmid pRF7. Deletion
of the start signal ATG for the 4.1 K polypeptide was obtained by
partially digesting pRF7 with MboI; this deletion had no effect on
the expression of incompatibility. More extensive deletions were
carried out in order to remove the start codon for the putative
3.4 K polypeptide and copies of the 22 bp direct repeats. Plasmid
pRF7, linearized with EcoRI, was partially digested with BAL31.
The extent of the deletions obtained by this treatment was determined
by Dde I restriction enzyme analysis. Deletion derivatives that lack
the DdeI site at 129 bp only (type A in Fig. 8) no longer contain the
start codon and retain a region that contains three to five repeats.
No decrease in the expression of incompatibility was observed with
these plasmid derivatives. But type B deletions (Fig. 8) that lack
the Dde I sites at both 129 bp and 184 bp exhibited markedly decreased incompatibility. These plasmids retained only two or three
of the direct repeats.

These data indicated that the direct repeat region is important
for incompatibility. To test directly whether it is the repeats
that express incompatibility, we cloned the 58 bp DdeI fragment (129
- 184 bp) containing two 22 bp repeats into pACYC184 that had been
linearized by partial DdeI digestion[25]. The 58 bp fragment was
inserted into various sites in pACYC184. These hybrid plasmids
expressed incompatibility not only with mini-F but also with F'*lac*.
When two copies of the fragment were inserted in tandem, expression
of incompatibility was considerably stronger. In fact, in this
case it was not possible to propogate host cells that contained both

the hybrid plasmid and the mini-F under conditions of selection for both plasmids.

While a role of the direct repeats in the expression of F incompatibility is established, the mechanism by which these repeat sequences function in this phenomenon remains to be determined. The sequence is clearly too small to code for a regulatory repressor polypeptide that inhibits the initiation of replication, but the possibility of expression from the direct repeat segment of an RNA molecule that functions in the incompatibility phenomenon is not ruled out.

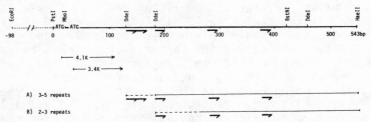

Figure 8. Prominent features of the *incC* region. The arrows show the location of the 22 bp repeats. The region shown by a dotted line is a ColEI DNA segment. Solid lines in (A) and (B) show the regions that are unambiguously present; dashed lines indicate the portions that may also be present[25].

CONCLUDING REMARKS

Direct nucleotide sequence repeats of 22 bp play a vital role in R6K γ origin activity. The region containing these repeats also is required for functional α and β origin activity. In addition, direct repeats play an important role in the expression of incompatibility by plasmids R6K and mini-F. When a 58 bp segment containing two copies of the 22 bp repeat sequences from the *incC* region of mini-F is inserted into plasmid pACYC184, which is normally compatible with the F plasmid, the hybrid plasmid is incompatible with mini-F derivatives and the F'*lac* plasmid. Similarly, the insertion of the 22 bp direct repeat region of R6K into the normally compatible plasmids pACYC184 and pBR322 renders these plasmids incompatible. Direct repeats of 17 bp also are a major feature of the replication origin region of plasmid RK2 and play a role in RK2 incompatibility. The biochemical nature of the role of these direct repeats in replication origin activity and incompatibility is unknown. Clearly the repeats can serve as binding sites for plasmid specific proteins involved in the replication and/or plasmid partitioning process. Indirect evidence has been obtained for the binding of the essential π protein to the R6K direct repeats. Alternatively or perhaps additionally, the direct repeats may facilitate association of the plasmid with a replication and/or plasmid partitioning membrane

site. Finally, it is possible that RNA transcripts of the direct
repeats account for their role in replication and/or incompatibility.

Considerable progress has been made towards an understanding
of R6K replication. The nucleotide sequence of the entire R6K λ-
origin replicon has been determined. Contained within this 1583 bp
sequence is the π protein structural gene and a 260 bp segment that
has been identified as the γ origin. No other protein is encoded
by this replicon. The π protein is required for the activity of
all three R6K origins of replication. Although it is required for
the initiation of replication, it is not a regulatory protein.
Clearly, however, there are constraints on the replication of
plasmid R6K since it is stably maintained at a copy number of 10-
15 per chromosome equivalent. The nature of the mechanism of
regulation of the R6K copy number remains to be determined.

ACKNOWLEDGEMENT

This work was supported by the National Institutes of Health
and the National Science Foundation. Avigdor Shafferman is a
recipient of J. E. Fogarty International Research Fellowship;
David M. Stalker is a recipient of an N.I.H. Postdoctoral Fellowship; Aslıhan Tolun is supported by a Damon Runyon-Walter Winchell
Cancer Fund (DR6-294-F).

REFERENCES

1. Meyer, R.J., Figurski, D. and Helinski, D.R. (1977),
       Mol. Gen. Genet. 152, 129-135.
2. Figurski, D. and Helinski, D.R. (1979), Proc. Natl. Acad.
       Sci. USA 76, 1648-1652.
3. Stalker, D.M., Thomas, C.M. and Helinski, D.R. (1981), Mol.
       Gen. Genet. 181 (in press).
4. Thomas, C.M., Stalker, D.M. and Helinski, D.R. (1981), Mol.
       Gen. Genet. 181 (in press).
5. Thomas, C.M. (1981), Plasmid (in press).
6. Kontomichalou, P., Mitani, M. and Clowes, R.C. (1970), J.
       Bacteriol. 104, 33-44.
7. Kolter, R. and Helinski, D.R. (1978), J. Mol. Biol. 124,
       425-441.
8. Crosa, J.H., Luttrop, L.K. and Falkow, S. (1978), J. Mol.
       Biol. 124, 443-468.
9. Inuzuka, N., Inuzuka, M. and Helinski, D.R. (1980), J.
       Biol. Chem. 255, 11071-11074.
10. Crosa, J.H. (1980), J. Biol. Chem. 255, 11075-11077.
11. Lovett, M.L., Sparks, R.B. and Helinski, D.R. (1975), Proc.
       Natl. Acad. Sci. USA 72, 2905-2909.
12. Crosa, J.H., Luttrop, L.K., Heffron, F. and Falkow, S.
       (1975) Mol. Gen. Genet. 140, 39-50.

13. Inuzuka, M. and Helinski, D.R. (1978), Biochemistry 17,
       2567-2573.
14. Inuzuka, M. and Helinski, D.R. (1978), Proc. Natl. Acad.
       Sci. USA 75, 5381-5385.
15. Kolter, R. and Helinski, D.R. (1978), Plasmid 1, 571-580.
16. Kolter, R., Inuzuka, M. and Helinski, D.R. (1978), Cell
       15, 1199-1208.
17. Stalker, D.M., Kolter, R. and Helinski, D.R. (1979), Proc.
       Natl. Acad. Sci. USA 76, 1150-1154.
18. Stalker, D.M., Kolter, R. and Helinski, D.R. (submitted
       for publication).
19. Kolter, R. and Helinski, D.R. (submitted for publication).
20. Shafferman, A., Kolter, R., Stalker, D.M. and Helinski,
       D.R. (submitted for publication).
21. Casadaban, M. and Cohen, S.N. (1980), J. Mol. Biol. 138,
       179-207.
22. Timmis, K., Cabello, F. and Cohen, S.N. (1975), Proc.
       Natl. Acad. Sci. USA 72, 2242-2246.
23. Lovett, M.A. and Helinski, D.R. (1975), J. Bacteriol. 127,
       982-987.
24. Manis, J.J. and Kline, B.C. (1978), Plasmid 1, 492-507.
25. Tolun, A. and Helinski, D.R. (submitted for publication).

CONTROL OF PLASMID REPLICATION AND ITS RELATIONSHIP

TO INCOMPATIBILITY

Robert H. Pritchard and Norman B. Grover*

Department of Genetics
University of Leicester
Leicester LE1 7RH, England

The mechanisms that determine plasmid copy number and the relationship between control of copy number and incompatibility are controversial topics. Since many people attending this conference do not have a day-to-day interest in them, it has been suggested to me that it would be useful to list the points on which there might be general agreement among those working on these related aspects of plasmid biology.

I propose to do this and then speculate a little about the nature of the control systems involved.

It is hazardous to generalise about plasmids. They are entrepreneurs of the bacterial world and different plasmids will no doubt have found different ways of securing their future. Nevertheless I believe that some generalisations can be made with reasonable confidence. Much of the experimental evidence upon which they are based is referred to in recent reviews by Gustafsson *et al*[1] and by Pritchard[2], and in various contributions to this meeting. It will not be listed exhaustively here.

I. The first point of agreement would be that plasmid replication is controlled at the level of initiation. What this means is that the concentration of plasmid origins is in some way sensed and maintained by regulation of the frequency of plasmid replication. Altering the size of a plasmid by inserting or removing DNA will not affect copy number unless it coincidentally interferes with the functioning of the control mechanism.

In apparent contradiction to this generalisation it has been
found that in some cases lengthening a plasmid by insertion of
additional DNA results in a compensating reduction in copy number
as if it were the total amount of plasmid DNA rather than the number
of plasmid copies that is controlled. In all of these exceptions,
however, the plasmids being studied were probably copy mutants (cop⁻)
in which the wild-type control system was defective. It has been
suggested that in such mutants copy number does not rise indefinitely
but plateaus when a cellular component involved in DNA chain elongation becomes rate limiting for plasmid replication. Increasing the
length of such a plasmid will inevitably lead to a reduction in copy
number. A direct test of this hypothesis has recently been made
with the plasmid ColE1. Deleting DNA of this plasmid does not affect
copy number of cop⁺ derivatives but increases the copy number of cop⁻
mutants[3].

The generalisation is thus only valid for plasmids with a
wild-type copy control genotype.

II. The rate of plasmid replication under steady state growth
conditions is determined by the concentration of an inhibitor which
is plasmid specified and acts in trans on all plasmids of the same
incompatibility group (see below). The inhibitor is an RNA species
in plasmids as different as ColE1[4] and R1[5] but is a protein in the
laboratory construct λdv (see ref. 2).

III. A third generalisation is that if a chimera is made between
plasmids with different copy numbers the copy number of the chimera
will not be less than that of the component plasmid with the higher
copy number. If the control system of the higher copy component
functions normally it will passively carry the copy number of the
low copy component to the same level. The control system of the
latter will sense this elevated copy number and respond by
reducing the probability of replication from its origin. This effect
has been termed switch-off[2]. The extent of switch-off will depend on
the sensitivity of the control system to enforced departure from the
copy number it freely determines.

Data conflicting with this generalisation also have been
reported. In the most fully analysed case[6] a chimera between ColE1
(average copy number about 20) and RK2 (average copy number about 5)
had a copy number of about 5. It was clearly demonstrated, however,
that the ColE1 component of the hybrid was incapable of initiating
replication and had even lost its capacity to express incompatibilit
against another ColE1 plasmid. Thus the conflict is only apparent.
Since the ColE1 component could be recovered from the cointegrate
as a functional replicon[6], its loss of function was probably due to
transcriptional read-through from an RK2 promoter across one of the

junctions between the two plasmids into the control region of ColE1.

IV. In the case of multicopy plasmids replication occurs at any
time during the cell cycle more or less randomly. Whether this
generalisation holds for plasmids like F, which have an exceptionally
low copy number (less than one plasmid per chromosome) is uncertain
because there is an unresolved conflict of evidence[7,8].

V.   This generalisation, which follows logically from IV, is that
plasmid replication is not correlated in time with (and therefore
not coupled to) any identifiable event in the cell cycle or chromosome replication cycle. This generalisation has been shown to be
valid for F despite the uncertainty about the timing of replication
of this plasmid[9].

VI. In the case of multicopy plasmids the choice of plasmid for
replication is approximately random. Thus a plasmid that has
recently replicated is as likely to replicate again as one that
has not[1].

VII. Incompatibility is the inevitable outcome of a copy control
system in which there is a random choice of plasmids for replication
and control of the total number of plasmid copies. This would be
true even if there were a perfect mitosis-like partitioning of
sister plasmids to daughter cells as was pointed out in the Sixties[10].
In cells initially containing an equal number of two phenotypically
distinguishable types of the same plasmid, random choice of plasmids
for replication would cause the proportions of each type to become
distributed randomly in the cell population. Some cells would
therefore contain only plasmids of one type. Since this sorting
out is irreversible, the whole population will ultimately consist
of pure clones containing one or other plasmid type. The severity
of incompatibility would be determined by the copy number. Low
copy plasmids will show strong incompatibility. High copy plasmids
will show weak incompatibility.

     It is not known whether sister plasmids do in fact undergo
mitosis-like partitioning of daughter cells. The alternative extreme
would be a completely random distribution of plasmids to daughter
cells[11]. If there were a random distribution some cells would be
born with no plasmid copies and the frequency of this zero class
is predictable[11]. For several low copy plasmids the zero class is
found to be too small to be consistent with random segregation
hence:

VII. There is a partitioning mechanism at least in low copy plasmids which ensures that cells are born with at least one plasmid copy. Plasmid mutants that are unstable (i.e. are lost from a significant proportion of the population at each cell doubling) are well known. Evidence that one class of unstable derivatives of the plasmid R1 is par^- is given by K. Nordström in his contribution to this meeting.

The nature of the copy number control system is beginning to emerge from molecular genetical analysis and from physiological studies of a number of plasmids.   Two observations from physiological studies providing useful insight into the properties of the control system will be mentioned here.

The concentration of all plasmids for which data are available (F, R1, P1, R6K, ColE1) is less at fast growth rates than it is at slow growth rates (e.g. Fig. 1).   The shape of the curve differs with different plasmids but the trend is the same suggesting that the relationship is a fundamental property of initiation control systems in plasmids.   The simplest relationship is that found for R1 where there appears to be a proportionality between doubling time and plasmid concentration[1].   What this means in the case of R1 is that the number of plasmid replications per minute is a constant independent of plasmid concentration.   This has lead Gustafsson and Nordström[12] to suggest that plasmid replication is controlled by a system that determines the frequency of replication without measuring the actual copy number, and that if initiation is controlled by an inhibitor there is no gene dosage effect on its concentration.

Another way of looking at this apparently paradoxical result is to consider the properties of a simple negative feedback loop

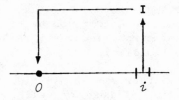

in which a plasmid gene i produces an inhibitor I which binds to the origin O of the plasmid to block initiation.   Assume that the probability of initiation at a plasmid origin is the same at all growth rates when the origin is 'open' (i.e. has no inhibitor bound to it).   Assume also that $[I] >>$ than K_b the binding constant of inhibitor.   Assume, finally, that I is produced constitutively

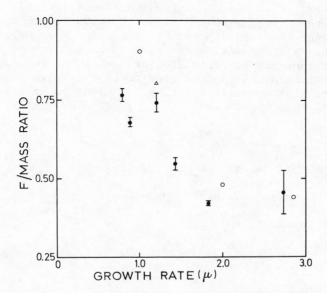

Figure 1.   The average concentration of F particles
in steady state exponential cultures of *Escherichia
coli* at different growth rates.   The figure is
modified from data presented in reference 9 which
gives details of the method of estimating F concentration.   One additional assumption made here is
that the average concentration of chromosome
origins is invariant.

and that the output of I per minute per i gene is proportional to the growth rate. (This relationship has been found for a number of constitutive genes in $E.coli$[13]). Using the first two assumptions:

$$\text{Replications/min/mass} \propto \frac{1}{[I]}\cdot[O] \qquad - \qquad - \qquad - \qquad (1)$$

or

$$= k\frac{1}{[I]}\cdot[O] \qquad - \qquad - \qquad (2)$$

In other words, the rate of replication in a unit of cell mass will be inversely proportional to the inhibitor concentration and directly proportional to the number of origins available for initiation. If the third assumption is correct then under steady state growth conditions the concentration of I will be proportional to the concentration of plasmid origins since every plasmid has an i gene and partially replicated plasmids with two origins and one i gene can be neglected. So:

$$[I] \propto [i] = [O] \qquad - \qquad - \qquad - \qquad - \qquad (3)$$

Therefore substituting for $[O]$ in (2) gives

$$\text{Replications/min/mass} = K. \qquad - \qquad - \qquad - \qquad (4)$$

where K is a constant, and

$$\text{Replications/generation/mass} = K.\tau \qquad - \qquad - \qquad (5)$$

or

$$[O] = K.\tau \qquad - \qquad - \qquad (6)$$

From this analysis it can be seen that the apparent constancy of the replication frequency independent of the origin concentration and the inhibitor concentration is due to the fact that they affect the probability of initiation in opposite directions. If the growth rate is raised $[O]$ falls, decreasing the rate of initiation, but $[I]$ falls proportionately increasing the rate of initiation by the same amount to give no net change of rate.

It is necessary to emphasise that a strict inverse proportionality between plasmid concentration and growth rate is not found for all plasmids (e.g. P1[14] and R6K[15]) indicating that the assumptions underlying equations (4)-(6) are not universally applicable.

The initial 'inhibitor dilution' model[10] proposed that initiation of chromosome and plasmid replication was under the control of a negatively acting inhibitor which was stable. In the same paper an alternative unstable inhibitor model was also considered. It is possible to distinguish between a stable inhibitor and an unstable inhibitor by determining the kinetics with which a plasmid equilibrates at its new concentration following a change of growth rate caused by a nutritional shift. Since the relationship in (3) can only hold during a transition if I has a rapid turnover the rate of replication can only remain constant during a transition if I is unstable. Gustafsson and Nordström[12] have found that equation (4) does hold during a transition indicating that $[I]$ is indeed unstable in R1.

Recent work[4] with the plasmid ColE1 suggests that in this plasmid initiation frequency is determined by a feedback loop with properties very similar to the unstable inhibitor model.

It might also be noted finally that in the case of ColE1 the copy number is not only higher at slow growth rates but also rises during the transition of a culture from exponential growth into stationary phase[3] as equation (6) predicts. The continued replication of ColE1 in the presence of chloramphenicol could also be predicted for a feedback loop of the type described. The fact that in more complex plasmids like F there is little run-on of plasmid replication during stationary phase or inhibition of protein synthesis suggests a more complex control of these plasmids or that other plasmid-coded or cellular products required for replication of these plasmids soon become limiting under these conditions.

R. H. P. especially wishes to acknowledge his appreciation of the many stimulating and challenging discussions he has had over many years with Kurt Nordström.

REFERENCES

1. P. Gustafsson, D. Dreisig, S. Molin, K. Nordström and B. E. Uhlin, *Cold Spring Harbor Symp. Quant. Biol.* 43:419-425 (1978).
2. R. H. Pritchard, *in* 'DNA Synthesis: Present and Future' Eds. I. Molineux and M. Kohiyama, Plenum, pp1-26 (1978).
3. B. Polisky, personal communication.
4. S. E. Conrad and J. L. Campbell, *Cell* 18:61-71 (1979).
5. K. Nordström, personal communication.
6. D. H. Figurski, R. J. Meyer and D. R. Helinski, *J. Mol. Biol.* 133:295-318 (1979).
7. J. Zeuthen and M. L. Pato, *Molec. Gen. Genet.* 111:242-255 (1971).
8. P. Gustafsson, K. Nordström and J. W. Perram, *Plasmid* 1:187-203 (1978).
9. R. H. Pritchard, M. G. Chandler and J. Collins, *Molec. Gen. Genet.* 138:143-155.
10. R. H. Pritchard, P. T. Barth and J. Collins, *Symp. Sco. Gen. Microbiol.* 19:263-298 (1969).

11. K. Nordström, S. Molin and H. Aagaard-Hansen, *Plasmid* 4:215-227
     (1980).
12. P. Gustafsson and K. Nordström, *J. Bacteriol.* 141:106-110 (1980)
13. B. M. Willumsen, *Cand. Scient. Thesis, University of Copenhagen.*
     (1975).
14. P. Prentki, M. Chandler, and L. Caro, *Molec. Gen. Genet.* 152:
     71-76 (1977).
15. M. R. Otten, M. Wlodarcyzk, B. C. Kline and R. Seelke, *Molec.
     Gen. Genet.* 177:495-500 (1980).

N.B. Grover's permanent address:
          Hubert H. Humphrey Centre for Experimental
            Medicine and Cancer Research,
          Hebrew University-Hadassah Medical School,
          Jerusalem 91000, Israel.

STRUCTURE AND FUNCTION OF THE REPLICATION ORIGIN REGION OF THE

RESISTANCE FACTORS R100 AND R1

Karen Armstrong, Jonathan Rosen, Thomas Ryder,
Eiichi Ohtsubo and Hisako Ohtsubo

Department of Microbiology, School of Medicine, State
University of New York at Stony Brook, Stony Brook
N.Y. 11794

R1 and R100 are large complex plasmids, approximately 90 kb in size, that code for multiple antibiotic resistance and functions involved in conjugal transfer of plasmid DNA.[1,2] Both R1 and R100 belong to the FII plasmid incompatability group,[3] indicating that the control of DNA replication in these plasmids is similar. Hetero-duplex studies have confirmed this relationship by showing that the regions of R1 and R100 that are required for autonomous DNA repli-cation have great sequence homology.[4] This region is about 2.5 kb in length for R100, and, in addition to the replication origin,[5,6,7] encodes at least one function that is required for replication. Part of this 2.5 kb replication region also encodes functions in-volved in plasmid incompatibility and copy number control.[6] Studies with R1 have led to very similar conclusions.[8]

pSM1 and pTR1 are small, high copy number plasmids that were derived from R100 and R1, respectively.[9,10,11] pSM1 and pTR1 share approximately 2.1 kb of homology, which is within the 2.5 kb repli-cation region. Part of the remainder of the replication region (about 250 bp) is non-homologous in R1 and R100 (Figure 1). We have determined the nucleotide sequence of the entire replication regions of both pSM1 and pTR1.[10,11] Here we will describe our analysis of this replication region with regard to the hypothetical coding frames, regions of possible secondary structure, RNA transcripts, and polypeptides that we have identified. This analysis has allowed us to formulate a model for DNA replication control in large drug resistance plasmids as exemplified by R1 and R100.

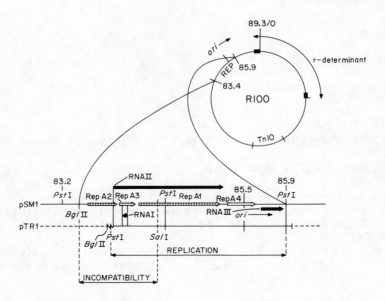

Figure 1.   A summary of some physical and genetic properties of
            plasmids R100, pSM1, and pTR1.. The open, crosshatched,
            and heavy arrows represent open reading frames predicted
            from nucleotide sequences, reading frames whose polypep-
            tide products have been identified, and RNA transcripts,
            respectively.

HYPOTHETICAL CODING FRAMES

     Four possible coding frames that are common to both pSM1 and
pTR1 have been identified from the nucleotide sequence of the replication regions of these two plasmids. These coding frames, which we
have designated RepA1, RepA2, RepA3 and RepA4, are all in the same
reading frame and are located within the nucleotide sequence as
shown in Figure 1. RepA1 is the longest common coding frame identified and encodes a polypeptide 33,000 daltons in size.[10,11] There
are 49 bp changes between the RepA1 coding frame of pSM1 and that of
pTR1. However, these changes result in only 8 amino acid substitutions because 39 of the bp changes occur in the third codon position.[10] Because the RepA1 coding frame crosses the junction of two
PstI fragments that is required in the original orientation for
autonomous plasmid replication,[6,7] it is likely that RepA1 is
required for replication.

     RepA2 and RepA3 are encoded within the region of R100 and R1
that specifies incompatibility and copy number functions.[6,7] (Figure 1) A part of this region (about 250 bases) is non-homologous

```
                                                                                        -500
5'-CCGGCGGTGAATÁCTGGCAACGTCAGAAGACGCÍTGCTGACAGAAAGGGAAGTCAGTTTTTATGAAAGGACTGTÍCAGAATTGTGGATATGAAGCGGTGGTATCTGTGTCCGCAG
                  PvuII                              PvuI                     -400
GTACGGGTCGCGGATATCGTCCAGCTGAACGGGAATAGTCCGGCCACGATCGCGCCAGTĜGTGGCAGTTATTCAGGATGGTGTCTCAGTGGCATGTTGATGTGGCATCGTTGAGCGGCGT
                                                     -300
TCGTTCAGTATTGTTGCAGCAGTAGAGCTGGATGATGCCAGCCATTTACGACCGGAACGCAGACGCCGGGATATTCTTCTGGAAGAGGTTCTGAGGCAGGCTGGTATTCCGTTGCTCAGA
              PstI        -200
AGCCACGATGCCAGAAAACTGCTGCAGATGACCGGAGAATGGCTGAATACAACAGGGGCTGATCAGCAGTCCCCGGAACATCGTAGCTGACGCCTTCGCGTTGCTCAGTTGTCCAACCCC
                                  -100
GGAAACGGGAAAAAGCAAGTTTTCCCCGCTCCCGGCGTTTCAATAACTGAAAACCCATACTATTTCACAGTTTAAATCACATTAAACGACAGTAATCCCCGTTGATTTGTGCGCCAACACA
  +1   BglII                                                                            100
GATCTTCGTCACAATTCTCAAGTCGCTGATTTCAAAAAACTGTAGTATCCTCTGCGAAACGATCCCTGTTTGAGTATTGAGGAGGCGAGATGTCGCAGACAGAAATGCAGTGACTTCCT
                                                                                MetSerGlnThrGluAsnAlaValThrSerS
erSerGlyAlaLysArgAlaTyrArgLysLysAsnProLeuSerSerAspAlaGluLysGlnArgLeuSerValAlaLeuArgAlaSerPheLysGluValGlnLysGluValPheLeuGluProL
CATCTGGCGCAAAACGAGCATACAGAAAGGGAATCCGCTTTCTGATGCAGAGAAACAAAGATTATCAGTGGCCCGTAAAAGAGCTTCGTTCAAGGAAGTAAAAGTATTTCTTGAACCAA
                                              200
yeTyrLysAlaMetGlnMetCysHisGlyLeuThrGlnAlaLeuGluValLeuThrAlaLeuIleLysSerGlnAlaLeuGlnAsnAspAlaCysAspAspGlyLeuThrPheL
AGTATAAGGCCATGCTCATGCAAATGTGTCATGAAGATGGTCTGACTCAGGCTGAAGTTCTGACCGCACTGATAAAAAGTGAAGCGCAAAACGATGCATGTGATGATGGGCTTACATTCT
                                              300
euSerValGlnLysIleSerAlaArgLeuLeuVal 400                                              MetTrpIleTyrArgArgGlnLysSerLysA
TGAGTGTTCAGAAGATTAGTGCTAGATTACTGATCGTTTAAGGAATTTTGTGGCTGGCCACGCGTAAGGTGGCAAGGACTGATTCTGATGTGGATTTACAGGAGCCAGAAAAGCAAAA
                              →RNA II                                              end RNA I
                                                                                      500
snProAspAsnLeuLeuGlnLeuLeuArgValArgLysArgTyrArgGlyProTyrSerGlnGlnPheSerTyrAlaGlySerIleValIleCysProGluLysPheLysT
ACCCCGATAATCTTCTTCAACTTTTGCGAGTACGAAAAGATTACCGGGGCCCACTTAAACCGTATAGCCAACAATTCAGCTATGCGGGGAGTATAGTTATATGCCCGGAAAAGTTCAAGA
                                                     600
hrSerPheCysAlaArgSerPheCysAlaLeu                    ValThrAspLeuHisGlnThrTyrTyrArgArgGlnValLysAsnProAlaProValGlyPheThrProAsnLeuGlyA
CTTCTTTCTGTCTGCTCGCTCCTTCTGCGCATTGTAAGTGCAGGATGGTGTGACTGATCTTCACCAAACGTATTACCGCCAGGTAAAGAAACCCGAATCCGGTGTTTACACCCCGTGAAGGTG
                                                     700
laGlyThrGluGlyPheLeuGluLysLeuMetGluLysAlaGluLeuAlaValGlnAspPhePheSerArgAspPhePheAlaIleHisValAlaHisGlyAlaArgSerArgGlyLeuArgArgArgMetProP
CAGGAACGCTGAAGTTCTGCGAAAAACTGATGGAAAAGGCGGTGGGCTTCACTTCCCGTTTTGATTTCGCCATTCATGTGGCGCATGCCCGTTCGCGTGGTCTGCGTCGACGCATGCCAC
                              SalI
roValLeuArgArgArgAlaIleAspAlaLeuLeuGlnGlyLeuCysPheHisTyrArgProLeuAlaAsnArgValGlnCysSerIleThrThrLeuAlaIleGluCysGluLeuAlaT
CAGTCTGCGTCGACGGGCTATTGATGCGCTCCTGCAGGGGCTGTGTTTCACTATGACCCGCTGGCCAACCGCGTCCAGTGCTCCATCACCACGCTGGCCATTGAGTGCGGACTGGCGA
                              PstI        900
hrGluSerValIleThrThrSerGlySerLeuThrAlaArgAlaThrArgAlaLeuThrPheLysAlaGlyLeuLeuGlyLeuIleThrTyrTyrGlnProLeuIleGlyCysTyrIleP
CGGAGTCTGCTGCCGGAAAAACTCTCCATCACCCGTGCCACCCGGGCCCTGACGTTCCTGTCAGAGCTGGGACTGATTACCTACCAGACGGAATAGACCCGCTTATCGGGTGCTACATTC
                              SmaI
roThrAspIleThrThrThrSerGlyLeuPheAlaAlaAlaLeuAspValSerGluGluAlaValAlaLeuAlaLaAlaArgArgSerArgValValTrpGlnAsnLysGlnArgLysGlnGlnGlyL
CGACCGATATCACGTTCACATCTGCACTGTTTGCTGCCCTCGATGTATCAGAGGAGGCAGTGGCCGCCGCGCCGCCGCAGCCGTGTGGTATGGGAAAACAAACAACGCAAAAAGCAGGGGC
                                                                             SmaI 1300
euAspThrArgLeuGlyMetAspGluLeuIleGluAlaIleAlaTrpArgAspPheValArgGluGluPheArgSerTyrGlnPheGluLeuLysSerArgGlyIleGluLysArgAlaArgAlaArgArgArgA
TGGATACCCTGGGCATGGATGAACTGATAGCGAAAGCCTGGCGTTTTGTTCGTGAGCGTTTTCGCAGTTATCAGACAGAGCTTAAGTCCCGGGGAATAAAGCGTGCCCGTGCGCGTCGTG
                              PvuII                HaeII
spAlaAspArgGluArgGluGlnAspIleValThrArgLeuValLeuLysArgGlnLeuThrArgGluIleAlaGluGlyTyrProThrArgAsnArgGluAlaValLeuArgGluValGlnValGluGluArgArgV
ATGCGGACAGGGAACGTCAGGATATTGTCACCCTGGTGAAACGGCAGCTGACGCGCGAAATCGCGGAAGGGCGCTTCACTGCCAATCGTGAGGCGGTAAAACGCGAAGTTGAGCGTCGTG
alLysGluArgGluMetIleLeuValSerArgAsnArgGluAsnTyrSerArgArgLeuAlaThrAlaSerPro
TGAAGGAGCGCATGATTCTGTCACGTAACCGTAATTACAGCCGGCTGGCCACAGCTTCCCCCTGAAAGTGACCTCCTCTGAATAATCCGGCCTGCGCCGGAGGCTTCCGCACGTCTGAAG
                                                                             1600
CCCGACAGCGCACAAAAAATCAGCACCACATACAAAAAACAACCTCATCATCCAGCTTCTGGTGCATCCGGCCCCCCCTGTTTTCGATACAAAACACGCCTCACGACGGGGAATTTTGC
                    1700                              HaeII
TTATCCACATTAAACTGCAAGGGACTTCCCCATAAGGTTACAACCGTTCATGTCATAAAGCGCCATCCGCCAGCGTTACAGGGTGCAATGTATCTTTTAAACACCTGTTTATATCTCCTT
                                              1900
TAAACTACTTAATTACATTCATTTAAAAAGAAAACCTATTCACTGCCTGTCCTGTGGACAGACAGATATGCACCTCCCACCGCAAGCGGCGGGCCCCTACCGGAGCCGCTTTAGTTACAA
                                                            2000
CACTCAGACACAACCACCAGAAAAACCCCGGTCCAGCGCAGAACTGAAACCACAAAGCCCTCCCTCATAACTGAAAAGCGGCCCCGCCCGCCGCCGAAGGGCCGGAACAGAGTCGCTTT
                                                     2100
TAATTATGAATGTTGTAACTACTTCATCATCGCTGTCAGTCTTCTCGCTGGAAGTTCTCAGTACACGCTCGTAAGCGGCCTGACGGCCCGCTAACGCGGAGATACGCCCCGACTTCGGG
                              2200
TAAACCCTCGTCGGGACCACTCCGACCGCGCACAGAAGCTCTCTCATGGCTGAAAGCGGGTATGGTCTGGCAGGGCTGGGGATGGGTAAGGTGAAATCTATCAATCAGTACCGGCTTACG
                    2300                                     PstI
CCGGGCTTCGGCGGTTTTACTCCTGTATCATATGAAACAACAGAGTGCCGCCTTCCATGCCGCTGATGCGGCATATCCTGGTAACGATATCTGAATTGTTATACATGTGTATATACGTGG
2400                    RNA III                                              →end RNAIII
TAATGACAAAAATAGGACAAGTTAAAAATTTACAGGCGATGCAATGATTCAAACACGTAATCAATATCTGCAGTTTATGCTGGTTATGCTGGCTGCATGGGGCATTAGTTGGGGAGCCAG
                                              2600
ATTTGTCATGGAGCAGGCCGTTCTGCTTTATGAATCAGGÁAAAAACTATTTGTTCTTCAGTCATGGACTACTGTTCTGATGTACCTGCTGTGTGTTTTCCTGGTATACCGGCCGTTGGATAGC
                    2700                              HaeII
TCCGCTACCGGTCGTTGGTCGCTGCGCAACGTTGGCGTACCGTGGCTGGTCGGTGCGATGGCCGTGGTGTATGTCGGTGTATTTCTGCTCGGTAAGGCGCPy-3'
```

Figure 2. Nucleotide sequence of one strand of the replication region of pSM1. Arrows below the sequence indicate the location of inverted repeat sequences. The sequences within the small boxes preceeding the open reading frames are nucleotides complementary to the 3' end of 16S rRNA. Replication proceeds rightward from the origin region, designated by the large boxes, which indicate one and two standard deviations from the position where the origin has been mapped. Bases corresponding to the 5' and 3' ends of the transcripts RNAI-III are shown by heavy arrows. The sequence in the origin region which is homologous to RNAI is underlined.

between mutually incompatible R100 and R1.[4,10,11] The non-homology
lies within the RepA2 coding frame and comprises 83% of the RepA2
sequence so it is unlikely that RepA2 plays a major role in determining incompatibility. In contrast to RepA2, the nucleotide
sequences for RepA3 in pSM1 and pTR1 have only two base pair differences, both of which would result in amino acid changes in the RepA3
polypeptide.[10,11] RepA4 is the fourth hypothetical coding region
common to pSM1 and pTR1 and encodes a polypeptide approximately
14,000 daltons in size.[10,11,12] The origin of replication is contained within RepA4.[10,11,12] However, because the nucleotide
sequence preceeding the RepA4 coding frame does not have the characteristics typical of polypeptide reading frames, we do not believe
that RepA4 encodes an actual polypeptide.[10,11]

SECONDARY STRUCTURES AT THE ORIGIN OF REPLICATION

The approximate location of the origin of replication of pSM1
has been determined by electron microscopic analysis,[5] and corresponds
to the region between nucleotides 1763 and 2456 allowing for two
standard deviations about this point, as shown in Figure 2.[10,11,12]
Replication proceeds unidirectionally to the right from this site.
[5,12] The origin and mode of replication used by pSM1 is the same as
that used by R100-1,[13] indicating that the control of replication of
the large plasmid is also present in pSM1, although most of the R100-
has been deleted in pSM1.[4,9]

Numerous sequences that are either direct or inverted repeats
can be found within the nucleotide sequence near the replication

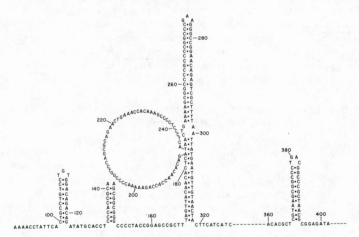

Figure 3.   Possible secondary structure at the pSM1 replication
            origin. Nucleotides 100 to 400 in this Figure corres-
            pond to nucleotides 1843 to 2143 in Figure 2.

origin of pSM1 and pTR1.[10,11,12] The stem–loop structures
that can be drawn using these repeated sequences is shown in Figure
3. The most striking feature of these structures is that they
occur in the region to which the origin has been mapped micro-
scopically. Although there are 12 bp changes in the region of these
structures between pSM1 and pTR1, none of these changes affect the
base pairing of any of the stem structures. The conservation of
this base pairing suggests that these structures are important for
DNA replication.[10,12] Complex secondary structures resembling
those shown in Figure 3 are also present at the replication origin
regions of other organisms such as E. coli,[14] Salmonella typhimurium,[15] and bacteriophage lambda.[16]

RNA TRANSCRIPTS

Three RNA transcripts are produced in vitro when superhelical
pSM1 and pTR1 DNA or the appropriate fragment from the replication
region of these plasmids are used as substrates. The smallest
transcript is 91 nucleotides in length and is designated RNAI. The
coding region for RNAI is contained totally within that of RepA3,
but RNAI is synthesized in the direction opposite to that of the
RepA3 transcript (Figures 1 and 2). Hypothetically, RNAI can form
two large, stable secondary structures as shown in Figure 4. There

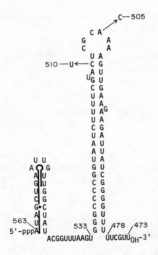

Figure 4. Possible secondary structure of RNAI. The two arrows
           at the top of the loop indicate the differences in the
           sequences of RNAI for pSM1 and pTR1. The line within
           the smaller hairpin shows the region complementary to
           the pSM1 origin region between nucleotides 2367 and
           2380 (See Figure 2).

are only two base changes in RNAI between pSM1 and pTR1, and both
changes occur at the top of the larger secondary structure loop
(Figure 4). In addition, 13 of the first 14 nucleotides of RNAI
are complementary to a sequence at the replication origin region
(Figure 2, refs. 11,17).

The second RNA transcript common to both pSM1 and pTR1 is very
large and is designated RNAII. This transcript begins 54 base pairs
to the 5' side of the initiation codon of RepA3. The location of
the 3' end of this transcript is presently not known; however, we
believe that RNAII is the mRNA for RepA1 and perhaps also for RepA3.
RNAII is synthesized in the direction opposite to that of RNAI and
the entire region encoding RNAI is contained within the RNAII coding
sequence (Figures 1 and 2).

The third RNA transcript, RNAIII,is synthesized in the same
direction as is RNAII from the region previously identified as the
replication origin of pSM1 and pTR1. RNAIII is found only when the
linear PstI fragment containing the replication origin is used as
a template (Figures 1 and 2) and not with superhelical pSM1 and pTR1
DNA. The 14 bp region of complementarity between RNAI and the replication is contained within RNAIII.[17]

POLYPEPTIDES SYNTHESIZED IN VIVO

When purified minicells containing pSM1 are incubated with
[35]S-methionine, thirteen labelled polypeptides are synthesized.
These polypeptides range in size from approximately 6,000 to 36,800
daltons, as determined by SDS polyacrylamide gel electrophoresis.[19]
The 36,800 dalton polypeptide is the only polypeptide produced by
pSM1 that is close to the size predicted for RepA1 (33,000 daltons,
ref. 10 and 11). Labeling with different amino acids to identify
the 36,800 dalton polypeptide definitively as RepA1 on the basis of
amino acid content is not possible because the DNA sequence predicts
that RepA1 contains all 20 amino acids.[10,11] Since no other coding
region for a polypeptide this large can be found in the nucleotide
sequence of the entire pTR1 plasmid and since the 36,800 dalton
polypeptide is produced by pTR1 as well as pSM1, we have identified
the 36,800 dalton polypeptide as RepA1.[19]

There are three polypeptides produced by pSM1 that are close
to the size predicted for RepA2, which is 11,400 daltons (Figure 5,
ref. 11). Since the nucleotide sequence predicts that RepA2 should
not contain tryptophan (Figure 2 and refs. 10,11), minicells containing pSM1 were labeled with radioisotopes of tryptophan, histidine and proline. Histidine and proline were incorporated in the
12,300 dalton polypeptide, but tryptophan was not.[19] In addition, the
12,300 dalton polypeptide is synthesized by the same PstI fragment
of pSM1 that encodes RepA2 and is not produced by pTR1, as predicted

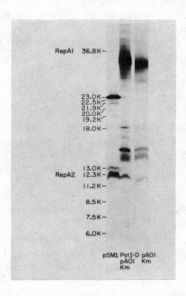

Figure 5.   Autoradiogram of Tris-borate polyacrylamide gel (ref. 8).
             Minicell strains derived from the E. coli K12 strain
             P678-54 (ref. 22) were purified by the method described
             by P. Matsumura (personal communication). Plasmids
             carried by the minicell strains are pSM1, pAO1-Km, a
             derivative of pML2 (ref. 24), and pAO1-Km carrying the
             PstI-D fragment of pSM1 (ref. 19).

by the nucleotide sequence (Figures 1 and 2. refs. 10 and 11).
Therefore, we have identified the 12,300 dalton polypeptide as RepA2
because of its size, amino acid content, map location, and lack of
production by pTR1.[19]

    RepA3 is a hypothetical polypeptide 6,700 daltons in size which
the nucleotide sequence predicts should not contain histidine.[10,11]
The RepA3 coding regions in pSM1 and pTR1 have only two bp differences and so are highly conserved.[10,11] However, no polypeptide
of this size and amino acid content has yet been identified in either
pSM1 or pTR1. In addition, no polypeptide close in size to 14,000
daltons (RepA4) has yet been identified. So, it is not clear at this
time whether polypeptides are actually made from the RepA3 and RepA4
coding frames.[19]

    Recently, a small polypeptide was identified that is produced
by the PstI fragment (fragment D) of pSM1 which encodes incompatibility and copy number functions. The size of this polypeptide
(approximately 6,000 daltons, Figure 5) is close to that predicted
by an extended RNAI transcript. Such an extended transcript actually

is synthesized in vitro in the presence of glycerol.[17] There does
not appear to be another open reading frame in the PstI-D fragment
that could code for a polypeptide of this size,[10,11] so we have tentatively identified the 6,000 dalton polypeptide as the product of the
extended RNAI transcript.

CONTROL OF DNA REPLICATION

We have used the DNA sites, coding frames, RNA transcripts, and
polypeptides identified from our studies of pSM1 and pTR1 to formulate a model for control of DNA replication. We have attempted to
emphasize only the most basic processes which might be involved in
this control.

From analysis of the replication origin sequences of pSM1 and
pTR1, we have identified a sequence that is capable of forming a
large secondary structure common to both plasmids and which is
similar to structures demonstrated at other replication origins.
We assume that the sequence at which this secondary structure occurs,
which is within the region previously identified as the replication
origin,[10,12] is essential for DNA replication.

One possible model for replication predicts that transcription
of RNAIII alters the conformation of this secondary structure. This
altered conformation would, in turn, allow an initiation complex,
which might include the positive effector polypeptide RepA1, to form
at the origin structure. DNA replication could commence after the
assembly of the initiation complex. Synthesis of the RNAIII transcript could be regulated by the binding of RNAI at the region of
complementarity between the 5' end of RNAI and the sequence of the
origin region between nucleotide 2367 and 2380 of the pSM1 nucleotide sequence, as shown in Figure 2. RNAI might function in this
way as a repressor molecule to control DNA replication.

However, another level of control of replication could also
exist. The bases of RNAI that are changed in pSM1 and pTR1 relative
to wild type R1, are found at the top of the large secondary structure in RNAI. These base changes are most likely responsible for
relaxation in replication control which results in the high copy
number phenotypes of pSM1 and pTR1.[10,11] Since it is unlikely that
the top of the stem-loop structure where these changes occur interacts directly with nucleotides at the replication origin, it seems
probable that the stem loop structure of RNAI would interact with
a polypeptide. RepA3 is a likely candidate for this polypeptide
since the RepA3 coding frame is so closely conserved in pSM1 and
pTR1, as would be expected of a controlling molecule. RNAI, then,
might not itself be a repressor but rather be required for initiatio
of DNA replication, which would occur in the absence of a repressor.

It is likely that some control is also exerted at the level of synthesis of RNAI and the postulated repressor polypeptide, RepA3. Since the coding regions for RNAI and RepA3 overlap, control of plasmid replication could be linked to cell growth by an attenuator-type mechanism,[20] as described in detail elsewhere.[17]

The model we have proposed here for control of replication of large drug resistance factors bears some resemblance to a model recently described for plasmid ColEl replication,[21] in that both models involve two RNA transcripts, one of which has nucleotide complementarity with the replication origin.

In summary, we have predicted from analysis of the replication region of pSM1 and pTR1 that three coding frames shared by both plasmids and one coding frame found only in pSM1 are most likely to encode actual polypeptides. To date, we have confirmed the existence of two of these polypeptides. (RepA1 and RepA2). We have also identified three RNA transcripts produced by the replication region of pSM1 and pTR1, one of which has a significant secondary structure. A model for control of DNA replciation that incorporates these features is proposed.

ACKNOWLEDGEMENTS

This work was supported by a National Needs Postdoctoral Fellowship (NSF) to K.A. (SPI-793986), by United States Public Health Service grants to E.O. (GM22007) and H.O. (GM26779), and by partial support to T.R. under an NIH training grant (CA-09176).

REFERENCES

1. E. Meynell, G.G. Meynell, and N. Datta, Phylogenetic relation-
        ships of drug resistance factors and other transmissible
        bacterial plasmids, Bact. Rev. 32:55 (1968).
2. R. Nakaya, A. Nakamura, and T. Murata, Resistance transfer
        agents in Shigella, Biochem. Biophys. Res. Commun. 3:654
        (1960).
3. N. Datta, Epidemiology and classification of plasmids, in
        "Microbiology 1974", D. Schlessinger, ed., American Society
        for Microbiology, Washington, D.C. (1974).
4. E. Ohtsubo, M. Rosenbloom, H. Schrempf, W. Goebel, and J. Rosen,
        Site-specific recombination involved in the generation of
        small plasmids, Mol. Gen. Genet. 159:131 (1978).
5. E. Ohtsubo, J. Feingold, H. Ohtsubo, S. Mickel, and W. Bauer,
        Unidirectional replication of three small plasmids derived
        from R factor R12 in Escherichia coli, Plasmids 1:8 (1977).
6. D.P. Taylor and S.N. Cohen, Structural and functional analysis
        of cloned segments containing the replication and incompa-

tibility regions of a miniplasmid derived from a copy number mutant of NR1, J. Bacteriol. 137:92 (1979).

7. T. Miki, A.M. Easton, and R.H. Rownd, Cloning of replication, incompatibility, and stability functions of R plasmid NR1, J. Bacteriol. 141:87 (1980).

8. R. Kollek, W. Oertel, and W. Goebel, Isolation and characterization of the minimal fragment required for autonomous replication ("basic replicon") of a copy mutant (pKN102) of the antibiotic resistance factor R1, Mol. Gen. Genet. 162:51, (1978).

9. S. Mickel and W. Bauer, Isolation by tetracycline selection of small plasmids derived from R-factor R12 in Escherichia coli K-12, J. Bacteriol. 127:644 (1976).

10. T.B. Ryder, J.I. Rosen, H. Ohtsubo, and E. Ohtsubo, Mechanisms of replication control based on nucleotide sequence comparison of two related plasmids of Escherichia coli, J. Bacteriol., In press (1981).

11. J. Rosen, T. Ryder, H. Inokuchi, H. Ohtsubo, and E. Ohtsubo, Genes and sites involved in replication and incompatibility of an R100 plasmid derivative based on nucleotide sequence analysis. Mol. Gen. Genet. 179:527 (1980).

12. J. Rosen, H. Ohtsubo, and E. Ohtsubo, The nucleotide sequence of the region surrounding the replication origin of an R100 resistance factor derivative, Mol. Gen. Genet. 171:277, (1979).

13. L. Silver, M. Chandler, E.B. delaTour, and L. Caro, Origin and direction of replication of the drug resistance plasmid R100 and of a resistance transfer factor derivative in synchronized cultures, J. Bacteriol. 131:929, (1977).

14. K. Sugimoto, A. Oka, H. Sugisaki, M. Takanami, A. Nishimura, Y. Yasuda, and Y. Hirota, Nucleotide sequence of Escherichia coli K-12 replication origin, Proc. Natl. Acad. Sci. U.S.A. 76:575 (1979).

15. J.W. Zyskind and D.W. Smith, Nucleotide sequence of the Salmonella typhumurium origin of DNA replication, Proc. Natl. Acad. Sci. U.S.A. 77:2460 (1980).

16. G. Hobum, R. Grosschedl, M. Lusky, G. Sherer., E. Scheartz, and H. Kössel, Functional analysis of the replicator structure of lambdoid bacteriophage DNAs, Cold Spring Harbor Symp. Quant. Biol. 43:165 (1978).

17. J. Rosen, T. Ryder, H. Ohtsubo, and E. Ohtsubo, Transcriptional involvement in replication, incompatibility, and copy number control of two resistance plasmid derivatives, Submitted (1981).

18. P. Tegtmeyer, M. Schwartz, J.K. Collins, and K. Rundell, Regulation of tumor antigen synthesis by Simian Virus 40 gene A, J. Virol. 16:168 (1975).

19. K. Armstrong and W. Bauer, Polypeptides produced by the mini-resistance plasmid pSM1, In preparation (1981).

20. F. Lee and C. Yanofsky, Transcription termination at the trp
     operon attenuators of Escherichia coli and Salmonella
     typhimurium RNA secondary structure and regulation of
     termination, Proc. Natl. Acad. Sci. U.S.A. 74:4365, (1977).
21. T. Itoh and J. Tomizawa, Formation of an RNA primer for initia-
     tion of replication of ColEl DNA by ribonuclease H, Proc.
     Natl. Acad. Sci. U.S.A. 77:2450 (1980).
22. H.I. Adler, W.D. Fisher, A. Cohen, and A.A. Hardigree, Minia-
     ture Escherichia coli cells deficient in DNA, Proc. Natl.
     Acad. Sci. U.S.A. 57:321 (1967).
23. V. Hershfield, H.W. Boyer, C. Yanofsky, M.A. Lovett, and D.
     Helinski, Plasmid ColEl as a molecular vehicle for cloning
     and amplification of DNA, Proc. Natl. Acad. Sci. U.S.A.
     71:3455 (1974).

PLASMID R1 INCOMPATIBILITY.

CONTRIBUTION FROM THE cop/rep AND FROM THE par SYSTEMS

Kurt Nordström, Søren Molin and Helle Aagaard-Hansen

Department of Molecular Biology, Odense University

Campusvej 55, DK-5230 Odense M
Denmark

INTRODUCTION

Plasmids are normally present in defined copy numbers; these can be expressed as number of plasmid molecules per cell, per protein, per chromosome equivalent, etc., but in the present paper we consequently use the baby cell as the unit. The copy number is determined by the plasmid, by the host, and by physiological conditions. Some plasmids are present in only a few (2–5) copies per cell. Nevertheless, these plasmids are completely stably inherited, loss of plasmid being a very rare event.

LIFE CYCLE OF PLASMIDS

Plasmid Replication and Partitioning

During the cell cycle, a baby cell grows until one generation time (τ) later its volume has been doubled. At that stage, the cell divides. In a plasmid-carrying cell population, the average number of plasmid copies in the cells also doubles during the time τ. At cell division, the plasmid copies are distributed to the daughter cells. Formally, this means that there are two plasmid events during the cell cycle, replication and partitioning (Fig. 1). If the copy number is n per newborn cell, this results in a plasmid cycle $n \rightarrow 2n \rightarrow n$. Let for example n be 2. Assume that one of the two plasmid copies in a newborn cell is mutated in a gene that is not involved in replication or partitioning, which gives rise to two variants of the plasmid, A and B. If the plasmid replication cycle were a mitotic one, the progeny of the cell where the

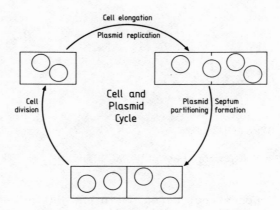

Fig. 1. Life cycles of bacteria and plasmids.

mutation occurred would be heterozygous (heteroplasmid) forever, i.e. would always carry A and B (Fig. 2a). However, heteroplasmid cells are known to segregate into pure A and B lines. What is the mechanism of this segregation? There are several possibilities. In case b (Fig. 2), all plasmid copies are replicated once and only once during the cell cycle, but there is a random assortment of the plasmid copies at cell division. This leads to the appearance of pure A and B lines (the frequency of these events is given within brackets in Fig. 2). Another possibility is that there is randomiza-

Case	Randomization		Pattern		LF (%)
	Rep	Par	Rep	Par	
a	−	−	AB ⟶ 2A2B ⟶ AB		0
b	−	+	AB ⟶ 2A2B	2A (1/6) AB (2/3) 2B (1/6)	33.3
c	+	−	AB < 2AB / A2B ; 3AB (1/3), 2A2B (1/3), A3B (1/3)	2A (1/12) A (1/12) 2AB (1/12) AB (1/2) A2B (1/12) B (1/12) 2B (1/12)	33.3
d	+	+	AB < 2AB / A2B ; 3AB (1/3), 2A2B (1/3), A3B (1/3)	2A (2/9) AB (5/9) 2B (2/9)	44.4

Fig. 2.   Effect of randomization during replication and/or partitioning on segregation of plasmids from a heteroplasmid population. A and B denote two genetically marked derivatives of a plasmid; the markers do not affect replication or partitioning. LF is the relative rate of reduction of the heteroplasmid population per generation of growth.

tion during replication but no assortment at partitioning (Fig. 2c). Again, pure A and B lines appear. Finally, randomization may occur at both replication and partitioning (Fig. 2d); in this case the frequency of pure A and B lines is higher than in cases b and c. The appearance of pure lines in a heteroplasmid population, i.e. segregation into heteroplasmid populations is operationally referred to as plasmid incompatibility. The exercise of Fig. 2 demonstrates how plasmid incompatibility is a logical consequence of randomization during replication and/or partitioning of the plasmid (cf. ref. 1).

Randomization Steps in the Plasmid Life Cycle

Randomization during replication has become evident from Meselson-Stahl (density-shift) experiments with many different plasmids[2,3,4]. The data are in agreement with the replication pattern of Figs. 2c-d. That there probably is randomization also at partitioning will be shown below.

Plasmid Incompatibility is a Quantitative Phenotype

Since cases a and b in Fig. 2 are ruled out by the Meselsohn--Stahl experiments, we will treat only cases c and d in more detail. In Fig. 2, we have schematically described the situation at the lowest possible heteroplasmid copy number ($n=2$). However, we have extended the analysis of the effect of plasmid replication and partitioning on incompatibility to higher n values (up to $n=8$). This analysis was performed by computer and the following assumptions were used[5]:

1) The partitioning (par) mechanism is distinct from the replication (rep) and replication control (cop) mechanism; a mutation abolishing partitioning does not affect the copy number of the plasmid[6].

2) Selection of plasmid copies for replication is random, i.e. replications occur one at a time and there is a time interval between consecutive replications, thus allowing the newly formed daughter plasmids the same probability as the rest of the plasmids in the cell to be selected for replication[3].

3) Two different replication control systems have been considered:
Model 1. The copy number is always set to $2n$ in all cells before cell division.
Model 2. Irrespective of copy number, exactly n copies are synthesized in each plasmid-carrying cell during one cell cycle.

4) A par mutation leads to random (binomial) distribution of

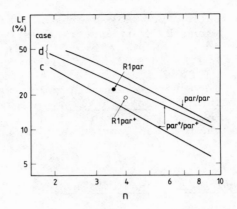

Fig. 3.   Theoretical calculation of LF values (see Fig. 2) at dif-
          ferent n values according to schemes c and d in Fig. 2.
          The circles represent experimental values obtained with
          plasmid R1.

plasmid copies between the daughter cells at cell division.

5) In the par^+ case, plasmid copies are equipartitioned, i.e. 50%
of the copies go to each daughter cell at cell division. Two cases
were considered in Fig. 2. In case c, the copies of each class (A
and B) are equipartitioned. This means that at even numbers the two
daughter cells get the same number of copies, whereas at odd

Table 1.   Effect of the par System on Incompatibility
           Theoretical Predictions

Par Function		LF (%)		Distribution of pure lines (%)	
A	B	$n = 4$	$n = 5$	A	B
I	I	23	18	50	50
None	None	27	22	50	50
I	None	21	16	62	38[a]
I	II	14	11	50	50
I	III	14	11	50	50
II	III	14	11	50	50

[a]Plasmid-free cells are included in the par group.

numbers one daughter cell gets one more copy than the other. In case d, the plasmid copies are selected randomly for partitioning (random assortment).

The computer analysis gave the following results: (i) The two replication models give virtually identical results. (ii) The rate of reduction of the relative size of the heteroplasmid population (i.e. the degree of plasmid incompatibility) is a function of the plasmid copy number (Fig. 3 and Table 1); this frequency (LF) is reduced by increasing copy number; plotting log(LF) against log(n) gives a straight line. The lowest LF value is obtained in case c, and case d gives a 50–100% higher LF value (the difference increases with the n value). Still slightly higher LF values are obtained in the absence of partitioning system.

PLASMID R1

Plasmid R1 Replication and Partitioning

We have for a long time been interested in control of plasmid R1 replication[7,8], and more recently in partitioning of this plasmid[5,6]. Plasmid R1 is inherited very stably, is present in a low copy number (about 1 per chromosome equivalent or 4 per baby cell when grown in broth). The genetic information for replication, including its control is located on a small part (about 3 kb, kilobases) clustered at the origin of replication (Fig. 4)[8,9]. However, plasmids only consisting of the basic replicon are not stably maintained but are lost in a frequency of 1–1½% per cell generation[6]. This is not due to a replication effect, since the copy number of these miniplasmids is the same as that of the full size plasmid (or 90% of that copy number). This has led to the definition of a region which is concerned with partitioning (par[6], repB[10], or stb[11]). These data show that replication and partitioning are independent processes. Similar data have been reported for plasmids pSC101[12] and P1[13].

The instability (loss rate) of par-deleted R1 replicons is consistent with random partitioning of the plasmids. By using pairs of par[+] or par derivatives of plasmid R1 it was possible to determine the degree of incompatibility (Table 2)[5]. The rate of reduction of the relative size of the heteroplasmid population was slightly higher for par/par than for the par[+]/par[+] combination and the data were in agreement with the model of Fig. 2d rather than that of Fig. 2c (Fig. 3). This was the first indication that there is randomization during partitioning as well as during replication.

Table 2. Effect of the par System on Incompatibility
          Experimental Results with the Basic Replicon of R1

| Par Function | | LF | Distribution in Colony (%)[a] | | | |
A	B	(%)	A + B	A	B	None
R1	R1	18	0.1	55	45	0
None	None	22	0.1	20	25	55
R1	None	16	1	95	3	2
R1	F	13	3	94	3	0
R1	pSC101	13	3	91	6	0

[a]Grown in absence of selection.

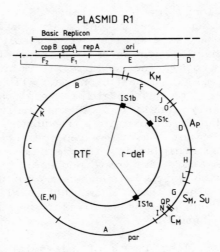

Fig. 4. Genetic and physical map of plasmid R1. Symbols: RTF,
         resistance transfer factor; r-det, resistance determinant;
         IS1a, b and c denote the three insertion sequences type 1
         located on the r-det; the capital letters inside the
         circle denote the 17 fragments generated by restriction
         endonuclease EcoRI; symbols outside the circle are Ap,
         ampicillin; Cm, chloramphenicol; Km, kanamycin; par, parti-
         tioning; Sm, streptomycin; Su, sulphonamides; The capital
         letters D, E, F_1 and F_2 on the linear part denote frag-
         ments generated by restriction endonuclease PstI.

Table 3.   Stability of Basic Replicons Carrying
Heterologous par Functions

Plasmid		Relative Copy Number	Inheritance
Basic Replicon	Par Function		
R1	R1	1.0	Stable
R1	None	0.9	Unstable (1.5%)[a]
R1	pSC101	1.0	Stable
R1	F	1.0	Stable
pSF2124-hybrid	R1	2.0	Stable
pSF2124-hybrid	None	1.8	Unstable (0.3%)[a]

[a]Loss Rate per Cell Generation.

Basic Replicons Carrying par from Other Plasmids

Hybrids between the basic replicon of plasmid R1 with rep(ts) derivatives of either plasmid pSC101 or miniF were stably inherited also at temperatures that were nonpermissive for the rep(ts) plasmids (Table 3). Since plasmids pSC101[12] and miniF[14] both are par+ this suggests that plasmid R1 can use par functions of other plasmids. The copy number of the hybrids was identical to that of R1 at the temperature that did not allow the other moiety to replicate. This adds to the conclusion that partitioning and replication are independent processes.

The ColE1 derivative pSF2124 was used as vector to clone the EcoRI fragment A (cf. Fig. 4), which harbours the par function of plasmid R1. The copy number of plasmid pSF2124 is fairly low and is reduced when large DNA fragments are inserted into the plasmid. This leads to a slightly unstable inheritance (Table 3). However, plasmid pSF2124 carrying the par fragment of plasmid R1 is completely stably inherited[5]. This suggests that plasmid pSF2124 does not carry any par function and that it can use that of plasmid R1.

Incompatibility Effects of the par System[5]

The construction of plasmid pSF2124 carrying the par region of R1 allowed a test of whether the partitioning process affects incompatibility. The result was that plasmid pSF2124 carrying parR1 was incompatible with plasmid R1 (Table 4)[5]. The copy number of either

Table 4. Incompatibility of Unrelated Replicons
that have the Same par Function.

Plasmid				Relative Copy Number		Plasmid Loss (% in a colony)[a]	
I		II		I	II	I	II
Rep	Par	Rep	Par	I	II	I	II
R1	R1	–	–	1.0	–	0	–
pSF2124	R1	–	–	2.0	–	0	–
pSF2124	R1	R1	R1	2.0	1.0	1	21

[a]Grown in absence of selection.

plasmid was not affected by the presence of the other plasmid. The
incompatibility was weak and plasmid R1 was being preferentially
lost which can be ascribed to the differences in copy number
between the two plasmids. Hence, there is (random) assortment
during partitioning and this randomization is specific to the par
system and not to the replicon type.

Incompatibility between R1 Derivatives Carrying Different par Functions

The construction of hybrid plasmids consisting of the basic
replicon of plasmid R1 and the par function of either plasmid F or
pSC101 enabled a test of the incompatibility effect of the par
system in a situation where assortment during partitioning is prohibited (case c, Fig. 2). On the assumption that replication and
partitioning are completely independent processes, the rate of
reduction of the relative size of the heteroplasmid population (the
LF value) was calculated (Table 1). The table also contains the expected distribution between the pure lines formed from the heteroplasmid population. We have also included the predicted outcome of
an incompatibility test involving a par[+] and a par derivative of
the same plasmid.

The corresponding experiments were then performed. As predicted, the rate of reduction of the heteroplasmid population was
reduced when the basic replicon of plasmid R1 carried different par
systems (Table 2). This adds to the conclusion that partitioning
involves randomization. However, the homologous pair had a clear
advantage over the heterologous one. Similarly, par[+] had a much

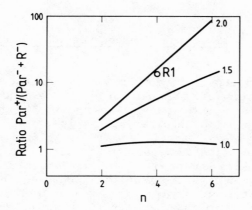

Fig. 5. Effect of different ratios in probability in selection for
replication of a par⁺ and a par derivative of a plasmid on
the formation of pure lines from a heteroplasmid population according to scheme d in Fig. 2. The lines represent
three different ratios as indicated at the lines. The
circle is the value found experimentally for plasmid R1.

stronger advantage over the par derivative than predicted. These
data suggest that the assumption used in the theoretical calculations are not completely correct. There seems to be a preferential
selection of the homologous plasmid during replication. Therefore,
we calculated the consequences of the different probabilities for
selection of the two plasmids during replication in a heteroplasmid
population (Fig. 5). The result was that only a minor bias in
selection for replication can explain the results of the incompatibility test shown in Table 2.

OTHER SYSTEMS

It seems to be a general phenomenon that chromosomes and
plasmids have partitioning functions that are independent of the
replication functions. Recently, this was shown for an eukaryotic
system; a minichromosome was constructed from a replicator and the
centromer of yeast[15]. This minichromosome behaved as a normal
chromosome in mitosis as well as in meiosis. Minichromosomes of E.
coli (oriC plasmids) are unstably maintained but are completely stabilized by the par region from plasmid F[16]. The par function most
likely is identical to incFI. Hence, different replicons having the
par function of plasmid F express a weak incompatibility, exactly
as those carrying the par function of plasmid R1 (cf. Table 4).

CONCLUSIONS

Plasmid Incompatibility is a Consequence of Replication and Partitioning of Plasmids

As discussed above, randomization either during replication or during partitioning of plasmids leads to segregation of hetero-plasmid populations into pure lines, i.e. to plasmid incompatibility. Hence, plasmid incompatibility is a logical consequence of these central events of the life cycle of plasmids[1]. Randomization at one stage (replication or partitioning) is enough to cause incompatibility. It has been shown that many (all) plasmids are selected randomly for replication[2,3,4]. However, randomization also seems to occur at partitioning. This is supported by (i) different replicons having identical par functions being incompatible, (ii) the relatively small difference in degree of incompatibility between a par$^+$/par$^+$ pair and a par/par pair, and (iii) the fact that the degree of incompatibility is reduced when two derivatives of the same basic replicon carry different par functions. Therefore, it seems fair to conclude that there is random selection for replication as well as random assortment during partitioning.

It should be stressed that plasmid incompatibility is a qualitative as well as a quantitative phenomenon. As has been pointed out by Novick and Hoppensteadt[1], plasmid incompatibility is caused by randomization during replication and/or partitioning. However, it is only possible to discuss degree of incompatibility in relation to the actual copy number.

In our opinion, plasmid incompatibility is basically (totally) a logical consequence of the properties of the replication and partitioning processes.

Replication and Partitioning are Independent Processes

Partitioning and replication are independent processes, since (i) deletion of the par region does not affect the copy number of the plasmid[6], and (ii) plasmids can use different par system to get stabilized without any effect on the copy number[5]. However, there seems to be an indirect linkage between these two processes, since a par$^+$ plasmid has a great selective advantage over its par deriva-tive. Similarly, a basic replicon carrying the homologous par$^+$ has a selective advantage over the same replicon with a heterologous par$^+$ function. This selective advantage most likely is exerted at the level of selection for replication. Since nothing is known about the mechanism of partitioning the reason for the bias in selection for replication can only be guessed. One possibility is that a replicon with the homologous par$^+$ function is kept in th vicinity of the replication site (if there is any) e.g. in the membrane. Similarly, a replicon carrying a heterologous par^+ function may be kept further apart from the replication site, i.e. in the vicinity of the replicon site that is normally used by the par function. A decision as to whether these thoughts are correct or not has to await further experimentation.

ACKNOWLEDGMENTS

The ideas presented above are the result of experiments but also to a great degree of conversation throughout the years with many colleagues. We particularly want to express our gratitude to Drs. Richard P. Novick and Robert H. Pritchard. The skilful technical assistance of Dorthe Dolleris Jensen, Marianne Hald Rasmussen, and Mona Andersen is gratefully acknowledged. The work was supported by grants from the Danish Medical Research Council (Grants Nos. 15367 and 20589).

REFERENCES

1. Novick, R.P. and Hoppensteadt, F.C. Plasmid 1:421–434 (1978).
2. Bazaral, M. and Helinski, D.R. Biochemistry 9:399–406 (1970).
3. Gustafsson, P., Nordström, K. and Perram, J.W. Plasmid 1:187–203 (1978).
4. Rownd, R. J. Mol. Biol. 44:387–402 (1969).
5. Nordström, K., Molin, S. and Aagaard-Hansen, H. Plasmid 5: (1981), in press.
6. Nordström, K., Molin, S. and Aagaard-Hansen, H. Plasmid 4:215–227 (1980).
7. Gustafsson, P., Dreisig, H., Molin, S., Nordström, K. and Uhlin, B.E. Cold Spring Harbor Symp. Quant. Biol. 43:419–425 (1978).
8. Molin, S., Stougaard, P. and Nordström, K. Microbiology, ASM (1981), in press.
9. Molin, S., Stougaard, P., Uhlin, B.E., Gustafsson, P. and Nordström, K. J. Bacteriol. 138:70–79 (1979).
10. Yoshikawa, M. J. Bacteriol. 118:1123–1131 (1974).
11. Miki, T., Easton, A.M. and Rownd, R.H. J. Bacteriol. 141:87–99 (1980).
12. Meacock, P.A. and Cohen, S.N. Cell 20:529–542 (1980).
13. Scott, J.R., Chesney, R.H. and Novick, R.P. Microbiology (1978) ASM, Washington, 74–77 (1978).
14. Kahn, M.L., Figurski, D. and Helinski, D.R. Cold Spring Harbor Symp. Quant. Biol. 43:99–103 (1978).
15. Clarke, L. and Carbon, J. Nature 287:504–509 (1980).
16. Ogura, T., Miki, T. and Hiraga, S. Proc. Natl. Acad. Sci. USA 77:3993–3997 (1980).

COPY NUMBER CONTROL AND INCOMPATIBILITY OF incFII R PLASMIDS

Robert H. Rownd, Alan M. Easton, and
Padmini Sampathkumar

Laboratory of Molecular Biology and Department of
Biochemistry
University of Wisconsin, Madison, Wisconsin 53706

INTRODUCTION

Bacterial plasmids are stably inherited even when present in low copy number in host cells. Thus, plasmid inheritance must be controlled by a mechanism which ensures that these extra-chromosomal elements are replicated during each cell division cycle and that at least one copy is segregated to each daughter cell at division. The molecular nature of the control of plasmid replication and segregation is presently not understood in any detail. Most available data are consistent with the negative control mechanism proposed by Pritchard (1978). This repressor dilution model postulates that an inhibitor or repressor specified by a gene on a replicon interacts with a specific receptor on the DNA to control the frequency of initiation of replication. This model can account for the control of plasmid copy number and also for the inability of two plasmids which share the same replication control mechanism to coexist stably in descendants of the same host cell (incompatibility). Mutations in either the repressor molecule or its binding site could lead to less stringent control so that plasmid copy number would be increased. A number of plasmid copy number mutants have been isolated and many, but not all, have been found to have altered incompatibility properties (Uhlin and Nordstrom, 1975; Miki et al., 1980; Rownd et al., 1980).

R plasmid NR1 (also called R100 and R222) is a 90 kilobase (kb), self-transmissible drug resistance plasmid which belongs to the FII incompatibility group (Rownd and Womble, 1978). The location of the resistance genes and the cleavage sites for several restriction endonucleases (Tanaka et al., 1976; Miki et al., 1978) and the transfer and replication functions on NR1 (Taylor et al., 1977; Taylor and Cohen, 1979; Miki et al., 1980; Rownd et al., 1980) have been determined previously. In this communication we describe more recent experiments on the copy number control (cop) and incompatibility (inc) genes of NR1. A region of less than 2.1 kb is sufficient for autonomous replication and plasmid incompatibility (exclusion) functions. The analysis of deletion mutants and hybrid plasmids formed from NR1 and a copy number mutant of NR1 have shown that the regions coding for copy number control, the ability to exclude an incompatible plasmid, and sensitivity to exclusion by an incompatible plasmid are all located within a 500 base pair (bp) segment located at least 1 kb from the origin of replication. When the inc/cop region of NR1 was cloned adjacent to a lacZ gene which lacks its own promoter, there was a stimulation in the level of synthesis of β-galactosidase which appears to result from transcription from a promoter in the inc/cop region. A greater stimulation was observed when the cloned inc/cop region was from copy number mutants of NR1, indicating an increased level of transcription. This production of β-galactosidase was found to be decreased by the introduction into the cells of plasmids carrying the inc/cop region having the same incompatibility phenotype. Transcription initiation sites have been mapped within the replicator region. A model is proposed in which the inc gene product is postulated to act within the 500 bp segment to repress initiation or extension of an RNA transcript originating within this segment and extending toward the origin of replication.

RESULTS AND DISCUSSION

Cloning of the Replication and Incompatibility Functions of R Plasmid NR1

Restriction fragments of NR1 capable of mediating autonomous replication were identified in sequential cloning experiments using different restriction endonucleases. In the initial experiments a miniplasmid was obtained which used EcoRI fragment B as the replicator (Fig. 1). Smaller miniplasmids were isolated from this derivative which contained two adjacent PstI fragments of size 1.1 and 1.6 kb. The incompatibility (inc) and copy number control (cop) functions have been shown to be located on the PstI 1.1 kb fragment (see below). The origin of replication (ori) is located on the PstI 1.6 kb fragment (Ohtsubo et al., 1977; Rownd et al., 1980). Non-essential Sau3A fragments have been deleted from these derivatives so that the replication region must be less than 2.1 kb. Since this smaller NR1 derivative has the same incompatibility properties as the wild type NR1, this function must lie within the 500 base pairs of the PstI 1.1 kb fragment which remain. In Fig. 1

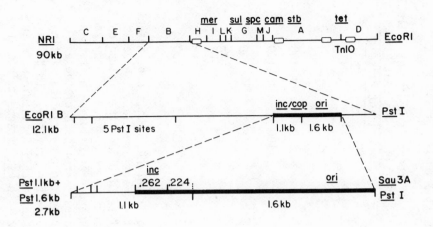

Fig. 1   Subcloning of the replication region of the incFII R plasmid
NR1

the thicker lines shown within the restriction fragments represent
the plasmid region which was found to be essential for replication
in the different cloning experiments.

Incompatibility Properties of Copy Number Mutants Derived from NR1

The PstI 1.1 kb and 1.6 kb fragments from NR1 and from a copy
number (cop⁻) mutant called pRR12 were cloned separately onto the
plasmid vector pBR322. The incompatibility properties of several
miniplasmids derived from NR1 and pRR12 and the pBR322 recombinant
plasmids have been examined using bacterial transformation. The
ability of donor plasmid DNA to exclude a resident plasmid was monitored when there was only selection for the donor plasmid in a
transformation experiment (Miki et al., 1980). Plasmids containing
the PstI 1.1 kb fragment of NR1 strongly excluded NR1 from the recipient cells, but did not exclude the cop⁻ mutant pRR12 which
therefore must also be an incompatibility (inc⁻) mutant (Table 1).
This was true irrespective of the copy number of the donor plasmid
carrying the PstI 1.1 kb fragment. The pBR322 derivatives carrying
only the PstI 1.6 kb fragment which contains the plasmid origin of
replication did not exclude either NR1 or pRR12 from the recipient
cells. Thus, the incompatibility function of NR1 lies on the PstI
1.1 kb fragment.

The corresponding plasmid derivatives of the cop⁻ pRR12 did
not exclude a resident cop⁺ NR1 from the cells which confirms the

Table 1. Incompatibility Properties of NR1 and the Copy Mutant pRR12

Donor Plasmid	Description	Percent of Recipient Cells Retaining Resident Plasmid	
		NR1	pRR12
pRR104	EcoRI B_{NR1} + kan	1	100
pRR933	PstI 1.1_{NR1} + PstI 1.6_{NR1} + cam	1	100
pRR935	pBR322 + PstI 1.1_{NR1}	0	100
pRR936	pBR322 + PstI 1.6_{NR1}	100	100
pRR114	EcoRI B_{cop12} + kan	96	96
pRR942	PstI 1.1_{cop12} + PstI 1.6_{cop12} + cam	100	100
pRR939	pBR322 + PstI 1.1_{cop12}	100	0
pRR937	pBR322 + PstI 1.6_{cop12}	100	100

Donor DNA was used to transform E. coli KP435 (recA) harboring either NR1 or its copy mutant pRR12 for drug resistance conferred by the donor plasmid. After transformation, the cells were cultured for 90 minutes in drug-free L broth and appropriate dilutions then spread on nutrient agar plates containing a single drug to which resistance was conferred only by the donor plasmid. Ten individual transformant colonies were suspended in dilution buffer and the suspensions were streaked onto drug-free Penassay agar plates. From each of these streaks 10 single colonies were picked and examined for drug resistance by replica plating (Miki et al., 1980). The donor plasmids were constructed as described previously (Miki et al. 1978;1980). The kan fragment is a 6.7 kb EcoRI fragment from the incFII R plasmid R6 which confers kanamycin/neomycin resistance. The cam fragment is a 2.1 kb PstI fragment from a deletion mutant of NR1 which confers chloramphenicol resistance.

inc⁻ phentotype of pRR12 previously observed (Table 1). The cop12
plasmid derivatives which were autonomously replicating miniplasmids (pRR114 and pRR942) did not exclude a resident pRR12 from the
recipient cells. Presumably a mixture of both donor and resident
plasmids can coexist in the host cells as a multicopy pool of
plasmids as long as the total plasmid copy number characteristic
of the cop12 mutation is not exceeded. However, the pBR322 derivative which carries the PstI 1.1 kb fragment of pRR12 (pRR939)
did exclude a resident pRR12 (but not a resident NR1) from the
cells. Presumably in this situation the high copy number of the
PstI 1.1cop12 kb fragment owing to its presence on pBR322 results
in the exclusion of the resident pRR12 plasmid. Thus, in addition
to increasing the plasmid copy number, the effect of the cop12
mutation is to change the incompatibility properties of the plasmid.
pRR12 is not incompatible with the wild type NR1 from which it was
derived but is incompatible with itself when there is a high copy
number of the inc12 region. Thus, pRR12 is an inc12/cop12 mutant
with respect to the inc⁺/cop⁺ NR1. It is interesting to note that
if NR1 and pRR12 had each been isolated as naturally occurring
plasmids, they would have been included in different incompatibility
groups.

Similar experiments were carried out with another copy number
mutant isolated from NR1 called pRR21. Although it was a cop⁻
mutant, pRR21 was found to be incompatible with NR1 and compatible
with pRR12 (data not shown). In this case the cop⁻ mutation did
not result in a change in the incompatibility properties of the
plasmid. Thus, pRR21 is an inc⁺/cop21 mutant.

Mapping of the Copy Number Control Gene and Incompatibility Recep-
tor Site

Since the PstI 1.1 and 1.6 kb fragments of NR1 and pRR12 have
been cloned separately onto pBR322, it was possible to construct
"hybrid" recombinant plasmids containing one PstI replicator fragment from NR1 and one from pRR12. The copy number and incompatibility properties of these hybrid plasmids were determined solely
by the source of the PstI 1.1 fragment (Table 2). When the hybrid
plasmids were used as the resident plasmid in recipient cells in
transformation experiments, hybrid plasmids containing the PstI 1.1
kb fragment from NR1 were excluded from cells only by transformation
with pBR322 carrying the PstI 1.1 kb fragment from NR1. On the
other hand, hybrid plasmids containing the PstI 1.1 kb fragment of
pRR12 were excluded from cells only by transformation with pBR322
carrying the PstI 1.1 kb fragment of pRR12. This exclusion specificity was maintained even if both the NR1 and pRR12 hybrid plasmid
derivatives were present simultaneously in the recipient cells
(data not shown). If incompatibility is due to the interaction of
a repressor with a receptor site on a plasmid molecule, these

Table 2. Properties of Hybrid Plasmids Containing PstI 1.1 and 1.6 kb Fragments of NR1 and pRR12

RESIDENT PLASMID COMMENT	NR1	pRR949	pRR955	pRR966	pRR957	pRR12
Source of PstI 1.1 fragment	NR1	NR1	NR1	pRR12	pRR12	pRR12
Source of PstI 1.6 fragment	NR1	NR1	pRR12	NR1	pRR12	pRR12
Copy Number	1.0	1.1	1.1	7.7	7.0	3
Percent of Transformants Harboring Resident Plasmids After Transformation by: pBR322 + PstI 1.1 (cop+)	0	0	0	100	100	99
pBR322 + PstI 1.1 (cop12)	100	41	42	0	0	0
pBR322	100	84	71	100	100	100

The PstI 1.1 kb and the 1.6 kb replicator fragments from NR1 and its copy mutant pRR12 and the 2.1 kb PstI cam fragment were cloned individually to the vector pBR322 at the PstI site. Appropriate combinations of the DNA of these recombinant plasmids were then mixed, digested with PstI, ligated, and used to transform a polA amber mutant of E. coli (JG112) to chloramphenicol resistance. Using this procedure, recombinant plasmids containing all four possible combinations of the PstI 1.1 and 1.6 kb fragments from NR1 and pRR12 were ligated to the cam fragment. The copy numbers (by assay of chloramphenicol acetyltransferase), ability to exclude a resident NR1 or pRR12 plasmid when used as the source of donor plasmid DNA in a transformation experiment (data not shown), and the ability to be excluded by NR1 or pRR12 when used as a resident plasmid in a transformation experiment were then examined.

results suggest that NR1 and pRR12 differ from one another in both the structural gene for the repressor and its receptor site. More-over both of these appear to be located on the PstI 1.1 kb frag-ment at a distance greater than 1 kb from the plasmid origin of replication. Since the copy number and incompatibility properties of pRR12 are both affected, the cop gene may be identical to the inc gene.

Since a cop⁻ mutation in the inc/cop region affects the frequency of initiation of replication when joined in cis to the origin of replication, it is possible that initiation is the result of a transcriptional event starting on the PstI 1.1 kb fragment which in some way activates the origin of replication on the PstI 1.6 kb fragment.

Mapping of RNA Polymerase Binding Sites and Transcription Initiation Sites

Using a nitrocellulose filter binding assay (Reznikoff, 1976; Taylor and Burgess, 1979), RNA polymerase binding sites were mapped on the Sau3A and HinfI fragments within the PstI 1.1 kb and 1.6 kb fragments from the replicator region. The thicker lines in Fig. 2 indicate the region essential for replication. When various com-binations of nucleoside triphosphates were added to the binding mixture, complexes which were resistant to high salt concentrations were formed between RNA polymerase and the restriction fragments with binding sites. This indicates that these binding sites can serve as sites for the initiation of transcription. There is only one RNA polymerase binding site and transcription initiation site located within the essential replication region within the PstI 1.1 kb fragment. It is possible that this site may represent the promoter for initiation of the transcription which regulates the expression of incompatibility and copy number control.

Construction of Lambda Phages Carrying the inc/cop Region Adjacent to the lacZ gene

Since a region involved in plasmid incompatibility and copy number control is located within a 500 bp segment of the PstI 1.1 kb fragment, it was of interest to examine whether transcrip-tion from this region was related to the copy number of a plasmid and whether the level of transcription could be controlled in trans by the presence of the inc/cop region which was cloned on a suit-able vector. The inc/cop region from NR1 (inc⁺/cop⁺) and from the copy number mutants pRR12 (inc⁻/cop⁻) and pRR21 (inc⁺/cop⁻) were cloned adjacent to a lacZ gene without its own promoter which was present on the lambda phage λRS205. The location of SalI and EcoRI cleavage sites on λRS205 and the miniplasmids constructed from NR1,

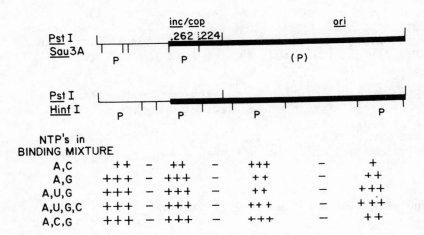

NTP's in
BINDING MIXTURE

A,C	+ +	−	+ +	−	+ + +	−	+
A,G	+ + +	−	+ + +	−	+ +	−	+ +
A,U,G	+ + +	−	+ + +	−	+ +	−	+ + +
A,U,G,C	+ + +	−	+ + +	−	+ + +	−	+ + +
A,C,G	+ + +	−	+ + +	−	+ + +	−	+ +

Fig. 2   RNA polymerase binding sites and transcription initiation
sites on the Sau3A and HinfI restriction fragments within
the replicator region. In these experiments RNA polymerase
was incubated with restriction enzyme-digested DNA in 0.1
M NaCl. The mixture was then filtered through a nitrocellulose filter and washed with 0.1 M NaCl. Under these
conditions restriction fractions which contain RNA polymerase binding sites (designated P) remain bound to the nitrocellulose filter. Filter-bound fragments were subsequently
eluted with 1.0 M NaCl or 0.2% SDS. Transcription initiation sites were analyzed by incubating RNA polymerase with
restriction enzyme-digested DNA in 0.1 M NaCl in the
presence of various combinations of CTP, ATP, GTP, and UTP.
The mixture was filtered through a nitrocellulose filter,
washed with 1.0 M NaCl, and the filter-bound fragments
were eluted with 0.2% SDS. Under both sets of conditions
the eluted fragments were analyzed on agarose or polyacrylamide gels to determine the distribution of RNA polymerase
binding sites or transcription initiation sites.

pRR12 and pRR21 using PstI cloning were convenient for this purpose
as diagrammed in Fig. 3. One of the SalI sites in the mini-
plasmids is about 50 base pairs from the PstI site between the
PstI 1.1 and 1.6 kb fragments. Lysogens were constructed using the
phages that carry the inc/cop region of NR1, of pRR12, or of pRR21.
In lysogens the expression of β-galactosidase from the lacZ gene
would be under the control of a promoter which in a plasmid would

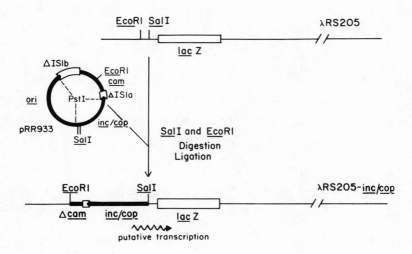

Fig. 3. Construction of lambda phages containing the inc/cop
region adjacent to a lacZ gene which lacks its own promoter.

direct transcription from the inc/cop region toward the origin of
replication. Lysogenic cells carrying a λ-inc/cop-lacZ phage
produced a higher level of β-galactosidase than the control strain
harboring a λ-lacZ phage without an inserted promoter (Table 3),
presumably due to transcriptional read-through from the inc/cop
region. There was a higher level of transcription from the
inc/cop region of the copy number mutants pRR12 and pRR21 than from
the inc/cop region of the wild type NR1. The introduction of a
pBR322 plasmid containing a cloned PstI 1.1 kb fragment of either
NR1, of pRR12, or pRR21 into the lysogenic cells reduced the level
of expression of β-galactosidase. The decrease was larger when
the λ-inc/cop-lacZ phage and the pBR322-inc/cop plasmid both had
the same incompatibility phenotype (i.e. both Inc⁺ or both Inc⁻),
irrespective of the copy number phenotype. This indicates that
the cloned PstI 1.1 kb fragment encodes a repressor which acts
in trans with a specificity which is determined by the incompatibility phenotype to reduce the level of transcription from a promoter in the inc/cop region. This specificity in control of the
level of transcription was not as remarkable as that observed in
the plasmid exclusion assays (Tables 1 and 2) in which there was
little or no interaction between the Inc⁺ NR1 and Inc⁻ pRR12.

Table 3. β-Galactosidase Production by Lysogens of λ-inc/cop-lacZ Phages

Control Strains[a]   β-Galactosidase Units[b]

NK5031 Δlac0 lacZ   0
NK5031 Δlac0 lacZ (λRS205)   67
NK5031 Δlac0 lacZ (λRS205-lacP$^+$)   1420

Source of inc/cop Region / Plasmid in Lysogen	NR1	pRR12	pRR21
None	220	504	1576
pBR322	245	563	1649
pBR322-inc$^+$/cop$^+$	52	152	232
pBR322-inc12/cop12	98	91	397
pBR322-inc$^+$/cop21	63	147	217

[a]The strain used for these tests was NK5031 which contains a lac0 lacZ deletion. This strain and the phage λRS205 were provided by Dr. K. Bertrand and Dr. W.S. Reznikoff.

[b]Assays were performed as described in Miller (1972).

If the decrease in the β-galactosidase levels in the λ-inc/cop-lacZ
lysogens is relevant to the plasmid incompatibility phenomenon, as
we propose, this new assay reveals a greater degree of cross reactivity between the incompatibility systems of NR1 and pRR12 than
the incompatibility assay used in this laboratory (Table 1).

It seems likely that the incompatibility repressor would also
be produced from the plasmid inc/cop region which was cloned into
the λ phages. In a lysogen which does not harbor a pBR322 plasmid
containing a cloned inc/cop region, the transcription emerging from
the inc/cop region in the λ phage which crosses the SalI site would
represent the level of transcription determined by the amount of
incompatibility repressor which exists in the cell. Since the
level of β-galactosidase in the lysogen containing the inc/cop
region from the copy number mutants was considerably higher than
observed for phages containing the inc/cop region from the wild
type NR1, it seems likely that the higher copy numbers of the cop⁻
mutants may be due to increased transcription from the inc/cop
region.

In Vitro Transcription from the Replicator Region

Using miniplasmid DNA which contains the PstI 1.1 and 1.6 kb
fragments linked to a PstI fragment containing the chloramphenicol
acetyltransferase gene in an in vitro transcription system, at
least five RNA transcripts have been identified from the two contiguous PstI fragments which form the replicator region of NR1
(data not shown). The largest of the RNA transcripts is greater
than 1100 bases in length and hybridizes to both the PstI 1.1 kb
(inc/cop) and the PstI 1.6 kb (ori) fragments, indicating that
there is transcription across the junction of these two PstI fragments. Preliminary data are available on the mapping of the other
RNA transcripts and the determination of their direction of transcription is currently in progress.

Model for Incompatibility and Copy Number Control of incFII Plasmids

Our experiments have shown that the copy number control gene,
the structural gene for incompatibility, and the incompatibility
receptor site are all located on a 500 base pair region within the
PstI 1.1 kb fragment of NR1. This region is located more than 1
kb from the origin of replication. Since a cop⁻ mutation on the
PstI 1.1 kb fragment affects the frequency of initiation of replication when joined in cis to the PstI 1.6 kb (ori) fragment from
either NR1 or pRR12 but not in trans when cloned on a pBR322 vector,
it is possible that the initiation of plasmid replication is the
result of a transcriptional event starting on the PstI 1.1 kb
fragment which in some way activates the origin on the PstI 1.6 kb

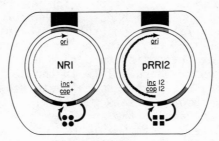

Fig. 4   Schematic illustration of a possible mechanism by which a
         cop⁻ mutation can affect both copy number control (cop) and
         incompatibility (inc). These two phenotypes are postulated
         to result from expression of the same gene (inc/cop) which
         specifies a diffusible repressor which regulates the fre-
         quency of initiation of transcription from a promoter
         located within or adjacent to the inc/cop gene. The re-
         pressor binding site (receptor) is located within the
         repressor structural gene. The inc⁻/cop⁻ mutation results
         in an alteration of both the repressor and its receptor
         site such that the inc⁻/cop⁻ repressor no longer recognizes
         the inc⁺/cop⁺ receptor site and the inc⁺/cop⁺ repressor no
         longer binds to the inc⁻/cop⁻ receptor site. As a result,
         the inc⁺/cop⁺ and the inc⁻/cop⁻ plasmids would be compat-
         ible. If the inc⁻/cop⁻ repressor regulates the frequency
         of transcription less stringently, there would be an in-
         crease in the inc⁻/cop⁻ plasmid copy number. Only one copy
         of the inc⁻/cop⁻ plasmid is shown in this schematic illustra-
         tion to avoid crowding. The origin of replication is shown
         attached to a cell surface structure (membrane?) to account
         for the cis-acting structural feature of the plasmid DNA
         which must be deleted in order to form a stable plasmid
         when two fragments containing the origin region are ligated
         together (Rownd et al., 1980).

fragment as indicated schematically in Fig. 4. According to this
interpretation, the frequency of the transcriptional event would be
controlled by repressor molecules specified by the inc/cop gene
which would determine the frequency of initiation of plasmid replication. The properties of the cop⁻ mutant pRR12 suggest that the
cop12 mutation(s) results in an alteration of the repressor and
its receptor site simultaneously such that the cop12 repressor
no longer recognizes the NR1 receptor (and vice versa), but
rather recognizes an altered cop12 receptor and regulates the
frequency of transcription less stringently (Fig. 4). As a
result, NR1 and pRR12 are compatible with each other and the pRR12
copy number is increased. These findings are consistent with the
view that the receptor site may lie within the repressor structural
gene such that both are affected simultaneously by the same mutation in the case of pRR12. Although there is relatively little
interaction between NR1 and pRR12 in terms of their ability to
exclude each other from host cells (incompatibility) (Tables 1
and 2), our experiments on the ability of the cloned inc/cop gene
to effect the level of transcription from the promoter in this
region indicate that there is still an interaction between the
controlling elements of the wild type and mutant plasmids (Table 3).

ACKNOWLEDGEMENTS

This work was supported in part by U.S. PHS Grants GM14398
and GM26527 and U.S. H.S., NIGMS Research Training Grants.

REFERENCES

Miki, T., Easton, A.M., Rownd, R.H.(1978) Mol. Gen. Genet. 158,217.
Miki, T., Easton, A.M., Rownd, R.H.(1980) J. Bacteriol. 141, 87.
Miller, J.H. (1972). Experiments in Molecular Genetics, Cold
    Spring Harbor Laboratory, New York.
Ohtsubo, E., Feingold, J., Ohtsubo, H., Mickel, S., Bauer, W.
    (1977). Plasmid 1, 8.
Pritchard, R.H. (1978) In DNA Synthesis:Present and Future, I.
    Molineux and M. Kohiyama, eds., Plenum Pub., NY
Reznikoff, W.S. (1976) In RNA Polymerase, R. Losick and M.
    Chamberlain, eds., Cold Spring Harbor, New York, p. 441.
Rownd, R.H., Easton, A.M., Barton, C.R., Womble, D.D., McKell, J.,
    Sampathkumar, R., Luckow, V.A. (1980) In Mechanistic Studies of
    DNA Replication and Recombination, B. Alberts, ed., Academic
    Press, New York, p. 311.
Rownds, R.H., Womble, D.D. (1978). In R Factor, Drug Resistance
    Plasmid, S. Mitsuhashi,ed., University of Tokyo Press, p. 161.
Tanaka, N., Cramer, J.H.,Rownd,R.H. (1976)J. Bacteriol. 127, 619.
Taylor,D.P.,Greenberg,J.,Rownd,R.H. (1977)J. Bacteriol. 132, 986.
Taylor, D.P., and Cohen, S.N. (1979). J. Bacteriol. 137, 92.
Taylor, W.E. and Burgess, R.R. (1979). Gene 6, 331.
Uhlin, B.E. and Nordstrom, K. (1975). J. Bacteriol. 124, 641.

REPLICATION AND INCOMPATIBILITY FUNCTIONS IN MINI-F PLASMIDS

Bruce Kline, Ralph Seelke and John Trawick

Department of Cell Biology/Section of Microbiology
Mayo Clinic
Rochester, MN   55905

INTRODUCTION

One common approach to building a model for plasmid maintenance is to identify, map and characterize the genes involved in
this process. The two major features of maintenance are plasmid
replication and partitioning to daughter cells. As depicted elsewhere in this text, the essential components of replication appear
to be at least a fixed origin of replication (*ori*), one to two
plasmid-specified gene products for replication (*rep*) and a copy
number control gene (*cop*) that appears to exert negative control.
So too, plasmid F, the classic conjugal plasmid of *Escherichia
coli*, appears to fit this general model of replication. However,
F may have a more complex genetic organization for this process
than other plasmids.

Our approach to characterizing F replication genes has been
to clone defined restriction fragments from mini-F plasmids. Plasmid
F is a 94.5kb molecule that is cut into 19 fragments by *Eco*RI.   One
fragment, f5, contains the 40.3 to 49.3kb sequences and the normal
maintenance genes of F (Timmis et al., 1975; Lovett and Helinski,
1976). Since F replication is a genetically controlled process,
we have also sought to map and clone wild type and mutant copy
number control and incompatibility genes. The incompatibility
response has been included in our analysis because the pioneering
work of Uhlin and Nordström (1975) indicated that copy number
control and incompatibility can be different aspects of the same
phenomenon.

Normal F maintenance, presumably replication, is inhibited
by the drug acridine orange (Hohn and Korn, 1969). We have also

317

examined our mini-F mutants derived from the EcoRI f5 fragment for
their sensitivity to this drug and have been able to identify a
region of F that is essential for a sensitive response to occur.
This region does appear to be involved in control of F replication.

The F Replication Region

Figure 1 depicts maps of various mini-F plasmids that we have
intentionally constructed or fortuitously isolated. They are all
derivatives of pMF21. The constructions and selections have been
described previously (Manis and Kline, 1977; Kline and Palchaudhuri,
1980) or are given in the Figure legend. The smallest plasmid
found is pBK138-2 which contains just 1.8kb of F DNA between

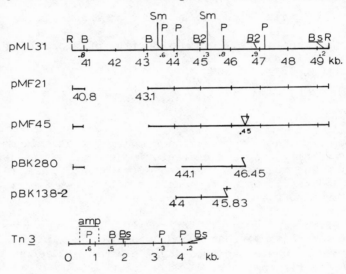

Fig. 1. Construction and characterization of mini-F plasmids.
          Plasmid pML31 contains the 9kb EcoRI f5 fragment 40.3 to
          49.3kb. We formed pMF21 from pML31 by *in vitro* deletion
          of the BamHI 40.8 to 43.1kb sequences (Manis and Kline,
          1977). Next, we isolated a pMF21::Tn3 plasmid, designated
          pMF45, in which the ampicillin resistance transposon, Tn3
          (∇) is inserted at coordinate 46.45kb (Manis and Kline, 1978
          Kline and Palchaudhuri, 1980). Note that the BamHI site in
          Tn3 is asymmetrically positioned on the Tn3 map and is des-
          ignated by a vertical mark on the inverted triangle. pBK280
          was formed from pMF45 by first deleting the sequences be-
          tween the BstEII Tn3 4.25kb coordinate and the BstEII F
          49.2kb coordinate and then by deleting the sequences be-
          tween PstI 43.6 and 44.1kb coordinates. The construction
          of pBK138-2 was as described by Kline and Palchaudhuri
          (1980). The restriction sites shown on pML31 and Tn3 are:
          (B) BamHI, (B2) BglII, (Bs) BstEII, (P) PstI, (Sm) SmaI and
          (R) EcoRI.

coordinates 44.0 and 45.83±0.03kb. However, control of pBK138-2 replication is not normal since the copy number of this plasmid is elevated about sevenfold and this plasmid is resistant to acridine orange curing. The smallest plasmid found that has a relatively low copy number (between 1.0 to 2.0 times the value of wild type F) and is sensitive to acridine orange is pBK280. This plasmid has the same F sequences as pBK138-2 plus the significant 45.83 to 46.45kb sequences (Seelke et al., in preparation). The other F sequences are without significance to replication control or acridine sensitivity.

Both pBK280 and pBK138-2 contain the origin of replication identified earlier at coordinate 44.4kb by Figurski et al. (1978). Therefore, it is of interest to know if a restriction fragment with the origin at 42.6kb (Eichenlaub et al., 1977) can form a plasmid or can complement *polA*-dependent ColE1 replication. The 42.6kb *ori* is contained on a 40.8 to 43.1kb *Bam*HI fragment. We have tried to make recombinants with this fragment that would form plasmids. For this purpose we used a 45.0 to 46.9kb *Bgl*II fragment with Tn*3* (Ap^r) inserted at 46.45kb or a *Bam*HI fragment containing the 46.45 to 49.3kb sequences as well as *amp* and *kan* genes. In no case were we successful at finding the expected recombinant plasmid. Likewise, Kahn et al. (1979) and Wehlmann and Eichenlaub (1980) have been unsuccessful in making F:ColE1 recombinants that are maintained in *polA* mutants when these recombinants contain the entire *Eco*RI f5 fragment but lack the 44.0 to 45.8kb sequences. From these results we conclude that the 44.0 to 45.8kb region contains *rep* information and that this information is more than just an *ori*.

Incompatibility Loci in Mini-F Plasmids

Results not shown identify the existence of an *inc*$^+$ function in pBK138-2. Kahn et al. (1979) have localized this function in the 45.0 to 45.8kb sequences. This function is termed *incB*. A recombinant plasmid containing the *incB* function on a *Pst*I fragment (44.1 to 45.8kb) has been cloned in our lab. This plasmid is designated pBK207 (Figure 2). A different *Pst*I fragment from pMF45 that has an *inc*$^+$ function has been cloned in pBR322. This fragment has the 45.8 to 46.45kb F sequences and 0.5kb of Tn*3* sequences. The recombinant plasmid is designated pBK232 (Figure 2) and the *inc* function is designated *incC*. Finally, as we described earlier (Manis and Kline, 1978), there is an *inc* function in the 46.4 to 49.3kb region. This function has been localized more precisely to somewhere within the 47.5 to 49.3kb sequences by making the F*inc*$^+$:pSC101 recombinant, pBK163, shown in Figure 2. Originally, we termed this function *incA*, but for reasons discussed elsewhere (Kline and Lane, 1980) the function is now called *incD*. Thus, there are at least three *inc*$^+$ functions in the mini-F region of 45.0 to 49.3kb.

An extensive genetic analysis by Tn*3* insertional mutagenesis has shown that the *incC* locus and acridine orange sensitivity locus

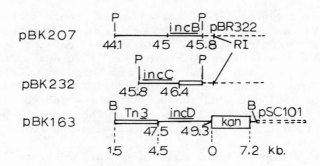

Fig. 2.   Identification of F sequences containing inc^+ genes. The
pBK207 and pBK232 plasmids were constructed by cloning the
indicated *Pst*I fragments from pMF45 into pBR322 (Bolivar
et al., 1977). The pBK163 plasmid was constructed from a
pMF21::Tn*3* plasmids (Tn*3* inserted at 45.83kb, Kline and
Palchaudhuri, 1980) in which Tn*3* had induced a deletion from
45.83 to 47.5kb. This deletion plasmid is known as pBK103.
The *Bam*HI fragment of pBK103 containing the sequences shown
above was cloned into the *Bam*HI site of pSC101 to form
pBK163. The pBK plasmids 163, 207 and 232 were each shown
to be incompatible with an F'*lac* plasmid contained in a *recA*
host. The incompatibility test used has been described by
Manis and Kline (1978). Restriction enzyme symbols are the
same as in Figure 1.

overlap at least within the coordinates 45.83 to 46.35kb (Wechsler
and Kline, 1980; Kline, unpublished). Remarkably, not only are *incC*
and *aos* functions in pMF21 destroyed by Tn*3* insertions at 45.83 and
46.35kb, but also these insertions cause about a sevenfold copy
number increase as well. The results indicate that *incC* is indeed a
complex locus. It would be easy to understand sensitivity to acridine if the dye blocked some essential function of *incC*; yet, as the
existence of pBK138-2 demonstrates, the *incC* locus is dispensible.
This paradoxical behavior is not understood.

Copy Number Control Loci in Mini-F

As described in the preceding paragraph, the *incC* locus is apparently involved in copy number control. Copy number mutants of
plasmid pMF45 have also been made by chemical mutagenesis with nitrosoguanidine or ethyl methane sulfonate (Manis and Kline, 1978; Seelke
Kline, Ritts and Trawick, in preparation). Bacteria harboring *cop*
mutant plasmids grow readily in the presence of 1.0 mg of ampicillin
ml whereas *cop*$^+$ plasmids do not permit this growth. This is the
basis for isolating *cop* mutants.

To map the chemically-induced *cop* mutations, we have made *in
vitro* recombinants between *cop*$^+$ and *cop* plasmids and then examined

the Cop phenotype of the recombinants. The maps of the recombinants showing a Cop⁻ phenotype (Fig. 3) indicate that the common sequences in all Cop⁻ recombinants are 45.3 to 45.8kb. This analysis has been done for five of the seven independently-generated *cop* mutants we have isolated. The *cop* loci that map within *incB* and *incC*, respectively, are called *copB* and *copC*. Thus far, chemically induced *cop* mutants have always been found to map in *incB* and Tn*3*-induced *cop* mutants to map in *incC* and no mutants isolated as phenotypically Cop⁻ have been found to map in *incD*.

To see if the *incD* locus influences F copy number, we have examined *incD* mutants. A leaky *incD*± mutant of pMF45 has been isolated and characterized. The mutant has the same copy number as pMF45 which is a value of two plasmids per chromosomal equivalent (Kline, 1979). Recently, we have successfully been able to delete *in vitro* the entire 46.4 to 49.25kb region of pMF45 by treating it with *Bst*EII which has only one recognition site in pMF21 at 49.25kb F and two recognition site in the Tn*3* sequences (Fig. 1). The

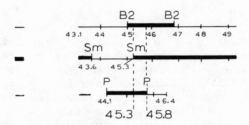

Fig. 3. Location of *cop* mutations in chemically induced Cop⁻ mutants of pMF45. To map the *cop* mutations, first the *Bgl*II (B2) 45.0 to 46.9kb fragment of each *cop* mutant was shown to contain the mutation by *in vitro* recombination of this fragment (━━━) to the complementary *Bgl*II fragment (───) from the *cop*⁺ pMF45 plasmid and subsequent examination of the copy number of the recombinant. To more precisely localize the *cop* mutation within the 45.0 to 46.9kb region, recombinant plasmids with structures shown above were formed from *Sma*I (Sm) fragments or from *Pst*I (P) fragments, then the copy numbers of the recombinants were examined. Note that the sequence within the 45.0 to 46.9kb region that is common to all *cop*⁻ recombinants is the 45.3 to 45.8 sequence. Therefore, the *cop* mutation from each of the five pMF45 *cop* mutants examined must map therein. These *cop* mutations are *cop48* and *50* (Manis and Kline, 1978) and *cop211*, *213* and *214* (Seelke, Kline, Trawick and Ritts, in preparation).

resulting mini-F plasmid with its *incD* deletion has the same copy
number as parental pMF45.

The low copy number and small size (12.4 megadaltons) of pMF45
makes it difficult to measure a small increase in copy number.
Therefore, we deleted the *incD* region (46.4 to 49.25kb) from one
copB-like mutant and three known *copB* mutants. In two of the deletion mutants we found no change and in two others we found a twofold
increase over the *copB⁻incD⁺* values; for example, the copy number increased from a value of 20 before deletion to a value of 40 plasmids
per chromosomal equivalent after deletion of *incD*. Moreover, we have
also made a recombinant of the *copB*-like mutant, *cop44*, that is, we
have made *cop44 incD⁻* double mutant. The double mutant has twice the
copy number of the *cop44* parental type. Hence, we suspect that *incD*
can influence F copy number although this influence may not be the
primary role for *incD*.

When all seven *copB* mutants were subsequently analyzed for the
status of their *inc* genes, they were found to be *incB⁺incC⁺incD⁺*.
By contrast, the *copC* mutants were found to be *incB⁺incC⁻incD⁺*.
These determinations were made by cloning each *inc* gene from each
cop mutant and testing the clones for incompatibility against F'*lac*.

DISCUSSION

Normal F replication results in a low copy number concentration
and is sensitive to the presence of acridine orange. The smallest
mini-F isolated by us with these properties has the F replication sequences 44.1 to 46.45kb. There is a smaller F plasmid, pBK138-2,
which contains just the 44.0 to 45.83 sequences, but its replication
control and sensitivity to drugs are abnormal. Recently, Kahn and
Helinski (personal communications) have been successful in making a
mini-F plasmid from the 44.1 to 45.8 *Pst*I fragment; but the properties of this plasmid have not been reported. Eichenlaub and Wehlmann
(1980) have successfully generated and mapped an amber mutant within
the 41.5 to 43.1kb coordinates that is defective in replication. Interestingly, they reported (Eichenlaub and Wehlmann, 1980) that when
the 40.8 to 43.1 *Bam*HI fragment is deleted from the amber mutant the
resultant plasmid is no longer replication defective. A clear explanation for this is not available, but the observation suggests
that it would be premature to conclude from our data that the 44.1
to 46.4kb region contains the sole *rep* determinants. However, this
region must play some essential role in replication since no one has
been able to show that the 40.3 to 44.1kb region or any part thereof
that contains the 42.6 *ori* can function as an independent plasmid
(Manis and Kline, 1978; Kahn et al., 1979; Wehlmann and Eichenlaub,
1980). Surprisingly, Wehlmann and Eichenlaub (1980) failed to find
any proteins produced by the 44.1 to 45.8kb region.

Kahn et al. (1979) and Kahn and Helinski (personal communication) first cloned *incB* (45.0 to 45.8kb) and *incC* (45.8 to 46.4kb)

and recognized them as such. However, Kahn et al. (1979) and
Wehlmann and Eichenlaub (1980) missed *incD* for reasons that are unclear; further, they initially confused the *incC* determinant with
incD. The structure of pBK232 (*incC*) and pBK163 confirms Kahn and
Helinski's observation that *incC* maps within 45.8 to 46.4 and estab-
lishes that *incC* and *incD* must be separate *inc* determinants.

Aside from the finding that *incB* and *incC* genes overlap *copB*
and *copC* genes, respectively, and that *copC* mutations result in loss
of the *incC*$^+$ function, there are no other results to indicate the
mechanism of incompatibility encoded by these genes. In fact, until
we produce point mutations or small deletions in *incC* and find a
corresponding increase in copy number, we must entertain the possibility that Tn*3* inactivation of *incC* is inconsequential for copy
number control. It might be that Tn*3* insertion has a polar effect
on the adjacent *copB* gene and that this effect is responsible for
the copy number increases.

One explanation for *incB* and *incC* gene products is that they
encode repressors of F replication. If this interpretation is
correct, then *copB* mutations have a property of operator mutations
in that the *copB* mutants remain *incB*$^+$.

Little is known about the *incD* mutants. At best only a twofold
increase in copy number can be seen with *incD* mutants and then it
can only be seen with some F plasmids that are in a high copy number
state before the *incD* mutation occurs. Clearly *incD* does not have
a profound effect on F copy number.

Another clear property of *incD* is that it is not essential for
plasmid maintenance; witness the existence of pBK280. Given this
observation, it is absolutely intriguing to find that when *incD* is
cloned into an unrelated plasmid such as pSC101 the pSC101:F *incD*
recombinant can be eliminated by *inc*FI plasmids and vice versa
(Kline, 1979). Moreover, IncFI plasmids are completely compatible
with pSC101. Thus, we have a situation in which an unrelated, non-
essential, *inc* gene can "poison" the normal maintenance of its
vector plasmid if the homologous *inc* gene is carried on another unrelated replicon. A very similar finding has been made by Timmis
et al. (1979) with an *inc* gene from R6-5 cloned in pBR322. These
situations are reminiscent of *incC* being a dispensible gene that
can "poison" the normal maintenance of its host plasmid in the presence of acridine orange. Whether or not this is merely a superficial similarity remains to be seen. In any event, the results suggest to us that both *incC* and *incD*, while they apparently make *trans*
functioning incompatibility substances, also likely have a *cis*
dominant role in maintenance. Put more simply, we feel that when
incC and *incD* are present in F they are quite important or become
essential for F maintenance.

The genetics of F replication and its control intertwined with the phenomenon of incompatibility is a complex subject about which more is probably unknown than is known. One approach to unravelling the complexities is to define the target sites for the *inc/cop* genes via incompatibility tests, mutant analysis and promoter identification, then to analyze promoter expression in the presence of various *inc*[+] genes. We are making substantial progress in this analysis, but at present it is incomplete. A summary of this paper is shown in Fig. 4.

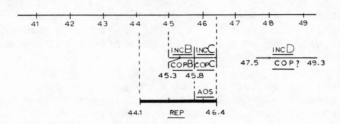

Fig. 4.   A map of the known replication, incompatibility, copy number and acridine orange sensitivity genes. Gene symbols are described in the text.

REFERENCES

Bolivar, F., Rodriquez, R. L., Greene, P. J., Betlach, M. C., Heynecker, H. L., Boyer, H. W., Crosa, J. H., and Falkow, S., 1977, Construction and characterization of new cloning vehicles. II. A multipurpose cloning system, *Gene*, 2:95.

Eichenlaub, R., Figurski, D., and Helinski, D. R., 1977, Bidirectional replication from a unique origin in a mini-F plasmid, *Proc. Natl. Acad. Sci. U.S.A.*, 74:1138.

Eichenlaub, R., and Wehlmann, H., 1980, Amber-mutants of plasmid mini-F defective in replication, *Mol. Gen. Genet.*, 180:201.

Figurski, D., Kolter, R., Meyer, R., Kahn, M., Eichenlaub, R., and Helinski, D. R., 1978, Replication regions of plasmids ColEl, F, R6K and RK2, *in*:"Microbiology-1978," D. Schlessinger, ed., American Society for Microbiology, Washington, D.C.

Hohn, B., and Korn, D., 1969, Cosegregation of a sex factor with the *Escherichia coli* chromosome during curing by acridine orange, *J. Mol. Biol.*, 45:385.

Kahn, M. L., Figruski, D., Ito, L., and Helinski, D. R., 1979, Essential regions for replication of a stringent and a relaxed plasmid in *Escherichia coli*, *Cold Spring Harbor Symp. Quant. Biol.*, 43:99.

Kline, B., 1979, Incompatibility between F*lac*, R386 and F:pSC101
    recombinant plasmids: the specificity of F incompatibility
    genes, *Plasmid*, 2:437.

Kline, B., and Lane, D., 1980, A proposed system for nomenclature
    for incompatibility genes of the *Escherichia coli* sex factor,
    plasmid F, *Plasmid*, 4:231.

Kline, B., and Palchaudhuri, S., 1980, Genetic studies of F plasmid
    maintenance genes, *Plasmid*, 4:in press.

Lovett, M. A., and Helinski, D. R., 1976, Method for the isolation
    of the replication region of a bacterial replicon: construction
    of a mini F'*km* plasmid, *J. Bacteriol.*, 127:982.

Manis, J. J., and Kline, B. C., 1977, Restriction endonuclease map-
    ping and mutagenesis of the F sex factor replication region,
    Mol. Gen. Genet., 152:175.

Manis, J. J., and Kline, B. C., 1978, F plasmid incompatibility and
    copy number genes: their map locations and interactions, *Plasmid*,
    1:492.

Timmis, K., Cabello, F., and Cohen, S., 1975, Cloning, isolation and
    characterization of replication regions of complex plasmid
    genomes, *Proc. Natl. Acad. Sci. U.S.A.*, 72:2242.

Uhlin, B. E., and Nordström, K., 1975, Plasmid incompatibility and
    control of replication: copy mutants of the R-factor R1 in
    Escherichia coli K-12, *J. Bacteriol.*, 124:641.

Wechsler, J., and Kline, B. C., Mutation and identification of the
    F plasmid locus determining resistance to acridine orange
    curing, *Plasmid*, 4:in press.

ACKNOWLEDGEMENT

    This research has been supported by a grant from the National
Institute of Health, GM25604, to B. Kline.

PLASMID MINI-F ENCODED FUNCTIONS INVOLVED IN

REPLICATION AND INCOMPATIBILITY

Rudolf Eichenlaub, Hermann Wehlmann, Jürgen Ebbers

Ruhr-Universität Bochum
Lehrstuhl Biologie der Mikroorganismen
Postfach 102148, 4630 Bochum, FRG

INTRODUCTION

The F factor of <u>Escherichia coli</u> is one of the most extensively studied plasmids. It belongs to the class of plasmids with a stringent mode of replication i.e. F is normally present in a cell in only 1-2 copies per chromosome[1]. In order to maintain the low copy number the replication must be tightly regulated, a notion which predicts that two different F'plasmids should not coexist in a bacterium. This has been experimentally proven and the phenomenon was termed incompatibility[2,3]. Thus incompatibility of two isogenic or related plasmids of the same incompatibility group may result from specific mechanisms engaged in the regulation of replication and partitioning during cell division.

In spite of intensive studies, so far there is no consensus on the nature of the regulatory mechanism controlling the initiation of plasmid DNA replication. Based mainly on studies with F two general models have been proposed which favour either positive or negative control[4,5].

In plasmid R6K an autoregulatory positive control element has been demonstrated[6]. While such a mechanism may function for a plasmid with a copy number of 10-15 per chromosome it is questionable whether a stringent regulation can be achieved by a positive control only. It is conceivable that negative control may be more efficient in stringent replication. Thus negative control, as first postulated by Pritchard et al.[5] has been favoured for the interpretation of copy number control in joined plasmid replicons[7] and Cop⁻ mutants of R1drd-19[8], although as yet there is no direct evidence for a repressor of replication.

The study of replication and maintenance of large complex plasmid genomes has been greatly facilitated by the recombinant

327

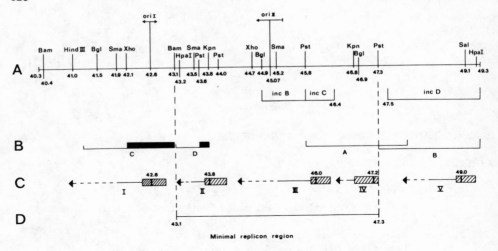

DNA technology which allowed the _in vitro_ construction of mini-plasmids exhibiting identical replication properties as the parental plasmid. Such a mini-F plasmid, the 9kb _EcoRI_ fragment f5[9,10] derived from F'_lac_, representing F-coordinates 40.3-49.3F[11,12] has become a useful model system for the study of plasmid replication.

Origins of Replication

Isolation of replicative intermediates of plasmid mini-F'_km_ (pML31) from _E. coli_ P678-54 revealed an unique origin of replication at 42.6F (oriI) with a predominantly bidirectional mode of replication[13]. Surprisingly, this origin located on a _BamHI_ fragment could be deleted without notable effect on replication and incompatibility[14,15]. Replicative intermediates from such a plasmid, pRE25 (mini-FΔBamtrp), linearized with _SalI_ showed an origin of replication at a distance of 30 ±2% of the total length from one of the _SalI_ restriction sites, with an unidirectional mode of replication (R. Eichenlaub, unpublished data;16). This second origin (oriII) was mapped at 44.4F[15]. However, based on more precise coordinates now available for the _SalI_ site (49.1F) and the _BamHI_ sites at 40.4F and 43.1F resulting in a total length of pRE25 of 13.4kb, oriII may rather map at 45.07F ±270 base pairs (Fig. 1A). This revised coordinate is also in better agreement with recent data showing that the region 44.8-45.8F carries sequences resembling the oriC of _E. coli_ (T. Murotsu, pers. communication) and that mini-F plasmids can be obtained deleted from 43.1F to 44.76F (D. Lane, pers. communication).

Fig. 1. Restriction map of plasmid mini-F and map positions of
◄━━━━━━━ mini-F encoded polypeptides and transcripts.
          (A) Mini-F restriction map with incompatibility loci incB,
          incC, and incD according to the nomenclature proposed by
          B. Kline and D. Lane[17]. Restriction sites in F-coordinates
          (kb). Bam = BamHI; Bgl = BglII; Sma = SmaI; Xho = XhoI;
          Pst = PstI; Kpn = KpnI; Sal = SalI.
          (B) Map location of mini-F encoded polypeptides, boxed
          regions in proteins C and D indicate the tentative loca-
          tion of the promoter. This mapping is based on the analy-
          sis of proteins obtained in minicells from restriction
          endonuclease generated deletion derivatives of mini-F:
          pBR322 hybrids as described by H. Wehlmann and
          R. Eichenlaub[18].
          (C) Map location of in vitro transcripts of plasmid mini-F
          obtained by R-loop analysis. Region of transcription
          starts (boxed), approximate start points in kb as calcu-
          lated from the distribution of starts within the boxed
          region, and direction of transcription (arrow). Length of
          the arrow corresponds to the longest transcript observed.
          (From H. Wehlmann and R. Eichenlaub, submitted for publi-
          cation.)
          (D) Minimal replicon region bordered by F-coordinates
          43.1F and 47.3F.

Conditional Replication Mutants

     Evidence whether plasmid encoded functions are involved in
plasmid replication can be obtained by the isolation of conditional
replication mutants.

     Using in vitro mutagenesis with hydroxylamine we isolated
mutants of mini-F thermosensitive in replication[19]. Although this
already suggested that a mini-F encoded polypeptide is involved in
replication further proof for the existance of such a protein may
come from the isolation of amber mutants. After in vitro mutagenesis of mini-F DNA and using an E. coli supFts as recipient in
transformation (which is su$^+$ at 28°C but su$^-$ at 42°C) two amber
mutants were obtained[20].

     A temperature shift from 28°C to 42°C resulted in rapid segre-
gation of the plasmid from the supFts host. When plasmid DNA synthesis was followed by the incorporation of tritiated thymidine no
label was incorporated into supercoiled mini-F DNA at 42°C[20].

     In order to identify the defective polypeptide, the proteins
synthesized in su$^-$ minicells of E. coli by wild type mini-F and
the amber mutants were compared. SDS-PAGE showed that a polypeptide
of 34K was missing in both amber mutants[20]. This documents that

replication of mini-F requires a mini-F encoded protein of 34K.
Experiments to map the amber mutation on the mini-F genome showed
that the am1-mutation maps on the 2.7kb BamHI fragment 40.4-43.1F
of mini-F (Fig. 1A,B). Deletion of this fragment which carries oriI
was accompanied by the loss of the mutant phenotype. From this observation it was concluded that the mutation am1 is only effecting
replication starting at oriI. It appears that in mini-Fam1 the
block of replication is not bypassed by initiation of replication
at oriII (45.07F). Thus the second replication system is only functioning when oriI together with the gene locus for the 34K protein
is deleted.

The other mutant mini-Fam3, however, behaved differently.
Upon deletion of the BamHI fragment 40.4-43.1F the amber phenotype
was retained indicating that mini-Fam3 carries two amber mutations,
effecting both replication systems. Although we have not yet identi-
ied the second defective polypeptide in mini-Fam3 it is suggested
that both replication system require mini-F encoded proteins.

Mapping of Polypeptides and Transcripts

Four proteins encoded by plasmid mini-F have been identified
in E. coli minicells and designated A-protein (44K), B-protein
(36K), C-protein (34K), and D-protein (25.3K)[18]. Mapping of the
polypeptides relatively to the mini-F genome has been achieved by
comparing the protein patterns of mini-F derivatives carrying deletions generated by restriction endonuclease cleavage[18]. The resulting map positions of the four polypeptides are shown in Fig. 1,B.

In order to correlate the corresponding transcripts to the
map position of the proteins we analysed R-loops formed with transcripts synthesized in vitro (Wehlmann and Eichenlaub, submitted
for publication) (Fig. 2). Five different transcription regions
can be distinguished (Fig. 2,3). Transcripts I, II, IV, and V
originate within the coding region of proteins A, B, C, and D
(Fig. 1B,C). Transcript III mapping between coordinates 43.9-45.9F
seems not to be translated, since we did not detect a polypeptide
in this region. The possible role of this transcript will be discussed later.

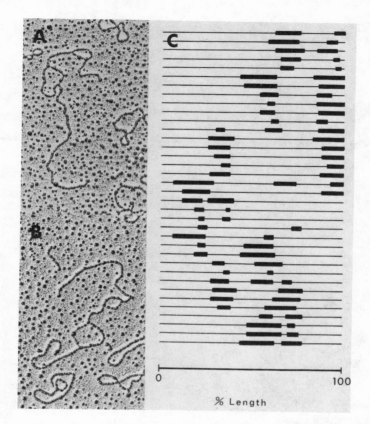

Fig. 2.   R-loop molecules of plasmid mini-F and plot.
Plasmid pJE401 (mini-F:pBR322)[20] was cleaved by restriction endonuclease EcoRI. After transcription the RNA was hybridized to the template DNA to form R-loop molecules which were analysed in the electron microscope as described by C. Brack[21]. Molecules with more than one R-loop (A and B) were exclusively evaluated. (C) Plot of R-loop molecules of the complete mini-F plasmid (40.3-49.3F) versus percent length. (From H. Wehlmann and R. Eichenlaub, submitted for publication.)

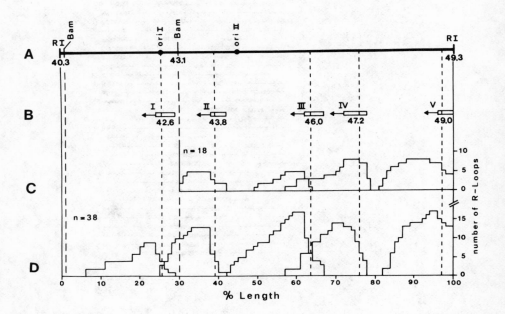

Fig. 3. Cumulative histograms of R-loop molecules.
         (A) Map of plasmid mini-F with relevant restriction
         endonuclease recognition sites and F-coordinates in kb.
         RI and Bam refer to EcoRI and BamHI, respectively.
         (B) Region of transcription starts (boxed), approximate
         start points in kb as calculated from the distribution
         of starts within the boxed region, and direction of
         transcription.
         (C) Cumulative histogram of R-loops of mini-F deleted
         for BamHI fragment 40.4-43.1F.
         (D) Cumulative histogram of R-loops of the complete
         mini-F plasmid (40.3-49.3F).
         Symbol n in C and D refers to the number of R-loop
         molecules evaluated. (From H. Wehlmann and R. Eichenlaub,
         submitted for publication.)

Complementation of Maintenance Deficient Deletion Derivatives

Although a plasmid reduced in size to a 2.8kb segment with coordinates 44.1-46.9F can be obtained[22], it is observed that deletions are often accompanied by instability of the plasmid. This may be due to the lack of certain polypeptides necessary for a stable maintenance of mini-F. Therefore we tested whether replication deficient mini-F plasmids deleted for restriction endonuclease generated fragments could be established in a bacterium provided that missing functions were supplied through complementation by another mini-F plasmid (Ebbers and Eichenlaub, submitted for publication).

In one such plasmid, pJE1001, the PstI fragment 45.7-47.3F was deleted resulting in the loss of the incC locus and the 44K A-protein (Fig. 4). This plasmid could only be established in E. coli in the presence of a wild type mini-F helper plasmid (pML31), indicating complementation of pJE1001 by the A-protein. Another plasmid, pJE2001, consisting of 44.0-45.7F and the trpED genes was constructed (Fig. 4) and was also only successfully established in E. coli in the presence of pML31. Since the mini-F segment present in pJE2001 does not encode a polypeptide[18] it appears that all F specific proteins required for replication and maintenance are supplied by the helper plasmid. However, pJE2001 and pJE1001 are still rather unstable, indicating that complementation is either only partially effective or that there is an incompatibility reaction between pML31 and pJE1001 and pJE2001, respectively.

By joining of the segment 44.0-45.7F to the PstI fragment 45.7-47.3F a plasmid was obtained (pJE3001) which encodes the oriII, the incB, and incC loci and the 44K protein (Fig. 4). Plasmid pJE3001 can be introduced into E. coli without the requirement for a helper plasmid, but segregation is observed at a rate of about 2 per cent per generation. The segregation indicates that pJE3001 lacks some function for total stability, although it has the A-protein which is required for plasmid maintenance. To test whether the lacking function could be supplied by complementation the stability of pJE3001 was examined in the presence of plasmids pJE421 and pHW30, respectively (Fig. 4). These two plasmids are compatible with other mini-F plasmids, they both lack the 44K protein and pHW30 also lacks the 25.3K protein. It was found that only pJE421 but not pHW30 complemented pJE3001 to total stability. Our interpretation of the complementation experiments is that two trans-acting proteins of 44K and 25.3K are involved in mini-F replication and maintenance.

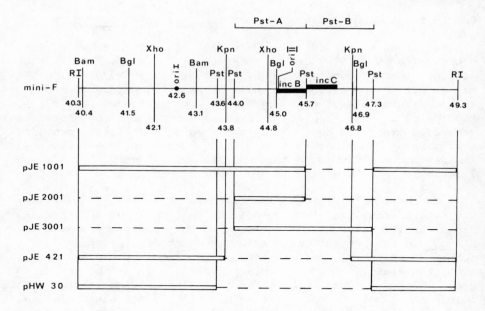

Fig. 4.   Restriction map of plasmid mini-F and map of its deriva-
          tives pJE1001, pJE2001, pJE3001, pJE421, and pHW30. Re-
          cognition sites for relevant restriction endonucleases
          are indicated with their corresponding F-coordinate in
          kilobases (kb). RI = EcoRI; Bam = BamHI; Xho = XhoI;
          Pst = PstI; Kpn = KpnI; Bgl = BglII. Dotted lines re-
          present the deleted part of the mini-F derivative. Plas-
          mids pJE1001, pJE2001, and pJE3001 carry an EcoRI or
          PstI fragment with the trpED genes as a selective marker.
          pJE421 and pHW30 represent mini-F: pBR322 hybrids with
          the mini-F derivative inserted into the EcoRI site of
          pBR322[18]. (From J. Ebbers and R. Eichenlaub, submitted
          to publication.)

Minimal Requirements for Plasmid Mini-F Replication and Maintenance

Within the 9kb mini-F genome two origins of replication[13,15],
four mini-F encoded proteins[18], five transcripts (Wehlmann and
Eichenlaub, submitted for publication), and three incompatibility
loci[22,23,24] have been identified. Therefore the question arises,
which of these components constitute the minimal replicon region
and which function they may have in the replication and maintenance of mini-F. It was shown that the oriI and the B-protein both
located within the BamHI fragment 40.4-43.1F can be deleted. The

stability and regulated replication of the remaining segment
43.1-49.3F indicates that besides oriII it posseses all control
functions required for such a status.

Based on the complementation experiments it becomes apparent
that two polypeptides are involved in the maintenance and replication control of mini-F. The D-protein mapping at 43.1-43.8F and
the A-protein mapping at 45.9-47.3F. Although the exact function
of these proteins is not known we have suggested that the A-protein
may act as a negative control element[18]. We further proposed that
the D-protein may then play a role as a positive control element
in the initiation of replication[18].

The region of 43.1-47.3F carries two adjacent incompatibility
loci, incB and incC[22], which can be cloned separately in pBR322.
Although, incompatibility is not impaired upon insertions at
XhoI (44.8F), BglII (44.9F), and PstI (45.7F) autonomous replication is always abolished (Ebbers and Eichenlaub, submitted for
publication; 22), indicating that continuity of the DNA sequence
between coordinates 44.8-45.7F is required for replication. Interestingly, this DNA sequence falls into the coding region for
transcript III. It is possible that this non-translated RNA may
serve as a primer for replication (o-RNA) possibly after being
processed by ribonucleases as has been described in another plas-
mitd system[25,26] or is produced during transcriptional activation
of oriII. Another possibility is that transcript III plays a role
in the association of F with the folded chromosome of E. coli[27]
which seems to be mediated by a rapidly metabolized, untranslated
RNA species[28].

The presented data indicate that the minimal region of mini-F
required for replication and stable maintenance of the plasmid
covers the region 43.1-47.3F (Fig. 1,D). Within this region two
polypeptides, two gene loci incB and incC expressing incompatibility[22] and an untranslated RNA species have been identified.
At present we can only speculate on the function of these components in F replication and maintenance, however, we exspect
that forthcoming experiments employing in vitro studies may eventually answer these questions.

ACKNOWLEDGEMENTS

    This work was supported by a grant from the Deutsche
Forschungsgemeinschaft. We are indepted to Rita Worttmann for
her skillful technical assistance and express our thanks to all
colleagues who have supplied us with bacterial strains, and
provided their unpublished data.

REFERENCES

1.   R. Frame and J. O. Bishop, Biochem. J. 121:93 (1971).
2.   R. Maas and W. K. Maas, Proc.Natl.Acad.Sci. USA 48:1887 (1962).
3.   R. Maas, Proc.Natl.Acad.Sci. USA 50:1051 (1963).
4.   F. Jacob, S. Brenner, and F. Cuzin, Cold Spring Harbor Symp.
     Quant. Biol. 28:329 (1963).
5.   R. H. Pritchard, P. T. Barth, and J. Collins, Symp.Soc.gen.
     Microbiol. 19:263 (1969).
6.   M. Inuzuka and D. R. Helinski, Proc.Natl.Acad.Sci. USA
     75:5381 (1978).
7.   K. N. Timmis, F. Cabello, and S. N. Cohen, Proc.Natl.Acad.
     Sci. USA 71:4556 (1974).
8.   B. E. Uhlin and K. Nordström, Molec.Gen.Genet. 165:167 (1978).
9.   M. A. Lovett and D. R. Helinski, J. Bacteriol. 127:982 (1976).
10. K. Timmis, F. Cabello, and S. N. Cohen, Proc.Natl.Acad.Sci.
     USA 73:2242 (1975).
11. M. S. Guyer, D. Figurski, and N. Davidson, J.Bacteriol.
     127:988 (1976).
12. S. Palchaudhuri and W. K. Maas, Proc.Natl.Acad.Sci. USA
     74:1190 (1977)
13. R. Eichenlaub, D. Figurski, and D. R. Helinski, Proc.Natl.
     Acad.Sci. USA 74:1138 (1977).
14. J. J. Manis and B. C. Kline, Molec.Gen.Genet. 152:175 (1977).
15. D. Figurski, R. Kolter, R. Meyer, M. Kahn, R. Eichenlaub, and
     D. R. Helinski, in: "Microbiology-1978", D. Schlessinger,
     ed., American Society of Microbiology, Washington,D.C.
     (1978).
16. R. Eichenlaub, R. B. Sparks, and D. R. Helinski, J.Bacteriol.
     138:257 (1979).
17. B. C. Kline and D. Lane, Plasmid 4:231 (1980).
18. H. Wehlmann and R. Eichenlaub, Molec.Gen.Genet. 180:205 (1980).
19. R. Eichenlaub, J.Bacteriol. 138:559 (1979).
20. R. Eichenlaub and H. Wehlmann, Molec.Gen.Genet. 180:201 (1980).
21. C. Brack, Proc.Natl.Acad.Sci. USA 76:3164 (1979).
22. M. L. Kahn, D. Figurski, L. Ito, and D. R. Helinski, Cold
     Spring Harbor Symp.Quant.Biol. 43:99 (1978).
23. J. J. Manis and B. C. Kline, Plasmid 1:492 (1978).
24. B. C. Kline, Plasmid 2:437 (1979).
25. S. E. Conrad and J. L. Campbell, Cell 18:61 (1979).
26. T. Itoh and J. Tomizawa, Proc.Natl.Acad.Sci. USA 77:2450
     (1980).
27. J. Miller, J. Manis, B. C. Kline, and A. Bishop, Plasmid
     1:273 (1978).
28. J. R. Miller and B. C. Kline, J.Bacteriol. 137:885 (1979).

NUCLEOTIDE SEQUENCE CHANGE IN A COLE1 COPY NUMBER MUTANT

Barry Polisky, Mark Muesing and Joseph Tamm

Department of Biology, Indiana University

Bloomington, Indiana 47405

INTRODUCTION

Despite a great deal of knowledge about the enzymology of DNA replication, the elements that regulate initiation of DNA replication are largely unknown. The definition and ultimate analysis of such elements depends initially on genetic identification of mutations affecting their function. In turn, the genetic analysis requires that the mutant be viable under certain conditions. For complex replicons such as the E. coli chromosome, such mutants have not been described. We have studied the multicopy plasmid ColE1 and its derivatives as a model system for the analysis of replication control elements. This plasmid is stably inherited and exists at a characteristic copy number of 10-15 copies per host chromosome. Our approach has been to perturb the control mechanism by isolating plasmid mutants which have altered copy number and then investigating the molecular consequences of the lesion. We have studied a high copy number mutant of the ColE1-derived cloning vehicle pBGP120 (Polisky, Bishop and Gelfand, 1976). The mutant plasmid, pOP1, and its derivatives, such as pOP1A6, comprise about 30% of intracellular DNA, compared to about 5% for the parent, pBGP120 (Gelfand et al., 1978). Previously, we localized the mutation to a 2kb region near the plasmid replication origin and demonstrated that the mutation was recessive, i.e., in cells containing both a copy number mutant and a wild-type plasmid, the copy number of the mutant was lowered to wild-type levels (Shepard, Gelfand and Polisky, 1979). The turn-down of copy number in trans was not observed when an unrelated plasmid co-resided with the mutant, suggesting the existence of a specific, plasmid-encoded, negative regulator of replication (Pritchard, 1978).

Here we describe more detailed mapping of the mutation in
deletion derivatives of pOP1 by DNA fragment recombination in
vitro. This approach enabled us to direct DNA sequencing efforts
to a small region of the plasmid genome. We have sequenced mutant
DNA fragments shown by recombination in vitro to contain the
overproducer mutation, as well as cognate wild-type fragments. We
have found the mutation to be a single GC→TA base-pair
transversion in a region of the plasmid genome which encodes two
RNA elements synthesized from opposite DNA strands. One of these
elements is a small, non-translated RNA, known as RNAl (Levine and
Rupp, 1978). The second element affected is the RNA primer
required for initiation of DNA replication in vitro (Itoh and
Tomizawa, 1980). RNAl has been reported to be 104 (Levine and
Rupp 1978) to 110 (Morita and Oka 1979) nucleotides in length and
is transcribed efficiently from supercoiled DNA templates in
vitro. It is located about 450 nucleotides upstream from the
replication origin and transcribed in the direction opposite to
that of replication fork movement of ColE1 (Chan, Lebowitz and
Bastia 1979; Morita and Oka, 1979). The mutation in pOP1 DNA
appears to promote readthrough transcription of RNAl in vitro,
generating a series of larger transcripts. We propose that RNAl
may be a negative modulator of ColE1 replication and that the
mutation in pOP1 DNA generates larger species of RNAl which are
unable to repress replication initiation. Campbell and Conrad
(1979a) have shown previously that an independently isolated copy
number mutant of ColE1, pFH118, was generated by insertion of
EcoR1 linkers in vitro into the region of the genome encoding
RNAl.

Mapping the Mutation in pOP1Δ6 DNA

Previously, we have shown that the mutation responsible for
high copy number in the mutant plasmid pOP1 is located within a
2kb region of the plasmid genome containing the origin of
replication and one structural gene, that specifying immunity to
colicin E1 (Shepard, Gelfand and Polisky, 1979). This 2kb region
is the only ColE1 DNA present in the identically sized,
Tn3-containing plasmids pOP1Δ6 and pNOP1 (Fig. 1). These plasmids
differ only in that pOP1Δ6 is Cop⁻ (copy number of 200-300 per
chromosome), while pNOP1 is Cop⁺ (copy number of 10-15 per
chromosome). pNOP1 is a Cop⁺ deletion derivative of pBGP120
constructed in vitro. pOP1Δ6 is a deletion derivative of pOP1
which arose spontaneously in vivo (Gelfand et al., 1978).

To further localize the mutation and minimize the size of the
DNA region we had to sequence, we carried out two general types of
recombination experiments in vitro. In one type, plasmids were
constructed with combinations of Cop⁺ and Cop⁻ purified
restriction fragments. In the second type, plasmids were
constructed with homologous Cop⁺ or Cop⁻ restriction fragments,

but deleted for a particular fragment. In these experiments, the
Cop phenotype of the resulting plasmids was determined
qualitatively both by a plate assay for β-lactamase production and
by analysis of cleared lysates by electrophoresis on agarose gels.
We screened the Cop phenotype of resident plasmids by adding a
chromogenic β-lactamase substrate to colonies on plates
(O'Callaghan et al., 1972). Due to gene dosage, more β-lactamase
is produced from colonies containing Cop⁻ plasmids than from
colonies containing Cop⁺ plasmids. Because β-lactamase is
exported from cells, such colonies are easily distinguished by the
size of the red halo surrounding them resulting from nitrocefin
cleavage.

Our mapping experiments began with the cognate 6.9kb Cop⁺ and
Cop⁻ plasmids pNOP1 and pOP1Δ6 (Fig. 1, A). Each of these
plasmids contains four PvuII sites, shown schematically in Fig. 1,
A. The relevent fragments are PvuIIC, which contains the
replication origin, and PvuIIB which contains the gene encoding
β-lactamase. The PvuII site immediately downstream from the
replication origin lies in ColE1 sequences in the HaeIIB fragment
about 200 nucleotides from the ColE1-Tn3 border. We purified the
PvuIIB and C fragments from both plasmids, ligated homologous
fragments, and transformed them into E. coli strain DG75. Apᴿ
transformants receiving PvuII B-C from pOP1Δ6 were Cop⁻. The
resulting new set of cognate Cop⁺ and Cop⁻ plasmids are 4.2kb and
designated pNOP42 and pOP42 respectively. These results indicate
that the mutation responsible for DNA overproduction does not lie
in the 200 bp region between the PvuII site and the ColE1-Tn3
border.

Analysis of colonies containing pNOP42 and pOP42 indicated
that both orientations of the PvuIIB and C fragments were
obtained. These are designated I and II and are shown
schematically in Fig. 1, B and C. Both plasmids have three HaeII
sites. The second recombination experiment was designed to map the
mutation with respect to the HaeII sites of pOP42, orientation I
(Fig. 1, B). In this orientation, the HaeIIA fragment contains
the β-lactamase gene and ColE1 sequences between the EcoRl site of
the ColE1 and the HaeIIA/C junction. The HaeIIC fragment contains
the origin of replication, and the HaeIIB fragment contains 285
nucleotides of ColE1 DNA downstream from the origin. The three
HaeII fragments of pOP42 and pNOP42 were isolated and ligated in
the combinations shown in Fig. 1, G. As before, ligated fragments
were transformed into DG75 and the Cop phenotype determined. The
results of these ligations and transformations are shown in Fig.
1, G. Lines 3 and 4 are homologous reconstructions generating a
new set of plasmids with molecular size of 3.6kb and which lack
any part of the HaeIIB fragment of ColE1. That these plasmids
differ in their Cop phenotype as did their parents means the
mutation does not lie in the HaeIIB fragment. These plasmids are

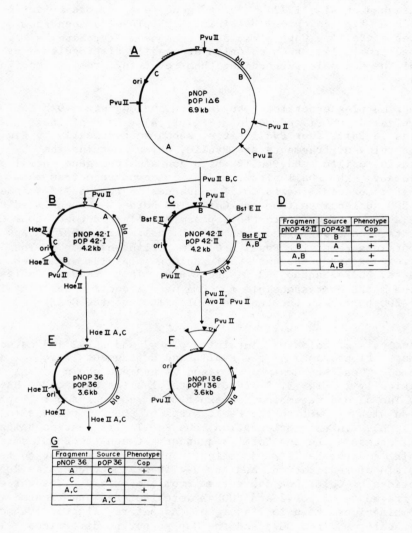

Fig. 1.   Construction and phenotypic analysis of plasmids used to map the <u>cop</u> mutation in pOP1Δ6 DNA. A, schematic diagram of the cognate Cop[+] and Cop[-] plasmids pNOP1 and pOP1Δ6. These plasmids are identical except for the mutation in the copy number control function. Each plasmid has four <u>PvuII</u> sites. The <u>PvuII</u> B fragment carries the β-lactamase gene (<u>bla</u>) while the <u>PvuII</u> C fragment contains the ColE1 replication origin and surrounding sequences. The bold segment in the diagram depicts ColE1-derived sequences while the narrow line shows sequences from the transposon Tn3, and a small segment (about 400bp) derived from the COOH-terminal region of the β-galactosidase gene which was present in pBGP120 (O'Farrell, Polisky, and Gelfand, 1978). <u>B</u>, <u>C</u>, <u>PvuII</u> B and C fragments from pNOP1 and pOP1Δ6 were purified from acrylamide gels, ligated homologously and transformed into DG75 with selection for Ap[R]. Four ligated plasmids were generated representing both orientations of <u>PvuII</u> fragments B and C. These plasmids are designated pNOP42·I and pOP42·I representing one orientation, and pNOP42·II and pOP42·II in the opposite orientation. Each plasmid is 4.2 kb and encodes Ap[R]. These opposite orientations were exploited to map the <u>cop</u> mutation. Both pNOP42·I and pOP42·I contain three <u>HaeII</u> sites as shown in B. These fragments are designated A, B, and C. Purified <u>HaeII</u> fragments A and C from both pNOP42·I and pOP42·I were ligated in all four possible combinations, transformed into DG75, and the Cop phenotype of the resulting Ap[R] transformants determined using the nitrocefin assay. The results are shown in Table G. The ligations resulted in the construction of two plasmids with identical orientation designated pNOP36 and pOP36, shown in part E. Each of these plasmids is 3.6kb, C; plasmids pNOP42·II and pOP42·II contain two <u>BstEII</u> sites. These fragments were isolated and ligated in the four combinations shown in <u>D</u> and the Cop phenotype of Ap[R] transformants determined as above. The Cop phenotype of the resulting transformants is shown in <u>D</u>. To demonstrate that ColE1 DNA sequences downstream from RNA1 were irrelevant to the <u>cop</u> mutation, plasmids pNOP136 and pOP136 were constructed from pNOP42·II and pOP42·II (C, F). In these constructions a DNA segment extending from an <u>AvaII</u> site 109bp downstream from the 3'-terminus of RNA1 to a <u>PvuII</u> site in the COOH-terminal region of the β-galactosidase gene (shown as an arc in F) was deleted from both pNOP42·II and pOP42·II. The isolated <u>AvaII</u>-<u>PvuII</u> fragments containing RNA1 and the replication origin from these plasmids were treated with T4 DNA polymerase to convert the <u>AvaII</u> end to a blunt end and these fragments were then ligated to a purified <u>PvuII</u> B

(Continued)

fragment (see 1A) which carries bla. We have previously
shown that the Tn3 moiety, from which the PvuII B
fragment derives, is devoid of copy number control
elements (Gelfand et al., 1978). Consequently, identical
results were obtained whether the PvuII B fragment was
derived from a Cop⁺ or Cop⁻ plasmid. The ligated
fragments were transformed into DG75 and the Cop
phenotype determined. These ligations created pNOP136
and pOP136, each 3.6 kb (F). pNOP136 is Cop⁺ while
pOP136 is Cop⁻ in DG75.

Δ denotes the EcoRl sites; ▲, AvaII: short
squiggled arrow denotes location of RNA1; ori is the
origin of replication with unidirectional fork movement
counter-clockwise; bla represents the gene encoding
β-lactamase, the arrow denoting the direction of its
transcription.

designated pNOP36 and pOP36. Lines 1 and 2 demonstrate that the
mutation lies in the HaeIIA fragment of pOP42, since the Cop
phenotype of the resulting plasmid depends on the source of the
HaeIIA fragment and not on the origin-containing HaeIIC fragment.

The HaeIIA fragment consists of 1014bp of ColE1 DNA and
contains three known genetic elements; the colicin immunity gene,
the promoter for the primer for DNA replication (Itoh and
Tomizawa, 1980), and RNA1. The DNA sequence for the entire region
has been determined (Oka et al., 1979). Since several groups have
constructed both point and deletion Col^{imm-} derivatives which are
not altered in plasmid copy number (see below), it seemed unlikely
that the mutation was in the immunity gene (Inselburg, 1977; Itoh
and Tomizawa 1980). On the other hand, the region of the genome
containing RNA1 has been implicated in replication control (Conrad
and Campbell, 1979). In addition to these elements, examination
of the sequence in this region (about 400-600bp upstream from the
replication origin) has revealed the existence of an open reading
frame, potentially capable of encoding a small, very arginine-rich
polypeptide. This sequence is highly conserved between ColE1 and
CloDF13 (Stuitje et al., 1980).

To distinguish whether the mutation was located in the region
containing RNA1 and the primer promoter, or the putative
polypeptide, we carried out the DNA fragment switch experiment
described schematically in Fig. 1 C, D. This experiment used
cognate Cop⁺ and Cop⁻ plasmids pNOP42 and pOP42, orientation II.
In this orientation we took advantage of a BstEII site located
between the open reading frame and RNA1 to generate two BstEII
fragments from both pNOP42 and pOP42. The BstEII site is 85bp
from the 5'-terminus of RNA1 (nucleotide 1 in Fig. 3). We

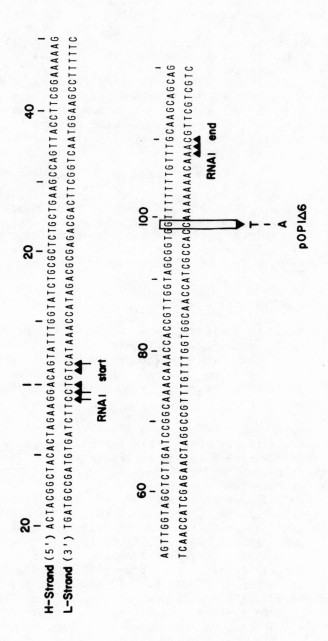

Fig. 2.   The DNA sequence in the region of ColE1 encoding RNA1.
          Triangles denote the A residues reported to be the
          initiating nucleotides of RNA1 (Chan, Lebowitz, and
          Bastia, 1979), and the 3' termination region of RNA1.
          Nucleotide numbers correspond to those of Morita and Oka
          (1979) for the RNA1 sequence. The mutation in pOP1Δ6 is
          shown at position 98. The initiating nucleotide of the
          ColE1 RNA primer has been reported to be the G at
          position 111 (Itoh and Tomizawa, 1980). Apart from the
          alteration in the mutant, the nucleotide sequence in the
          region shown and the region between the BstEII site and
          the RNA1 start site agrees exactly with that reported by
          Oka et al. (1979).

purified these fragments and ligated them together in various
combinations, transformed DG75, and determined the Cop phenotype
of the resulting Ap^R transformants. The ligation combinations and
results are shown in Fig. 1, D. The results demonstrate that the
Cop phenotype of the plasmids constructed in vitro depends on the
source of the BstEIIB fragment, which encodes RNA1 and the primer
promoter.

The Nucleotide Sequence Alteration in pOP42 DNA

     We determined the nucleotide sequence of the region encoding
RNA1 in pNOP42 and pOP42 DNAs. We found a single alteration--a
GC→TA transversion located in the structural gene for RNA1 (Fig.
3). In RNA1, this alteration is located in a GC-rich region
immediately preceding the uridylate run at the 3'-terminus of the
transcript (see Fig. 3).

     To demonstrate that the sequence alteration detected in the
RNA1 sequence was directly responsible for the Cop phenotype of
pOP1Δ6 and its derivatives, it was necessary to establish that the
670bp sequence between the 3'-terminus of RNA1 and the EcoRI site
was irrelevant to the Cop⁻ phenotype (see Fig. 1, C). To show
this, we constructed plasmid derivatives of pNOP42II and pOP42II
in vitro that were deleted for sequences between an AvaII site
109bp downstream from the 3'-terminus of wild-type RNA1, and the
EcoRI site of pNOP42II and pOP42II (Fig. 1, C). This region is
known to encode the gene conferring immunity to colicin E1. The
construction of these cognate derivatives, called pNOP136 and
pOP136, is shown in Fig. 1, C and F. We found that the Cop
phenotype of the deletion derivatives depended on the Cop
phenotype of the parent plasmid used in the construction (results
not shown). In addition, we determined the nucleotide sequence of
both pNOP42 and pOP42 DNAs between the AvaII site and the
3'-terminus of RNA1. No sequence changes between the two plasmids
were detected in this region (not shown). These results

demonstrate that the sequence alteration detected in the RNA1
region of pOP1Δ6 is necessary and sufficient for its
Cop⁻ phenotype.

The role of RNA1 in ColE1 replication has been the subject of
considerable speculation. Backman et al. (1978) proposed that
RNA1 was a "nomadic primer" which hybridized to the replication
origin and served as a primer for elongation by DNA polymerase I.
In this model, RNA1 was viewed as a positive element in
replication control. Comparison of the nucleotide sequence of
RNA1 with the replication origin indicated that RNA1 contains a
sequence of 10 nucleotides complementary to the region where the
first deoxyribonucleotide is incorporated (Chan, Lebowitz and
Bastia, 1979). Moreover, Conrad and Campbell (1979) have detected
weak hybridization between RNA1 and DNA fragments containing the
replication origin. On the other hand, it is clear that RNA1 is
not obligatory for replication since Oka et al. (1979) and others
(B.P. unpub. data) have constructed ColE1 deletion mutants lacking
the entire template for RNA1 and the primer promoter. The results
reported here and those reported previously for the copy number
mutant pFH118 (Conrad and Campbell, 1979) implicate RNA1 as a
potential element in plasmid copy number control.

How might RNA1 negatively modulate ColE1 replication?
Recently, Itoh and Tomizawa (1980) have demonstrated that
initiation of ColE1 DNA replication in vitro involves a large RNA
molecule which is processed at or near its 3'-terminus by
ribonucleaseH to generate a primer approximately 550 nucleotides
in length to which deoxyribonucleotides are subsequently added.
The involvement of RNaseH in the processing of the primer implies
that some portion of the primer remains associated with its
template strand after synthesis by RNA polymerase. These results
indicate that formation of the primer RNA-DNA hybrid is an
obligatory step for successful initiation in vitro, since very
little replication occurs in vitro if RNaseH is omitted from the
reaction (Itoh and Tomizawa, 1980). The addition of RNA1 to the
in vitro replication system inhibits formation of the primer (Itoh
and Tomizawa, 1980). This inhibition of primer formation by RNA1
could be a result of displacement of the primer RNA-DNA hybrid and
reformation of the DNA duplex. With respect to this possibility,
it is intriguing that both the ColE1 primer RNA and RNA1 originate
from the same template region of ColE1. RNA1 is entirely
complementary to the first 100 nucleotides of the 5'-terminal
region of the primer. Conceivably, RNA1 could act by formation of
an RNA-RNA duplex with the primer leading to displacement of the
primer from its template strand. However, this idea seems
inconsistent with our observation that a single nucleotide change
in RNA1 generating a longer RNA1 species increases the copy
number.

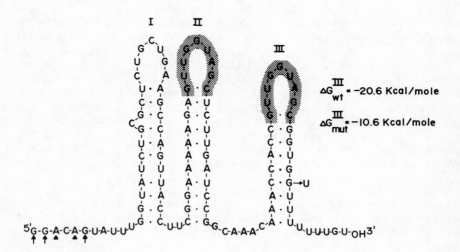

Fig. 3.   A model for the secondary structure of RNA1, modified
          slightly from that proposed by Morita and Oka (1979).
          Loops II and III are 9bp direct repeats (shaded areas).
          The arrow denotes the location of the mutation in pOP1Δ6
          encoded RNA1.   Free energy estimates for the stability of
          stem III in wild-type and mutant RNA1 are shown.   These
          were determined by the rules proposed by Tinoco et al.
          (1973).   Triangles denote the two A residues from which
          initiation of RNA1 has been reported to occur (Chan,
          Lebowitz and Bastia, 1979; Morita and Oka, 1979).

The nucleotide sequence of RNA1 suggests a high degree of secondary structure (Fig. 3). Morita and Oka (1979) have obtained evidence by partial T1 ribonuclease digestion that a substantial degree of secondary structure exists in RNA1 and have proposed a model shown in Fig. 3. Especially striking is the presence of two 9bp direct repeated sequences which comprise loops II and III (Fig. 3). We estimate that the mutation in pOP1Δ6 lowers the stability of stem III from approximately -20.6 kcal/mole to -10.6 kcal/mole. However, at present, we do not know whether the mutation in pOP1Δ6 affects RNA1 function by altering the stability of stem III per se, by the altered secondary structure of the readthrough transcript relative to wild-type RNA1, or by altering the stability of RNA1 itself.

Acknowledgements

H.M.S. was supported by a postdoctoral fellowship from the Damon Runyon-Walter Winchell Cancer Fund. This work was supported by NIH grant GM24212 to B.P.

REFERENCES

Backman, K., Betlach, M., Boyer, H.W., and Yanofsky, S. (1978). Genetic and physical studies on the replication of ColE1-type plasmids. Cold Spring Harbor Symp. 43, 69-76.

Chan, P.T., Lebowitz, J., and Bastia, D. (1979). Nucleotide sequence determination of a strong promoter of the colicin E1 plasmid. Analysis of restriction sites protected by RNA polymerase interactions before and after limited transcription. Nuc. Acids Res. 7, 1247-1262.

Conrad, S.E., and Campbell, J.L. (1979). Role of plasmid-coded RNA and ribonuclease III in plasmid DNA replication. Cell 18, 61-71.

Gelfand, D.H., Shepard, H.M., O'Farrell, P.H., and Polisky, B. (1978). Isolation and characterization of a ColE1-derived plasmid copy number mutant. Proc. Natl. Acad. Sci. USA 75, 5869-5873.

Inselburg, J. (1977). Studies of colicin E1 plasmid functions by analysis of deletions and TnA insertions of the plasmid. J. Bacteriol. 132, 332-340.

Itoh, T., and Tomizawa, J. (1980). Formation of an RNA primer for initiation of replication of ColE1 DNA by ribonuclease H. Proc. Natl. Acad. Sci. USA 77, 2450-2454.

Levine, A.D., and Rupp, W.D. (1978). Small RNA product from the in vitro transcription of ColEl DNA. In Microbiology—1978. D. Schlessinger, ed. (Washington, D.C., American Society for Microbiology), pp. 163–166.

Maxam, A.M., and Gilbert, W. (1980). Sequencing end–labeled DNA with base–specific chemical cleavages. In Methods in Enzymology, Vol 65, L. Grossman and K. Moldave, eds. (New York: Academic Press), pp. 499–580.

Miller, J.H. (1972). Experiments in molecular genetics. Cold Spring Harbor Laboratory, Cold Spring Harbor, N.Y.

Morita, M., and Oka, A. (1979). The structure of a transcriptional unit on Colicin El plasmid. Eur. J. Biochem. 97, 435–443.

O'Callaghan, C.H., Morris, A., Kirby, S., and Shingler, A.H. (1972). Novel method for detection of β–lactamases using a chromogenic cephalosporin substrate. Antimicrobial Agents and Chemotherapy 1, 283–288.

O'Farrell, P.H., Polisky, B., and Gelfand, D.H. (1978). Regulated expression by read–through translation from a plasmid–encoded β–galactosidase. J. Bacteriol. 134, 645–654.

Oka, A., Nomura, N., Morita, M., Sugisaki, H., Sugimoto, K., and Takanami, M. (1979). Nucleotide sequence of small ColEl derivatives: Structure of the regions essential for autonomous replication and colicin El immunity. Mol. Gen. Genet. 172, 151–159.

Polisky, B., Bishop, R.J., and Gelfand, D.H. (1976). A plasmid cloning vehicle allowing regulated expression of eukaryotic DNA in bacteria. Proc. Natl. Acad. Sci. USA 73, 3900–3904.

Pritchard, R.H. (1978). Control of DNA replication in bacteria. In DNA Synthesis, I. Molineaux and M. Kohiyama, eds. (Plenum Press: New York), pp. 1–26.

Shepard, H.M., Gelfand, D.H., and Polisky, B. (1979). Analysis of a recessive plasmid copy number mutant; evidence for negative control of ColEl replication. Cell 18, 267–275.

Stuitje, A.R., Veltkamp, E., Maat, J., and Heynecker, H.L. (1980). The nucleotide sequence surrounding the replication origin of the Cop 3 mutant of the bacteriocinogenic plasmid CloDF13. Nuc. Acids Res. 8, 1459–1473.

Tinoco, I., Borer, P., Dengler, B., Levine, B., Uhlenbeck, O., Crothers, D., and Gralla, J. (1973). Improved estimation of secondary structure in ribonucleic acids. Nature New. Biol. 246:40–41.

TRANSPOSITION AND REARRANGEMENTS IN PLASMID EVOLUTION

C. J. Muster, L. A. MacHattie, and J. A. Shapiro

Department of Microbiology
University of Chicago
Chicago, Illinois 60637

SUMMARY

Transposable elements participate in two classes of replicative recombination events: (i) full transposition; and (ii) genome rearrangements. Transpositions mobilize DNA sequences <u>internal</u> to the transposable element, while rearrangements also mobilize sequences <u>external</u> to the transposable element. We will illustrate several ways in which rearrangements mediated by IS1 and mutant Tn1 elements lead to the formation of new plasmid replicons. The effect of the Tn1/Tn3 <u>tnpR</u>$^+$ gene product leads to dissolution of new replicons formed by Tn1-mediated rearrangements. Replicons formed by IS1-mediated rearrangements are much more stable. This result indicates that IS1 employs a different pathway to full transposition. Thus, there are at least two classes of transposable elements in bacteria which play different roles in plasmid evolution.

INTRODUCTION

Structural rearrangements in plasmids play a key role in the history of bacterial populations. These rearrangements include insertions, deletions, and inversions. They occur spontaneously in nature and can be selected in the laboratory. Frequently, one rearrangement in a previously stable plasmid structure leads to further reorganizations until a new stable molecule has evolved. Many workers have observed such instability followed by stabilizing changes after <u>in vitro</u> insertion of DNA fragments into cloning vectors. When studying plasmid rearrangments it is advisable to remember that several recombinational events may have intervened between the first structural change and the final stable molecule.

349

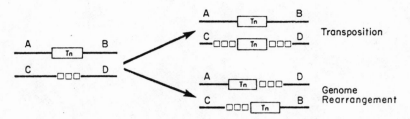

FIGURE 1.   Replicative recombination events involving transposable elements (Tn) and target oligonucleotide sequences (boxes).[2]

Transposable elements constitute a group of highly developed agents for inducing plasmid rearrangements.   Figure 1 shows two alternative recombinant structures arising from the activity of transposable elements.   In full transposition, the element is inserted into the target DNA without otherwise grossly altering the linkage relationships of DNA sequences external to the transposable element.   This recombination event is frequently seen with the acquisition of new drug resistance markers by plasmids.   In genome rearrangements, the element serves as a kind of recombination sequence to join different regions of the genome and form two "reciprocal" recombinant structures.   Such recombination events are responsible for replicon fusions and adjacent deletions (Figure 2).

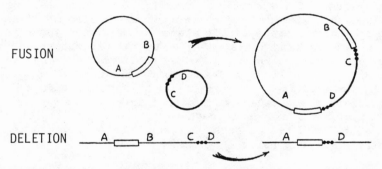

FIGURE 2.   Replicon fusion (top) and adjacent deletion (bottom)— two particular examples of genome rearrangement[10].

As other papers in this collection document, replicon fusion plays an important role in conjugal mobilization of some Tra⁻ plasmids and in the formation of new hybrid plasmids.   Both full transposition and genome rearrangements involve duplication of two sequences: the transposable element itself, and a short segment of the target DNA[1,2].   Sequence analysis has shown that the target duplication occurs by de novo replication and not by recombination with an homologous oligonucleotide adjacent to the transposable element (data summarized in reference 3).   We have similarly shown that transposable element duplication is inherent to the recombination event and does not result from prior theta replication of the donor replicon[4].

Two important questions concern the relationship of full transposition to genome rearrangements: (i) Are the two recombination events related? And, if so, (ii) Is one event a precursor of the other? The answer to the first question is yes. For all elements where it has been studied, mutants defective in transposition are also defective in fusions, deletions, and inversions (see 2, 3 for summaries of the data). In the case of Tn3 and other related transposons, the answer to the second question is also yes because the rearrangement product is clearly a precursor to the full transposition product[2,5] (Heffron et al., Reed, and Schmitt et al. in this volume). Figure 3 illustrates the Tn3 pathway to full tranposition: the rearrangement is catalyzed by the tnpA gene product activity at transposon termini, and the rearrangement products recombine at an internal site, tnpS, in a Rec-independent event catalyzed by the tnpR gene product[6,7] (Heffron et al. and Reed in this volume). Thus, mutants lacking either tnpS or the tnpR gene product yield only rearrangement products in Rec⁻ cells. When tnpR⁻ mutant cointegrates (from replicon fusion) encounter tnpR gene product they resolve to yield full transposition products.

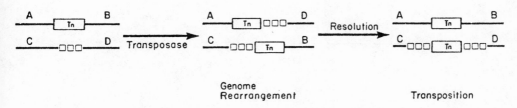

FIGURE 3.   Pathway of Tn3 transposition.

Thus, we can discern two classes of transposable elements depending on whether they mediate one or the other class of recombination event. Elements that usually go through full transposition mobilize DNA internal to the transposable element. Elements that usually participate in genome rearrangements also mobilize DNA external to the transposable element. For elements similar to Tn3, the difference between these classes resides in the presence or absence of the second resolution step (Figure 3).

In this paper we concentrate on elements which mediate rearrangements and summarize studies tracing the formation of novel complex plasmid replicons by transposable element-specific recombination events.

CONVERSION OF A BACTERIOPHAGE INTO A PLASMID BY ADJACENT DELETION

    The origin of the self-encapsidating plasmid pλCM is an example of adaptively significant genetic change brought about in vivo by a transposable element. In this case, the DNA molecule of temperate bacteriophage λcI857 was converted into a plasmid as a result of natural interactions with the composite transposon Tn9. Tn9 consists of two parallel copies of IS1 bracketing the structural gene for chloramphenicol acetyl transferase: IS1-cat-IS1.

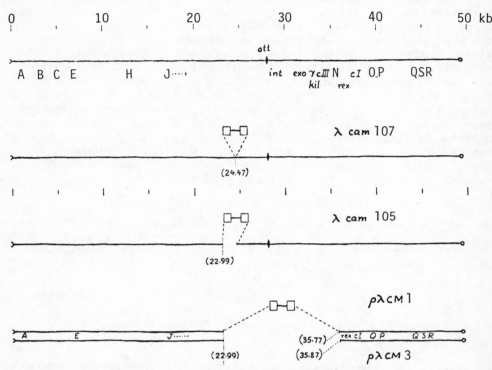

FIGURE 4. Origin of pλCM from λ (top) by Tn9 insertion (λcam107) and successive adjacent deletions (λcam105 and pλCM). Two independent isolates are shown. The coordinates of deletion end-points are given in kilobase positions on the λ map.

    The initial insertion of Tn9 into a dispensable region of the λ sequence (Figure 4) produced a plaque-forming chloramphenicol resistant (Cm^r)-transducing phage λ cam107. A short adjacent deletion leftward from Tn9 increased the stability of Cm^r about threefold (λcam105). These phages transduce Cm^r with efficiencies around 10^{-3} per particle, consistent with normal expectations for λ. However, in λcam105 lysates, about one particle in 10^5 is found to transduce about 10^3 time more efficiently than the majority, that is at about 1

transductant/such particle. These particles are sensitive to antiserum, are lower in density than λcam105, impart neither λ immunity
nor temperature sensitivity to the transduced cell, and do not form
plaques on normal E. coli (Muster, MacHattie, Shah and Shapiro,
manuscript in preparation). However, they can be grown to high
titers in the presence of a "helper" λ phage, and helpers incapable
of excising or packaging their own DNA can be used to produce pure
transducing lysates.

Physical characterization of the particle DNA shows that the
increased transduction efficiency results from a second adjacent
deletion which removes all λ sequences rightward from Tn9 into the λN
gene (Figure 4; Muster et al., manuscript in preparation). The rest
of the λ sequence from cI through DNA synthesis, lysis and structural
genes remains intact. Covalently closed circular DNA of the same
sequence can be extracted from transductants by standard plasmid DNA
extraction methods. The high transducing efficiency is a property of
λ phage particles which inject a stably-maintained plasmid DNA into
the host cells. This entity has been named pλCM, as a λ-derived
chloramphenicol resistance plasmid.

We have used pλCM as a convenient system to study transposition-
related events. The plasmid can be synchronously introduced into a
population of cells by infection and subsequently recovered free of
other cellular DNAs by packaging. The pλCM DNA is 21% shorter than
wild-type λ DNA, allowing it to accommodate insertions up to 13 kb
and still remain packageable. In the case of composite structures of
larger sizes, λ packaging serves as a powerful method to produce and
select derivatives that have suffered deletions which reduce them to
packageable size.

When pλCM and the defective Tn3-containing plasmid RSF1596[5] are
together in the same cell, fusions between the two plasmids can be
produced by two different mechanisms (Figure 5). When the system is
complemented by a source of tnpA gene product, the most frequent
fusion event is Tn3 mediated. In this case the novel joint of the
fusion product is between direct repeats of the Tn3Δ596 and various
points in pλCM (Muster et al., manuscript in preparation). The
target sites are not entirely random, however: of four structures
analyzed, two show the Tn3 inserted at or very close to one end of
the Tn9 in pλCM. When the source of tnpA gene product is a
derepressed tnpA (such as that in the Tn1ΔAp carried by RSF103)[5,6],
Tn3-promoted fusions with pλCM are frequent: about 2% of the
available pλCM molecules become carbenicillin resistant (Cb^r) per
cell division cycle. The fusion activity is temperature sensitive,
as expected, since tnpA gene product is temperature sensitive[9],
dropping more than three logs in frequency between 32° and 42°.

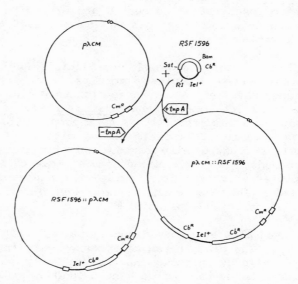

FIGURE 5.   Pathways of replicon fusion between pλCM and RSF1596 mediated by IS1 (-tnpA) and Tn3Δ596 (+tnpA).

In the absence of Tn1/3 transposase, pλCM becomes Cb^r at much lower frequencies; between 10^{-7} and 10^{-8} per cell division at 32°. Structural analysis of these $Cm^r Cb^r$ molecules shows that fusion is mediated by IS1 activity. The novel joints are between the endpoints of one of the IS1s in Tn9 and various points in RSF1596, and a copy of IS1 is present at each joint between the pλCM and RSF1596 sequences (Figure 5; Muster et al., manuscript in preparation).

The cointegrate replicons produced by the two kinds of fusion events carry two distinct DNA replication systems: that of phage λ, and that of RSF1596 (the ColE1 replicator). The transduction behavior of pλCM::RSF1596 cointegrates demonstrates that both of these replication systems are functional: in contrast to pλCM, whose transduction efficiency drops to about 10^{-4} in the presence of λ repressor under Rec⁻ Red⁻ conditions, the pλCM::RSF1596 transduce lysogens as readily as nonlysogens. In contrast to RSF1596, whose ColEl replicator requires DNA polymerase I, the cointegrates transduce <u>polA</u>⁻ strains with about the same efficiency as <u>polA</u>⁺ strains.

INCORPORATION OF A RESISTANCE GENE BY ADJACENT TRANSPOSITION

TnlΔAp is a deletion mutant whose genotype is <u>tnpA</u>⁺, <u>tnpS</u>⁺, <u>tnpR</u>⁻ <u>bla</u>⁻ [5,6,7]. We expect TnlΔAp to participate in rearrangements, but not full transposition events in Rec⁻ cells. The plasmid RSF103 contains TnlΔAp inserted into the sulfa resistance (Su^r) gene of RSF1010 adjacent to the streptomycin (Sm^r) gene[5,6] (Figure 6). This plasmid, RSF103, was used to search for "adjacent transposition"[10] of the Sm^r gene mediated by TnlΔAp. We envision adjacent transposition to occur by (i) adjacent deletion in RSF103 resulting in excision of a TnlΔAp-Sm^r DNA circle followed by its replicon fusion with a second plasmid, or (ii) replicon fusion of RSF103 with a second plasmid followed by an adjacent deletion of RSF1010 material. In either case, the final product should be the TnlΔAp-Sm^r-TnlΔAp composite "transposon" structure illustrated in Figure 6.

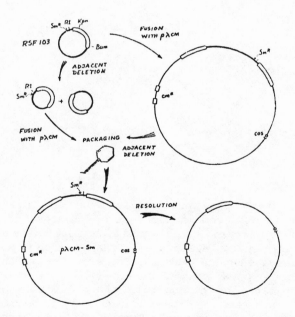

FIGURE 6.   Adjacent transposition of Sm^r from RSF103 to pλCM by successive fusion and deletion events.

We used pλCM to infect <u>recA</u>⁻ strains carrying RSF103 (or an RSF103–R388 cointegrate) and recovered pλCM by superinfection with a <u>red</u>⁻ <u>cI</u>857 helper phage. These lysates were used to transduce <u>recA</u>⁻ recipients. Cm^{r}Sm^r transductants were isolated (about 0.1–7% of all Cm^r transductants), and the Sm^r transposons were named Tn417–426 and are here referred to collectively as Tn-Sm. Physical characterization of pλCM::Tn419, pλCM::Tn422, and pλCM::Tn424 revealed the expected TnlΔAp-Sm^r-TnlΔAp structure inserted in pλCM (Figure 6; Muster et al., <u>manuscript in preparation</u>). pλCM::Tn421 appears to have the Sm^r transposon inserted into one of the IS1 sequences of Tn9. This illustrates a general tendency of transposable elements to insert in other transposable elements.

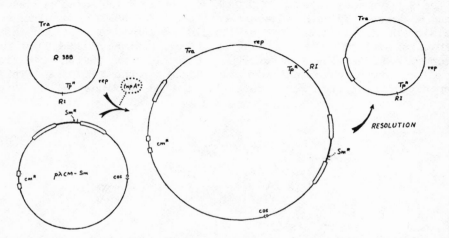

FIGURE 7. Formation and resolution of pλCM::Tn-Sm::R388 cointegrates in λ immune cells.

Since no <u>tnpR</u> gene product is made in Tn417–426, no full transposition is expected in Rec$^-$ hosts. To test this expectation, <u>recA</u>⁻ λ lysogens carrying the plasmid R388 were infected with lysates containing pλCM::Tn419, 422 and 424. Sm^r transductants were recovered. These transductants should represent pλCm::Tn-Sm insertions into R388 since pλCM cannot replicate in the presence of a λ prophage. Transfer by conjugation of the trimethoprim resistance (Tp^r) of R388 into <u>recA</u>⁻ recipients resulted in the cotransfer of Cm^r and Sm^r. Physical analysis of plasmid DNA from these exconjugants revealed structures consistent with replicon fusions of pλCM::Tn-Sm and R388 (Figure 7; Muster et al., <u>manuscript in preparation</u>). These plasmids appear stable in <u>recA</u>⁻ hosts and are free to express λ immunity.

EFFECT OF RESOLUTION ACTIVITY ON Tn1ΔAp CONSTRUCTS

In the presence of tnpR resolution function, the pλCM::Tn-Sm structures are expected to resolve to give a single Tn1ΔAp insertion. RP1 and pMB8::Tn3 are plasmids carrying wild type Tn1 or Tn3 where tnpR$^+$ is expressed. When these plasmids are introduced into cells carrying pλCM::Tn-Sm or R388::pλCM::Tn-Sm, the expected resolution occurs. In the case of pλCM::Tn-Sm, addition of TnpR$^+$ results in the loss of Sm^r, and physical analysis reveals the expected pλCM::Tn1ΔAp structure (Figure 6). Likewise, in the case of R388::pλCM::Tn-Sm, addition of tnpR$^+$ results in loss of pλCM and Tn-Sm DNA, and the product recovered was R388::Tn1ΔAp (Figure 7). When pREG118 (tnpA$^+$ tnpS$^+$ tnpR$^-$ bla$^+$)[11] is added to strains harboring pλCM::Tn-Sm in a recA$^-$ background, no loss of Sm^r is noted. This experiment shows that the resolution is specific for the tnpR gene product. Resolution is extremely rapid (>95% complete in 40 minutes at 42°C), and complete (<10^{-4} pλCM::Tn-Sm retained the Sm^r determinant after infection of a tnpR$^+$ cell) (Muster et al., manuscript in preparation). The observation that the resolution function does not establish an equilibrium between resolved and rearrangement structures is consistent with Reed's observations that only physically linked parallel tnpS sites are efficient recombination substrates for tnpR gene product (Reed, this volume)

DISCUSSION

We have described several in vivo isolations of plasmids/cosmids/phasmids generated by nonhomologous replicative recombination events mediated by transposable elements. Adjacent deletions and/or replicon fusions, not full transpositions, are the bases for these plasmid rearrangements. Our results therefore suggest that rearrangements rather than full transpositions mediate the formation of hybrid replicons.

In the case of Tn1/3 where tnpR gene product resolves hybrid molecules rapidly, transposon-bounded DNA such as Tn1ΔAp-Sm^r-Tn1ΔAp is highly unstable and cannot be mobilized. Here, we see that mobilization of internal sequences by full transposition and stable mobilization of external sequences by replicon fusion or adjacent transposition are mutually exclusive depending on the presence or absence of a functional tnpR gene.

Some other transposons do not exhibit the resolution-determined distinction between transposition and rearrangements. IS1-flanked sequences are highly stable, even in Rec$^+$ cells, compared to Tn1/3 flanked DNAs[12] (Muster et al., manuscript in preparation). Compound transposons such as Tn5 and Tn10 which are flanked by long inverted repeats do not show a high inversion rate even in Rec$^+$ cells (D. Berg, personal communication; N. Kleckner, personal communication).

These differences in character suggested that there must be more than
one biochemical pathway for full transposition. It remains to be
established whether the pathways to genome rearrangements are similar for these two classes of transposable elements.

ACKNOWLEDGMENTS

We thank Carol L. Burck for excellent technical assistance and
Chan Stroman for assistance in the preparation of this manuscript.
We also thank Ron E. Gill for sending us strains containing pREG118,
RSF103, and RSF1596. This research was supported by a grant from the
U.S. Public Health Service (NIGMS 24960).

REFERENCES

1. N. D. F. Grindley and D. Sherratt, Cold Spring Harbor Symp.
      Quant. Biol. 43:1257 (1979).
2. J. A. Shapiro, Proc. Natl. Acad. Sci. USA 76:1933 (1979).
3. M. P. Calos and J. H. Miller, Cell 20:579 (1980).
4. C. J. Muster and J. A. Shapiro, Cold Spring Harbor Symp.
      Quant. Biol. 45:(in press).
5. R. Gill, F. Heffron, G. Dougan, and S. Falkow, J. Bacteriol.
      136:742 (1978).
6. F. Heffron, B. J. McCarthy, N. Ohtsubo, and E. Ohtsubo, Cell
      18:1153 (1979).
7. A. Arthur and D. Sherratt, Mol. Gen. Genet. 175:267 (1979).
8. L. A. MacHattie and J. B. Jackowski, in:"DNA Insertion Elements,
      Plasmids, and Episomes," A. I. Bukhari, J. A. Shapiro, and
      S. L. Adhya, eds., Cold Spring Harbor Laboratory, Cold Spring
      Harbor (1977).
9. P. J. Kretschmer and S. N. Cohen, J. Bacteriol. 139:515 (1979).
10. S. N. Cohen and J. A. Shapiro, Sci. Am. 242:40 (1980).
11. R. Gill, F. Heffron, and S. Falkow, Nature 282:797 (1979).
12. L. A. MacHattie and J. A. Shapiro, Proc. Natl. Acad. Sci. USA
      75:1490 (1978).

COMPLEMENTATION OF TRANSPOSITION FUNCTIONS ENCODED BY

TRANSPOSONS Tn501(Hg^R) AND Tn1721(Tet^R)

Rüdiger Schmitt[a], Josef Altenbuchner[a] and John Grinsted[b]

[a]Lehrstuhl für Genetik, Universität Regensburg
D-8400 Regensburg, FRG
[b]Department of Bacteriology, University of Bristol
Bristol BS8 1TD, U.K.

INTRODUCTION

Recent experiments have demonstrated that the two transposons Tn501 and Tn1721, which code for diverse resistance characters, have a continuous sequence of approximately four kilobases (kb) in common (Altenbuchner et al., 1981). This communication contains (i) descriptions of Tn501 and Tn1721 and (ii) an analysis of the four kb-homology region indicating that it encodes functions required for transposition.

THE Hg^R-TRANSPOSON Tn501

The 8.1 kb-transposon Tn501, originally found in Pseudomonas aeruginosa, confers inducible resistance to mercuric ions (Hg^R) and organomercurials on host cells (Bennett et al., 1978). The element is flanked by 38 base-pair inverted repeats and generates a five base-pair direct repetition of a recipient sequence at the site of insertion (Brown et al., 1980). Three EcoRI restriction sites, two located within the terminal repeats and one at 2.2 kb, divide Tn501 into a large (5.9 kb) and a small (2.2 kb) EcoRI fragment (Fig. 1).

The genes responsible for the Hg^R phenotype are probably homologous to the Hg^R determinant of plasmid R100-1 (R. Rownd, pers. communication). This latter has been studied in more detail by Nakahara et al.(1979) and by Foster et al.(1979). It comprises three genes: a regulatory gene (merR), which exerts positive control over two structural genes responsible for the transport (merT) and reduction (merA) of mercuric ions. The minimum length of the

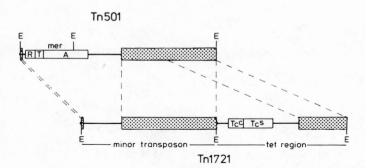

Fig. 1.   Diagram of Tn501 and Tn1721 superimposed with respect to
          the four kb-homology region derived from Fig. 2. Shaded
          boxes connected by dashed lines indicate portions common
          to both elements. The location of resistance genes, as
          described in the text, is shown (mer operon: R=regulation,
          T=transport, A=reductase; tet genes derived from pheno-
          types of insertion mutants: Tc^C=constitutive expression
          of resistance, Tc^S=sensitive to tetracycline). The extent
          of the minor transposon and the repetitious tet region of
          Tn1721 and positions of EcoRI sites (E) are marked.

complete region is 2.6 kb; a single EcoRI site is located in merA
and inactivation of merA renders cells supersensitive to mercurials
(Hg^{SS}). Assuming that the mer operon of R100-1 is homologous to the
Tn501-specified system, these results together with the previously
established insertion map of Tn501 (Grinsted et al., 1978) locate
the mer operon of Tn501 relative to the EcoRI site at 2.2 kb: merR
is close to the left-hand inverted repeat (Fig. 1) and transcriptional polarity is from left to right. This assignment is corroborated by the presence of an AUG start codon at 0.2 kb followed by an
open reading frame of at least 21 triplets with an "upstream" promoter containing Pribnow and Shine-Dalgarno sequences (Brown et al.,
1980 and unpublished observations of these authors). Moreover, cloning of the small EcoRI fragment of Tn501 leads to the Hg^{SS} phenotype indicating, that this fragment contains merT and that cleavage
with EcoRI inactivates merA. Since practically all of the small
EcoRI fragment codes for Hg^R, transposon-coded transposition functions must reside in the large EcoRI fragment.

THE TET^R-TRANSPOSON Tn1721

　　　Tn1721, originally identified as a constituent of R-plasmid
pRSD1 in Escherichia coli, confers inducible tetracycline resistance
(Tet^R) on its host (Mattes et al., 1979; Schmitt et al., 1979). The
11 kb transposable element consists of two distinct portions, the
"tet region" (5.6 kb), which encodes resistance, and the "minor
transposon" (Tn1722; 5.4 kb), which is capable of transposing independently of the rest of Tn1721 (Schmitt et al., 1981). The two
portions are defined by three 38 base-pair repeats, two in direct
and one in inverted orientation, as shown in Fig. 3. Each repeat
contains an EcoRI restriction site. Translocation of Tn1721 leads
to five base-pair direct repeats at the site of insertion (Schöffl
et al., 1981). The inverted repeats are practically identical to
those of Tn501 and are 50% homologous to those of Tn3 (Altenbuchner
et al., 1981).

　　　Heteroduplex analysis and Southern hybridisation have shown,
that the Tet^R determinants of Tn1721 are homologous to those of RP1
and RP4, respectively (Mendez et al., 1980; Schmitt et al., 1981).
Insertion mutagenesis using TnA has been applied to the tet genes
of RP1 and mutants sensitive to tetracycline (structural genes) or
constitutive for the expression of resistance (repressor gene) have
been mapped in an 1.8 kb region (P.M. Bennett, pers. communication).
These results and the presence of a single SalI and two SmaI sites
in the respective regions permitted location of the tet genes on the
map of Tn1721 (Fig. 1). Using a minicell system, we have identified
two polypeptides of 34K and 26K, respectively, produced by Tn1721
after induction with tetracycline (K. Schmid, J. Altenbuchner and
R.Schmitt, in preparation). Deletions leading to smaller derivatives
of 34K are tetracycline sensitive indicating a major role of this
species in tetracycline resistance. The function of the 26K polypeptide is still unclear.

　　　The tet genes of Tn1721 are flanked by 1.9 kb direct repetitions, which provide the structural basis for recA-dependent amplification of the tet region (Schmitt et al., 1981). Up to nine tandem
repeats of this region have been isolated from rec$^+$ cells. The amplified forms can be stably maintained in a rec$^-$ background. This
property of Tn1721 has been used to analyse the relationship between
gene dosage and tetracycline resistance of this particular system.
The resistance levels conferred by plasmids containing from one to
nine copies of the tet region have thus been tested in a recA host.
It has been found, that in exponentially growing cells the uninduced
level of resistance increases with gene dosage. Moreover, the rate
at which maximum resistance is attained upon induction with tetracycline is proportional to the number of tet genes present in a cell.
This positive gene dosage effect is a feature distinguishing the Tet^R
determinants of Tn1721 and Tn10 (Jorgensen and Reznikoff, 1979;
Coleman and Foster, 1981).

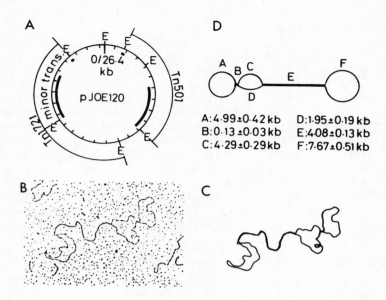

Fig. 2.   Heteroduplex analysis of Tn501 and Tn1721. The double-re-
          combinant plasmid pJOE120, which contains the two trans-
          posons in inverted orientation, was used for re-annealing
          experiments. (A) Physical map of pJOE120 showing position's
          of the transposons and indicating the regions of homology
          derived from Fig. 2B (E=EcoRI sites). (B) Electron micro-
          graph of re-annealed single-stranded circular molecule of
          pJOE120 showing two duplexed regions of homology and three
          single-stranded loops. (C) Tracing of B (—— single-strand-
          ed, ▬▬ double-stranded DNA). (D) Diagram of C with assig-
          ments of single- and double-stranded regions. Their contour
          lengths (averaged from 20 independent molecules) are given
          below ± standard deviations.

        Since the minor transposon can transpose independently of the
rest of Tn1721 (Schmitt et al., 1981), transposon-encoded transposition function(s) must be part of this segment. The large EcoRI
fragment of Tn501 contains the genes that encode the equivalent
function(s) of this element (see above). This fragment and the minor
transposon have a continuous sequence of about 4 kb in common, as
demonstrated by heteroduplex formation within a double-recombinant
plasmid containing both elements in opposite orientation (Fig. 2).
Thus, the genes responsible for transposition coded for by Tn501 and
Tn1721 are closely related suggesting to us the complementation experiments described below.

COMPLEMENTATION BETWEEN Tn501 AND Tn1721

The ampicillin resistance transposon Tn3 is one of the best-studied transposable elements (Heffron and McCarthy, 1979). Genetic analysis and sequence data have revealed, that the transposition of Tn3 requires the integrity of the terminal repeats and at least two transposon-encoded functions, "transposase" (coded for by tnpA) and "resolvase" (coded for by tnpR; Heffron and McCarthy, 1979). Cointegrate structures of the donor and recipient replicons containing directly repeated copies of Tn3 have been identified as intermediates in transposition; their resolution yields the two constituent replicons and requires site-specific recombination at an internal target sequence (the "internal resolution site" of IRS; Shapiro, 1979; Arthur and Sherratt, 1979). Transposition of Tn501 follows a similar sequence of events and the data below show, that there are similar genes coding for the functions required on Tn501 and Tn1721.

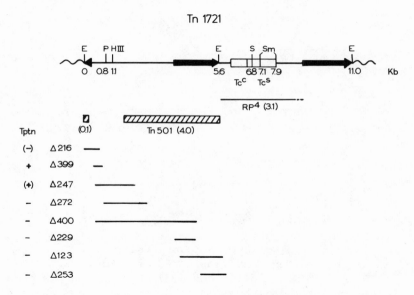

Fig. 3.   Diagram of Tn1721 showing terminal and central repeats (arrowheads), extent of internal homology (heavy bars), approximate location of tetracycline resistance genes (Fig. 1) and restriction coordinates (E=EcoRI, HIII=HindIII; P=PstI; S=SalI; Sm=SmaI). Regions of homology with plasmid RP4 (line) and Tn501 (hatched boxes) are shown in kb. A set of deletions was constructed from pJOE105 (a Tn1721 recombinant with a derivative of pBR322; Schmitt et al., 1981). The extent of deletions is shown and their respective transposition profienciencies (Tptn) are indicated (transposition positive:+, reduced:(+), low:(-), negative:-).

Partial HaeII-digestion and subsequent ligation of pJOE105, a
derivative of the high-copy vector pBR322 (Schmitt et al., 1981),
were used to generate a set of deletions which extend into Tn1721 to
various degrees, as diagramed in Fig. 3. The transposition proficiency of these deletions has been tested according to the scheme shown
in Fig. 4B. Transposition products were analysed by genetic and restriction mapping. The following results were obtained (also indicated in Fig. 3):

(i) A deletion of the left-hand terminal repeat (Δ216) reduces trans-
    position frequencies about 100-fold. In the ensuing rare trans-
    position events the tet region is translocated alone. This indi-
    cates that the 38 base-pair repeats, which flank this region in
    direct orientation, serve as "secondary substrate" for the ini-
    tial, transposase-catalysed step.

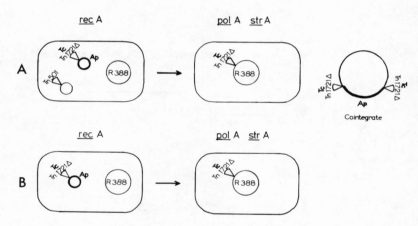

Fig. 4.   Diagram of donor and recipient cells used in conjugal
          crosses to test the transposition proficiencies of various
          Tn1721(pJOE105) deletions (Tn1721Δ) in the presence (A) and
          absence (B) of Tn501 (Tc=tetracycline resistance; Ap=ampi-
          cillin resistance). The frequency of inter-replicon trans-
          position of Tn1721Δ to R388 was determined in each experi-
          ment. Left: recA donor cells containing the conjugative
          plasmid R388 and transposons Tn501 (part of pACYC184 re-
          combinant) plus various Tn1721Δ (from pJOE105; see Fig. 3)
          inserted into different compatible, non-conjugative high-
          copy vectors. Right: Selected exconjugant recipient cell
          containing R388 with Tn1721Δ inserted (polA mutation pre-
          vents the autonomous replication of high-copy vectors trans
          ferred as cointegrates). Far right: Structure of a cointe-
          grate shown to be an intermediate of transposition.

Table 1. Complementation of Tn1721-Encoded Transposition
Functions by Tn501[a]

Donor[b]	Tn501	Hg^{++}[c]	Transposition Frequency[d]	% Cointegrates[e]
pJOE105	-	-	5 x 10^{-3}	O (8)
(wild type	+	-	1 x 10^{-2}	O
Tn1721)	+	+	3 x 10^{-2}	O (12)
	-	-	1.6 x 10^{-3}	100
Δ247	+	-	4 x 10^{-3}	98
	+	+	1.5 x 10^{-2}	100
	-	-	O	-
Δ229	+	-	4 x 10^{-4}	O (4)
	+	+	4.6 x 10^{-2}	O (2)
	-	-	O	-
Δ272	+	-	3.6 x 10^{-3}	100
	+	+	3.5 x 10^{-2}	100
	-	-	O	-
Δ400	+	-	1 x 10^{-5}	100
	+	+	1.5 x 10^{-4}	100

[a] Conjugal crosses according to Fig. 4. Overnight cultures (30°) subcultured at 37° were mated during exponential growth for two hours and plated onto selective media.

[b] Plasmid designations according to Fig. 3.

[c] Where indicated, 60 μg/ml of merbromin were added to overnight cultures.

[d] Determined as the quotient of Tet^R transconjugants and total number of trimethoprim resistant transconjugants.

[e] Fraction of Tet^R transconjugants also showing ampicillin resistance (see Fig. 4).

(ii) With the exception of Δ247, deletions extending into the four kb-homology region cause a complete loss of transposition proficiency. Deletion 247, which extends between O.5 and O.7 kb into the homology region, reduces transposition frequencies about fourfold and leads to 100% cointegrates.

In a second series of experiments (illustrated in Fig. 4A) the possibility that Tn501 (supplied in trans) complements the deleted transposition function(s) of Tn1721 was tested (Table 1). The following results were obtained:

(i)   Transposition frequencies of Tn1721 (pJOE105) and Δ247 are increased two- to threefold in the presence of Tn501. The transposition-deficient deletion mutants Δ229, Δ272, and Δ400 regain proficiency indicating that Tn501 is capable of complementing the deleted Tn1721-specified function(s).

(ii) The high proportion of unresolved cointegrates observed with Δ247, Δ272, and Δ400, but not with Δ229, suggests that the former three derivatives have lost a locus for site-specific recombination (IRS) and/or a gene coding for resolvase (tnpR) or that the resolvase of Tn501 does not complement that of Tn1721. This latter possibility is unlikely (experiments in progress).

It becomes obvious that the diffusible function(s) furnished by Tn501 in complementing Δ229, Δ272, and Δ400, respectively, is analogous to the tnpA product (transposase) of Tn3 (see above). The boundaries of the corresponding gene(s) are located between Δ247 (2.3 kb) and the central inverted repeat of Tn1721 (5.6 kb), with its left-hand terminus located within Δ272 (endpoint coordinate: 3.0 kb). The length of this region thus ranges between 2.6 and 3.3 kb, a size similar to that of the tnpA gene sequence of Tn3 (3 kb; Heffron and McCarthy, 1979).

A three- to 100-fold increase in transposition frequencies was observed, if donor cells were preinduced with mercurials (Table 1). Sherratt and coworkers (Kitts et al., 1981) have shown, that Tn501-specified resolvase requires the presence of Hg^{++}. This two sets of data are consistent with the following model: Hg^{++}-induced stimulation of the transposition functions involves transcriptional readthrough from the mer operon into the tnp genes (Fig. 5). This assume the gene order mer operon - tnpR - tnpA, all with the same polarity (left to right), so that the promoter activated by the merR gene product upon induction with Hg^{++} (Foster et al., 1979) would also be responsible for the transcription of tnp genes. Without induction, the tnpA gene is expressed, but to a much lesser extent (Table 1). It is therefore proposed, that the tnpA gene has a secondary promoter, which becomes apparent when the more efficient promoter of the mer system is inoperative. This would be reminiscent of the E.coli tryptophan operon (Jackson and Yanofsky, 1972).

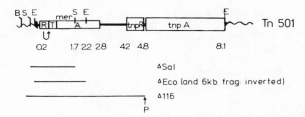

Fig. 5. Diagram of Tn501 with the mer operon located as in Fig. 1 and the transposition genes (tnpR=resolvase, tnpA=transposase) located in the homology region (see text). Relevant restriction sites and coordinates (in kb) are marked (B= BamHI, E=EcoRI, P=PstI, S=SalI). The extent and configuration of three deletions (ΔSal, ΔEco, Δ116) are indicated.

Table 2. Complementation of Δ229 with Deletions of Tn501[a]

Donor	Tn501 Derivative[b]	Transposition Frequency
	Tn501	4×10^{-4}
	ΔSal	3.3×10^{-3}
Δ229	ΔEco	3.5×10^{-4}
	Δ116	2.5×10^{-3}

[a]Test conditions as described in Table 1.

[b]Deletions shown in Fig. 5.

Based on these assumptions, we have tested three deletions that lack the mer control region. These are shown in Fig. 5. The transposition frequencies of Δ229 promoted by these Tn501 deletions are listed in Table 2. Two of these deletions (ΔSal and Δ116) show an unexpected six- to eightfold stimulation of transpositon proficiency compared to the control (Tn501), whereas a third deletion (ΔEco) with an additional inversion of the large EcoRI fragment shows a frequency close to that of the control. In line with the model above, these data are interpreted in terms of an external promoter to the left of Tn501 fused to the tnp genes by deletions ΔSal and Δ116, respectively, but ineffective upon inversion of the fragment containing the tnp genes (ΔEco). A pACYC184::Tn501 recombinant has been used in these experiments, and the tet promoter on pACYC184 (Chang an Cohen, 1978) is in the right relative position to act as transcriptional start.

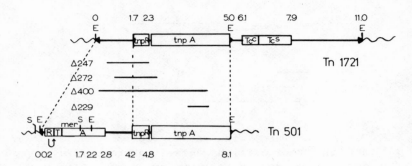

Fig. 6.   Diagram showing a comparison of Tn1721 and Tn501. Resistance
          determinants and genes required for transposition are locat-
          ed as in Figs. 1, 3 and 5, respectively. Regions common to
          both elements are indicated by dashed lines. Relevant dele-
          tions in Tn1721 used to define the location of resolvase
          (tnpR) and transposase (tnpA) are drawn as in Fig. 3 (see
          text for details).

        A view of Tn501 and Tn1721 in line with the experimental evi-
dence is diagramed in Fig. 6. It shows the two transposable elements
superimposed with respect to their homology regions. Genes specifying resolvase (tnpR) and transposase (tnpA) comprise this region,
their dimensions being in close agreement with the data published
for the corresponding genes specified by Tn3. Unlike Tn3, the tnpR
and tnpA genes of Tn501 and Tn1721 are thought to have identical
transcriptional polarity. It should be noted, that Tn3 is unable to
promote transposition of Tn501 (D.J. Sherratt, pers. communication).
Whereas Tn501-specified tnpR is transcribed from an external mer
promoter, the tnpR gene of Tn1721 has its own promoter, presumably
located outside the homology region. Deletion mapping places the IRS
sequence into the left-hand portion of this region, possibly between
genes tnpR and tnpA.

ACKNOWLEDGEMENTS

        One of us (R.S.), who spent three months as a guest at the
University of Bristol, thanks Mark Richmond for his generous
hospitality and support. The skilled technical assistance of Heather
Champion, Liz Hann and Sabine Unsin is appreciated. This investigation was supported by grants from MRC and from the Deutsche Forschungsgemeinschaft.

REFERENCES

Altenbuchner, J., Choi, C.-L., Grinsted, J., Schmitt, R. and Rich-
    mond, M.H., 1981. The transposons Tn501(Hg) and Tn1721(Tc)
    are related. Genet. Res., (in press).
Arthur, A. and Sherratt, D.J., 1979. Dissection of the transposition
    process: a transposon-encoded site-specific recombination
    system. Molec. gen. Genet., 175: 267.
Bennett, P.M., Grinsted, J., Choi, C.-L. and Richmond, M.H., 1978.
    Characterisation of Tn501, a transposon determining resist-
    ance to mercuric ions. Molec. gen. Genet., 159: 101.
Brown, N.L., Choi, C.-L., Grinsted, J., Richmond, M.H. and White-
    head, P.R., 1980. Nucleotide sequences at the ends of the
    mercury transposon, Tn501. Nucl. Ac. Res., 8: 1933.
Chang, A.C.Y. and Cohen, S.N., 1978. Construction and characteriza-
    tion of amplifiable multicopy DNA cloning vehicles derived
    from the P15A cryptic miniplasmid. J. Bacteriol., 134: 1141.
Coleman, D.C. and Foster, T.J., 1981. Analysis of the reduction in
    expression of tetracycline resistance determined by trans-
    poson Tn10 in the multicopy state. Molec. gen. Genet.,
    (submitted).
Foster, T.J., Nakahara, H., Weiss, A.A. and Silver, S., 1979. Trans-
    poson A-generated mutations in the mercuric resistance genes
    of plasmid R100-1. J. Bacteriol., 140: 167.
Grinsted, J., Bennett, P.M., Higginson, S. and Richmond, M.H., 1978.
    Regional preference of insertion of Tn501 and Tn802 into RP1
    and its derivatives. Molec. gen. Genet., 166: 313.
Heffron, F. and McCarthy, B.J., 1979. DNA sequence analysis of the
    transposon Tn3: three genes and three sites involved in
    transposition of Tn3. Cell, 18: 1153.
Jackson, E.N. and Yanofsky, C., 1972. Internal promoter of the
    tryptophan operon of Escherichia coli is located in a
    structural gene. J. Mol. Biol., 69: 307.
Jorgensen, R.A. and Reznikoff, W.S., 1979. Organization of structur-
    al and regulatory genes that mediate tetracycline resistance
    in transposon Tn10. J. Bacteriol., 138: 705.
Kitts, P., Symington, L., Burke, M. and Sherratt, D., 1981. Trans-
    poson-specified recombination. Proc. Natl. Acad. Sci. USA,
    (in press).
Mattes, R., Burkhardt, H.J. and Schmitt, R., 1979. Repetition of
    tetracycline resistance determinant genes on R plasmid pRSD1
    in Escherichia coli. Molec. gen. Genet., 168: 173.
Mendez, B., Tachinaba, C. and Levy, S.B., 1980. Heterogeneity of
    tetracycline resistance determinants. Plasmid, 3: 99.
Nakahara, H., Silver, S., Miki, T. and Rownd, R.H., 1979. Hypersen-
    sitivity to Hg^{2+} and hyperbinding activity associated with
    cloned fragments of the mercurial resistance operon of
    plasmid NR1. J. Bacteriol., 140: 161.

Schmitt, R., Bernhard, E. and Mattes, R., 1979. Characterization of Tn1721, a new transposon containing tetracycline resistance genes capable of amplification. Molec. gen. Genet., 172: 53.

Schmitt, R., Altenbuchner, J., Wiebauer, K., Arnold, W., Pühler, A. and Schöffl, F., 1981. Basis of transposition and gene amplification by Tn1721 and related tetracycline resistance transposons. Cold Spring Harbor Symp. Quant. Biol., (in press).

Schöffl, F., Arnold, W., Pühler, A., Altenbuchner, J. and Schmitt, R., 1981. The tetracycline resistance transposons Tn1721 and Tn1771 have three 38-base-pair repeats and generate five-base-pair direct repeats. Molec. gen. Genet., 181: (in press).

Shapiro, J.A., 1979. A molecular model for the transposition and replication of bacteriophage Mu and other transposable elements. Proc. Natl. Acad. Sci. USA, 76: 1933.

THE STRUCTURE OF TN5

W. S. Reznikoff, S. J. Rothstein, R. A. Jorgensen,
R. C. Johnson, J. C. P. Yin
Department of Biochemistry, University of Wisconsin

Madison, WI, U.S.A.   53706

INTRODUCTION

Tn5 is a transposable genetic element which encodes resistance
to aminoglycoside antibiotics such as kanamycin and neomycin. This
resistance results from the synthesis of the enzyme neomycin phosphotransferase type II (NPTII, also named aminoglycoside 3'-phos-
photransferase-II)(Berg et al., 1978). Its structure is in general
similar to other transposons with two inverted repeats 1534 bp
long (Auerswald and Schaller, 1980) flanking a unique central
region approximately 2700 bp long (Berg et al., 1975; Jorgensen
et al., 1979).

Tn5 is a possible model system for studying the genetic control of antibiotic resistance and for examining the transposition
process. With this in mind, my laboratory has pursued studies
aimed at defining the genetic organization of Tn5. Our experiments (some of which have been described elsewhere; Jorgensen
et al., 1979; Rothstein et al., 1980a; Rothstein et al., 1980b;
Rothstein and Reznikoff, 1981; Johnson and Reznikoff, manuscript
in preparation) were directed at asking the following questions:
(1) How many proteins does Tn5 encode?
(2) Where is the gene for NPTII (subsequently called "neo")?
(3) Where is the neo promoter?
(4) Where is (are) the gene(s) for the diffuseable transposition
function(s)?
(5) Where is (are) the transposition function(s) promoter(s)?
(6) Are either of these two sets of promoters regulated and, if
so, how?

Although these questions have not been answered in full, the
analyses have generated an overall picture of the genetic
organization of Tn5 which is schematically presented in Fig. 1.
Our approach towards elucidating this structure has been to:

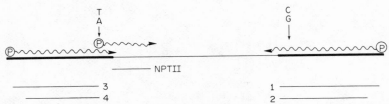

Fig. 1.   The Genetic Organization of Tn5. The location of the in-
          verted repeat and neo promoters, the proteins encoded by
          Tn5 and the single bp mismatch are presented. Protein
          #1 and possibly protein #2 are required for the trans-
          position process. This figure was first presented in
          Rothstein et al., 1980b.

(1) Determine the restriction enzyme cleavage map of Tn5.
(2) Knowing this map, use recombinant DNA techniques to derive
Tn5 mutations (some of these are shown in Fig. 2).
(3) Analyze the neomycin resistance, transposition and protein
coding properties of these mutant DNA's.
(4) Analyze RNA polymerase binding and transcription properties
of defined restriction fragments.
(5) Perform specific sequence analyses.
The results of these studies are described below.

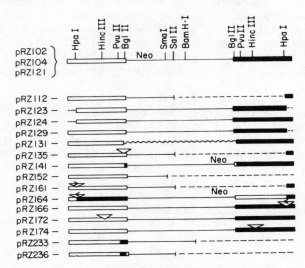

Fig. 2.   Tn5 Mutants. The constructions and analyses of these
          mutants are described in Jorgensen et al. (1979), Rothstei
          et al. (1980 a & b) and Rothstein and Reznikoff (1981).
          The symbols are defined as follows: ☐ = "left" inverte
          repeat DNA, ■ = "right" inverted repeat DNA, ∿ =
          substitution, ▽ = insertion (with arrowhead indicating
          orientation of promoter if present), and - - - - = deletion

RESULTS

I.   The NPTII Gene.

The gene for NPTII can be localized to a 960 bp region between the left inverted repeat BglII site and the SmaI site in
the unique central region. This was determined by examining the
neomycin resistance phenotype and NPTII protein coding properties
of various mutant Tn5 DNA molecules (see Jorgensen et al., 1979;
Rothstein et al. 1980a & 1980b). The particular mutants of
interest for this determination are pRZ112, pRZ135, pRZ152 and
pRZ172 described in Fig. 2. The relevant results are presented
in Table 1. Plasmids which contain mutations defining the 1275
bp HincIII–Sma I fragment (pRZ112, pRZ152 and pRZ172) encode normal levels of neomycin resistance and the NPTII protein. Plasmid
pRZ135 (which carries an insertion in the BglII site) encodes
very low but significant levels of both. Its properties can most
easily be explained by hypothesizing that the BglII insertion
mutation has separated the neo gene from its promoter; a hypothesis
which will be verified below. This genetic placement for the
NPTII structural gene has been confirmed by the Auerswald-
Schaller sequence analysis which localized the NPTII translation
initiation codon 34 bp inside from the BglII cut site (Auerswald and Schaller, 1980).

The neo promoter is located between the PvuII and BglII sites
in the left inverted repeat and the equivalent sequence from the
right inverted repeat can not perform this function when correctly
positioned (Rothstein et al., 1980 a & b; Rothstein and Reznikoff,
1981). The results which first suggested that the neo promoter
was located within this region were the observations that
insertions into the BglII site or deletions up to the BglII site
drastically reduced the level of neomycin resistance and the synthesis of the NPTII protein (for example see the results for plasmid pRZ135 in Table 1 which were mentioned above), whereas comparable mutations at the left HincIII site (pRZ172) had no affect.
Furthermore, the HincIII–BglII fragment which precedes this cut

Table 1.   Neomycin Resistance Levels of Tn5 Mutants.

Plasmid	EOP_{50} (µg/ml neo)
pRZ102	90
pRZ112	75
pRZ135	2
pRZ141	10
pRZ172	130
pRZ236	<1/6 of $Tn5^+$ in same vector

(Results are from Rothstein et al (1980 a & b) and
Rothstein and Reznikoff (1981). pRZ236 is carried
on a different vehicle and its EOP_{50} is indicated
relative to wild type Tn5 in the same vehicle.)

site binds RNA polymerase in a specific, heparin resistant
fashion as would be expected for a fragment which contains a
promoter (Rothstein et al., 1980a).

The dissimilarity between the two inverted repeats was discovered by analyzing the neomycin resistance properties of mutants
such as a BglII inversion mutation (the neomycin resistance level
of pRZ141 is drastically reduced, see Table 1), and a construct
which substitutes the right PvuII-BglII region for the left PvuII-
BglII region (pRZ236 encodes a low level of neomycin resistance).
These results not only suggested that the two inverted repeats
are different in this region, but also indicated that this was
an important target for DNA sequence analysis. A DNA sequence
determination of 130 bp containing this region was performed (and
was independently confirmed by Auerswald and Schaller, 1980) and
a single base pair difference between the two inverted repeats was
detected (see Fig. 3). In Fig. 4 a portion of this sequence is
compared to the model promoter sequence of Rosenberg and Court
(1979). A good match can be achieved if one assumes that the
single bp mismatch occurs in the highly conserved "Pribnow Box"
region of the promoter.

II. Inverted Repeat Functions.

Each inverted repeat is known to encode two proteins with
different N termini but otherwise largely shared sequences although
the two repeats differ from each other in that the right inverted
repeat proteins extend further at their C termini than the left
proteins. As shall be shown below this difference in the C termini
has a functional affect (one or both of the right inverted repeat
proteins is (are) required for transposition while neither of the
left proteins are required for transposition), and is due to the
single bp mismatch described above. (Rothstein et al., 1980 a & b;
Rothstein and Reznikoff, 1981).

Fig 5 presents an example of several minicell experiments in
which the protein coding properties of different Tn5 mutations were
examined. These are summarized in Table 2. In the particular

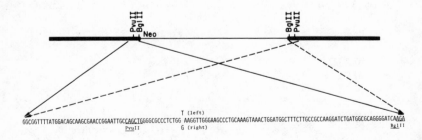

Fig. 3.   DNA Sequence of Left and Right Inverted Repeat PvuII-Bgl
Regions. This 130 bp sequence was determined by both Ma
-Gilbert (1977) and Sanger et al. (1977) protocals as wa
described in Rothstein and Reznikoff (1981).

Proposed Neo Promoter

CCGGAATTGCCAGCTGGGGCGCCCTCTGGTAAGGTTGGGAAGCCCTGCAA

↓ bp 1442 difference

G

Model Promoter Sequence

```
tt--tgTTGACA-ttt-------atttgtTATAATg---cat------aa
aa   c        cca        g gtg  ag a   tg        gt
cc            aa         t cc      t
```

Fig. 4.   Proposed neo Promoter. Within the sequence described
           in Fig. 3 is a sequence which resembles the model
           promoter sequence described by Rosenberg and Court
           (1979). This model sequence is indicated and its si-
           milarities to the proposed neo promoter is shown by
           underlinings.

experiment shown in Fig. 5, deletions up to the left inverted repeat HpaI site and up to the right HpaI site are compared to the
protein coding functions of normal Tn5. This type of experiment
reveals that Tn5 encodes 5 proteins; NPTII and proteins 1, 2, 3
and 4. Deletion up to the left HpaI site (or insertions into that
site) abolishes synthesis of protein 3 and reduces synthesis of
protein 4. This is similar to all other left inverted repeat mutations in that only these two proteins are affected but is different in that the other mutations abolish synthesis of both proteins (see Table 2). The deletion mutation up to the right
inverted repeat HpaI site (or insertion into that site) abolishes
synthesis of protein 1 and reduces synthesis of protein 2 (other
right inverted repeat mutations abolish synthesis of both 1 and 2).
The results of this and other similar experiments indicate the
coding localization for proteins 1, 2, 3 and 4 shown in Figs 1 and
6, and suggest that their genes are oriented in the following
manner. Genes for proteins 1 and 3 have their N terminal coding
sites situated between the outside Tn5 edges and the HpaI sites
and proteins 2 and 4 have their N terminal coding sites located
slightly inside of the HpaI sites.

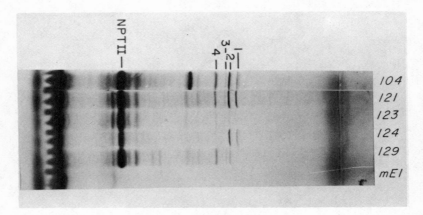

Fig. 5.   Proteins Encoded by Tn5 Deletion Strains. Minicells
            containing the indicated plasmids were labeled with
            35-S-methionine and their extracts were analyzed by
            polyacrylamide gel electrophoresis as described pre-
            viously (Rothstein et al., 1980). Plasmid mE1 is pVH51.

Table 2.   Inverted Repeat Coding Properties.

| Plasmid | Tn5 Inverted Repeat Proteins Found | | | | % W.T. Transposition |
	1	2	3	4	
pRZ102	+	+	+	+	100
pRZ112	–	–	+	+	<0.5
pRZ112(SupB)	n.d.	n.d.	n.d.	n.d.	103
pRZ121	+	+	+	+	n.d.
pRZ123	–	<	–	<	n.d.
pRZ124	+	+	–	<	n.d.
pRZ129	–	<	+	+	n.d.
pRZ131	–	–	+	+	n.d.
pRZ164	–	<	+	+	<0.5
pRZ166	–	<	+	+	<0.5
pRZ172	+	+	–	–	27
pRZ174	–	–	+	+	<0.5
pRZ233	+	+	–	–	n.d.

(The minicell protein coding properties (+=normal levels,
<=reduced levels, -=non detectable) and transposition
frequency data come from Rothstein et al (1980 a & b) and
Rothstein and Reznikoff (1981). Transposition data for
pRZ131 is available in Berg et al 1980. n.d. means not
determined.)

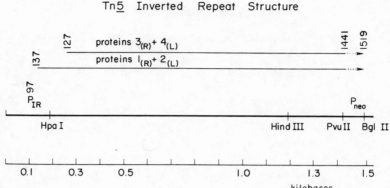

Fig. 6.   Structure of Tn5 Inverted Repeats. The locations of
           the promoters and translation start and stop signals
           were positioned on the Auerswald-Schaller (1980) se-
           quence using results summarized in the text.

The DNA sequences outside of the HpaI sites are known to
contain promoters because fragments from these regions specifically bind RNA polymerase and program transcription which proceeds
inward towards the unique region (Rothstein et al., 1980a). From
size measurements of full length transcripts made from restriction
fragments which carry this region, an RNA start point was approximately located at 95 bp from the end of each inverted repeat. The
exact start point has been identified as bp 97 (Johnson and
Reznikoff, in preparation) based upon the following types of
evidence. The transcript initiates with a 5' pppA residue (transcription requires a high concentration of ATP but not GTP, CTP or
UTP and the transcript is labeled with $\gamma^{32}P$ labeled ATP). RNase
T1 digestion of $\gamma^{32}P$ ATP labeled mRNA indicates that the first G
is at position 8. The oligoribonucleotides synthesized during the
abortive initiation process (described in Munson and Reznikoff,
1981) are pppApA, pppApApC and pppApApCpU. The inverted repeat
promoter sequence (for both left and right inverted repeat
promoters) is shown in Fig 7.
     Knowledge of the promoter location allows one to unambigu-
ously select the correct translation start sites for the inverted
repeat proteins in the Auerswald-Schaller (1980) sequence. Proteins
1 and 3 must start with the GUG codon corresponding to bp 137-139.
This is the only translation initiation codon subsequent to the
transcription start site which is in the open reading frame and
which is prior to the HpaI cut site. Proteins 2 and 4 must start
with the AUG on the other side of the HpaI site at positions bp
257-259. These assignments fit with the apparent molecular weight

Tn5 Inverted Repeat Promoter Sequence

```
TCTGACTTCCATGTGACCTCCTAACATGGTAACGTTCATGATAACTTCTGCT
••••••                                          AACUUCUGCU
CTGACTCTT outer end                             IR mRNA
CTGTCTCTT inner end
```

Model Promoter Sequence

```
tt--tgTTGACA-ttt-------atttgtTATAATg-----cat------aa
aa   c       cca       g gtg ag a        tg       gt
cc           aa        t cc        t
```

Fig. 7. The Inverted Repeat Promoter. The exact inverted
         repeat mRNA start point was determined as described
         elsewhere (Johnson and Reznikoff, in preparation).
         Also described are the similarities to the Rosen-
         berg and Court (1979) model sequence and to the
         small inverted repeats found at the ends of each
         Tn5 inverted repeat.

estimates for the proteins and explain why mutations at the HpaI
sites prevent synthesis of proteins 1 and/or 3 but not 2 and 4.
A detailed picture of the Tn5 inverted repeat structure is
presented in Fig 6.
     The protein coding properties of Tn5 derivatives carrying
substitutions of the internal BglII fragment (such as pRZ131)
suggest that the C termini of proteins 1 and 2 are encoded beyond
the right BglII cut sites (this substitution fails to synthesize
proteins 1 and 2 instead making fusion peptides) while the C
termini of proteins 3 and 4 is before the BglII cut site (Rothstein
et al 1980 a & b, Rothstein and Reznikoff, 1981). The observation
that plasmid pRZ233 (see Table 2 and Fig 2) encodes proteins 1 and
2 (Rothstein and Reznikoff, 1981) localizes the C terminus of
proteins 3 and 4 to the region substituted in this plasmid, the
region between the left inverted repeat PvuII and BglII sites.
     These conclusions have been confirmed by the DNA sequence
analyses (Auerswald and Schaller, 1980; Rothstein and Reznikoff,
1981). The single bp T/A → G/C difference at bp 1442 (see Fig. 3)
creates an in phase ochre codon in the left inverted repeat
missing on the right where the first in phase nonsense codon is
at position 1520-1522 (with the BglII cut site being between bp
1517 and 1518).

The differences in the inverted repeat protein C termini
have interesting functional implications. This is apparent
from the transposition tests summarized in Table 2. Mutations in
the right inverted repeat (pRZ112, pRZ174, pRZ166) prevent transposition while those in the left repeat (pRZ172) lower the level
of transporition but do not prevent its occurrence. In these and
all other mutants discussed below, the failure to synthesize protein 1 is always correlated with a failure to transpose. This important functional difference between the two inverted repeats can
be localized to the same region in which the neo promoter, the
difference in C terminal coding capacity and the single bp mismatch
are located by virtue of the following types of observations:
(1) Mutations which substitute the left inverted repeat PvuII-
BglII region for the right PvuII-BglII region and vice versa
always invert the functional polarity of the inverted repeats. For
instance plasmid pRZ164 carries a HpaI inversion and a HpaI site
insertion in the "new" left inverted repeat. This mutant Tn5
fails to transpose and fails to synthesize protein 1 as would be
expected for right inverted repeat HpaI site insertion.
(2) Introduction of some right inverted repeat mutant plasmids
(such as pRZ112) into an supB (ochre suppressor) genetic background suppresses the transposition defect (Table 2).
     Thus the twenty six additional amino acid residues at the C
terminus of protein 1 (or of proteins 1 and 2) must play an
essential role in some transposition related function.

DISCUSSION AND CONCLUSION
     Our analysis of Tn5 structure has led to a fairly complete
picture as is summarized in Fig. 1 and for which details are presented in Figs 4, 6 and 7. In spite of this general understanding, several rather obvious questions are outstanding such as:
(1) How did the overlap of the neo promoter and the left inverted
repeat evolve?
(2) What is the enzymatic function of protein #1 in transposition?
(3) Does protein #2 play a role in this process?
(4) Why do left inverted repeat mutations have a partial affect
on transposition?
     There are also some less obvious questions that have arisen
from our studies which I shall describe below.
     The studies of Biek and Roth (1980) have suggested that the
Tn5 transposition process may be regulated. The sequence of the
inverted repeat promoter (Fig 7) suggests a possible mechanism of
autoregulation for inverted repeat protein biosynthesis. Doug
Berg's laboratory (Berg et al., 1980) has discovered that the right
inverted repeat can transpose by itself and that the two ends of
the inverted repeat are related by a small inverted repeat
(CTGACTCTT...AAGAGACAG) (D. Berg, personal communication; note that
this implies that the "true" or "functional" end of the large

inverted repeat is at bp 1533 not 1534) with only 1 mismatch.
Presumeably this is a sequence which must be recognized by the
Tn5 transposase (protein 1 or 1+2). As indicated in Fig 7, the
inverted repeat promoter sequence contains a 6 out of 9 bp match
with this sequence offering a target site at which the transposase
could block the transcription of its own mRNA.

The ochre suppressor studies mentioned above yielded a positive suppression result for most but not all right inverted repeat mutations. Specifically, the transposition defect in
pRZ166 was not suppressed. This raises the possibility that the
fusion peptide made in pRZ166 acts as a negatively complementing
protein or that the production of proteins 1 and 2 must be in the
correct ratio for a positive transposition phenotype and this
suppressed mutant provides an excess of protein 2.

ACKNOWLEDGEMENTS
        This research was supported by grants from the NIH (GM19670)
and the NSF (PCM7910686) to W.S.R. R.C.J. and J.C-P.Y. were
supported by training grants from the NIH.

REFERENCES
Auerswald, E.A. and Schaller, H. (1980). Cold Spring Harbor
        Symp. Quant. Biol., in press.
Berg, D. E., Davies, J., Allet, B. and Rochaix, J. (1975).
        Proc. Nat. Acad. Sci. USA 72, 3628-3632.
Berg, D.E., Jorgensen, R. and Davies, J. (1978). In:
        Microbiology - 1978, D. Schlessinger, ed. ASM
        Publications, Washington, D. C. pp. 13-15.
Berg, D.E., Egner, C., Hirschel, B.J., Howard, J., Jorgensen,
        R.A., Johnsrud, L. and Tlsty, T.D. (1980). Cold
        Spring Harbor Symp. Quant. Biol., in press.
Biek, D. and Roth, J. R. (1980). Proc. Nat. Acad. Sci. USA
        77, 6047-4051.
Jorgensen, R.A., Rothstein, S.J. and Reznikoff, W.S.
        (1979). Molec. Gen. Genet. 177, 65-72.
Maxam, A. and Gilbert, W. (1977). Proc. Nat. Acad.
        Sci. USA 74, 560-564.
Munson, L.M. and Reznikoff, W.S. (1981). Biochemistry
        in press.
Rosenberg, M. and Court, D. (1979). Ann. Rev. Genetics
        13, 3A-353.
Rothstein, S.J., Jorgensen, R.A., Postle, K. and Reznikoff,
        W.S. (1980a). Cell 19, 795-805.
Rothstein, S.J., Jorgensen, R.A., Yin, J.C.-P., Zhang, Y.,
        Johnson, R. and Reznikoff, W.S. (1980b) Cold
        Spring Harbor Symp. Quant. Biol. in press.
Rothstein, S.J. and Reznikoff, W.S. (1981). Cell, in
        press.
Sanger, F.S., Nicklen, S. and Coulson, A.R. (1977). Proc.
        Nat. Acad. Aci. USA 74, 5463-5467.

TRANSPOSITION OF THE INVERTED REPEATS OF Tn5

Douglas E. Berg, Chihiro Sasakawa, Bernard J. Hirschel,
Lorraine Johnsrud, Lyn McDivitt, Carol Egner and Rajani
Ramabhadran

Departments of Microbiology and Immunology and of
Genetics
Washington University Medical School
St. Louis, Missouri 63110

INTRODUCTION

The defining characteristic of bacterial transposons is their
ability to move to new loci in the absence of extensive DNA
sequence homology. Some, designated IS elements, contain only
the genes and sites necessary for their own transposition; other
transposons are composites of genes necessary for transposition
and genes for auxiliary traits (such as antibiotic resistance or
virulence)[1]. Although the mechanism of transposition is
unknown, plausible models involving breakage and reunion[2] or
replication[3,4] have been proposed.

We are studying kanamycin resistance transposon Tn5 (Fig. 1)
because this element transposes at high frequency, exhibits low

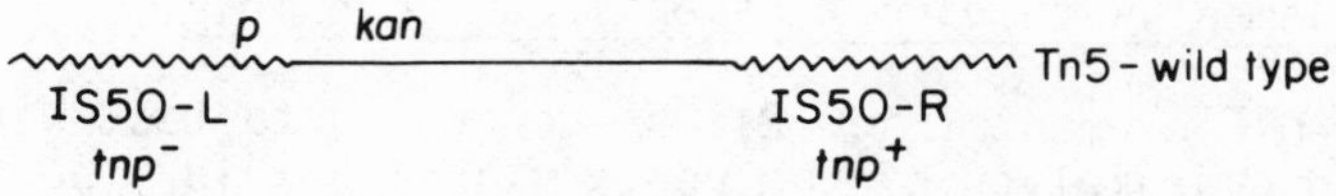

Fig. 1.   The functional organization of transposon Tn5. Tn5's
inverted repeats are indicated by serrated lines. The
gene for transposase (designated tnp+) is present in
Tn5's right repeat (IS50-R). A single base pair change
1442 bp from the outer end of the left repeat renders
the left repeat's tnp gene nonfunctional and creates a
pro moter (p) used for expression of the kanr
gene[5,10-12].

specificity in the choice of new insertion sites, serves as a good
model for analyses of transposition mechanisms, and is a useful
molecular genetic research tool[2,5-9]. It is 5700 bp long,
contains 1534 bp long inverted repeats[5,10], and is not
homologous to any sequences normally present in the chromosome
of Escherichia coli K12[13]. A gene whose product is necessary
for transposition (transposase) is present in Tn5's right
repeat. The left repeat contains a nonfunctional allele of the
transposase gene, inactivated by a single base pair
change[10-12,14,15].

The mutations Tn5 creates when it inserts into new sites are
polar regardless of Tn5's orientation[6]. These insertion
mutations revert by excision of Tn5 in recA⁻ as well as in
recA⁺ cells. Excision of Tn5 is unrelated to transposition,
depends on the inverted orientation of Tn5's repeats, but not
Tn5's tnp gene, and has been hypothesized to occur by copy errors
during DNA synthesis[15,16].

Because of Tn5's structural similarity to several transposons
known to contain terminal repeats of IS elements[1] we had
hypothesized that each of Tn5's repeats might be transposable[13].
The analyses summarized here confirm that each of Tn5's repeats
is an IS element which we have named IS50. Our analyses also
suggest functional differences between the two ends of the IS50
element, and spatial constraints on the action of transposase.

RESULTS

We tested three predictions of the hypothesis that each of
Tn5's repeats is an IS element: 1. The inverted orientation of
Tn5's repeats should not be essential for transposition. 2. Each
of Tn5's repeats should transpose from Tn5 to other DNA
segments. 3. Tn5 should mediate "inverse transposition".

1. A Tn5 element with direct repeats can transpose.

The Tn5-DR2 element (Fig. 2) was generated to test whether
the inverted orientation of the repeats in Tn5-wild type is
essential for transposition. We reversed the orientation of
Tn5's right repeat in a pBR322::Tn5 plasmid DNA molecule because
only the right repeat encodes a functional transposase, and thus
might have evolved less than Tn5's left repeat. The plasmid used
(Fig. 2) contains Tn5 inserted near position 3,200 bp of pBR322,
oriented such that Tn5's right repeat is nearest pBR322's amp[r]
gene[15,17,18]. Its DNA was digested with BamHI, and the DNA
fragments were ligated, and used to transform competent cells to
a Amp[r] Kan[r] Tet[s] phenotype. The structure expected (Fig. 2)

was verified by restriction endonuclease analysis. Studies
reported elsewhere indicate that Tn5-DR2 transposes with a
frequency and specificity similar to that of Tn5 wild
type[15],[17]. Thus a Tn5 derivative with direct repeats can
transpose, and the inside end of Tn5's right repeat can join to
other DNA sequences, as predicted by the view that these repeats
are IS elements.

2.   Detection of the IS50 transposon.

The transposition of one of Tn5's repeats to pBR322 would
provide a direct demonstration that the repeat is a transposon.
Our selection for insertion of IS50 into pBR322 was based on the
finding that conjugal transfer of pBR322 mediated by fertility
factor F is associated with the insertion of the $\gamma-\Delta$ IS sequence
of F into pBR322[19]. We found that FΔ::Tn5, an F derivative
lacking all transposons except Tn5, mediated the transfer of
pBR322's amp^r tet^r traits at a frequency of about 10^{-10}.
Approximately two-thirds of the transfered plasmids encoded
kan^r, were 10 kb long, and contained new restriction
endonuclease cleavage sites indicative of the insertion of the
5.7 kb Tn5 element into 4.4 kb pBR322. Although most of the
remainder contained no detectable insertion, one fourth of them
were 5.8 kb in size. Restriction endonuclease analyses of six
independent 5.8 kb isolates showed that each contained an
insertion of one of Tn5's repeats at a different site in
pBR322[20]. We have named this new transposon IS50[15],[20].

We constructed λ lysogens of strains carrying each
pBR322::IS50 plasmid, induced phage development in these
lysogens, and found λ Amp^r Tet^r transducing phage at a
frequency of 10^{-8}. Genetic and restriction endonuclease

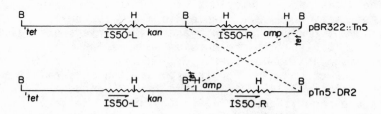

Fig. 2.   Construction of a Tn5 derivative with direct repeats by
BamHI digestion and ligation of pBR322::Tn5. The
plasmid DNA molecule is depicted in linear fashion,
arbitrarily cut at the BamHI site (B) in pBR322's tet^r
gene[17].

analyses showed that these phages contained insertions of pBR322
bracketed by direct repeats of IS50. DNA sequence analysis of
one of the pBR322::IS50 plasmids demonstrated that it contained
IS50-R (the Tn5 repeat which encodes transposase)[15,20]. In
control experiments in which pBR322 lacking IS50 was used, the
frequency of λ transducing phage containing pBR322 sequences was
less than 10[-10]. These results are in accord with findings
that the presence of Tn3 and of IS1 in plasmids converts these
plasmids to transposons[20,21].

We determined the junction sequences at three sites of IS50
insertion into pBR322, and found the following: (i) The transposed IS50 element extends from nucleotide position 1 to position
1533 in the 1534 bp long sequence[10] of Tn5's inverted repeats;
(ii) no pBR322 sequences are deleted by insertion; (iii) 9 bp of
pBR322 target sequence are duplicated directly by insertion of
IS50; (iv) the ends of IS50 consist of a 8 bp interrupted
inverted repeat (Fig. 3)[20].

```
5'CTGACTCTTATACACAAGTA·····AGATCTGATCAAGAGACAG
  GACTGAGAATATGTGTTCAT·····TCTAGACTAGTTCTCTGTC5'
```

         outside end   inside end

Fig. 3. The termini of IS50. The 7 bp interrupted inverted
         repeats are indicated by horizontal lines[20].

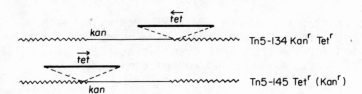

Fig. 4. The sites and orientations of tet[r] insertions in Tn5.
         These tet[r] genes are present in a 2700 bp BglII
         fragment derived from Tn10 and are inserted into BglII
         sites 1515 bp from the outside ends of Tn5[10].
         Although in Tn5-134 the insertion appears to be within
         the structural gene for transposase (which terminates
         at position 1519)[10,11,15], the Tn5-134 encoded
         transposase is active[15,16]. In Tn5-145 the tet[r]
         segment is inserted between the kan[r] gene and its
         promoter, and causes a partially Kan[S] phenotype.
         However, cells carrying Tn5-145 become Kan[r] when
         grown in 1 μg/ml tetracycline, apparently because of
         induction of transcription in the tet[r] segment and
         readthrough the kan[r] gene[15,20].

To determine if Tn5's left repeat could transpose, as predicted from the finding that the IS50 sequence is contained within the left as well as the right repeat, we marked Tn5's repeats by insertion of tet[r] genes (Fig. 4), and selected the transposition of tet[r] to phage λ; the resulting λ Tet[r] phage were scored for Kan[r]. Six percent of the Tet[r] phage resulted from transpositions involving Tn5-145 (tet[r] left repeat), and 22% of the Tet[r] phage which resulted from transpositions involving Tn5-134 (tet[r] right repeat) were Kan[s]. Restriction endonuclease digestions confirmed that Tet[r] Kan[s] phage resulted from transposition of just the marked IS50 element, and that Tet[r] Kan[r] phage resulted from transposition of the entire Tn5 element[20]. Thus, although each repeat can transpose as a separate unit, transposition of the entire Tn5 element seems to be preferred.

3. Tn5 mediated inverse transposition.

Inverse transposition in which the inside termini of a transposon's repeats join to new DNA sequences[23] would provide another demonstration that Tn5's repeats are IS elements. We have detected inverse transposition in two ways:

First, we induced λ::Tn5 prophages in cells carrying pBR322 plasmids, and selected Amp[r] Tet[r] transducing phages. They were Kan[s], and restriction endonuclease anayses showed that they had resulted from the insertion of λ into pBR322 using the inside ends of Tn5's inverted repeats (Fig. 5).

In the reciprocal approach, we induced phage development in a lysogen harboring pBR322::Tn5 as a stable dimer (Fig. 6). Amp[r] Tet[r] transducing phage were selected, and fell into

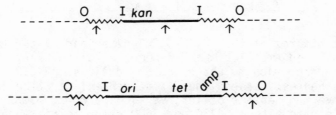

Fig. 5.   λ::Tn5, and the product of its insertion into pBR322. Dashed lines represent λ sequences; O and I represent "outside" and "inside" ends respectively of IS50; Vertical arrows indicate XhoI cleavage sites.

three classes: The Kan^S Amp^r Tet^r phage expected following
simple inverse transposition comprised approximately 1% of the
selected phage. The remaining 99% of Amp^r Tet^r phage were
Kan^r, and contained three copies of IS50 in either of two
arrangements (Fig. 6).

We used restriction endonuclease digestion to determine if
the insertion of pBR322::Tn5 sequences into λ could use IS50-L
as well as IS50-R. As shown in Fig. 6, BamHI digestion should
generate internal fragments whose size (4450 or 5600 bp)
indicates which IS50 element had been used. The results of
these digestions showed that in 20 of 21 cases analyzed IS50-R
mediated the joining of pBR322::Tn5 sequences to the λ genome;
in only one of 21 cases was the insertion mediated by IS50-L
(see Fig. 7). Thus, IS50-R appears to transpose much more
efficiently than IS50-L.

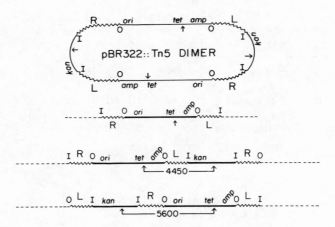

Fig. 6.   Structures of the pBR322::Tn5 dimer and of the Amp^r
           Tet^r and Amp^r Tet^r Kan^r genomes resulting from
           transposition to phage λ. Solid lines, pBR322
           sequences; dashed lines, λ sequences; serrated lines,
           inverted repeats of Tn5; vertical arrows, BamHI
           cleavage sites. 4450 and 5600 refer to distances in
           base pairs between the indicated BamHI cleavage
           sites[17].

DISCUSSION

Our experiments establish that each of Tn5's long terminal inverted repeats is a transposon which we have named IS50. The ends of IS50 comprise an interrupted 8 bp inverted repeat likely to constitute at least part of the transposase recognition site. Like Tn5[10], IS50 inserts into many sites and generates duplications of 9 bp of target DNA sequences. Pairs of IS50 elements often transpose together, carry with them any intervening genes, and thus are the building blocks of composite transposons such as Tn5.

The transposition of Tn5-DR2, of pBR322 bracketed by direct repeats of IS50-R, and of pBR322::Tn5 sequences containing direct repeats of IS50 all show that composite elements with direct repeats can transpose. Thus, there is no longer reason to suspect[24] that the inverted orientation of Tn5-wild type's repeats might play a specal structural role in transposition.

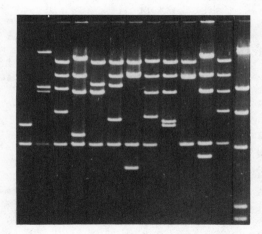

Fig. 7.   BamHI digestion of λ Amp[r] Tet[r] Kan[r] phage DNAs
           generated by pBR322::Tn5 transposition. The left most
           lane contains BamHI digested pBR322::Tn5. The right
           most lane contains a HindIII digested λ DNA standard
           (fragment sizes 22.8, 9.8, 6.4, 4.2, 2.2 and 1.8
           kilobases). The λ Amp[r] Tet[r] Kan[r] genomes
           replicate in cells as plasmids, and were extracted
           from recA−, immune transductants as described
           previously[15,17]. The phage genomes in lanes 2-8 and
           10-12 resulted from transposition involving IS50-R
           (Fig. 6, line 3). The phage in lane 9 resulted from
           transposition involving IS50-L (Fig. 6, line 4).

Although our data show that each of Tn5's repeats can transpose, the data also indicate that the outside end of IS50 (see Fig. 5) is more active than the inside end, and that IS50-R which encodes transposase (see Fig. 1), is more active than IS50-L which does not encode a functional transposase. The strongest indication of inequality of IS50's ends comes from experiments with tet[r] insertion elements Tn5-134 and Tn5-145 (see Fig. 4). Even though IS50-R is used in preference to IS50-L, (see Fig. 6 and 7) we found that IS50-R (tet) transposed at only one-third the efficiency of the entire Tn5-134 element. Thus IS50-R's inside end is less active than IS50-L's outside end. The inequality between IS50's two ends can be understood by postulating that the 8 base pairs common to both ends (Fig. 3) constitute a weak transposase recognition site, and that additional sequences unique to the outside end make it a strong recognition site.

The analysis of Amp[r] Tet[r] Kan[r] phages resulting from pBR322::Tn5 transposition showed that IS50-R was used more frequently than IS50-L in transposition (Fig. 6 and 7). Although control experiments to show that preferential use of IS50-R is independent of the position and orientation of Tn5 in pBR322 remain to be completed, we believe that these results indicate that transposase acts preferentially on the DNA segment which encodes it. Independent support for this interpretation comes from findings that the complementation of transposition deficient derivatives of Tn5 by Tn5-wild type is inefficient[25]. Preferential action of transposase on the IS50 element which encodes it can be understood if recognition of IS50's ends is a property of a domain in the amino terminal region of transposase, and if the growing transposase polypeptide generally folds to form this domain prior to completion of transcription and translation of the tnp message. A similar cis action of transposase on the unrelated Tn903 transposon has also been postulated[26]. We suspect that the tendency of IS50's transposase to act on the DNA segment encoding it may have minimized selective pressures to evolve a stronger recognition site at IS50's inside end.

ACKNOWLEDGEMENT

We are grateful to Dr. C.M. Berg for critical reading of the manuscript, to J. Howard for skilled technical assistance, and to Drs. H. Schaller and W.S. Reznikoff for communicating DNA sequencing data in advance of publication. L.J. is the recipient of the RHO prize in Microbiology from Washington University. C.S. is the recipient of Public Health Service International Research Fellowship 1 F05 TWO2940. This work was supported by Public Health Service research grant 5 RO1 AI 14267 to DB from the National Institute of Allergy and Infectious Disease.

REFERENCES

1. Calos, M., and Miller, J.H., Cell 20: 579-595 (1980).
2. Berg, D.E., in "DNA Insertion Elements, Plasmids and
      Episomes." (ed. Bukhari, A.I., Shapiro, J.A. and
      Adhya, S.K.) pp.205-212. Cold Spring Harbor Press.
3. Grindley, N., and Sherratt, D., Cold Spring Harbor. Symp.
      Quant. Biol. 43: 1257-1261 (1978).
4. Shapiro, J.A., Proc. Natl. Acad. Sci., USA 76: 1933-1937 (1979).
5. Berg, D.E., Davies, J., Allet, B., and Rochaix, J.-D., Proc.
      Natl. Acad. Sci., USA 72: 3628-3632 (1975).
6. Berg, D.E., Weiss, A., and Crossland, L. J. Bact. 142: 439-
      446 (1980).
7. Shaw, K., and Berg, C.M., Genetics 92: 741-747 (1979).
8. Miller, J.H., Calos, M.P., Galas, D., Hofer, M., Buchel, D.,
      and Muller-Hill, B., J. Mol. Biol. 144: 1-18 (1980).
9. Berg, C.M., and Berg, D.E., in: "Microbiology 1981". (ed. D.
      Schlessinger) ASM Publications (in press).
10. Auerswald, E., Ludwig, G., and Schaller, H., Cold Spring
      Harbor Symp. Quant. Biol. 45, in press.
11. Rothstein, S., Jorgensen, R., Postle, K., and Reznikoff,
      W.S., Cell 19: 795-805 (1980).
12. Rothstein, S.J., Jorgensen, R.A., Yin, J.C.P., Yong-di, Z.,
      Johnson, R., and Reznikoff, W.S., Cold Spring Harbor
      Symp. Quant. Biol. 45: in press.
13. Berg, D.E., and Drummond, M.H., J. Bacteriol. 136: 419-
      422 (1978).
14. Meyer, R., Boch, G., and Shapiro, J., Molec. Gen. Genet.
      171: 7-13 (1979).
15. Berg, D.E., Egner, C., Hirschel, B.J., Howard, J., Johnsrud,
      L., Jorgensen, R.A., and Tlsty, T.D., Cold Spring
      Harbor Symp. Quant. Biol. 45: 115-123 (1980).
16. Egner, C., and Berg, D.E., Proc. Natl. Acad. Sci., USA 78:
      459-463 (1981).
17. Hirschel, B.J., and Berg, D.E., submitted.
18. Sutcliffe, J.G., Cold Spring Harb. Symp. Quant. Biol. 43:77-
      90 (1978).
19. Guyer, M., J. Mol. Biol. 126: 347-365 (1978).
20. Berg, D.E., Johnsrud, L., McDivitt, L., and Hirschel, B.J.,
      submitted.
21. Gill, R., Heffron, F., Dougan, G., and Falkow, S., J.
      Bacteriol. 136: 742-756 (1978).
22. Ohtsubo, E., Zenilman, M., and Ohtsubo, H., Proc. Natl.
      Acad. Sci., USA 77: 750-754 (1980).
23. Chandler, M., Roulet, E., Silver, L., Boy de la Tour, E.,
      and Caro, L., Molec. Gen. Genet. 173: 23-30 (1979).
24. Davies, J., Berg, D., Jorgensen, R., Fiandt, M., Huang,
      T.-S.R., Courvalin, P., and Schloff, J., in: "R
      Factors: Their Properties and Possible Control, (ed.
      Drews and Hogenauer), pp. 101-110 (1977).

25. Berg, D.E., and Stamberg, J., <u>Genetics</u> <u>91</u>: s7 (Abstract),
        (1979).
26. Grindley, N., and Joyce, C., <u>Cold Spring Harb. Symp. Quant.</u>
        <u>Biol.</u> <u>45</u>: in press (1980).

HOST FUNCTIONS REQUIRED FOR TRANSPOSITION OF Tn5 FROM λ b221 cI857 rex::Tn5

Masanosuke Yoshikawa, Chihiro Sasakawa and Yuko Uno

Institute of Medical Science, University of Tokyo
4-6-1, Shiroganedai-machi, Minato-ku, Tokyo

SUMMARY

By assaying transposition of Tn5 from λ b221 cI857 rex::Tn5
(Berg,1977)(abbreviated as λ::Tn5) in PolA-proficient and deficient
cells, both DNA polymerase and 5' to 3' exonuclease activities of
DNA polymerase I of Escherichia coli K12 have been shown to be
required for transposition of Tn5. Such a requirement could not
clearly be observed in three other experiments in which the transposon donor replicon had existed in cells before transposition
was assayed presumably because a hypothetical repressor-regulated
protein encoded by the transposon itself rather than DNA polymerase
I became rate-limiting in the overall transposition process. One
polA mutant was found among more than 50 transposition-deficient
mutants isolated by the λ::Tn5 method. Preliminary experiments also
suggested that several host functions related to DNA repair or
recombination were involved in determining the frequency of transposition of Tn5.

INTRODUCTION

DNA segments which move to various sites are defined as transposable elements. The insertion sequence,IS, is the most simple
and contains no known determinants unrelated to insertion function.
The transposon is more complex than IS and contains genes such as
antibiotic resistance or toxin determinants in addition to those
for transposition or its regulation(see reviews by Kleckner,1977;
Starlinger,1980; Calos and Miller,1980). Considering the genetical
as well as medical importance of these elements the transposon has
extensively been studied. Among many observations reported the
following two seem to be the most important. First, DNA sequencing

technology has demonstrated that insertion of a transposable element
into a new site results in duplication of a 5 to 12-base pair
sequence at the target site (Calos et al.,1978; Grindley,1978;
Johnsrud et al., 1978; Oka et al.,1978; Schaller,1978; Cohen et al.,
1978; Kühn et al.,1979; Ghosal et al.,1979; Habermann et al.,1979).
Secondly, transposition accompanies duplication of the transposable
element itself, leaving one at the original site(Ljungquist and
Bukhari,1977; Bennett et al.,1977; Gill et al.,1978; Klaer et al.,
1980). Although the functions encoded by the element itself have
been shown necessary for transposition and to be under repression
control in several representative transposons(Gill et al.,1979;
Chou et al., 1979; Meyer et al., 1979; Rothstein et al., 1980), these
two observations suggest that host-encoded DNA repair and replication
functions may also play important roles.

In this paper we describe that both DNA polymerase and 5' to
3' exonuclease activities of DNA polymerase I in E. coli seem to be
important determinants of the frequency of transposition of Tn5 from
λ::Tn5 to the chromosome. A similar requirement could not be observed
in any experiment in which the transposon donor replicon had existed

Table 1. Reduced Transposition Frequencies of Tn5
         from λ::Tn5 to the Chromosome in DNA
         Polymerase I Deficient Cells

Strain Code	polA	Transposition Frequencies (X 10^{-3})
YC256	+	3.4 $\pm$ 1.1
WA5023	polA1	0.3 $\pm$ 0.1
W3623	+	0.42
HI97	polA11	0.051
KS463	+	0.20
RS5064	polA ex2 (Ts)	0.004

Stationary cultures of the strains listed were
infected with λ::Tn5, allowed 15 min at 30C for
adsorption followed by 30 min for phenotypic
expression and then plated on agar containing
kanamycin sulfate at 75 mcg/ml. Incubation of
plates was at 30C for 2 days. For the thermosensitive 5' to 3' exonuclease mutant and its parent,
growth was at 37C before phage addition to minimize the residual activity.

in cells before transposition event was assayed. The reason will
also be discussed why the requirement could be shown only in the
former but not in the latter methods to assay the frequency of transposition.

RESULTS

PolA – Mutation Decreases the Frequency of Tn5 Transposition from λ::Tn5 to the Chromosome

Three DNA polymerase I mutants and their respective parents
were examined for their ability to produce kanamycin resistant
colonies when infected with λ ::Tn5. Mutants polA1 and polA11 are
defective only in their polymerase with about 1 % residual activity,
whereas the mutant polA ex2 (Ts) is thermosensitive with respect to
5' to 3' exonuclease remaining 3 % of the wild type activity at 30 C.
For the DNA polymerase mutants, incubation was at 30 C, whereas the
5' to 3' exonuclease mutant was grown at 37 C before the λ::Tn5
infection to minimize the residual activity but subsequently kept
at 30 C to prevent thermal induction of the phage due to thermosensitive cI repressor. Under the conditions employed, the frequencies of
appearance of kanamycin resistant colonies per viable cell were
always lower with polA mutants than with their wild type parents
after 2 days incubation (Table 1).

In order to exclude the possibility that the rate with which
cells express the kanamycin resistance phenotype is dependent on
DNA polymerase I activity, the time of shaking at 30 C for phenotypic expression after λ::Tn5 infection and before selection on
kanamycin plates was altered within the range of 0 to 60 min. In
all other experiments phenotypic expression was allowed by shaking
for 30 min at 30 C after adsorption. As shown in Fig.1A, the number
of kanamycin resistant colonies per viable cell was larger in PolA-
proficient cells shaken for 30 min than in PolA-deficient cells
shaken for 60 min. Thus, such a possibility seems to be unlikely.

During prolonged incubation of kanamycin agar plates the number
of kanamycin resistant colonies increased but those derived from
PolA-proficient strains were always more than those from PolA-deficient (Fig.1B). As the growth rate of these strains, YC256(polA$^+$)
and WA5023(polA1) were similar without kanamycin, we believe that
comparisons may be made at the same period of incubation time for
kanamycin resistant colonies too.

As described by Berg(1977), the majority of these kanamycin
resistant colonies was not immune to λ , indicating that they had
been formed by transposition of Tn5 to the chromosome. This was also
verified by our previous observation of various chromosomal locations
of Tn5 among these colonies(Sasakawa and Yoshikawa,1980).

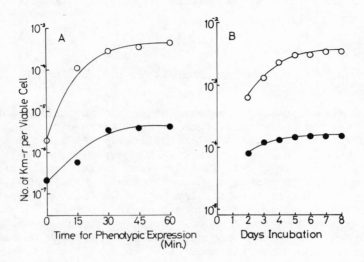

Fig.1. The Effect of the Time for Phenotypic Expression and for
       Incubation of Selective Agar Plates

Fig.1A; After cells were infected with λ::Tn5, 15 min incubation at
30 C was allowed for adsorption followed by shaking at 30 C for
various periods of time to rule out a possibility that PolA-defici-
ency affects the time required for the phenotypic expression of
kanamycin resistance. Fig.1B; Experiments were performed as described
in Table 1 but the plates were continued to observe for 8 days. Each
circle represents averages of two independent experiments. Open and
closed circles are for YC256(polA⁺) and WA5023(polA1),respectively.

     To rule out the possibility that λ multiplication rather than
transposition is dependent on DNA polymerase I, adsorption rate,
relative efficiency of plating, host cell killing and burst size as
determined by the one step growth experiment by the use of λ::Tn5
at 30 C were examined and no difference was detected between PolA-
proficient and deficient strains in any of these parameters, indicating that phage λ::Tn5 produced progeny at a similar rate in both
of them.

     When the multiplicity of infection of λ::Tn5 was changed to
infect a constant number of bacteria, kanamycin resistant colonies

Table 2. Effect of <u>polA</u> Mutation in Three Established Experimental
        Systems of <u>Tn5</u> Transposition

Expt.	Transposon Donor Replicon	Transposon Target Replicon	<u>polA</u>	Frequencies of <u>Tn5</u> Transposition	
I	Established R100-1::<u>Tn5</u>	Exogenously Infected λbb	+	4.6 ± 1.0	$(\times 10^{-10})$
			–	3.3 ± 1.0	
	Established R388::<u>Tn5</u>	Exogenously Infected λbb	+	3.9 ± 1.1	$(\times 10^{-10})$
			–	3.1 ± 0.3	
II	Prophage λbb::<u>Tn5</u>	Established R100-1	+	1.3	$(\times 10^{-5})$
			–	1.3	
III	pSC101::<u>Tn5</u>	R100-1	+	4.1	$(\times 10^{-6})$
			–	6.2	
		pMY1011	+	2.3	$(\times 10^{-6})$
			–	1.1	

Expt.I; <u>Tn5</u> transposition from plasmids to exogenously infected
phage λ <u>b515 b519 cI857</u> Sam7 (abbreviated as λbb). λbb grown and heat
induced in PolA-proficient and deficient strains carrying R100-1::
<u>Tn5</u> or R388::<u>Tn5</u> were used to transduce C600 to kanamycin resistance.
Expt.II; <u>Tn5</u> transposition from a prophage λ bb::<u>Tn5</u> to R100-1. PolA-
proficient and deficient λ bb::<u>Tn5</u> lysogens were infected with R100-1
and the plasmid was transferred by selection with either kanamycin
or chloramphenicol. Expt.III; <u>Tn5</u> transposition from a nonconjugative to conjugative plasmids. To T6 resistant, PolA-proficient and
deficient intermediate recipients carrying pMY0019(pSC101::<u>Tn5</u>),
R100-1 or pMY1011 was transferred followed by lysis from without by
T6 and subsequent re-transfer by the membrane filter method to the
final recipient resistant to rifampicin and T6. Selection was on
agar containing both rifampicin and either kanamycin or tetracycline.
It was later confirmed that the majority of kanamycin resistant
colonies did not show incompatibility phenotype to pSC101::<u>Tn3</u>,
indicating that they were unlikely to be formed by mobilization of
the nonconjugative plasmid or by co-integration of the donor and
the target replicons.

appeared at a constant frequency per phage and always lower in PolA-deficient than in proficient strains.

Unclear Effect of PolA-Deficient Mutation When Examined in Cells Established with the Transposon Donor Replicon

For convenience we describe the following three experiments as established experimental systems because we believe the difference between these and the λ::Tn5 method described above being due to the repressor encoded by the transposon itself, although separate regulatory protein has not yet been identified for Tn5.

The first established experiment(Expt.I, Table 2) was to grow λbb(abbreviation see Table 2) in PolA-proficient and deficient strains carrying R100-1::Tn5 or R388::Tn5 and resulting lysates were used to transduce C600 to kanamycin resistance. There was no clear difference in the frequencies of transposition from preexisting conjugative plasmids to exogenously infected λ bb between PolA-proficient and deficient hosts.

The second established experiment(Expt.II, Table 2) was to lysogenize PolA-proficient and deficient cells with λ bb::Tn5 to which R100-1 was transferred. The resulting strains were used as the donor to transfer the plasmid to the final recipient. No difference was observed in the frequencies of transposition from the prophage λ bb::Tn5 to R100-1 between PolA-proficient and deficient lysogens.

The third established experiment(Expt.III, Table 2) was to transform PolA-proficient and deficient cells with pMYOO19(pSC101 ::Tn5), to which R100-1 or pMY1011(a super-derepressed mutant of an IY plasmid R621a(Sasakawa and Yoshikawa,1978) was transferred as the target. After killing the initial donor by lysis from without by T6, the mixture was used as the secondary donor to the final recipient by the membrane filter method. No appreciable difference was observed between PolA-proficient and deficient hosts in the frequencies of transposition from a nonconjugative to a conjugative plasmid.

A Transposition-Deficient Mutant Is Phenotypically Similar to PolA-Deficient Mutants

By a method essentially based on the λ::Tn5 method more than 50 transposition-deficient mutants were isolated and characterized (Uno,Sasakawa and Yoshikawa, manuscript in preparation). One of them was shown to be similar to polA mutants as judged by the phenotypes listed in Table 3.

DISCUSSION

The results reported here seem to indicate that both DNA poly-

Table 3. Characteristics of a Transposition-Deficient Mutant
         Isolated by the λ::Tn5 Method

Strain Code	Transposition[b] Frequencies	Sensitivity		E.O.P.[c] of λ::Tn5	Transformation[d] of	
		UV	λ red3		pMY1113	pMY0019
C600	1.0	1.0	S	1.0	1.0	1.0
118-3[a]	$< 1.2 \times 10^{-3}$	10^{-4}	R	0.78	$< 10^{-3}$	0.41
YC256	1.0	1.0	S		1.0	
WA5023	8.8×10^{-2}	10^{-4}	R		$< 10^{-4}$	

[a]A mutant 118-3 is one of more than 50 transposition deficient
mutants of C600. Results on YC256 and WA5023 were added in the Table
for comparison.
[b]Transposition frequencies were calculated based on the experiment
as shown in Table 1.
[c]Efficiency of plating of λ::Tn5 relative to the parent as the indicator cells.
[d]pMY1113(Sasakawa and Yoshikawa,1980) is a mini-ColE1, pAO3(Oka et
al.,1978) inserted by Tn5. pMY0019 is a Tn5 inserted derivative of
pSC101.
All the figures were expressed in relative to the respective parents.
S and R represent sensitivty and resistance to the phage indicated.

merase and 5' to 3' exonuclease activities of DNA polymerase I are
important determinants of the frequency of Tn5 transposition from
λ::Tn5. However, there was no effect of polA mutation in the
established experiments where a transposon donor replicon had
existed before introduction of the target. The frequency of Tn5
transposition to the chromosome has been known to be 10^{-2} to 10^{-3}
and the highest among any method so far reported(Berg,1977). These
observations may be explained as follows.

    It has been well known that the transposon codes for at least
two transposition-related proteins by itself(Gill et al.,1979; Chou
et al.,1979;Meyer et al.,1979; Rothstein et al.,1980). The most
extensively investigated transposon is Tn3 which codes transposase,
another enzyme responsible for site-specific recombination for
resolution of the cointegrate composed of the donor and target

replicons(personal communication) and an autoregulatory repressor controlling transcription of the transposase operon. Similar regulatory mechanisms have recently been reported for Tn5(Biek and Roth, 1980), Tn10(Beck et al.,1980),Tn1721(this meeting) and an IS-like element, γδ(this meeting). Under established system as defined above, the transposase operon, if any, is repressed and hence the transposase activity itself may be rate-limiting in overall transposition process. This is in accord with the observation, for example, in Tn3 that a mutation within the repressor locus is phenotypically expressed as the actual increase in the frequency of transposition(Gill et al.,1979;Chou et al.,1979).

On the other hand, polA mutants ordinarily have some residual activity and no polA deletion mutants have so far been isolated (Kornberg,1980). Furthermore, there may be compensation of PolA functions by other related enzymes, although our preliminary results have shown that a polB mutation in addition to polA exhibits no additional effect on transposition. These factors may result in apparent inability of the polA mutation to be rate-limiting in overall transposition process and transposase may still be rate-limiting.If the transposase operon is derepressed phenotypically, as in classical examples of zygotic induction of λ repressor(Jacob and Wollman, 1956) or the lactose operon repressor(Pardee et al.,1959) and high frequency of plasmid transfer in conjugation(Stocker et al.,1963), then the consequence may be the same as a genetically derepressed mutation within the repressor locus of a transposase. Infection of bacteria with an integration-defective λ::Tn5 may result in the phenotypic derepression of the transposase operon although transiently. Under such a condition the transposase activity is no longer rate-limiting in overall transposition process in a polA mutant and the effect of the polA mutation is now manifested.

What is then the role of DNA polymerase I ? The current models for transposition(Grindley and Sherratt,1978; Shapiro,1979;Arthur and Sherratt,1979) assume DNA repair synthesis for gap filling and DNA replication for duplication of the transposable element itself. In this connection it is interesting that both polymerase and 5' to 3' exonuclease activities of DNA polymerase I seem to be required for transposition of Tn5. In our preliminary experiments several known mutants related to DNA repair or recombination, such as uvr, recB and lon(capR) have been shown to be concerned with transposition of Tn5 in the λ::Tn5 system. Furthermore, among more than 50 transposition-deficient mutants isolated we found one polA mutant. This supports our view that DNA polymerase I is an important determinant of the frequency of transposition of Tn5. It is also intersting that the majority of these mutants are not thermosensitive in spite of the fact that we isolated them at 30 C. This indicates that many functions coded by the chromosome are involved in transposition but not essential for cell growth.

Financial supports for this investigation and for participating this meeting provided by the Ministry of Education, Science and Culture, the Japanese Government are gratefully acknowledged.

REFERENCES

Arthur,A., and Sherratt,D.1979. Dissection of the transposition process:A transposon-encoded site-specific recombination system, Mol. Gen. Genet.,175:267.

Beck,C.F., Moyed,H., and Ingraham,J.L.1980. The tetracycline-resistance transposon Tn10 inhibits translocation of Tn10, Mol. Gen. Genet.,179:453.

Bennett,P.M.,Grinsted,J., and Richmond,N.H.1977. Transposition of TnA does not generate deletions. Mol. Gen.Genet.,154:205.

Berg,D.E.1977, Insertion and excision of the transposable kanamycin resistance determinant Tn5,in:"DNA insertion elements, plasmids and episomes,"A.I.Bukhari, J.A.Shapiro, and S.L.Adhya, ed., Cold Spring Harbor Laboratory,Cold Spring Harbor.

Biek, D., and Roth,J.R.1980.Regulation of Tn5 transposition in Salmonella typhimurium,Proc. Natl. Acad. Sci.,U.S.A.,77:6047.

Calos,M.P.,Johnsrud,L., and Miller,J.H.1978. DNA sequences at the integration sites of the insertion element IS1,Cell,13:411.

Calos, M.P., and Miller,J.H.1980.Transposable elements,Cell,20:579.

Chou,J.,Lemaux,P.G.,Casadaban,M.J., and Cohen,S.N.1979.Transposition protein of Tn3:identification of an essential repressor-controlled gene product,Nature(London),282:801.

Cohen,S.N.,Casadaban,M.J.,Chou,J., and Tu,C.P.D.1978.Studies of the specificity and control of transposition of the Tn3 elements, Cold Spring Harbor Symp. Quant. Biol.,43:1247.

Ghosal,D.,Sommer,H., and Saedler,H.1979.Nucleotide sequence of the transposable element IS2, Nucleic Acid Res.,6:1111.

Gill,G.,Heffron,F., Dougan,G., and Falkow,S.1978.Analysis of sequence transposed by complementation of two classes of transposition-deficient mutants of Tn3,J. Bacteriol.,136:742.

Gill,R.E., Heffron,F., and Falkow,S.1979. Identification of the protein coded by the transposable element Tn3 which is required for its transposition, Nature(London),282:797.

Grindley,N.D.F.1978. IS1 generates duplication of a nine base sequence at its target site, Cell,13:419.

Grindley,N.D.F., and Sherratt,D.J.1978.Sequence analysis at IS1 sites:models for transposition,Cold Spring Harbor Symp.Quant. Biol.,43:1257.

Habermann,P.,Klaer,R.,Kühn,S., and Starlinger,P.1979.IS4 is formed between eleven or twelve base pair duplication, Mol.Gen.Genet., 175:363.

Jacob,F., and Wollman,E.L.1956. Sur les processus de conjugaison et de recombinaison chez Escherichia coli.I. L'induction par conjugaison ou induction zygotique,Ann. Inst. Pasteur,91:486.

Johnsrud,L.,Calos,M.P., and Miller,J.H.1978.The transposon Tn9 gene-
    rates a 9 bp repeated sequence during integration,Cell,13:1209.
Klaer,R.,Pfeiffer,D., and Starlinger,P.1980.IS4 is still found in
    its chromosomal site after transposition to galT,Mol.Gen.
    Genet.,178:281.
Kleckner,N.1977.Transposable elements in procaryotes,Cell,11:11.
Kornberg,A.1980."DNA replication,"Freeman,San Francisco.
Kühn,S.,Frits,H.J., and Starlinger,P.1979.Close vicinity of IS1
    integration sites in the leader sequence of the gal operon of
    E.coli, Mol.Gen.Genet.,167:235.
Ljungquist,E.,and Bukhari,A.I.1977.State of prophage Mu DNA upon
    induction,Proc.Natl.Acad.Sci.,U.S.A.,74:3143.
Meyer,R.,Boch,G.,and Shapiro,J.1979.Transposition of DNA inserted
    into deletions of the Tn5 kanamycin resistance element,Mol.Gen.
    Genet.,171:7.
Oka,A.,Nomura,N.,Sugimoto,K.,Sugisaki,H.,and Takanami,M.1978.Nucleo-
    tide sequence at the insertion site of a kanamycin transposon,
    Nature(London),276:845.
Pardee,A.B.,Jacob,F., and Monod,J.1959.The genetic control and cyto-
    plasmic expression of "inducibility" in the systhesis of β-
    galactosidase by E.coli. J. Molec. Biol.,1:165.
Rothstein,S.J.,Jorgensen,R.A.,Postel,K.,and Reznikoff,W.S.1980. The
    inverted repeates of Tn5 are functionally different;Cell,19:795.
Sasakawa,C.,and Yoshikawa,M.1978. Requirements for suppression of a
    dnaG mutation by an I-type plasmid,J.Bacteriol.,133:485.
Sasakawa,C.,and Yoshikawa,M.1980.Transposon (Tn5)-mediated suppress-
    ive integration of ColE1 derivatives into the chromosome of
    Escherichia coli K12(dnaA), Biochem.Biophys.Res.Communs.,96:
    1357.
Schaller,H.1978.The intergenic region and the origins for filament-
    ous phage DNA replication,Cold Spring Harbor Symp.Quant.Biol.,
    43:401.
Shapiro,J.A.1979.A molecular model for the transposition and replica-
    tion of bacteriophage Mu and other transposable elements,Proc.
    Natl.Acad.Sci.,U.S.A.,76:1933.
Starlinger,P.1980.IS elements and transposons,Plasmid,3:241.
Stocker,B.A.D.,Smith,S.M.,and Ozeki,H.1963.High infectivity of
    Salmonella typhimurium newly infected by the colI factor,J.Gen.
    Microbiol.,30:201.

PLASMID MOBILIZATION AS A TOOL FOR IN VIVO GENETIC ENGINEERING

J. Leemans¶, D. Inzé°, R. Villarroel°, G. Engler°,
J.P. Hernalsteens¶, M. De Block° and M. Van Montagu°¶

°Laboratory of Genetics, Rijksuniversiteit Gent, Belgium
¶Laboratory GEVI, Vrije Universiteit Brussel, Belgium

K.L. Ledeganckstraat 35, B-9000 Gent (Belgium)

INTRODUCTION

Mutagenesis through the insertion of transposons has proved to be an invaluable technique for mapping the genes of complex plasmids[1]. No selection for a mutant phenotype has to be devised, but a straightforward selection for the antibiotic resistance markers, encoded by the transposon, is sufficient to identify the presence of a mutant plasmid.

One general method[2] for performing this type of mutagenesis uses plasmid conjugation, one of the techniques used originally to identify transposons[3]. Transformation and transduction also are efficient methods for isolating mutant plasmids, but are primarily restricted to small plasmids in Enterobacteriaceae. Conjugal transfer remains the method of choice for large plasmids and for most Gram-negative bacteria. Since all plasmid cloning vector and the majorities of naturally occurring plasmids are autotransferable (tra⁻) or are repressed for transfer, we assessed to possibilities of plasmid mobilization. It is possible to transfer such plasmids to a new host with the aid of some conjugative episomes.

This mediated transfer may take place by any one of three mechanisms[4].
(a) The nonconjugative plasmid may contain an origin of transfer (oriT) and an activation site (bom) but lack trans-acting functions necessary to activate these genes. These functions can be provided by an appropriate conjugative plasmid.

401

(b) Both conjugative and nonconjugative plasmids may contain region homologous to each other. Homologous recombination may fuse these plasmids transiently. Both plasmids then transfer as a cointegrate.

(c) When one of the plasmids of the pair contain a transposable element, a recA$^+$ independent plasmid fusion can occur and the plasmids transfer as a cointegrate. However, upon resolution of the cointegrate, a copy of the transposable element remains in both plasmids.

These three methods of mediating plasmid transfer were used extensively in experiments in which plasmids are transferred between different species of bacteria. The third method was of particular interest, since it provided a general tool for mutagenizing nonconjugative plasmids.

RESULTS

Mobilization of plasmid cloning vectors by transactivation of oriT transfers these plasmids without any alteration to their new hosts. This technique has limited application, since one rarely has all necessary complementation functions combined in a single helper plasmid[5].

The recA$^+$ dependent fusion of a conjugative and a nonconjugative plasmid also allows the original plasmids to be recovered after transfer.

The main advantage of this method is that the sole requirement for cotransfer is a single region of DNA homology between the plasmids. Furthermore, broad host range plasmids with homology to any portion of the cloning vector can be used to transfer this cloning vector to numerous Gram-negative bacteria.

For example, we have recloned sections of the Ti plasmids of Agrobacterium tumefaciens in nonconjugative broad host range cloning vehicles derived from the W-type plasmid Sa[6,7]. The transfer of these chimeric plasmids to Agrobacterium can be mediated by the N-type plasmids RN3 and R128. These plasmids[8,9] cannot establish themselves in Agrobacterium[3] but can be maintained as cointegrates so long as selection for the drug markers of the N-plasmids is applied. RN3 (Sm^{R}Su^{R}Tc^R) recombined within the streptomycin sulphonamide resistance locus of the Sa derivative (pGV1106) and transferred to Escherichia coli with a frequency of 10^{-3} and to Agrobacterium with a frequency of 10^{-6}. R128 (Su^{R}Tc^{R}Ap^R) transfers one tenth as efficient, presumably due to smaller regions of homology. The lower transfer efficiency of pGV1106 and derivatives to Agrobacterium might be explained by the instability of the RN3 in Agrobacterium and not to inefficient conjugation. In fact, RN3 probably conjugates as efficiently as RP4 since both RN3 and the "suicide plasmid"[10] RP4::Mu::Tn7 introduce the Tn7 transposon at an equal frequency, 10^{-5}. Indeed, RN3 is a preferable "suicide plasmid" for the introduction of transposons into Agrobacterium because the entire RN3 is invariably lost whereas portions of RP4::Mu can remain[7].

Transposon-mediated tansfer

The broad host range plasmid RP4 has been widely used to "mobilize" plasmids between different species. A study of the cointegrates between RP4 and a nontransferable plasmid demonstrated that these cointegrates harbored a directly repeated sequence at the junction sites of the two replicons[11]. This repeat had the properties of an insertion sequence and was denoted IS8. Since the cointegrate had the structure of a proposed intermediate in the transposition of an IS-element, we determined whether "mobilization" by RP4 invariably resulted in an insertion of IS8 in the transmitted plasmids. This was indeed the case as was shown by Southern blot analysis : the "mobilization" by RP4 in Agrobacterium always involves transposition of IS8.

In order to demonstrate the generality of this phenomenon, we tested the ability to mediate transmission of other P-type plasmids. From the P-type plasmids listed in Table 1, only pUZ8 was unable to transmit pACYC184 between E. coli strains. The cotransfer-proficient plasmids listed in Table 1 all contained either IS8 or an other transposable element. The relationship between RP4 and those plasmids, as determined by electron microscopy heteroduplex analysis[12], is shown in Table 2.

Table 1. Transmittance of pACYC184 by several conjugative

plasmids in E. coli

Conjugative plasmid	Compatibility	recA character of donor	Transmission frequency
RP4(KmTcAp)	P	+	1.2×10^{-6}
RP4(KmTcAp)	P	-	1.0×10^{-6}
R934(KmTcApHg)	P	-	10^{-6}
R702(KmTcSmSuHg)	P	-	5.0×10^{-6}
pUZ8(KmTcHg)	P	-	$< 10^{-8}$
pUZ8::Tn7(KmTcHgSmTp)	P	-	$< 10^{-8}$
R483(SmTp)	Iα	-	$< 10^{-8}$
R483::Tn1(SmTpAp)	Iα	-	10^{-6}

Table 2. Electron microscopic heteroduplex analysis of the relationship among several P-type plasmids

Plasmid	Ref.	% RP4 sequences in common	Size (Md)	Position on RP4 map[17] (Md)	Insertions Markers	Remarks and ref.
RP4	1	100%	3.6	3.2 to 5.8	Ap	Tn1 [1]
			1.2	21.5 to 22.7		IS8 [11]
R702	18	83%	10	1.2	Sm Su Hg	Tn1831 [15]
			4.8	7.0	---	---
R934	19	90%	6.0	9.8	Ap Hg [16]	not transposable[16]
			1.2	21.5 to 22.7		IS8[11]
pUZ8	20	83%	2.4	1.2	Hg	not transposable[7]
R1033	21	100%	3.6	3.2 to 5.8	Ap	Tn1[1]
			10.7	8.4	Sm Su Hg Cm Gm	Tn1696[24]
			1.2	21.5 to 22.7	---	IS8[11]
R26	22	100%	4.8	3.2 to 5.8	Ap	Tn1 with insertion
			10.7	8.4	Sm Su Hg Cm Gm	
			1.2	21.5 to 22.7	---	IS8[11]
R938	23	90%	9.4	7.8	Sm Ap	TAβ[23]
			1.2	21.5 to 22.7	---	IS8[11]
			9.2	33.4	Sm Su Hg Cm	---

Table 3. Transposon-mediated transmission of pACYC184-derivatives
         in E. coli

Conjugative plasmid	pACYC184 derivative	Transmission freq./ pUZ8 transfer
pUZ8	pACYC184	$< 8.0 \times 10^{-9}$
pUZ8	pACYC184::Tn1	5.0×10^{-7}
pUZ8	pACYC184::IS8	1.0×10^{-6}
pUZ8::Tn1	pACYC184	2.0×10^{-6}

The requirement for an insertion element in the process of
transmission was systematically examined using the pairs of
plasmids listed in Table 3. From these data we may conclude that
the transmission of the nonconjugative plasmid is dependent on
the presence of a transposable element in either one of the
participants. Therefore, every case of plasmid transmittance
shown in Table 2 should have resulted in the insertion of a
transposable element into pACYC184. This was indeed shown to be
the case (Table 4).

Table 4. Identity of transposable elements inserted
         in pACYC184 after transmission with the
         indicated conjugative plasmids in E. coli

Conjugative plasmid	Transposable element	Frequency
RP4 }	Tn1	35%
	IS8	65%
R702	Tn1831	100%
R934	IS8	100%
pUZ8::Tn1	Tn1	100%
R483::Tn1	Tn1	100%

RP4 contains Tn1 and IS8, either of which could participate in a transmittance event. In E. coli they are equally effective (Table 4) but in Agrobacterium only IS8 is active. This indicates that the failure of a plasmid to be transmitted does not mean neither of the plasmids contain a transposable element. Tn7, for example, is an efficient transposable element in E. coli, yet it cannot promote transmission in this host (Table 1). A plausible and testable explanation is that resolution of the cointegrates is exceptionally efficient.

Transmission-mediated mutagenesis

It is apparent at this point that this type of plasmid transmission mutates one of the participants.

We have systematically applied this technique for mutagenizing portions of the Agrobacterium Ti plasmid, cloned in pGV1106. In a typical experiment, pGV1106 containing a 15-16 Kb fragment of the pTiC58 Ti plasmid (fragment EcoRI-1)[13] was transmitted by R483::Tn1 at of frequency of 5×10^{-6}. Of the 34 transmitted plasmids examined, 26 carried a Tn1 inserted into the Ti fragment and this in at least 16 different locations. These mutated Ti plasmid fragments were subsequently introduced into Agrobacterium by a recA$^+$ dependent mobilization with RN3. Homologous recombination allowed afterwards the exchange of the mutated fragment with the corresponding segment of the Ti plasmid and hence the construction of a new set of mutant Ti plasmids[14].

CONCLUSION

Transmission-mediated mutagenesis has decided advantages over "classical" transposon mutagenesis. For example, it is not possible to select for the insertion of IS sequences in genes that do not have an assayable phenotype. The technique presented here can be used conveniently to provide a large collection of such mutants. The use of the classical technique is primarily limited to the Enterobacteriaceae since it is presently difficult to transform or transduce in most other families. Transmission-mediated mutagenesis has no such limitations. This is important, since it allows the mutagenesis in the host in which the assay for gene expression has to be conducted. Finally, many large plasmids, common in nature, and important to agriculture or industry, have not been analyzed genetically. Transmission-mediated mutagenesis will be the method of choice for mutagenizing these unstudied plasmids.

ACKNOWLEDGEMENT

We thank Dr. A. Caplan for his help with assembly of this manuscript. This research was supported by grants from the "A.S.L.K.-Kankerfonds", the "Instituut tot aanmoediging van het Wetenschappelijk Onderzoek in Nijverheid en Landbouw" (I.W.O.N.L., # 2481A), the "Fonds voor Geneeskundig Wetenschappelijk Onderzoek" (F.G.W.O., # 30052.78) and the "Onderling Overlegde Akties" (O.O.A., # 12052179) to J.S and M.V.M.

REFERENCES

1. M. Holsters, B. Silva, F. Van Vliet, C. Genetello, M. De Block, P. Dhaese, A. Depicker, D. Inzé, G. Engler, R. Villarroel, M. Van Montagu and J. Schell, The functional organization of the nopaline A. tumefaciens plasmid pTiC58, Plasmid 3:212 (1980).
2. N. Datta, R.W. Hedges, E.J. Shaw, R.B. Sykes and M.H. Richmond, Properties of an R-factor from Pseudomonas aeruginosa, J. Bacteriol., 108:1244 (1971).
3. J.P. Hernalsteens, R. Villarroel-Mandiola, M. Van Montagu and J. Schell, Transposition of Tn1 to a broad host range drug resistance plasmid, in: "DNA Insertion Elements, Plasmids, and Episomes", A.I. Bukhari, J.A. Shapiro, and S.L. Adhya, eds., Cold Spring Harbor Laboratory, New York (1977).
4. A.J. Clark and G.J. Warren, Conjugation transmission of plasmids, Ann. Rev. Genet. 13:99 (1979).
5. G.J. Warren, A.J. Twigg and D.J. Sherratt, ColE1 plasmid mobility and relaxation complex, Nature 274:259 (1978).
6. M. De Wilde, A. Depicker, G. De Vos, M. De Beuckeleer, E. Van Haute, M. Van Montagu and J. Schell, Molecular cloning as tool to the analysis of the Ti-plasmids of Agrobacterium tumefaciens, Ann. Microbiol. (Inst. Pasteur) 129B:531 (1978).
7. Unpublished results of the authors.
8. T. Watanabe, H. Nishida, C. Ogata, T. Arai and S. Sato, Episome mediated transfer of drug resistance in Enterobacteriaceae : VII. Two types of naturally occurring R factors, J. Bacteriol. 88:716 (1964).
9. N.D.F. Grindley, J.N. Grindley and E.S. Anderson, R factor compatibility groups, Molec. Gen. Genet. 119:287 (1972).
10. J.P. Hernalsteens, M. Holsters, A. Silva, F. Van Vliet, R. Villarroel, G. Engler, M. Van Montagu and J. Schell, A technique for mutagenesis by transposon insertion, applicable to most Gram-negative bacteria, Arch. Intern. Physiol. Biochim. 86:432 (1978).

11. A. Depicker, M. De Block, D. Inzé, M. Van Montagu and J.
     Schell, IS-like element IS8 in RP4 plasmid and its
     involvement in cointegration, Gene 10:329 (1980).
12. J. Leemans, R. Villarroel, R. Maenhaut, G. Engler, R.W.
     Hedges and M. Van Montagu, Heteroduplex analysis of
     P-type plasmids : the role of insertion and deletion of
     transposable elements, (submitted).
13. A. Depicker, M. De Wilde, G. De Vos, R. De Vos, M. Van
     Montagu and J. Schell, Molecular cloning of overlapping
     segments of the nopaline Ti-plasmids pTiC58 as a means
     to restriction endonuclease mapping, Plasmid 3:193
     (1980).
14. M. Van Montagu, J. Schell, M. Holsters, H. De Greve, J.
     Leemans, J.P. Hernalsteens, L. Willmitzer and L. Otten,
     Transfer, maintenance and expression of genes intro-
     duced into plant cells via the Ti plasmid, in:"Molecu-
     lar Biology, Pathogenicity and Ecology of Bacterial
     plasmids," S.B. Levy, ed., Plenum Press, New York
     (1981).
15. P.J.J. Hooykaas, H. Den Dulck-Ras and R.A. Schilperoort,
     Molecular mechanism of Ti-plasmid mobilization by
     R-plasmids. Isolation of Ti-plasmids with transposons
     insertion in Agrobacterium tumefaciens, Plasmid 4:64
     (1980).
16. Dr. R.W. Hedges, personal communication.
17. A. Depicker, M. Van Montagu and J. Schell, Physical map of
     RP4, in: "DNA Insertion Elements, Plasmids, and Episome
     s", A.I. Bukhari, J.A. Shapiro, and S.L. Adhya, eds.,
     Cold Spring Harbor Laboratory, New York (1977).
18. R.W. Hedges, A. Jacob and J.T. Smith, Properties of an R
     factor from Bordetella bronchiseptica, J. Gen.
     Microbiol. 84:199 (1974).
19. R.W. Hedges, V. Rodriguez-Lemoine and N. Datta, R factors
     from Serratia marcescens, J. Gen. Microbiol. 86:88
     (1975).
20. R.W. Hedges and M. Matthew, Acquisition by Escherichia coli
     of plasmid-bone β lactamases normally confined to
     Pseudomonas spp., Plasmid 2:269 (1979).
21. D.I. Smith, R. Gomez Lus, M. Rubio Calvo, N. Datta, A.E.
     Jacob and R.W. Hedges, Third type of plasmid conferring
     gentamicin resistance in Pseudomonas aeruginosa,
     Antimicrob. Agents Chemother. 8:227 (1975).
22. V.A. Stanisich and J.M. Ortiz, Similarities between plasmids
     of the P incompatibility group derived from different
     bacterial genera, J. Gen. Microbiol. 94:281 (1976).
23. R.W. Hedges, M. Matthew, D.I. Smith, J.M. Cresswell and A.E.
     Jacob, Properties of a transposon conferring resistance
     to pennicillins and streptomycin, Gene 1:241 (1977).

24. C.E. Rubens, W.F. McNeill and W.E. Farrar, A transposable
         plasmid DNA sequence in Pseudomonas aeruginosa which
         mediates resistance to gentamicin and four other anti-
         microbial agents, J. Bacteriol. 139:877 (1979).

PROINSULIN FROM BACTERIA

Karen Talmadge and Walter Gilbert

Biological Laboratories
Harvard University
Cambridge MA 02138

One problem we face in the cloning and expression of a small hormone like insulin, is that the normal hormone is made in the pancreas through a series of precursors. Preproinsulin is a molecule some 100 amino acids long that has on its amino terminal end a hydrophobic presequence of 24 amino acids which is cleaved off as that molecule is passed through the cell membrane (1, 2). The resulting fragment, proinsulin, folds up; disulphide bonds form, and then a portion of the peptide chain, the C peptide, is cleaved out between two pairs of basic amino acid residues to produce the final molecule, insulin itself. When we make insulin in bacteria, we can do the final maturation ourselves with a mixture of trypsin and carboxypeptidase B. However, how can we arrange that the amino terminus will be the correct one for insulin rather than bearing some other amino acid or the presequence?

Originally, in collaboration with Villa-Komaroff et al. (3), we synthesized proinsulin attached to a special long precursor. We thought that it would be best to synthesize this molecule not by leaving it inside the bacterial cell but by arranging for it to be secreted to the periplasm. We did that cloning by taking plasmid pBR322, which has a Pst site in the middle of the ampicillin resistance gene, opening it at this Pst site, and inserting into it cDNA for preproinsulin. The ampicillin resistance gene product, the beta-lactamase, is a secreted protein. Three times larger than preproinsulin, it has a presequence of 23 amino acids, that leads to the transport of this protein through the E. coli membrane and to the cleavage of this presequence (4, 5; for a review of protein secretion, see ref. 6). The original fusion we had made inserted proinsulin at amino acid 182 in the prepenicillinase molecule, and we could show by antigenic techniques that that combined molecule made in a small amount in the bacterial cell was transported through the membrane and could be recovered from the periplasmic space (3). To examine that transport more closely, we altered this construction to remove the material that separated the presequence from the proinsulin. We made a set of cloning vehicles which enabled us

easily to create a series of fusions of proinsulin to the
prepenicillinase leader (7).

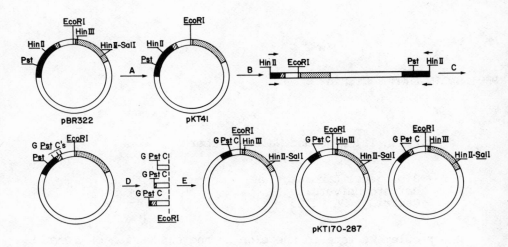

Fig. 1.   Scheme by which signal sequence plasmids were constructed.
           Each step is described in ref. 7. Pst=PstI, HinII=HincII,
           HinIII=HindIII, G Pst C=an inserted PstI linker, whose
           sequence is 5'-GCTGCAGC- 3', where CTGCAG defines the PstI
           restriction site. Certain gene regions are represented as
           follows: prepenicillinase signal sequence, shaded; mature
           penicillinase, black; tetracycline resistance, dotted.

        Figure 1 shows the procedure. We first removed a few
restriction cuts in the tetracycline resistance gene, which could
have gotten in our way, by simply mutagenizing the plasmid and
selecting for a functional tetracycline gene on a plasmid resistant
to the restriction enzyme. We then opened the plasmid at the Hind
II cut in the middle of the ampicillin resistance gene, trimmed back
the ends with Bal 31 (an enzyme that cuts back on both strands of
DNA), inserted a Pst linker and closed the plasmid up again. That
produced a shrunken plasmid that still had a tetracycline
resistance. If we isolate the Eco Rl to Pst pieces, size them, and
combine them with the large Eco Rl to Pst fragment of pBR322, we
eventually make a series of plasmids which bear deletions between
various points in the leader sequence and the Pst cut. By
sequencing we can know what we have. Figure 2 shows this set of
plasmids, a set of cloning vehicles with a single Pst cut either
right after the leader or inside the leader; enough to have the cut
occur in all possible translation reading frames. Similarly, Figure
3 shows we took the cDNA for preproinsulin and trimmed back the end,
added a Pst linker, and thus obtained a series of structures in
which the hydrophobic leader sequence for preproinsulin has been
either extended by a series of glycines (from the original cloning)
or shrunk by a series of enzymatic nibblings to provide a set of

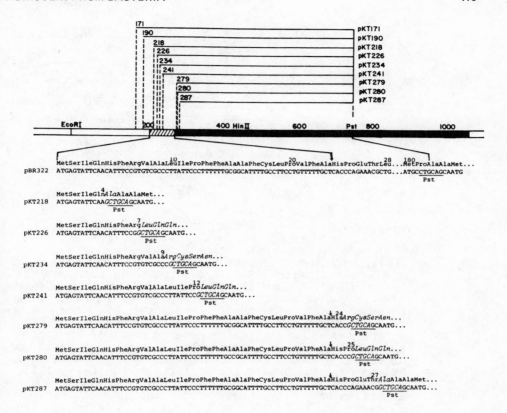

Fig. 2.   Deletion map of pBR322 penicillinase gene and sequence of
derivative plasmid signal sequence regions (7). DNA
regions that encode proteins are represented as follows:
penicillinase signal sequence, hatched; mature
penicillinase protein, black. The derivatives were deleted
from the Pst to the signal sequence coding region and the
Pst site (C-T-G-C-A-G) was re-created by insertion of a
Pst linker whose sequence is G-C-T-G-C-A-G-C. The bases
donated by the linker on that strand are indicated in
italics. The last wild-type penicillinase amino acid is
indicated by the number of is wild-type position above it.
The amino acids encoded by the inserted Pst linker are in
italics. The arrows indicate the site of cleavage for
maturation of wild-type prepenicillinase to penicillinase.

molecules in which we have either an essentially complete proinsulin
hydrophobic leader sequence, a middle-sized, 7 amino acid long
hydrophobic leader sequence, or a molecule with no hydrophobic
leader sequence at all but just a series of glycines going to the
fourth amino acid of proinsulin (8).

For each combination of proinsulin and cloning vector we could

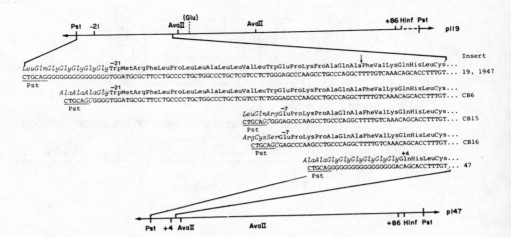

Fig. 3.   Restriction map of rat preproinsulin (pI19) and proinsulin
           (pI47) Pst inserts (1947 is a recombinant between the
           19-insert 5' end and the 47-insert 3' end at the first Ava
           site to remove a mutant glycine encoded in the 19 insert);
           sequences at the 5' end of these inserts and the digested
           derivatives of 1947 insert. Bases in the digested 1947
           insert sequences in italics have been donated by an
           inserted Pst linker. The first wild-type amino acid is
           indicated by the number of its wild-type position above
           it. Amino acids in italics were created by G-C-tailing
           during the original isolation of pI19 and pI47 or by the
           insertion of a Pst linker. Arrows indicate the site of
           cleavage for maturation of preproinsulin to proinsulin.

measure how much proinsulin was inside the bacterium or in the
periplasmic space (defined as a space external to a lysozyme
spheroplast) by a standard radioimmune assay, competing labelled
proinsulin with cold insulin. We got three characteristic answers:
either most of the proinsulin is secreted and only about ten percent
is inside, or most is inside the cell, or half is in the cell and
half in the periplasmic space (8). Table 1 shows that if there is no
hydrophobic leader sequence, we find the molecule inside the
bacterium. If we have a full length bacterial leader sequence, the
molecule is transported by the bacterial sequence and we find 90% on
the outside. We were surprised and delighted, however, that in
these cases in which we have very few amino acids from the bacterial
sequence but have mainly a eucaryotic signal sequence, again 90% of
the molecule has moved to the periplasm. Thus the eucaryotic signal
sequence serves in bacteria to transport the preproinsulin throught
the membrane to the periplasmic space. The 50% effect molecules we
don't understand fully; they do have a complete bacterial sequence,
and there is an appreciable amount of transport, however, they have
other charges inserted because of the nature of the linker sequence;
these charges may interfere with the transport.

     Now the general secretion phenomenon is not only that a protein
sequence is transported from the cytoplasm to the periplasm but also
that, in all but one case, the sequence that does that transporting

is at the amino terminus of the protein and is cleaved off of the protein either at the moment of transport or after it. Obviously if we are transporting preproinsulin through the cell membrane with

```
                    PENICILLINASE-PREPROINSULIN SIGNAL FUSIONS
                                              ↓
pen'ase      MSIQHFRVALIPFFAAFCLPVFA   HPETLVK.......


i27/+4       MSIQHFRVALIPFFAAFCLPVFA   HPETL  AAGGGGGG                         QHLC...   >90%

i25/-21      MSIQHFRVALIPFFAAFCLPVFA   HP     LQGGGGG   WMRFLPLLALLVLWEPKPAQA  FVKQHLC... >90%

i12/-21      MSIQHFRVALIP                     LQGGGGG   WMRFLPLLALLVLWEPKPAQA  FVKQHLC... >90%

i4/-21       MSIQ                             AAAG      WMRFLPLLALLVLWEPKPAQA  FVKQHLC... >90%


i25/-7       MSIQHFRVALIPFFAAFCLPVFA   HP     LQR                 EPKPAQA      FVKQHLC... 50%

i24/-7       MSIQHFRVALIPFFAAFCLPVFA   H      RCS                 EPKPAQA      FVKQHLC... 50%


i12/-7       MSIQHFRVALIP                     LQR                 EPKPAQA      FVKQHLC... <10%

i9/-7        MSIQHFRVA                        RCS                 EPKPAQA      FVKQHLC... <10%

i4/+4        MSIQ                             AAGGGGGG                         QHLC...   <10%


preproinsulin                                 MALWMRFLPLLALLVLWEPKPAQA ↓ FVKQHLC...
```

Table 1. Each sequence begins at the penicillinase fMet and ends at amino acid 7 of proinsulin (8). Each line represents one continuous sequence which has been grouped to emphasize similarities and differences as follows: first group, penicillinase signal sequence amino acids; second group, matured penicillinase amino acids; third group, amino acids created by the inserted Pst linker (italics) or by poly(G,C) tailing (glycines); fourth group, preproinsulin signal sequence amino acids; fifth group, matured proinsulin amino acids through amino acid 7. The arrows above the prepenicillinase and preproinsulin sequences indicate sites of cleavage for maturation. A, Ala; R, Arg; C, Cys, Q, Gln; E, Glu; G, Gly; H, His; I, Ile; L, Leu; K, Lys; M, Met; F, Phe; P, Pro; S, Ser; T, Thr; W, Trp; V, Val.

each of these constructions, the immediate question is are these secretory leader sequences cleaved off the molecule or not? We could try to answer that question by inserting a radioactive label into each of these molecules (in fact we used radioactive sulpher and labelled the methionines and the cystines) and recovering from the periplasm of the labelled cells the radioactive molecule by binding it to antibody and isolating the antibody complex with the staph A protein (10). Figure 4 shows what these first four molecules look like. There are three constructions in which there is a full length preinsulin secretory sequence; each of these produces a protein molecule of the same size (Fig. 4, lanes b–d). The construction with a full length bacterial presequence and a few amino acids of the bacterial protein attached to a proinsulin structure creates a slightly larger molecule (Fig. 4, lane a). The size of these molecules is what one would expect, if they had been correctly processed in the bacteria. However, this is not sufficient evidence to show correct processing; we went to a more explicit experiment. We isolated each of these proteins and, using the sequenator, cut in amino acid after amino acid from the amino terminus to ask where are the labelled cystines (10).

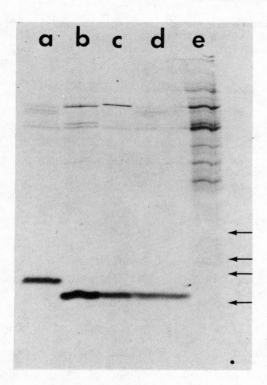

Fig. 4.   Immunoprecipitated insulin antigen from E. coli bearing
           insulin plasmids electrophoresed on a 15%
           SDS-polyacrylamide gel (10). Lane a, i27/+4; b, i25/-21;
           c, i12/-21; d, i4/-21; e, PR13 bearing pKT41, a control
           plasmid without an insulin insert (see table 1). The
           molecular weight markers (arrows) are: sperm whale
           myoglobin (17,200), chicken lysozyme (14,400), human
           Beta2-microglobulin (11,600), and bovine proinsulin
           (8700). The molecular weight of authentic rat proinsulin
           is 9100. The dye front is indicated by a dot. The amount
           of material in each lane corresponds to an input of 0.5
           mCi in the labeling. The dry gel was exposed for 12 hours.

Figure 5 (left) shows data for three molecules in which the insulin
eucaryotic hydrophobic leader sequence is used for the transport:
we find the cleavage is exactly at the beginning of proinsulin. As
we sequence along these molecules, label appears only in cystine at
position 7 and the cystine at position 19, in all three cases. Not
only is the insulin hydrophobic leader sequence, the eucaryotic
presequence, being recognized sufficiently well in the bacteria to
transport the protein to the periplasm but furthermore the bacteria
enzymes recognize the end of that hydrophobic leader sequence, or
some property of it, and cleave it off to make a correct proinsulin
molecule. Fig. 5 (right) also shows that in the fourth case, with
the penicillinase leader, the cleavage occurs at the usual place at
the end of the penicillinase sequence.

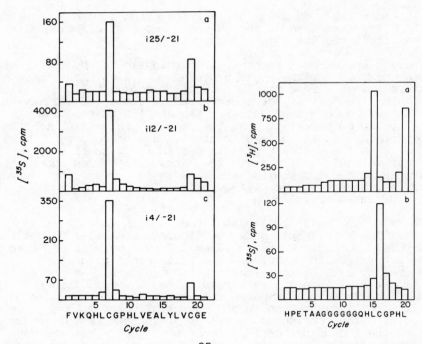

Fig. 5   (left).   Location of ^{35}S-containing residues in the amino
          terminal region of the insulin products of three
          constructions containing the DNA encoding the
          preproinsulin signal sequence (10). The antigen was
          purified from H_2SO_4-labeled cells by
          immunoprecipitation and SDS/polyacrylamide gel
          electrophoresis and then subjected to automated Edman
          degradation. The amount of radioactivity released by each
          cycle of degradation was determined by liquid
          scintillation counting. The amino-terminal sequence of
          authentic rat proinsulin is presented for comparison. (A)
          i25/-21: 20,000 cpm loaded, double-coupled at steps 1, 2
          and 10, double-cleaved at step 9, 10% of each cycle
          analyzed. (B) i12/-21: 150,000 cpm loaded, double-coupled
          at step 1, 50% of each cycle analyzed. (C) i4/-21: 50,000
          cpm loaded, double-coupled at step 1, double-cleaved at
          step 9, 50% of each fraction analyzed.
          (right).   Location of the ^{35}S-containing and
          (^{3}H)leucine residues in the amino-terminal sequence of
          i27/+4. The insulin antigen was purified from cells
          labeled with both H_2SO_4 and (^{3}H)leucine by
          immunoprecipitation and SDS/polyacrylamide gel
          electrophoresis and then subjected to automated Edman
          degradation. (A) 300,000 cpm loaded; (B) 85,000 cpm
          loaded. Double-coupling was done at step 1, ^{35}S and
          double-cleaving at steps 2 and 18. The amount of ^{35}S and
          ^{3}H radioactivity released at each cycle of degradation
          was determined by liquid scintillation counting, with the
          crossover into the ^{3}H channel subtracted. Ten percent of
                                                      (Continued)

each fraction was analyzed. The amino-terminal sequence of
i27/+4 matured at the correct bacterial clipping site is
presented for comparison.

The cleavage enzyme must recognize something in the sequence rather
than some property of the whole protein. One might have thought
that the cleavage enzyme simply recognizes some little tail sticking
out from the boundary of the protein and it comes and cleaves that
off. That would be a reasonable interpretation of the cleavage of
the eukaryotic sequence, because the result, proinsulin, is the
mature protein. In the case of penicillinase of course, the
cleavage forms the mature protein. But in the case of this
particular molecule, there are a few extra amino acids and a string
of glycines on the proinsulin; there is no reason for the cleavage
to occur at the end of the presequence, unless the sequence at this
position dictates the cleavage (10).

We have gone on to pulse label the insulin made in these
bacteria. The experiments shown in Figure 4 use material built up
over several generations of labelling. If we pulse label, we can
see the preproinsulin precursor, the full length precursor
synthesized by each of these constructions, as well as the matured
product. We see, in a thirty second pulse, the full length
molecule, and in several minutes the processing of that molecule.
The results of that processing are essentially the ones that we had
inferred from the continuous label: that is that the cleavages are
either at the end of the penicillinase presequence, in the case in
which there is only the penicillinase presequence, or they are at
the end of the eukaryotic presequence.

These experiments show that we can make a mature molecule
cleaved correctly using the bacterial system to do all the work for
us. This does argue that there is a common feature in the
eucaryotic and the bacterial systems involving the transport of
proteins, which was unsuspected. That feature may be that the
transport involves nothing other than the existence of the
hydrophobic leader sequence, and its interaction with a membrane,
which is a perfectly general structure, rather than the existence
highly specific receptors involved in the transport of these
proteins. Furthermore, the enzyme that does the cleavage is
general. Either the cleavage has something to do again with the
shape of the presequence that has to do with the transport, or else,
just accidentally, that the enzymes recognize the same sequences.

We originally put the proinsulin molecule into penicillinase,
to move it outside the bacterium both because we wanted to study its
secretion and also because we expected that the molecule,
synthesized within the bacterium, would not be terribly stable.
Insulin is a somewhat floppy protein hormone; protein hormones are
often subject to proteolytic degradation. We have been able to
study the stability problem, using these same strains, by pulse
labelling the insulin and asking what happens to the insulin
molecule in those bacteria in which it is being rapidly secreted or
in those bacteria in which it is not secreted at all and remains in
the periplasm. In all the cases in which the molecule remains in
the cytoplasm, we recover very much less insulin. If we pulse
label, we can follow the degradation of the insulin: in the

cytoplasm there is a one minute half-life for insulin; while in the periplasm there is a twenty minute half-life for insulin. In fact, the molecule is very dramatically stablized, protected against proteases in the cell, by being moved through the cell membrane.

Acknowledgement

The work described here was supported in part by Biogen, N.V. and in part by the National Institutes of Health. W.G. is American Cancer Society Professor of Molecular Biology. K.T. is a postdoctoral fellow funded by Biogen, N.V. Both authors gratefully acknowledge the collaboration of Jim Kaufman and Stephen Stahl.

Bibliography

(1) Chan, S.J., Keim, P. and Steiner, D. Proc. Natl. Acad. Sci. USA 73, 1964-1968 (1976).

(2) Chan, S.J. and Steiner, D. Trends Biochem. Sci. 2, 254-256 (1978).

(3) Villa-Komaroff, L., Efstradiatis, A., Broome, S., Lomedico, P., Tizard, R., Naber, S.P., Chick, W.L. and Gilbert, W. Proc. Natl. Acad. Sci. USA 75, 3727-3731 (1978).

(4) Sutcliffe, J.G. Proc. Natl. Acad. Sci. USA 75, 3737-3741 (1978).

(5) Ambler, R.P. and Scott, G.K. Proc. Natl. Acad. Sci. USA 75, 3732-3736 (1978).

(6) Blobel, G., Walter, P., Chang, C.N., Goldman, B.M., Erikson, A.H. and Lingappa, V.R. Symp. Soc. Exp. Biol. 33, 9-36 (1979).

(7) Talmadge, K. and Gilbert, W. Gene 12, 235-241 (1980).

(8) Talmadge, K., Stahl, S. and Gilbert, W. Proc. Natl. Acad. Sci. USA 77, 3360-3373 (1980).

(9) Lomedico, P., Rosenthal, N., Efstradiatis, A., Gilbert, W., Kolodner, R. and Tizard, R. Cell 18, 545-558 (1979).

(10) Talmadge, K., Kaufman, J. and Gilbert, W. Proc. Natl. Acad. Sci. USA 77, 3988-3992 (1980).

Construction and Properties of Plasmid Vectors Containing the

trp Regulatory Region Suitable for Expressing Foreign Genes

Robert A. Hallewell and Howard M. Goodman

Department of Biochemistry & Biophysics

University of California, San Francisco 94143

Structure and Regulation of the trp Operon

The E. coli tryptophan (trp) operon consists of a regulatory region followed by five structural genes (trpE through trpA)[1,2]. The trp structural gene products, which are co-ordinately synthesized in equimolar amounts, catalyze the conversion of chorismate to tryptophan[1,3]. Transcription of the operon is repressed by tryptophan by two mechanisms. Tryptophan binds trp repressor (trpR) resulting in an increase in the affinity of the repressor for the trp operator[4]. Since the trp operator sequence overlaps the trp promoter sequence (see Fig. 1) binding of repressor prevents binding of RNA polymerase. Secondly, in the presence of tryptophan about 90% of the RNA polymerase molecules which are able to initiate, terminate transcription about 140 base pairs (bp) from the transcription start (see Fig. 1). The ability of the transcription terminator to function is determined by the level of tryptophanyl tRNA[9].

Methods of Inducing the trp Promoter

Both mechanisms for repressing trp transcription described above can be antagonized by lowering the levels of intracellular tryptophan. The two methods described below for achieving this have the disadvantage that they depend on limiting the availability of intracellular tryptophan which in turn may prevent efficient expression of cellular proteins. However, tryptophan is a rarely used amino acid[10] and substantial amounts of proteins containing tryptophan residues can be synthesized by the mthods described here.[15]

In the first method trp⁻ cells[11] are grown to stationary

421

```
                                              -35 region
        Hhal                                  AlulHindll               T
   1    GCGCCGACATCATAACGGTTCTGGCAAATATTCTGAAATGAGCTGTTGACAATTAATCAT
        CGCGGCTGTAGTATTGCCAAGACCGTTTATAAGACTTTACTCGACAACTGTTAATTAGTA


        trp(po)PB
        aql      Hpal      RsaI   mRNA start    trpL SD Taql  MetLysAlaIleP
   60   CGAACTAGTTAACTAGTACGCAAGTTCACGTAAAAAGGGTATCGACAATGAAAGCAATTT
        GCTTGATCAATTGATCATGCGTTCAAGTGCATTTTTCCCATAGCTGTTACTTTCGTTAAA
        Hindll


        RsaI                     Hhal
        heValLeuLysGlyTrpTrpArgThrSerOP                     Hph
   120  TCGTACTGAAAGGTTGGTGGCGCACTTCCTGAAACGGGCAGTGTATTCACCATGCGTAAA
        AGCATGACTTTCCAACCACCGCGTGAAGGACTTTGCCCGTCACATAAGTGGTACGCATTT


                             TT                              trpE SD
   180  GCAATCAGATACCCAGCCCGCCTAATGAGCGGGCTTTTTTTTTGAACAAAATTAGAGAATA
        CGTTAGTCTATGGGTCGGGCGGATTACTCGCCCGAAAAAAAACTTGTTTTAATCTCTTAT


                             HinflHindlll
        MetGlnThrGlnLysProThr
   240  ACAATGCAAACACAAAAACCGACTCAAGCTTACT
        TGTTACGTTTGTGTTTTTGGCTGAGTTCGAATGA
                             Alu
```

Figure 1.   DNA sequence of the trp regulatory region (Ref. 5 and our unpublished results) cloned in ptrpE2-1 (see Figure 3).   Regulatory features are in bold type.   PB, Pribnow Box[6]; SD, Shine-Dalgarno sequence[7]; TT, transcription terminator[8].

---

phase in repressing concentrations of tryptophan (40 µg/ml). They are then diluted 20-fold into medium lacking tryptophan so that tryptophan is present at a nearly derepressing concentration (about 1 µg/ml). After a few hours growth in this medium tryptophan levels will fall and all trp promoters will become fully active. The medium for dilution is usually M9 salts, glucose[12], supplemented with 0.2% casamino acids, which contains no tryptophan but all the other amino acids used in proteins. A trp strain is required to ensure that the cells do not synthesize any tryptophan de novo which would result in partial repression of the trp promoters[1]. This method can be readily adapted for use on agar plates. Colonies are initially grown on nitrocellulose filters overlaid on plates containing excess tryptophan and then transferred on the nitrocellulose to plates containing 1 µg/ml tryptophan.

In the second method trp^+ cells are grown to stationary phase in a repressing concentration of tryptophan, diluted in medium lacking tryptophan so that tryptophan is present at a derepressing concentration (1 μg/ml) resulting in partial derepression of trp promoters[1]. After a few hours growth the tryptophan analog 3β-indolylacrylic acid (IA) is added so that trp transcription becomes maximal[13,14,15].

Non-regulated maximal expression of the trp promoter can be obtained using a $trpR^-$ strain[16]. This method requires a vector molecule such as ptrpL1 (see Fig. 3) which lacks the trp attenuator[17]. This method has the advantage that cells can be grown in excess tryptophan in complex media; its disadvantage is that expression is constitutive and thus if the over-produced gene product confers a disadvantage on cells synthesizing it, such strains may be unstable or impossible to construct[14].

Levels of trp Mediated Expression Compared with Other Systems

The trp promoter is a relatively powerful E. coli promoter with an efficiency comparable to the phage λ P_L promoter[18,19,20]. Some T-phage promoters are considerably stronger than trp[21] but no vectors containing them are yet available. A comparison of the levels of expression of human interferon and growth hormone from vector systems based on the lac and trp regulatory regions indicates that the fully derepressed trp system is 5-10 times more efficient than lac[22]. It is not known if this is due to higher transcriptional or translational efficiency of trp.

Figure 2 shows the induction kinetics of cells containing the plasmid ptrpED5-1 induced with IA as analyzed by a sodium dodecyl sulfate-polyacrylamide gel stained with coomassie blue[14]. The plasmid contains the trp regulatory region and the first structural gene (trpE). Note that the trpE protein is synthesized in small amounts in the absence of inducer but that 3 hrs after induction the trpE protein represents about 30% of cellular protein. Eucaryotic gene products appear to be synthesized in much smaller amounts[22,23] (unpublished results) but the reason for this is not yet known.

Function of the trp Regulatory Regions on Multicopy Plasmids

The chromosomal trp genes are regulated over approximately a 500-fold range; 50-fold at the operator[24] and 10-fold at the attenuator[25]. This regulation appears to function normally on multicopy plasmids[14,26]. In contrast the lac promoter cannot be regulated on a multicopy plasmid because of insufficient numbers of lac repressor molecules[27]. Recent evidence leads one to expect that trp regulation would be normal on a multicopy plasmid; the trpR gene is autogenously regulated[28] and the trp attenuator is rho-independent and probably depends only on transcription and translation for its function[8]. Thus, none of the

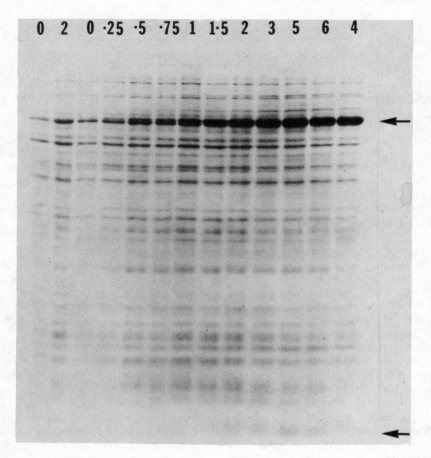

Figure 2. Kinetics and levels of synthesis of trp proteins in cells containig ptrpED5-1[14]. After cells were derepressed for trp transcription with IA, samples were removed at the times indicated above the gel in hrs. A plasmid free culture was similarly induced as a control as shown on the two tracks (Ø and 2) on the left of the gel. The SDS-polyacrylamide gel was stained with coomassie blue. The upper arrow indicates the position of the trpE gene product and the lower arrow that of the trpD protein fragment.

---

molecules involved in trp regulation should be overtitrated when the trp regulatory region is amplified on a multicopy plasmid.

Construction and Properties of Plasmid ptrpL1

To construct a vector molecule lacking the trp attenuator and suitable for constructing hybrid ribosome binding sites using

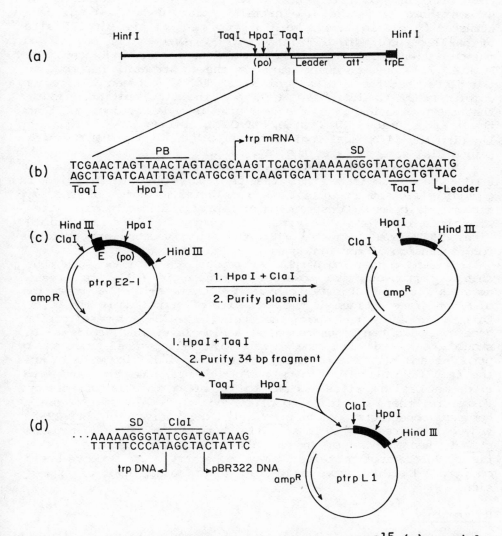

Figure 3. Construction of expression vector ptrpL1[15] (a) partial restriction map of the 492 bp HinFI fragment. The genetic regions promoter-operator, (po); leader region; attenuator, att; and trpE structural gene are shown in their approximate locations[5]. (b) DNA sequence of promoter-operator and proximal portion of the leader region. Regulatory features are as in Figure 1. (c) and (d) construction of ptrpL1 and the DNA sequence at the newly formed ClaI site, respectively.

the initiator codon of eucaryotic cDNAs[15,29] we followed the scheme shown in Figure 3. Initially, plasmid ptrpE2-1 was constructed by cloning a 492 bp HinfI fragment at the HindIII site of pBR322[30] using HindIII linkers[15,31]. One end of the cloned molecule lies 7 codons from the N-terminus of the trpE gene (see Figure 1). The subsequent steps in the construction depended on the facts that there is a TaqI site, T/CGA, between the region complementary to 16S rRNA[7] (SD) and the trpL initiator codon, that the nucleotide 5' to the TaqI site is a dA residue, and that there is a unique ClaI site, AT/CGAT, in ptrpE2-1. Thus, by ligating the 34 bp HpaI-TaqI fragment to HpaI/ClaI cut ptrpE2-1 a unique ClaI site replaces the TaqI site.

Studies of gene fusions between trpL and the trpE[32] or trpC[33] genes indicate that the trpL ribosome binding site is equally efficient at initiating translation as those of the trp structural genes. Construction of hybrid ribosome binding sites with human interferons[22], human growth hormone[23], and hepatitis B virus (HBV) core antigen[15] show that such vectors are suitable for expression of foreign genes.

Strains containing ptrpL1 overproduce β-lactamase such that when trp transcription towards this gene is fully derepressed about 20% of cellular protein is β-lactamase[15]. The insertion of HBV surface antigen at the PstI site of ptrpL1 using the dG/dC tailing procedure has shown that this fused β-lactamase/foreign gene construct can be expressed at a high level in E. coli[15]. It should be noted that the levels of β-lactamase produced by ptrpE2-1 and ptrpL1 containing cells after induction with IA are the same (unpublished results). Furthermore, the trpL and trpE ribosome binding sites appear to be of comparable efficiency. Therefore, there should be no difference in levels of expression between constructs using ptrpL1 or derivatives of ptrpE2-1[31] (unpublished results). Thus, while there are advantages in using ptrpL1 (see Methods of Induction), for the expression of potentially deleterious proteins it may be better to use vectors based on ptrpE2-1, which have a 10-fold lower basal level of expression.

References

1. J. Ito and I.P. Crawford, Regulation of the enzymes of the tryptophan pathway in Escherichia coli, Genetics 52:1303 (1965).
2. C. Yanofsky, V. Horn, M. Bonner, and S. Stasiowski, Polarity and enzyme functions in mutants of the first three genes of the tryptophan operon of Escherichia coli, Genetics 69:409 (1971).
3. J. Ito and C. Yanofsky, Anthranilate synthetase, an enzyme specified by the tryptophan operon of Escherichia coli: Comparative studies on the complex and the subunits, J. Bacteriol. 97:734 (1969).

4. C.L. Squires, F.D. Lee, and C. Yanofsky, Interaction of the
    trp repressor and RNA polymerase with the trp operon, J.
    Mol. Biol. 92:93 (1975).
5. F. Lee, K. Bertrand, G. Bennett, and C. Yanofsky, Comparison
    of the nucleotide sequences of the initial transcribed
    regions of the tryptophan operons of Escherichia coli and
    Salmonella typhimurium, J. Mol. Biol. 121:193 (1978).
6. D. Pribnow, Nucleotide sequence of an RNA polymerase binding
    site at an early T7 promoter, Proc. Nat. Acad. Sci. USA
    72:784 (1975).
7. J. Shine and L. Dalgarno, The 3'-terminal sequence of Escher-
    ichia coli 16S Ribosomal RNA: complementarity to nonsense
    triplets and ribosome binding sites, Proc. Nat. Acad.
    Sci. USA 71:1342 (1974).
8. G. Zurawski, D. Elseviers, G.V. Stauffer, and C. Yanofsky,
    Translational control of transcription termination at the
    attenuator of the Escherichia coli tryptophan operon,
    Proc. Nat. Acad. Sci. USA 75:5988 (1978).
9. C. Yanofsky and L. Soll, Mutations affecting tRNA^{Trp} and its
    charging and their effect on regulation of transcription
    termination at the attenuator of the tryptophan operon,
    J. Mol. Biol. 113:663 (1977).
10. R. Grantham, C. Gautier, M. Gouy, R. Mercier, and A. Pavez,
    Codon catalog usage and the genome hypothesis, Nucleic
    Acids Res. 8:49 (1980).
11. B. Ratzkin and J. Carbon, Functional expression of cloned
    yeast DNA in Escherichia coli, Proc. Nat. Acad. Sci. USA
    74:487 (1977).
12. J.H. Miller, in "Experiments in Molecular Genetics, Appendix
    I, Cold Spring Harbor Laboratory, Cold Spring Harbor, New
    York (1972).
13. D.E. Morse, R.D. Mosteller, and C. Yanofsky, Dynamics of
    synthesis, translation, and degradation of trp operon
    messenger RNA in E. coli, Cold Spring Harbor Symp. Quant.
    Biol. 34:725 (1969).
14. R.A. Hallewell and S. Emtage, Plasmid vectors containing the
    tryptophan operon promoter suitable for efficient regu-
    lated expression of foreign genes, Gene 9:27 (1980).
15. J.C. Edman, R.A. Hallewell, P. Valenzuela, H.M. Goodman, and
    W.J. Rutter, The synthesis of hepatitis B surface and
    core antigens in E. coli, Nature, in press.
16. W. Roeder and R.L. Somerville, Cloning the trpR gene, Molec.
    gen. Genet. 176:361 (1979).
17. D.L. Oxender, G. Zurawski, and C. Yanofsky, Attenuation in
    the Escherichia coli tryptophan operon: Role of RNA
    secondary structure involving the tryptophan codon
    region, Proc. Nat. Acad. Sci. USA 76:5524 (1979).
18. J. Davison, W.J. Brammar, and F.F. Brunel, Quantitative
    aspects of gene expression in a λ-trp fusion operon, Mol.
    gen. Genet. 130:9 (1974).

19. D.F. Ward and N.E. Murray, Convergent transcription in bac-
     teriophage λ: Interference with gene expression, J. Mol.
     Biol. 133:249 (1979).

20. H.-U. Bernard, E. Remaut, M.V. Hershfield, H.K. Das, and
     D.R. Helinski, Construction of plasmid cloning vehicles
     that promote gene expression from the bacteriophage
     lambda P_L promoter, Gene 5:59 (1979).

21. A. von Gabain and J. Bujard, Interaction of Escherichia coli
     RNA polymerase with promoters of several coliphage and
     plasmid DNAs, Proc. Nat. Acad. Sci. USA 76:189 (1979).

22. D.V. Goeddel, H.M. Shepard, E. Yelverton, D. Leung, and R.
     Crea, Synthesis of human fibroblast interferon by E.
     coli, Nucleic Acids Res. 8:4057 (1980).

23. J.A. Martial, R.A. Hallewell, J.D. Baxter, and H.M. Goodman,
     Human growth hormone: complementary DNA cloning and
     expression in bacteria, Science 205:602 (1979).

24. D.E. Morse and C. Yanofsky, Amber mutants of the trpR regu-
     latory gene, J. Mol. Biol. 44:1855 (1969).

25. E.N. Jackson and C. Yanofsky, The region between the opera-
     tor and first structural gene of the tryptophan operon of
     Escherichia coli may have a regulatory function, J. Mol.
     Biol. 76:89 (1973).

26. V. Hershfield, H.W. Boyer, C. Yanofsky, M.A. Lovett, D.R.
     Helinski, Plasmid ColEl as a molecular vehicle for clon-
     ing and amplification of DNA, Proc. Nat. Acad. Sci. USA
     71:3455 (1974).

27. P.H. O'Farrell, B. Polisky, and D.H. Gelfand, Regulated
     expression by readthrough translation from a plasmid-
     encoded β-galactosidase, J. Bacteriol. 134:645 (1978).

28. C.K. Singleton, W.D. Roeder, G. Bogosian, R.L. Somerville,
     and H.L. Weith, DNA sequence of the E. coli trpR gene and
     prediction of the amino acid sequence of Trp repressor,
     Nucleic Acids Res., in press.

29. T.M. Roberts, I. Bikel, R.R. Yocum, D.M. Livingston, and M.
     Ptashne, Synthesis of simian virus 40 t antigen in
     Escherichia coli, Proc. Nat. Acad. Sci. USA 76:5596
     (1979).

30. J.G. Sutcliffe, Complete nucleotide sequence of the Escheri-
     chia coli plasmid pBR322, Cold Spring Harbor Symp. Quant.
     Biol. 43:77 (1979).

31. W. Tacon, N. Carey, and S. Emtage, The construction and
     characterization of plasmid vectors suitable for the
     expression of all DNA phases under the control of the E.
     coli tryptophan promoter Molec. gen. Genet. 177:427
     (1980).

32. G.F. Miozzari and C. Yanofsky, Translation of the leader
     region of the Escherichia coli tryptophan operon, J. Bac-
     teriol. 133:1457 (1978).

33. G.E. Christie and T. Platt, A functional hybrid ribosome
     binding site in tryptophan operon mRNA of E. coli, J.
     Mol. Biol., in press.

ISOLATION AND ANALYSIS OF A COSMID HYBRID CONTAINING THE HUMAN GENOMIC INTERFERON GENE, HuIFNβ1

Gerhard Gross, Ulrich Mayr, Frank Grossveld*
Henrik M.Dahl* Richard A.Flavell* & John Collins

Gesellschaft für Biotechnologische Forschung

Mascheroder Weg 1, D3300 Braunschweig-Stöckheim
F.R.Germany

*National Institute for Medical Research

The Ridgeway, Mill Hill, London, U.K.

INTRODUCTION

Human fibroblast interferon HuIFNβ has an anti-viral activity and can also stimulate natural killer cell action against neoplastic cells[1] [2] [3]. The IFNβ-gene belongs to a rare class of eukaryotic genes for which the immediate induction of transcription in response to certain inducers such as poly I:poly C has been demonstrated[4] [5] [6]. Recent findings indicate that two IFNβ mRNAs exist which are at the most only distantly related, but are co-ordinately induced in human fibroblasts[7]. It therefore seemed of great interest to isolate the chromosomal region for the IFNβ1 gene so as to study the structure of the transcription unit, the possible adjacent transcription units, and the later application of this information to the production of interferon ß in eukaryotic cells.

The initial impetus to isolate an IFNß cDNA clone came primarily from the wish to produce an IFNß-producing E.coli strain, as has recently been demonstrated by three other groups[8] [9] [10]. The isolation of a clone containing part of the IFNß1 cDNA and the use of this DNA as a probe for the isolation of a genomic hybrid is described here. Evidence was found that the transcribed region and most of the 3′-tail region of the IFNß gene has no intron.

METHODS

Production of a cDNA Gene Bank

Human fibroblast FS4 cells were cultured and super-
induced for the production of interferon according to
the method of Raj and Pitha[4], except that a lower polyI:
poly C concentration was used. For the extraction of mRNA
a number of methods were employed including the polysome
isolation method of Palmiter[11], phenol-SDS[7], or guanidine
hydrochloride extraction[12]. Clones derived from various
batches of DNA were pooled for screening.

mRNA purified by two passages through oligo-dT cellulose columns was used for cDNA synthesis without size fractionation. Reverse transcriptase reactions were carried
out as described by Ullrich et al.[13], after denaturation
of the mRNA with methyl mercury hydroxide[14]. Terminal
transferase reactions were carried out according to Nelson
and Brutlag[15] using an excess of terminal transferase, and
a 100-fold ratio of dNTP to DNA ends for five minutes at
room temperature. Annealing of dC-tailed cDNA to dG-tail-
ed pBR322 was carried out by slow cooling from 65°C to
37°C over a 12 hour period. Starting with 50μg of mRNA
some 500ng of appropriately tailed cDNA was obtained.
This yielded an initial bank of 600 hybrid colonies. The
flow chart for the individual steps is shown in figure 1.

Initial attempts to use pools of plasmid DNA for mRNA
enrichment or for hybrid arrest translation experiments
in Xenopus oocytes were found to yield erratic results.
The screening finally was carried out as shown in the
figure 2. The later part of this screening depended very
much on the sequence data already available from Taniguchi
et al.[16].

Production and Screening of a Genomic Cosmid Gene Bank

The detailed description for the production of the
cosmid gene bank will be presented elsewhere (F.Grossveld
H.M.Dahl, R.A.Flavell et al., manuscript in preparation).
A scheme for the production of the bank is given in figure
2, which essentially follows the protocol and recommendations of Hohn and Collins[17]. The bank consisted of 1.5
x 10[5] colonies, maintained on 15 fifteen cm diameter
nitrocellulose filters. Screening of the bank by colony
hybridisation was according to Hanahan and Meselson[22],
with the following modifications. Filters were boiled
before sterilisation. Filters were not dried between
consecutive steps of the washing procedure and excess cel
debris was wiped off the filter during the wash in 1M
Tris, pH 8, 1.5M NaCl. This wiping step was followed
by an additional wash in the same buffer.

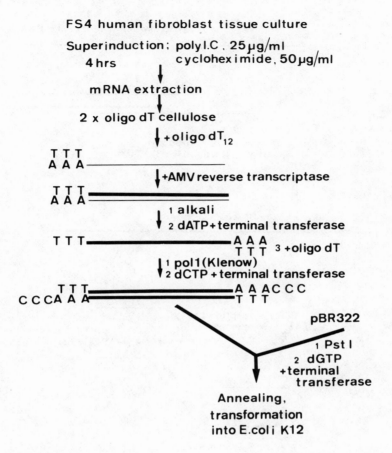

Fig. 1. Scheme for the production of the cDNA gene bank.

cDNA gene bank→1. Screening by colony hybridisation
with cDNA from:
a) polyI:C-induced
or b) non-induced FS4 cell mRNA
2. Restriction maps (PstI, BgIII, RsaI)
3. DNA-sequencing

Fig. 2. Scheme for the screening of the cDNA gene bank.

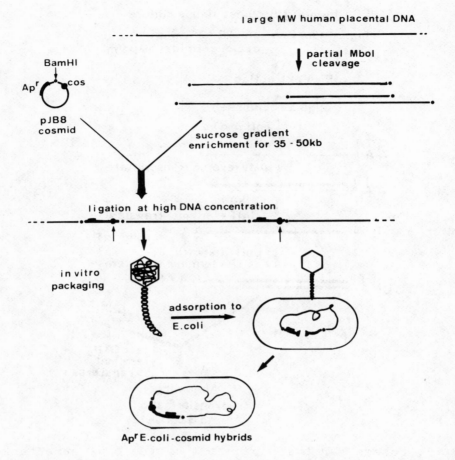

Fig. 3. Scheme for the production of the human genomic
       cosmid gene bank.

DNA and RNA Blot-Hybridisation

DNA blotting and hybridisation was carried out according
to Southern[18]. RNA blotting was carried out as described
by Thomas[19], except that the RNA gel-electrophoresis was
made in 2% agarose containing 2.2M formaldehyde in the
buffer. Nick-tranlation to make ^{32}P-labelled DNA probes
was carried out according to Maniatis et al.[20].

RESULTS

Isolation of a Clone Containing IFNß1-DNA

Following the screening of the initial 600 hybrid cDNA clones, as outlined above, a single clone was identified as containing IFNß1 DNA. The structure of this clone is shown in figure 4.

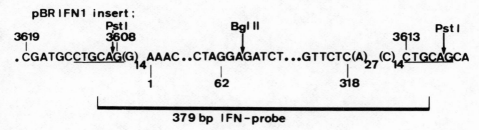

Fig. 4. The structure of the insert in pBRIFN1. The cDNA is inserted at the PstI site of pBR322 by GC-tailing such that two PstI sites are preserved at the boundaries of the insert. The numbering above the sequence indicates pBR322 coordinates and the numbering below, the cDNA homology to IFNß mRNA, homopolymer stretches not included. Bases 1 to 150 and 250 to 318 as well as the homopolymers were sequenced from the PstI and BglII sites using the Maxam and Gilbert method.

By comparison of the sequenced regions with the sequence of Toniguchi et al.[16], bases 1 to 68 were seen to constitute part of the 3'-non-translated tail and 69-318 the C-terminal coding region for IFNß1. The 379 base pair fragment was used as a nick-translated probe to isolate the genomic clone from the cosmid gene bank, and as a probe against mRNA from induced and non-induced cells (figure 5). As can be seen from this "Northern " blot a single band hybridises at 11S in agreement with the observations of Sehgal and Sagar[7]. Moreover, this band is only observed when mRNA from poly I:C induced cells is used (comparison of slots A and B), indicating that no mRNA having homology to this probe is present in non-induced cells.

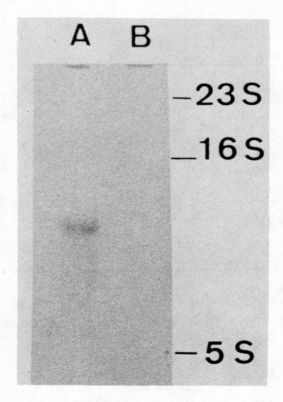

Fig. 5.   Hybridisation of an RNA blot with nick-translated
           379-fragment (figure 4). A: mRNA from poly I:C
           induced FS4 cells ; B: mRNA from non-induced
           cells at 10µg per slot. 3 x 10^7 c.p.m./µg DNA.

Isolation of a Genomic IFNß1 Clone from the Cosmid bank

        The cosmid gene bank was simultaneously screened
with three different labelled probes of which only one
will be discussed here. One hundred suspected colonies
were picked and screened with the individual probes. One
colony gave a strong hybridisation with the 379 bp-probe.
After two further dilutions and repicking of hybridising
colonies, a single colony was isolated and designated
pCosIFNß (pCosIF). Using single and double digests of this
cosmid DNA with BglII, BamHI, HpaI and HindIII in combination with Southern blot hybridisation with labelled 379
fragment or pBR322 DNA (which designated pJB8 fragments)
as shown for example in figure 6, a map of the whole
cosmid was constructed with an estimated length of 46.5kb
The pJB8 vector is shown (1.8 to 6.8) as a thick line.
Extending the Southern blot analysis with SstI, PstI and

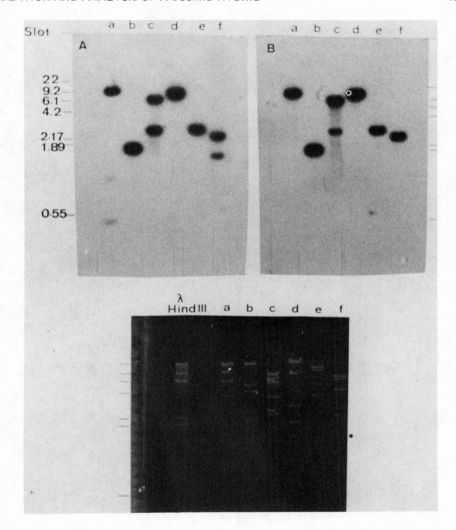

Fig. 6.   Restriction mapping of pCosIFNß. A UV-photograph
          of an agarose gel of the following digests is
          shown in the lower part of the figure : a,HindIII,
          b, EcoRI, c, BglII, d,HpaI, e, SstI, f, PstI with
          λ HindIII fragments as markers. Southern hybrid-
          isations are shown to the same scale: A,with the
          1.9kb EcoRI fragment, or B, the 379bp fragment
          as hybridisation probe.

EcoRI a more detailed map of the IFN region was produced.
This also gave the orientation of the BglII and PstI sites
and hence the orientation of the gene. The genomic clone
therefore contains 36kb to the 5' end of the IFNß gene and

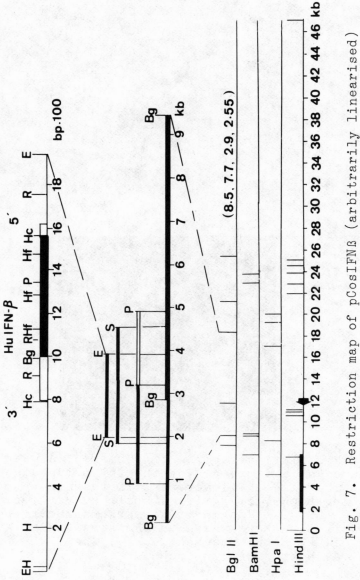

Fig. 7. Restriction map of pCosIFNß (arbitrarily linearised)

5kb to the 3'-end. The 1.9kb EcoRI fragment was isolated
preparatively by electroelution and subjected to further
detailed mapping as well as being used as a hybridisation
probe for Southern blots (figure 6). It is of particular
interest that when the EcoRI fragment is used in this
manner only one band lights up on the Southern blot, thus
indicating the absence of "pseudo-genes" or adjacent duplications of the same gene. Fine mapping with RsaI(R),
HinfI(Hf), SstI(S), HindIII(H), BglII(Bg), PstI(P) and
HincII(Hc), yielded a map of the 1900bp EcoRI fragment as
shown at the top of Fig.7.A box representing the position
of the IFNß gene has been positioned according to the fact
that: a 179bp RsaI , 167 and 197bp HinfI, and a 570bp
BglII fragments are present as predicted from the sequence
of the IFNß cDNA [16]. This is interpreted as indicating
that no intron exists between the left-most RsaI site
and the right-most HincII site of this map, a region which
includes all of the translated region and half of the 3'-
tail region. Sequencing studies are still in progress.
This EcoRI fragment has been subcloned as well as overlapping PstI fragments.

DISCUSSION

        The experiments described here are a further demon-
stration of the use of the cosmid cloning system to isolate very large regions from complex genomes, and in particular is the first application of cosmid cloning of the
the human genome.
        The IFNß1 gene region was isolated in entirety. It
was concluded that the gene was present as a single copy
in this hybrid and that no related sequences are present.
The translated region and at least half of the 3' non-
translated tail region contain no intron, on the basis of
restriction mapping.
        The presence of some 36kb of DNA 5-prime to the IFNß
gene in this clone, make it an interesting subject for
studies of gene expression in vivo in eukaryotic cells.
        The isolation of at least 8 distinct genomic regions
coding for IFNα interferons by Nagata et al.[21] and the
publication of the sizes of BglII, EcoRI, HindIII and
BamHI fragments allows us to conclude that none of the
alpha interferon coding regions are present in pCosIFNß.
Nagata et al. also conclude that the IFNα1 gene contains
no intron.

ACKNOWLEDGEMENTS

        We are gratefull to Julian Berg and David Ish-
Horowisch for the cosmid pJB8. F.G. and H.M.D. are grate-

full for an EMBO fellowship to initiate this work in
Braunschweig.

REFERENCES

1. W. E. Stewart II, The Interferon System, Springer, New
   York (1979).
2. U. Mayr, Forum Mikrobiol. 5, 269-279 (1980).
3. B. R. Bloom, Nature, 284, 593-595 (1980).
4. N. B. K. Raj and P.M. Pitha, Proc. Natn.Acad.Sci.U.S.A.
   74,1483-1487 (1977).
5. P. B. Sehgal, B. Doberstein and I. Tamm, Proc.Natn.Acad
   Sci.U.S.A., 74,3409-3413 (1977).
6. R. L. Cavalieri, E. A. Havell, J.Vilcek and S. Pestka,
   Proc.Natn.Acad.Sci.U.S.A.,74,4415-4419 (1977).
7. P. B. Sehgal and A. D. Sagar, Nature, 288,95-97 (1980).
8. T. Taniguchi, L. Guarente, T. M. Roberts, D. Kimelman,
   J. Douhan III and M. Ptashne, Proc. Natn.Acad.Sci.
   U.S.A.,77, 5230-5233 (1980).
9. R. Derynck, J. Content, E. Declercq, G. Volckaert, J.
   Tavernier, R. Devos and W. Fiers, Nature, 285, 542
   -547 (1980).
10. D. V. Goeddel, H. M. Shepard, E. Yelverton, D. Leung,
    R. Crea, A. Sloma and S. Pestka, Nucleic Acid Res.
    8, 4057-4074 (1980).
11. R. D. Palmiter, Biochemistry, 13, 3606-3615 (1974).
12. R. G. Deeley, J. I. Gordon, A. T. H. Burns, K. B.
    Mullinix, M. Bina-Stein and R. F. Goldberger, J.Bio
    Chem., 252, 8310-8319 (1977).
13. A. Ullrich, J. Shine, J. Chirgwin, R. Pictet, E.
    Tischer, W. J. Rutter, and H. M. Goodman, Science,
    196, 1313-1318 (1977).
14. F. Payvar and R. T. Schimke, J.Biochem.Chem., 254,
    7636-7642 (1979).
15. T. Nelson and D. Brutlag, Methods Enz.68, 41-49 (1980
16. T. Taniguchi, S. Ohno, Y. Fujii-Kuriyama and M.
    Muramatsu, Gene, 10, 11-15 (1980).
17. B. Hohn and J. Collins, Gene, 11, 291-298 (1980).
18. E. Southern, Methods Enz., 68, 152-176 (1980).
19. P. S. Thomas, Proc.Natn.Acad.Sci.U.S.A., 77, 5201-
    5205 (1980).
20. T. Maniatis, A. Jeffrey and D. G. Kleid, Proc.Natn.
    Acad.Sci.U.S.A., 72, 1184-1188 (1975).
21. S. Nagata, N. Mantei and C. Weissmann, Nature, 287,
    401-408 (1980)
22. D. Hanahan and M. Meselson, Gene, 10, 63-67 (1980).

DEVELOPMENT OF BROAD HOST-RANGE PLASMID VECTORS

Peter T. Barth*, Lyn Tobin* and Geoffrey S Sharpe**

*ICI Corporate Laboratory, The Heath, Runcorn, Cheshire
England
**ICI Joint Laboratory, University of Leicester
Leicester, England

INTRODUCTION

The majority of cloning vectors developed so far are based on plasmids or phages with a narrow host-range such as ColEI(pBR322[1]), P15A(pACYC184[2]),pSC101[3] or phage λ[4]. These are limited to *Escherichia coli* or closely related enterobacterial species. For the genetic analysis and manipulation of a wider range of micro-organisms, including those of agricultural, medical, environmental or industrial importance, use has been made of plasmids belonging to the IncP group such as RP4 or RK2. For example RP4 has unique cloning sites for *Eco*RI, *Bam*HI, *Hind*III,*Hpa*I and *Bgl*II[5,6] and has been converted into a *Sal*I cloning vector pRP301[7,8]. From RK2 a two vehicle system: pRK290 plus pRK2013, has been constructed[9]. But such vectors remain relatively large, have a low copy number and are therefore unsuitable for some cloning purposes. For ease of manipulation and high gene dosage of the cloned material we need small, high copy number, broad host-range plasmids.

The non-conjugative plasmids have mostly not been given incompatibility group designations, although several types have been reported to be compatible with one another[10,11]. These are shown in Table 1 although many more groups probably exist. Only one of these groups, as represented by R300B, has been given an Inc designation viz IncQ[12]. This seems to be the only one of these plasmid groups with an extended host range as judged by attempts to mobilize members of these groups from *E.coli* into *Pseudomonas aeruginosa* or *Methylophilus methylotrophus* using RP4 (unpublished observations). We used plasmid mobilization because, in contrast to transformation, it is little affected by restriction systems in the host. IncQ plasmids are very commonly found[10], over a broad geographical and bacterial

Table 1. Incompatibility Groups of Non-conjugative Plasmids

Plasmid	Size (kb)	Phenotype[a]	Inc group	References
P15A	2.0	cryptic	–	2
ColE1-K30	5.3	ColE1$^+$	–	10,11
ColE2-P9	6.9	ColE2$^+$	–	10
ColK-235	6.9	ColK$^+$	–	13
pHH509	8.4	Ap^R	–	11
NTP2,R300B	8.5	SmSu^R	Q	10,11
pSC101	9.3	Tc^R	–	11
R831a	13.8	SmKm^R	–	11

[a]Phenotypic symbols are according to Novick et al[14]. The references give information on incompatibility relationships.

species range[15] and thus represent a particularly successful plasmid type. Members of this group that have been studied in recent years are R300B[15], NTP2[10], RSF1010 (which is identical to NTP2[16]) and R1162[17]. All these plasmids are indistinguishable at present[15,18].

Apart from their broad host-range, the other characteristics that might make IncQ plasmids suitable as cloning vectors are: 1) the are relatively small (the majority of those studied were 8.5kb[15]), 2) they have a relatively high copy number (in *E.coli*, measured as supercoiled DNA, we found 8-12 copies per chromosome[15,11]) and 3) they are non-conjugative but efficiently mobilized by conjugative plasmids of various groups (see below).

In this paper we describe further studies on R300B including th derivation of a restriction map, a genetic map by Tn3 mutagenesis, polypeptide synthesis in mini-cells and the creation of various derivatives useful in cloning.

MATERIALS AND METHODS

Growth media. Growth media were as previously described[19]. For *M.methylotrophus* we used M9 salts medium supplemented with 1% methanol plus FeCl3,10 mg/l.

Plate-mating. Plasmids were generally transferred on solid media: a colony of the recipient strain was spread with a little sterile saline onto half the surface of a selective medium plate and coloni of the donor strains were then streaked in one direction across the plate into the recipient. For transfer into a variety of different (usually prototrophic) species, we used a *thy* donor which can be counterselected on Isosensitest (Oxoid) medium.

Plasmid DNA Isolation. Plasmid DNA was isolated after sarkosyl lysi

of cells in ethidium bromide-CsCl gradients in a scaled-up version of
the previously described method[15].

DNA Restriction Analysis. Plasmid DNA was restricted and analysed by
gel electrophoresis as previously described[7]. Bands were cut out of
gels and the DNA isolated by electroelution into dialysis tubing. DNA
ligations overnight at 10°C and subsequent transformation were carried
out by standard methods.

Analysis of Polypeptides in Minicells. Plasmids were mobilized or
transformed into the minicell producing strain χ1411 trpEΔ. Minicells
were isolated in freeze-thaw generated sucrose gradients[5], radiolabelled,
the polypeptides electrophoresed through polyacrylamide gels and autoradiographed approximately as described by Dougan et al[20].

Isolation of Tn3 derivatives of R300B. Cultures of C600 (R1drd19/R300B)
were grown overnight at 30°C to facilitate transposition[21] and then
plated out on media containing 1 mg ampicillin/ml. Clones containing
R300B::Tn3 are selected because the increase in copy number of the bla
gene produced by transposition from the low copy number R1drd19 to the
high copy number R300B leads to a corresponding increase in ampicillin
resistance[22].

RESULTS

The Host-range of IncQ Plasmids

     We have previously reported[15] that the host-range of IncQ plasmids
includes E.coli, Salmonella typhimurium, S.senftenberg, S.dublin,
Proteus mirabilis, P.morganii, Providencia sp. and Pseudomonas
aeruginosa. Since then they have also been reported to replicate
stably in Ps. phaseolicola[23] Rhizobium meliloti[24], Rhodopseudomonas
sp[25] and Acinetobacter calcoaceticus[26]. Experiments in this laboratory
have shown that R300B or its derivatives can also stably inhabit
Methylophilus methylotrophus, Alcaligenes eutrophus, Ps.putida,
Klebsiella aerogenes and Serratia marcescens. We have used conjugative
plasmids of the following groups to mobilize IncQ plasmids into some
of the above species:- IncFI: F104[15]; IncFII: R1drd19, JR72; IncIα:
R144drd3[12], R483, JR66a; IncN: N3T; IncP: RP4, R751, R702; IncW: R7K.
Not all of these plasmids are effective in all crosses except for RP4.
This host-range list is not complete, merely those tested so far.
However we have not yet found a Gram negative species that IncQ
plasmids do not inhabit.

A Restriction Map of R300B

     The construction of broad host-range cloning vectors from R300B
depends upon knowing its restriction and genetic maps. A simple map
of R300B was published recently[7]. Figure 1 shows our present restriction map. Although the EcoR1 and HpaI sites are not distinguishable

by restriction analysis we have shown that deletion of DNA to the left of the *Eco*R1 site (as in the construction of pGSS8, see below) does not remove the *Hpa*I site. A genetic map of RSF1010 relative to the *Eco*RI has been produced in Falkow's laboratory[16,18]. We have superimposed it onto our map in the orientation shown because removal of the 0.8kb *Pst*I fragment from R300B led to loss of sulphonamide resistance[7] whereas the cloning of random *Sst*I-cut fragments of *M.methylophilus* chromosomal DNA into the *Sst*I site always led to loss of streptomycin resistance.

In addition to the sites shown in Figure 1 there are also several sites on R300B susceptible to *Bgl*I[27], *Hae*II, *Hae*III, *Hinf*I[27] and *Sau*3A and a single site for *Sst*II[28]. But we found no cleavage sites for *Bam*HI, *Bgl*II, *Cla*I, *Hind*III, *Kpn*I, *Pvu*I, *Sal*I, *Sma*I, *Xba*I, *Xho*1 or *Xma*I. A similar map has been published for RSF1010[29] and two simple maps for R1162 are also consistent with it[17,30].

A Genetic Map of R300B

We have begun a genetic analysis of R300B using Tn3 mutagenesis, Figure 2 shows some of the Tn3 insertions we have mapped using restriction endonucleases. These data confirm the hypothesis first proposed by Heffron et al[18,31] that the two genes giving sulphonamide (*sul*) and streptomycin (*aphC*) resistance are in a single operon with *sul* proximal and *aphC* distal to the promoter : thus, pLT108 has lost

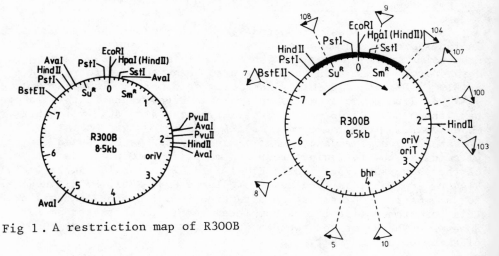

Fig 1. A restriction map of R300B

Fig.2. A Tn3 insertion map of R300B. The arrow heads on the Tn3 symbols are at the *bla* end and show the direction of transcription out of the transposon[31] when Tn3 is in its normal repressed (*tnp*R+) state[32]. The arrow within the circle shows the proposed start and direction of transcription of the operon giving drug resistances.

both Su^R and Sm^R whereas pLT9 has lost only Sm^R. The promoter is
presumably to the left of the *Pst*I site at 7.6 kb since, as noted
above, removal of the *Pst*I fragment does not lead to loss of Sm^R,
although the level of resistance is somewhat reduced.

        Insertions of Tn3 at around 4kb affect the broad host-range
(bhr) properties of R300B. Such plasmids are still mobilizable into
E.coli but not into *M.methylotrophus*. We do not know whether this is
an effect on their transfer into, or maintenance in, the latter species.
We also include in Figure 2 the approximate site of the presumed
transfer origin *(ori*T). Nordheim and Timmis[33] have shown that the
relaxation nick site of RSF1010, presumed to be *ori*T, is close to, but
not at, the site of the replication origin *(ori*V).

Transcription of the *sul aph*C Operon

        We have examined the polypeptides expressed by R300B and some of
its Tn3 derivatives in minicells. As *sul* and *aph*C are in the same
operon, their expressed polypeptides are likely to be present in about
equal amounts. In Figure 3 it can be seen that band E is reduced to
approximately half intensity by the Tn3 insertion of pLT9 (Sm^S),showing
that the eliminated polypeptide (the amino-glycoside 3" phosphotransferase) bands at this position and suggesting that the remaining polypeptide in band E is the dihydropteroate synthase *(sul)*. Dougan et
al[34] have also deduced the identity of the former polypeptide. These
polypeptides have a molecular weight of a little under 30,000 which
require a coding capacity of just less than 900 base pairs each. The
sul and *aph*C genes have therefore been drawn as this size on Fig.2.
Their positions come from various considerations: (i) the Tn3
insertion in pLT104 does not affect the level of Sm^R, (ii) genes in an
operon are normally adjacent and (iii) cleavage at the *Eco*RI site of
R300B separated but did not inactivate the genes giving Su^R and Sm^R in
the construction of pGSS8 and 9 from pGSS6 (next section). The *Eco*RI
and probably the *Hpa*I sites therefore appear to be cloning sites
within a transcription unit that would not give rise to fused proteins.
This *sul aph*C operon appears to be highly expressed from a comparison
of band E with the β-lactamase bands F and G.

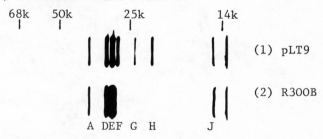

Fig.3. Autoradiogram of ^{35}S-labelled polypeptides from minicells
       containing (1) pLT9 (see Fig 2) and (2) R300B. Molecular
       weight markers are indicated above.

Construction of new Cloning Vectors from R300B

R300B has few sites for the restriction enzymes normally used for cloning. We therefore generated new derivatives by introducing genes from other plasmids. As pBR322 has been sequenced and is well understood, we used it as a source. By *Hae*II partial cleavage of both R300B and pBR322, followed by ligation, we generated a series of cointegrate plasmids such as pGSS6 (Figure 4). In this figure we have designated the origin of pBR322 as *ori*E and that of R300B as *ori*Q. Replication from *ori*E is dependent on *pol*A[+35] whereas from *ori*Q it is not[36]. We have used this difference to distinguish between the two types of origin in the cointegrates and the subsequent cleavage products. We next cleaved pGSS6 and similar cointegrates with *Eco*RI and self-ligated the two fragments formed. From pGSS6, the ApSu[R] plasmid (pGSS9) produced was found to be *pol*A[+] dependent and not mobilizable into eg *M.methylotrophus* whereas the TcSm[R] plasmid (pGSS8) shown in Figure 4 is *pol*A[+] independent and has the broad host-range of the parental R300B. It also has the *Cla*I, *Hind*III, *Bam*HI and *Sal*I cloning sites in the gene conferring Tc[R]. Transcription of the gene conferring Sm[R] is however dependent on a backward reading promoter near the beginning of the *tet* gene. Cloning into the *Cla*I or *Hind*III sites can therefore cause loss of both markers.

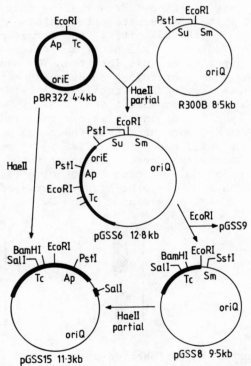

Fig. 4   Construction of R300B derivatives using DNA from pBR322.

Because of this, we decided to introduce the *bla* gene, which has its own promoter, from pBR322. *Hae*II cleavage of pBR322 and pGSS8 followed by ligation and transformation into a *pol*A host led to the recovery of pGSS15. In this plasmid the *bla tet* boundary of pBR322 has been reconstructed but the plasmid has the replication and host-range properties of R300B. (Unfortunately, an extra *Hae*II fragment carrying the *Sal*I site was also introduced. We are at present attempting to remove it).

Another series of vectors was made by addition rather than substitution of genes: these retain the strong *sul aph*C promoter of R300B. We restricted pACYC184[2] and pMK20[38] plasmid DNAs to completion with *Hae*II, ran them on a gel and then electroeluted the 1.3kb band from the former and the 1.5kb band from the latter. These contain the genes conferring CmR and KmR respectively from the two plasmids as shown in Figure 5. These were separately ligated to partially *Hae*II cut R300B DNA eluted from a gel at the whole linear plasmid (8.5kb) position and transformed into *E.coli* selecting for CmR or KmR clones. Few of the CmR clones proved to contain R300B::CmR plasmids like the example pTB86 in Figure 5: the majority had plasmids consisting of

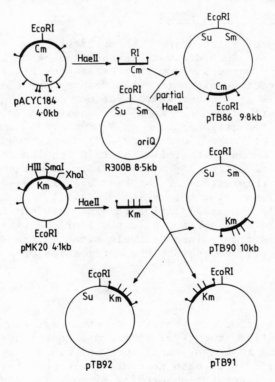

Fig.5. Construction of the CmR and KmR derivatives of R300B. The *Hae*II sites are marked thus ↑.

the two largest, adjacent *Hae*II fragments of pACYC184 which can form a replicon[39]. The original *Eco*RI site needs to be removed from pTB86 and its sisters in order to use the one in the gene conferring Cm^R as an insertional inactivation site.

The Km^R clones were found to contain R300B::Km^R plasmids. Of 78 examined so far, 62 were $SuSmKm^R$ like pTB90, 6 were Km^R only, like pTB91 and 10 were $SuKm^R$ like pTB92. The latter two classes are consistent with the model that R300B has a single *sul aph*C operon with *sul* being proximal to the promoter and suggest that the inserted *Hae*II fragment blocks transcription in either orientation. Each of these plasmids has gained a *Hind*III, *Sma*I and *Xho*I cloning site. R300B has about 20 *Hae*II sites so we would expect insertion of the Km^R fragment at several of these sites causing other changes in phenotype apart from the loss of $SuSm^R$ or Sm^R already noted. We have therefore tested these 62 clones for such changes. Two have a reduced and one an increased, plasmid copy number (as determined by the Km and Sm resistance levels), 13 are non-mobilizable and 10 have a reduced host-range. We are mapping the inserts in these plasmids at present to complement our Tn3 mutagenesis mapping.

Transposon Derivatives of R300B

Another way of introducing cloning sites into plasmids is by using transposons. Such derivatives can then be further adapted by excising specific segments from them using pre-existing and newly-introduced restriction sites (as we have done for the RP4::Tn7 system[5,7]). This is another reason for our isolating the R300B::Tn3 derivatives described above. A Tn5 derivative of R300B (pTB70) has been used by us recently to clone gdh^+ from *E.coli* into a glutamate synthase mutant of *M.methylotrophus*[8]. By the consequent switch in the pathway for ammonium assimilation this has led to a significant improvement in the efficiency of conversion of methanol to single-cell protein by this organism. We have also isolated a Tn1771[40] derivative of R300B. The *tet* region of Tn1771 (and the indistinguishable Tn1721) can be amplified to give multiple tandem repeats[41] Genes cloned into this portion will therefore be similarly amplified Furthermore genes cloned into suitable sites on transposon derivativ of R300B can be transposed into the chromosomes of a wide range of organisms.

DISCUSSION

We have described the genetic structure and properties of R300E and the construction from it of some broad host-range cloning vecto which are proving to be very useful in our cloning systems. Bagdasarian et al[29] have also generated IncQ vectors, with *Bgl*II an *Xba*I insertional inactivation cloning sites. Meyer and Shapiro[37] a Bagdasarian et al[29] have reported the construction of cointegrates between a ColE1 and an IncQ plasmid using the *Eco*RI or *Pst*I sites respectively, but these plasmids do not stably inhabit *Pseudomonas*, or if selected, delete part of the ColE1[37]. (Gautier and Bonewald[30] also made such cointegrates via *Eco*RI but they do not report any reduction in host-range). It seems there may be a region of ColE1 that is inimical to broad host-range maintenance. If so, it must have been disrupted in the construction of pGSS6, as this plasmid (and its derivatives pGSS8 and 15) do not suffer this handicap: they are stable in at least *E. coli, P. aeruginosa, M. methylotrophus* and *A. eutrophus*.

There is some confusion in the literature about whether or not IncQ plasmids require polymeraseI for replication. Our data confirm the painstaking data of Grindley and Kelley[36] that they do not. Gautier and Bonewald[30] however, have drawn the opposite conclusion. This may be due to the slight instability of these plasmids in some *pol*A mutants[36].

There is clearly plenty of scope for the further development of these broad host-range cloning vectors. We do not know at present whether they can be reduced in size without loss of valuable functions. But we can introduce or select stronger promoters and put in cloning sites suitably down-stream from ribosome binding sites with perhaps a secretion leader sequence between. We also hope that our genetic analysis of R300B will lead to an understanding of how this fascinating plasmid functions.

ACKNOWLEDGEMENTS

We are grateful to T C Hodgman for his analysis of the polypeptides synthesised in minicells and to S A Withe for his help with the restriction analysis of R300B and the photography. We would also like to thank D R Helinski for his hospitality to one of us (PTB) in his laboratory recently, during which time the Cm^R and Km^R derivatives of R300B were isolated with the particular help of D Stalker.

REFERENCES

1   F Bolivar, R L Rodriguez, P J Greene, M S Betlach, H L Heyneker, H W Boyer, J H Crosa and S Falkow, Gene 2:95 (1977).
2   A C Y Chang and S N Cohen, J Bacteriol 134:1141 (1978).
3   S N Cohen and A C Y Chang, J Bacteriol 132:734 (1977).
4   N E Murray, W J Brammar and K Murray, Molec Gen Genet 150:53(1977)
5   P T Barth and N J Grinter, J Mol Biol 113:455 (1977)
6   A DePicker, M Van Montagu and J Schell in "DNA Insertion Elements, Plasmids and Episomes" Bukhari, Shapiro and Adya, eds, 678 (1977), Cold Spring Harbor Laboratory.
7   P T Barth, in "Plasmids of Medical, Environmental and Commercial Importance", K N Timmis and A Pühler eds, 399 (1979), Elsevier/ North Holland.
8   J D Windass, M J Worsey, E M Pioli, D Pioli, P T Barth, K T Atherton, E C Dart, D Byrom, K Powell and P J Senior, Nature 287:396 (1980).

9   G Ditta, S Stanfield, D Corbin and D R Helinski, Proc Natl Acad Sci in press.

10   H R Smith, G O Humphreys and E S Anderson, Molec Gen Genet 129:229 (1974).

11   P T Barth, H Richards and N Datta, J Bacteriol 135:760 (1978).

12   N J Grinter and P T Barth, J Bacteriol 128:394 (1976).

13   G J Warren, A J Twigg and D J Sherratt, Nature 274:259 (1978).

14   R P Novick, R C Clowes, S N Cohen, R Curtiss III, N Datta and S Falkow, Bacteriol Rev 40:168 (1976).

15   P T Barth and N J Grinter, J Bacteriol 120:618 (1974).

16   J De Graaff, J H Crosa, F Heffron and S Falkow, J Bacteriol 134:1117 (1978).

17   R Meyer, G Boch and J Shapiro, Molec Gen Genet 171:7 (1979).

18   F Heffron, C Rubens and S Falkow, Proc Natl Acad Sci 72: 3623 (1975).

19   P T Barth, N J Grinter and D E Bradley, J Bacteriol 133:43(1978)

20   G Dougan, M Saul, A Twigg, R Gill and D Sherratt, J Bacteriol 138:48 (1979).

21   P J Kretschmer and S N Cohen, J Bacteriol 139:515 (1979).

22   J A Nowak and A J Clark, Lunteren Lectures on Molecular Genetics (1979).

23   N J Panopoulos, B J Staskawicz and D Sandlin in "Plasmids of Medical, Environmental and Commercial Importance", K N Timmis and A Pühler eds, 365 (1979), Elsevier/North Holland.

24   Gary Ditta, personal communication.

25   JoAnne Williams, personal communication.

26   Tom Schmidthauser, personal communication.

27   Wolfgang Schuch, personal communication.

28   Kim Ellis, personal communication.

29   M Bagdasarian, M M Bagdasarian, S Coleman and K N Timmis, in "Plasmids of Medical, Environmental and Commercial Importance", K N Timmis and A Pühler eds., 411 (1979), Elsevier/North Holland

30   F Gautier and R Bonewald. Molec Gen Genet 178:375 (1980).

31   C Rubens, F Heffron and S Falkow, J Bacteriol 128:425 (1976).

32   F Heffron, B J McCarthy, H Ohtsubo and E Ohtsubo, Cell 18:1153 (1979).

33   A Nordheim and K N Timmis, Lunteren Lectures on Molecular Genetics (1979).

34   G Dougan, M Saul, A Twigg, R Gill and D J Sherratt, J Bacteriol 138:48 (1979).

35   D T Kingsbury and D R Helinski, Biochem Biophys Res Comm 41:153 (1970).

36   N D F Grindley and W S Kelley, Molec Gen Genet 143:311 (1974).

37   R Meyer and J Shapiro, EMBO Workshop on Control of Replication and Partitioning of Bacterial Chromosomes and Plasmids, Leicester (1

38   M Kahn and D R Helinski, Proc Natl Acad Sci 75:2200 (1978).

39   David Stalker, personal communication.

40   F Schöffl and A Pühler, Genet Res Camb. 33:253 (1979).

41   R Mattes, H J Burkardt and R Schmitt, Molec Gen Genet.168:173 (1979).

THE SURVIVAL OF EK1 AND EK2 SYSTEMS IN SEWAGE TREATMENT PLANT

MODELS

Bernard P. Sagik, Charles A. Sorber, Barbara E. Moore

Drexel University: University of Texas at Austin
Cart, University of Texas at San Antonio

PREFACE

In March 1977 the National Academy of Sciences (USA) convened
a Forum on Research with Recombinant DNA. It was clear to participants that this potentially was an opportunity to affect national science policy. In trying to assess the benefits and risks
inherent in recombinant DNA technology, some argued the risks were
not different than any in the microbiology laboratory; others
warned that such research was the first step towards the manipulation of human genetics, that it could contaminate the biosphere
irrevocably.

The decision to support work determining the potential for
survival of EK1 and EK2 hosts and vectors in sewage treatment processes (as well as the vectors' capacity to be transmitted to
secondary hosts indigenous to sewage) must be understood in this
1977 context rather than in the triumphant editorial in Science
Recombinant DNA Revisited (1).

What was proposed in these studies was (a) to monitor the
survival of EK1 and EK2 hosts and vectors and (b) to monitor the
transmission of vectors to secondary hosts during sewage treatment.
The importance of risk assessment was underlined by such reports
as the interbacterial transfer of inter-E. coli-Drosophilia
melanogaster recombinant plasmids (2) and the mathematical analysis of the probability of establishing these or other chimeric
plasmids in natural populations of bacteria (3). Work subsequent
to that reported here has resulted in a technique for expressing
eukaryotic genes in bacteria (4) and the converse, the expression
of a bacterial gene in mammalian cells (5). In addition, Peden

449

et al. (6) have used the plasmid pBR322 to clone Simian Virus 40 in E. coli.

Levy et al. (7) have attempted a preliminary assessment of the probability of survival of an E. coli host-vector system in mouse and human intestines. In their report, no recoveries of E. coli K12, strain χ1776 were made from mice or human subjects 24 hours after ingestion. However, where the same strain bearing plasmid pBR322 was fed, recoveries were made for four days (6/10^6 ingested). The non-disabled E. coli K12 strain χ1666 (with or without pBR322) survived in $\overline{10^4}$ greater number and was recovered for six days. No evidence for intestinal colonization was obtained, nor was there any evidence for plasmid transfer to indigenous aerobic fecal bacteria.

Abelson (8) discussed the risk problem in terms of the inadvertent creation of a pathogen. The example he used was a "worst case" model in which E. coli carrying polyoma DNA would be found to induce tumors in mice. Less dramatic, but equally important examples of recombination among E. coli plasmids were cited (9-11). Striking in this context were the results of Gyles and his co-workers (12) who reported that genes for drug resistance are spread in nature not only by being part of an R factor but also by becoming incorporated into other plasmids. Almost at the same time, Williams (13) reported on self-transmissable plasmid transfer in the human alimentary tract. He found that in the absence of selective pressure, transfer of col V plasmids to indigenous fecal coliforms occurred in the human intestine after the ingestion of E. coli K12. These results are not completely consistent with the recent report of Levy et al. (7) discussed above.

In the U.S., municipalities generally use either primary settling coupled with lagooning or secondary biological treatment before disinfection and discharge to surface waters or irrigant ponds. The primary and secondary sludges may be dewatered and buried or incinerated or -- occasionally -- used as soil emendation agents with or without further treatment. (Alternatively these sludges may be digested anaerobically, and then dewatered, etc.)

Large cities, where land for lagooning is less available and far more costly, are likely to use some form of activated sludge treatment by which solid human organic wastes are solubilized. A significant by-product of this microbial degradation process is a large mass of biologically-generated secondary sludge. This often is subjected to anaerobic digestion at elevated temperatures with the production of methane as a potentially useful product. The stabilized product of such anaerobic digestion is then dewatered and/or incinerated, buried in sanitary landfills, or used as a soil emendation agent.

In small communities with inexpensive available land, treatment plants may use only primary settling followed by more or less prolonged lagooning prior to releasing the primary effluent (with or without disinfection) to receiving surface waters or land to be irrigated.

Foster and Engelbrecht (14) have noted the high level of removal of enteric viruses by biological secondary treatment. This is consistent with Schaub and Sagik's report (15) of the high efficiency of association of such viruses with clay particulates and colloidally-suspended organics. Removal was not synonomous with inactivation and such adsorbed viruses were still infectious in cell culture and in animals. K.R. Ranganathan and his colleagues (16) demonstrated in bench-scale models that viruses were protected by occlusion in the secondary sludge biomass. Moore et al. (17) in their analysis of a 10 mgd contact stabilization treatment plant found that well over 90% of enteric viruses entering the plant were concentrated into the mixed liquor suspended solids. This observation was confirmed in studies of virus distribution in other activated sludge treatment plants. Further studies by Moore (see Sagik ref. 18) and by Sanders et al. (19) showed the relative longevity in anaerobic digesters of sludge-associated viruses as compared to free viruses.

Analyses of wastewater grab samples for possible pathogenic bacteria were performed by Sagik et al. (20). Among the organisms isolated, enumerated, and identified were several which could serve as potential secondary hosts for plasmid vehicles.

MODEL TREATMENT PLANT RESULTS

The Treatment Plant. The wastewater treatment system used in this study was a bench-scale model incorporating all of the widely-used conventional treatment modalities (see Figure 1). As designed and operated, the system was fed with approximately 55 liters of raw sewage daily. The central treatment train was an activated sludge system which utilized primary and secondary (activated sludge) unit processes. There were three additional unit processes ancillary to this system: lagooning of both primary and secondary effluents and anaerobic digestion of wasted sludges. For simplicity, the unit processes are not described here, but details may be found in Eckenfelder's text (21) and in Sagik and Sorber (22).

During the course of this study, the unit processes comprising the model treatment plant were operated within the usual limits of loading and generally functioned as efficiently as do the field installations being simulated. Operational characteristics of the model treatment plant for the first six operational studies compared well with data typical of full-scale field installations (22).

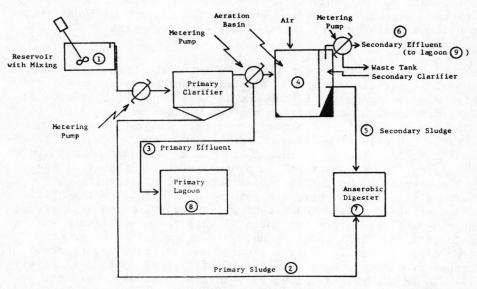

Figure 1.   Schematic of Model Wastewater Treatment Facility and
            Sampling Points

Organism Survival. To provide a basis for the interpretation of
the survival of EK1 and EK2 hosts within the treatment model, a
series of operational studies were undertaken using a genetically
marked sewage isolate, E. coli GF 215. Raw wastewater was seeded
at a level of approximately 5 x 10^7 cfu/ml with sampling continued over 120 hours. The survival of E. coli GF 215 in the wastewater reservoir (0-48 hr) and in the primary and secondary lagoons
(48-120 hr) is summarized in Table 1. Similar results were obtained using two marked prototypes of parental E. coli K12. The
results obtained all show a high degree of correlation (r^2) between
microbial inactivation and time. The k value (decay constant) of
about 2 observed for parental E. coli K12 GF 29 was quite similar
to that demonstrated for indigenous E. coli GF 215. The fate of
these three prototypic E. coli strains during anaerobic digestion
at 37°C is summarized graphically in Figure 2.

TABLE 1   Correlation Coefficients and Decay Constants
          for Survival of an Indigenous E. coli (GF215)

Unit	mean BOD_5 (ml/1)	r^2	k
Raw Wastewater Reservoir	140	.95	2.2
Primary Lagoon	21	.89	1.9
Secondary Lagoon	<10	.85	.96

Of the EK2 hosts, strain Dp50supF demonstrated survival analogous to parental E. coli strains while E.coli χ1776 was inactivated more rapidly in raw wastewater and primary effluent with a maximum decay constant of 3.6. The effectiveness of anaerobic digestion of sludges can be inferred by the rapid disappearance of E. coli χ1776 to a level of nondetectability within 20 hours (5 $\log_{10}$ loss). The survival of E. coli Dp50supF in an anaerobic digester was closer to parental K12 strains, with a 90% reduction evident after 20 hours.

Two plasmid-bearing hosts also were evaluated as part of this study. Survival data for E. coli χ2656, carrying pBR322, and E. coli GF2174, carrying pBR325, are given in Table 2. It is seen that E. coli GF2174 was more

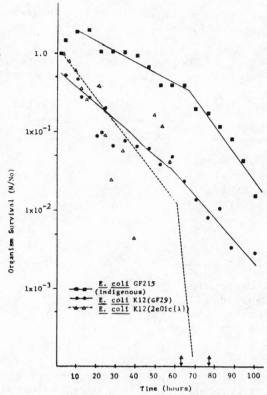

Figure 2.   Inactivation of Prototypic and Paremtal E. coli strains during Anaerobic Digestion

labile than either E. coli χ2656 or total coliforms in raw sewage. Similarly, strain GF2174 was inactivated rapidly during anaerobic digestion with only sporadic recovery of viable organisms 20 hours after introducing seeded-sludges into the digester. E. coli χ2656(pBR322) was more stable in this unit process, with an observed 90% reduction within 30 hours. From these results it is not evident that the presence of a plasmid within a host cell confers any unique survival capabilities to an organism.

The only cloning vector used during this study was the lambda phage, Charon 4A. Its correlation coefficient is near 1.0, as is that of indigenous E. coli, indicating a linear relationship between organism decay and time. As in previous studies the decay constant (k) for total coliforms was about 1.5. The Charon 4A phage displayed a similar decay constant in both lagoons. In raw wastewater, however, the vector disappeared much more rapidly as evidenced by a k value exceeding 5. A plausible explanation for this extreme discrepancy may be viral adsorption to particulate

matter present in raw sewage at a greater concentration than in
lagooned effluents.

TABLE 2   Correlation Coefficients and Decay Constants for
Survival of Total Coliform and Plasmid-Bearing EK2 Hosts

Unit	mean BOD_5 (mg/l)	Total Coliforms r^2	k	E. coli r^2	2656(pBR322) k
Raw Wastewater Reservoir	280	.60	.38	.89	1.2
Primary Lagoon	28	.89	1.4	.91	1.9
Secondary Lagoon	2	.71	.79	.93	1.5

Unit	mean BOD_5 (mg/l)	Total Coliforms r^2	k	E. coli r^2	GF2174(pBR325) k
Raw Wastewater Reservoir	400	.83	.62	.90	2.7
Primary Lagoon	26	.85	1.8	.89	1.9
Secondary Lagoon	6	.24	.70	.26	.67

Organism Removal. The treatment effectiveness of the primary and
secondary unit processes were evaluated using BOD_5 and TSS values.
The reduction of organisms within either unit was viewed in relation to the removal of the physical/chemical parameters. For
purposes of this presentation, secondary treatment was handled
as an independent unit process. Mean removals were calculated
using only positive values; that is, when effluent values were
lower than influent values. This approach was used in order to
compensate for treatment system upsets. The small model plant
operated during this study had very little buffer capacity when
compared to the field treatment plants which seldom lose their
ability to affect some degree of wastewater treatment.

Studies using genetically identifiable indigenous E. coli
K12 GF 215 and parental E. coli K12 GF29 demonstrated similar
reductions of 20% to 30% as a result of primary treatment and
95% to 99.9% removal as a result of secondary treatment. Comparable results were obtained with EK2 hosts during primary and
secondary treatment. The removal of both E. coli Dp50supF and
E. coli $_\chi$1776 was compared to the behavior of indigenous bacteria
as measured by total coliform organisms and similar results were
obtained.

Results in Table 3 demonstrate the behavior of the lambda phage, Charon 4A, within the treatment train. While bacterial levels in primary effluent are decreased, very little effective removal of the Charon phage occurred during primary treatment. However, phage removal from sewage during secondary treatment was quite effective.

Overall, the removal of EK1 and EK2 hosts and the Charon phage during the process of conventional sewage treatment paralleled the behavior of indigenous wastewater bacteria. Not unexpectedly, more variability was observed during primary treatment. This unit process essentially represents passive settling of particular matter that has a higher specific gravity than water and is too large to remain in suspension due to convection. Indigenous bacteria may be associated with solids to a variable extent depending upon their source (fecal material or other) and the degree of solids dispersion due to turbulence in transmission lines and, in the case of this study, mixing within the wastewater reservoir. Test organisms were added to the wastewater as a suspension and initially were unassociated with particulates. Even so, organism removal occurred during primary treatment and was confirmed by the detection of viable seed bacteria and phage within the primary sludge.

TABLE 3   Treatment Effectiveness for the Removal
of Charon 4A Phage

Time (days)	Primary Treatment (% removal)				Secondary Treatment (% removal)			
	BOD_5	TSS	Total Coliform	Charon 4A	BOD_5	TSS	Total Coliform	Charon 4A
0	55	64	91	–	53	29	89	–
1.0	50	66	36	-165	70	50	98	97
2.0+	78	66	67	41	70	9	77	93
5.0	38	55	**	**	64	39	96	α
mean β	50	62	53	41	69	46	90	96

α organism concentration below detection levels
β calculated from positive removals
* not analyzed
** not calculated after cessation of seeding
+ organism seeding discontinued at 48 hr., fresh sewage placed
   in reservoir
++ not calculated after cessation of seeding

Secondary treatment of wastewater by activated sludge processes involves the active development of bacterial floc utilizing the soluble organics in sewage as a nutrient source. Organisms entering the aeration basin become entrapped within the mixed liquor suspended solids (MLSS). This association with MLSS does not immediately lead to organism inactivation. For secondary treatment to achieve effective organism removals, therefore, separation of the liquid and solid phases (MLSS) must be achieved within the secondary clarifier. Because of this, the correspondence between TSS removal and organism removal is more evident during secondary treatment.

As with the primary treatment process, the biomass generated by secondary treatment carries viable test organisms. Seventy-two hours after the cessation of seeding the raw wastewater reservoir, relatively high levels of selected host bacteria were still being recovered from secondary sludge in these studies. The accumulation of viable organisms in sewage sludges and their persistence in this mileau reiterate the need for adequate sludge handling prior to terminal disposal of these solids. Efficient high-rate anaerobic sludge digestion can provide a useful buffer for this purpose.

Mass Balance of Test Organisms With the Primary Clarifier. In an attempt to ascertain the potential for EK1 and EK2 host colonization within the central treatment plant model, a limited mass balance approach was used. The primary treatment process was assumed to be the ideal unit to study, in that the organisms were subjected to relatively quiescent conditions with maximum organic load (nutrient source). The data documenting influent and effluents (sludge and primary effluent) of the primary clarifier were readily available.

A mass balance ration (MBR) relates the level of test organisms transferred out of the primary clarifier to the number of test organisms entering the primary clarifier over a 12 hour period:

$$MBR = \frac{\Sigma(E + S + Cap)}{\Sigma(I + Cip)}$$

where: E = total cfu leaving the clarifier in primary effluent
S = total cfu in primary sludge wasted from the clarifier
I = total cfu entering the clarifier in influent wastewater
Cap = average cfu in primary clarifier
Cip = instantaneous cfu in primary clarifier at the end of the preceding 12 hour period.

If organism colonization (as evidenced by growth) occurred, the
MBR value should be significantly greater than unity.

As evidenced by MBR values of approximately one, no significant colonization of the primary clarifier could be documented
for any of the E. coli hosts tested.

Plasmid Transfer Studies. Laboratory studies using pure cultures
of test organisms were conducted to ascertain the most favorable
conditions under which the transfer of plasmid DNA might occur.
Based on the results of these controlled laboratory studies, it
was expected that the transfer of either pBR322 or pBR325 to
indigenous organisms in sewage would be quite low. Addition of a
mobilizer strain such as E. coli χ1784 would be expected to increase the frequency of plasmid transfer to a more readily
detectable level.

Initial testing was conducted by mixing equal volumes of E.
coli χ2656 with raw sewage or primary sludge. Stationary cultures
were held at 37°C and sampled at times 0, 5, and 25 hours. A
rapid disappearance of χ2656 was observed along with an increase
of 3 - 4 $\log_{10}$/24 hr of indigenous organisms showing resistance
to tetracycline (12.5 μg/ml) and carbenicillin (500 μg/ml). Subsequent experiments demonstrated that this increased antibiotic
resistance of sewage bacteria was attributable solely to the test
conditions promoting growth of this population. No transfer of
pBR322 could be demonstrated in this system.

Plasmid transfer of pBR325 from E. coli GF2174 to indigenous
sewage bacteria was evaluated in both the presence and absence of
the mobilizer strain, E. coli 1784. Representative results from
such an experimental series are shown in Table 4. In the absence
of either donor or mobilizer strains, levels of indigenous wastewater bacteria resistance to tetracycline (12.5 μg/ml), carbenicillin (100 μg/ml) and chloramphenicol (25 μg/ml) increased by a
factor of 4.7 at 24 hours. When E. coli GF2174 (pBR325) was added
to wastewater, the level of this resistant indigenous population
was observed to increase 8.1 over the same time interval. Interestingly, with both donor and mobilizer E. coli strains present
in the test system, a 25-fold increase in the level of antibiotic
resistant indigenous wastewater bacteria was measured. Such
observations are suggestive of plasmid transfer.

SUMMARY AND CONCLUSIONS

We proposed in 1978 to monitor (a) the survival of EK1 and
EK2 hosts and vectors and (b) the transmission of such vectors to
secondary hosts during sewage treatment. In order to do (a)
meaningfully, we carried out comparative studies with indigenous

bacteria modified so as to permit their selective observation against the background of unaltered microbiota.

These studies have shown a good linear relationship between organism decay and time in the raw wastewater reservoir, and in the primary and secondary lagoons for both the strain derived from indigenous flora and that derived from a non-debilitated E. coli K12. During anaerobic digestion, the indigenous strain showed greater stability than did the K12 (1 $\log_{10}$ reduction in 70 hours for the former vs 30 hours for the latter). The EK2 host E. coli Dp50supF showed survival characteristics similar to the non-debilitated K12 derived strain. E. coli χ1776 was inactivated far more rapidly in raw wastewater and primary effluent and could not be recovered from anaerobic digestors by 20 hours after seeding. In contrast, Dp50supF suffered only a one $\log_{10}$ reduction in 20 hours (being similar to the non-debilitated parental E. coli K12 strain). There is no evidence that the presence of a plasmid within the host cell confers any differential survival.

TABLE 4

Frequency of $_p$BR325 Plasmid Transfer to Indegenous Wastewater Bacteria

Flask	Sampling Time (hr)	E. coli GF2174		E. coli χ1784		Tet^R Carb^R Cm^R Wastewater Bacteria	
		cfu/ml	N/No	cfu/ml	N/No	cfu/ml	N/No
A	0	None	–	None	–	5.5×10^6	1.0
	0.5					6.5×10^6	1.2
	1.5					5.5×10^6	1.0
	24					2.6×10^7	4.7
B	0	5.5×10^8	1.0	None	–	8.0×10^6	1.0
	0.5	6.0×10^8	1.1			6.5×10^6	0.8
	1.5	6.5×10^8	1.2			6.0×10^6	0.8
	24	3.5×10^8	0.6			6.5×10^7	8.1
C	0	5.7×10^8	1.0	1.6×10^{10}	1.0	8.3×10^6	1.0
	0.5	7.5×10^8	1.3	1.8×10^{10}	1.1	8.3×10^6	1.0
	1.5	8.3×10^8	1.5	2.0×10^{10}	1.3	7.4×10^6	0.9
	24	6.0×10^8	1.1	1.6×10^{10}	1.0	2.1×10^8	25

The lambda phage Charon 4A was studied as one example of a
cloning vector. With the exceptions of raw wastewater and the
anaerobic digestor, the data indicate a linear relationship between
organism decay and time (correlation coefficient equal to 1.0).
In raw wastewater, however, disappearance of this phage was very
rapid (with $K > 5$). In contrast, recovery of Charon 4A was excellent in anaerobic digestors with about a one $\log_{10}$ reduction in
40 hours. These data suggest the importance of continuing studies
on plasmid transfer to indigenous flora.

In laboratory studies using E. coli χ2656 (pBR322) as a donor
strain and other strain χ1784 (R – $\overline{100^+}$ drd) – derepressed, for
transfer – or F 101/C600 as mobilizer strain, conditions for
transmission of the plasmid to strain χ1997 were examined. In
untreated wastewater, in the absence of either donor or mobilizer
strains, indigenous organisms resistant to tetracycline (12.5 μg/
ml), carbenicillin (100 μg/ml) and chloramphenicol (25 μg/ml)
increased by a factor of 4.7 in 24 hours. With the addition of
E. coli GF2174 (pBR325), the recovery of such multiply resistant
possibly indigenous organisms increased 8.1-fold in the same time.
With both the donor and mobilizer E. coli strains present in the
raw wastewater, there was a 25-fold increase in the level of
multiply resistant organisms recovered. This observation is consistent with plasmid transfer during initial contact with indigenous flora, with the recipients then replicating in the next 24 hours
of monitoring.

Acknowledgement: This work was supported by Grant #N01-AI
                  82566 to Dr. Bernard Sagik from the
                  National Institutes of Health.

REFERENCES

1.   Singer, M. 1980. Science 209:4463:1317.
2.   Hamer, D.H. 1977. Science 196:4286:220-221.
3.   Levin, B.R. and F.M. Stewart. 1977. Science 196:4286:218-220.
4.   Guarente, L., T.M. Roberts and M. Ptashne. 1980. Science
       209:4463:1428-1430.
5.   Mulligan, R.C. and P. Berg. 1980. Science 209:4463:1422-1427.
6.   Peden, K.W.C., J.M. Pipas, S. Pearson-White and D. Nathans.
       1980. Science 209:4463:1392-1396.
7.   Levy, S.B., B. Marshall and D. Rowse-Eagle. 1980. Science
       209:4454:391-394.
8.   Abelson, J. 1977. Science 196:4286:159-160.
9.   Cooper, P. 1971. Genet. Res. 17:151-159.
10. Nisioka, T., M. Mitani and R.C. Clowes. 1970. J. Bacteriol.
       103:1:166-177.

11.   Palchaudhuri, S., W.K. Maas and E. Ohtsubo. 1976. Molec. Gen.
      Genet. 146:215-231.
12.   Gyles, C.L., S. Palchaudhuri and W.K. Maas. 1977. Science
      198:4313:198-199.
13.   Williams, P.H. 1977. FEMS Microbiol. Letters 2:91-95.
14.   Foster, D.H. and R.S. Engelbrecht. 1973. In Recycling
      Treated Municipal Wastewater and Sludge through Forest
      and Cropland. W.E. Sopper and L.T. Kardos (ed.) The
      Penn State University Press, University Park, PA.
15.   Schaub, S.A. and B.P. Sagik. 1975. Appl. Microbiol. 30:
      212-222.
16.   Malina, J.F., Jr. K.R. Ranganathan, B.P. Sagik and B.E. Moore,
      1975. J. Water Pollut. Control Fed. 47:2178-2183.
17.   Moore, B.E., L. Funderburg, B.P. Sagik and J.F. Malina, Jr.
      1975. In Virus Survival in Water and Wastewater Systems,
      J.F. Malina, Jr. and B.P. Sagik (ed.) Water Resources
      Symposium No. 7, Center for Research in Water Resources,
      University of Texas, Austin, TX.
18.   Sagik, B.P. 1975. In proceedings, Williamsburg Conference
      on Management of Wastewater Residuals. J.L. Smith and
      E.H. Bryan (ed.). Colorado State University, Ft. Collins,
      CO.
19.   Sanders, D.A., J.F. Manina, Jr., B.E. Moore, B.P. Sagik and
      C.A. Sorber. 1979. J. Water Pollut. Control Fed. 51:
      333-343.
20.   Sagik, B.P., B.E. Moore and C.A. Sorber. 1979. In Utiliza-
      tion of Municipal Sewage Effluent and Sludge on Distri-
      buted Land, W.E. Sopper and S.N. Kerr (ed.). The Penn.
      State Univ. Press. University Park, PA.
21.   Eckenfelder, W.W. 1970. Water Quality Engineering for
      Practical Engineers. Barnes and Noble, Inc., N.Y.
22.   Sagik, B.P. and C.A. Sorber. 1979. Recombinant DNA Technical
      Bulletin, 2:55-61.

cos PLASMID IN BACILLUS SUBTILIS

R. Marrero, F.A. Chiafari, and P.S. Lovett

Department of Biological Sciences
University of Maryland Baltimore County
Catonsville, Md. 21228

INTRODUCTION

The genome of temperate phage λ is a linear duplex DNA molecule with single stranded termini. The single ends contain complementary base sequences allowing λ DNA to circularize in vitro. Treatment of such hydrogen bonded circles with DNA ligase produces a covalently-closed circle. In vivo λ DNA replicates via the rolling circle model (1) and the viral DNA is packaged into phage heads as linear molecules. The cohesive ends of λ DNA appears to serve as initiation sites for packaging the λ genome (2). Insertion of the cohesive ends (cos) of λ DNA into a plasmid, by recombinant DNA technology, confers on the resulting cos plasmid susceptibility to packaging by λ in vivo or in vitro, if the size of the plasmid approximates that of the viral genome (3). Insertion of cos into a small plasmid, such as pBR322, generates a cos plasmid that can only be packaged into mature phage particles if additional DNA is cloned into the small cos plasmid to increase its molecular size. Thus, λ cos plasmids or cosmids serve as excellent vectors for cloning rather large DNA segments (3).

Two relatively well studied Bacillus subtilis temperate phages, Ø105 and SPO2 (4), were chosen to determine if the cohesive ends could be cloned on a plasmid in B. subtilis, and the biological properties of such a chimera.

CLONING RESTRICTION FRAGMENTS OF Ø105 and SPO2 DNA IN B. subtilis.

We previously reported that the B. pumilus temperate phage Ø75 was capable of transduction of plasmid pPL10 (5). In contrast,

461

Ø75 did not mediate transduction of many other plasmids including
pUB110 and pCM194. Subsequent studies demonstrated that the Ø75
genome shared extensive homology with pPL10 (R. Taylor, unpublished).
Thus we tested whether insertion of segments of the genomes of Ø105
and SPO2 into plasmids would render the resulting chimeras
susceptible to transduction by the phage whose DNA was cloned into
the plasmid. The resulting method, called transductional cloning,
allows one to directly select for plasmids containing phage DNA
inserts (6). In practise, phage DNA (e.g., Ø105) is digested with
a chosen restriction endonuclease such as EcoR1, which generates
cohesive termini. A vector plasmid such as pUB110 which specifies
neomycin-resistance (Neo^R) and has a single EcoR1 sensitive site,
is similarly digested and ligated with the phage DNA fragments (7).
The mixture is used to transform a B. subtilis 168 derivative that
is lysogenic for Ø105 [BR151 (Ø105)]. Neo^R transformants are
selected in liquid culture, and the cells are treated with mitomycin
C to induce the Ø105 prophage. The resulting Ø105 lysate is used
to transduce BR151 (Ø105) to Neo^R. Each transductant contains a
pUB110 derivative with a phage DNA insert (6).

     Cloning EcoR1 fragments of SPO2 DNA into pUB110 with selection
by the transductional cloning procedure allowed recovery of only a
single type of chimera designated pPL1010. pPL1010 (4.6 Md)
consists of the 1.6 Md segment of SPO2 DNA corresponding to the
cos region of the phage genome previously identified by Yoneda
et al (8) joined to pUB110 (3 Md).

BIOLOGICAL PROPERTIES OF pPL1010

     pPL1010 is not detectably transduced by Ø105 whereas the plasmid
is transduced by SPO2 at a frequency of 1 transductant per 100 PFU.
This frequency is about 100-fold greater than that of other chimeras
constructed (6) and is presumably the reason for pPL1010 being the
only detected product of cloning EcoR1 SPO2 DNA fragments.
Hybridization of nick translated pUB110 to Southern blots of
undigested DNA from SPO2 (pPL1010) transducing particles subjected
to agarose gel electrophoresis, demonstrated that pPL1010 was carried by the phage in a form whose molecular weight approximated
that of the SPO2 genome (6). Accordingly, pPL1010 was thought to
be carried by transducing particles either as a multimer or as a
recombinant between plasmid and the SPO2 genome. If the plasmid
were carried as a multimer then the transducing activity of SPO2
(pPL1010) lysates should be more resistant to ultraviolet irradiation than if the plasmid were carried as a single copy per phage
particle due to complementation and/or recombination among the
plasmid subunits in the multimer. As shown in Table 1, SPO2
transduction of pPL1010 is more resistant to ultraviolet irradiation
than is inactivation of PFU when the recipient is recombination-
proficient. This apparent resistance to inactivation is lost when

Table 1.   Effect of ultraviolet irradiation on transduction
by SPO2 (pPL1010)

Time of irradiation	PFU	Neo^R Transductants Recipient	
		recE$^+$	recE$^-$
0 min	100%(1.6x10^{8}PFU/ml)	100%(1.6x10^6/ml)	100%(1.4x10^6/ml)
1	60%	98%	30%
2	11%	94%	9%
4	2%	88%	0.9%
5	0.4%	72%	0.4%

the transduction recipient is recombination-deficient (Table 1).

pPL1010 has a buoyant density of 1.699 whereas SPO2 DNA has a
buoyant density of 1.702.   If the plasmid were carried as a multimer,
then the transducing particles should have a reduced buoyant density
relative to SPO2 infectious particles.   In fact, nearly complete
resolution of transducing particles from infectious particles can
be achieved in a CsCl equilibrium gradient (Fig 1).   DNA isolated
from such enriched transducing particles and centrifuged to
equilibrium in CsCl (using an analytical ultracentrifuge) contained
predominately the 1.699 DNA species (pPL1010) and a second species
of 1.702 (SPO2 DNA).   Thus, the plasmid isolated from enriched
transducing particles retained its characteristic buoyant density,
which would not be the case if the plasmid were carried as a
recombinant with the SPO2 genome.

RESTRICTION ENZYME ANALYSIS OF DNA FROM ENRICHED TRANSDUCING
PARTICLES

pPL1010 and SPO2 DNA can be distinguished by their sensitivity
to BamH1 and Sst-1 restriction endonucleases (9).   BamH1 cuts
pPL1010 once but does not cut SPO2 DNA, and Sst-1 digests SPO2 DNA
into seven fragments but does not cut pPL1010.   Hybridization of
nick translated pUB110 to Southern blots of electrophoretically
separated products resulting from Sst-1 digestion of DNA from
enriched transducing particles demonstrated homology only with DNA
migrating at the approximate position of intact SPO2 DNA (9).
Thus, pPL1010 is likely carried as a multimer.   Substituting BamH1
for Sst-1 resulted in an autoradiogram demonstrating that pUB110
hybridized predominently to 4.6, 3.3, and 1.3 Md linear digest
products (9).   These data suggest that pPL1010 is carried by SPO2
as a linear multimer with the 3.3 and 1.3 Md linears representing
the BamH1 ends of the multimer.

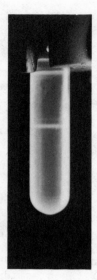

Fig. 1.   An SPO2 (pPL1010) lysate centrifuged to equilibrium in
           CsCl. Upper band contains approximately 10^{10} tranducing
           particles and 10^{10} PFU, while the lower (main) band
           contains approximately 10^{12} PFU and 10^9 transducing
           particles.

DISCUSSION

     The evidence presented indicates that pPL1010 is carried by
SPO2   transducing particles as a linear multimer. A diagram
of the proposed structure of pPL1010 as isolated from SPO2
transducing particles is shown in Figure 2. The number of plasmid
monomers in the multimer (probably seven) is inferred from the
molecular weight of pPL1010 (4.6 Md) and the molecular weight of
the SPO2 genome (approx 31 Md; ref 9).

     Transducing particles carrying a plasmid containing the cohesive
ends of λ DNA harbor the plasmid as a monomeric linear (10). The
ends of the linear contain the cohesive ends of λ. A plausable
explanation for the origin of the multimeric linear form of pPL1010
detected in SPO2 particles requires pPL1010 to replicate according
to the rolling circle model (1). It is not essential that the
normal mode of replication for pPL1010 follow the rolling circle
model; this replication mechanism could be induced by infection of
a cell carrying pPL1010 by SPO2. The product of this mode of
replication is a linear concatamer from which head full pieces,
starting and finishing with <u>cos</u> can be packaged by SPO2. The key
features of the pPL1010 multimer that are consistent with its
origin from such a replication mechanism include the similarity in
molecular weight of the plasmid multimer and the SPO2 genome, the

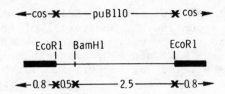

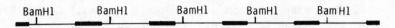

Fig. 2.   Diagram of pPL1010 (opened at the cohesive ends) and
the proposed structure of the multimeric linear carried
by SPO2 transducing particles. The multimer is shown
as a pentamer for diagrammatic purposes only. The
multimer is more likely a heptamer since its molecular
weight approximates that of the SPO2 genome.

organization of the subunits in the multimer in the same polarity,
and the 3.3 and 1.3 Md <u>BamHl</u> generated ends of the multimer which
suggest the ends contain the cohesive ends of SPO2.

ACKNOWLEDGEMENTS

    This investigation was supported by Public Health Service
grant AI-10331 from the National Institute of Allergy and
Infectious Diseases, National Science Foundation grant PCM 78-05755,
and grant VC-296 from the American Cance Society. P.S.L. is
recipient of Public Health Service Research Career Development
Award AI-00119 from the National Institute of Allergy and Infectious
Diseases.

REFERENCES

1. W. Gilbert, and D. Dressler. DNA replication: the rolling
circle model. Cold Spring Harbor Symposium 33: 473 (1968).
2. S.W. Emmons. Bacteriophage lambda derivatives carrying two
copies of the cohesive end site. J. Mol. Biol. 83: 511
(1974).
3. J. Collins and B. Hohn. Cosmids: a type of plasmid gene-clon-
ing vector that is packageable <u>in vitro</u> in bacteriophage λ
heads. Proc. Natl. Acad. Sci. U.S.A. 75: 4242 (1978).
4. H.E. Hemphill and H.R. Whitely. Bacteriophages of <u>Bacillus
subtilis</u>. Bacteriol. Rev. 39: 257 (1975).

5. M.G. Bramucci and P.S. Lovett. Selective plasmid transduction
    in Bacillus pumilus. J. Bacteriol. 131: 1029 (1977).
6. R. Marrero and P.S. Lovett. Transductional selection of cloned
    bacteriophage Ø105 and SPO2 deoxyribonucleic acids in
    Bacillus subtilis. J. Bacteriol. 143: 879 (1980).
7. P.S. Lovett and K.M. Keggins. Bacillus subtilis as a host for
    molecular cloning. Methods Enzymol. 68: 342 (1979).
8. Y. Yoneda, S. Graham and F.E. Young. Restriction-fragment map
    of temperate Bacillus subtilis bacteriophage SPO2. Gene 7:
    51 (1979).
9. R. Marrero, F.A. Chiafari, and P.S. Lovett. SPO2 particles
    mediating transduction of a plasmid containing the SPO2
    cohesive ends. J. Bacteriol in press.
10. H.J. Vollenweider, M. Fiandt, E.C. Rosenvold, and W. Szybalski.
    Packaging of plasmid DNA containing the cohesive ends of
    coliphage lambda. Gene 9: 171 (1980).

A MUTATIONAL AND TRANSCRIPTIONAL ANALYSIS OF A TUMOR INDUCING

PLASMID OF AGROBACTERIUM TUMEFACIENS

E.W. Nester, D.J. Garfinkel, S.B. Gelvin, A.L. Montoya
and M.P. Gordon*
Departments of Microbiology and Immunology and
Biochemistry*
University of Washington
Seattle, Washington   98195

INTRODUCTION

The large tumor inducing (Ti) plasmids (Zaenen et al., 1974) of Agrobacterium tumefaciens are the causitive agents of gall tumors on dicotylendonous plants. The plant cell transformation is brought about by the stable integration of a portion of the bacterial Ti-plasmid into plant nuclear DNA (Chilton et al., 1978a; Thomashow et al., 1980a; Thomashow et al., 1980b; Lemmers et al., 1981; Chilton et al., 1980; Yadav et al., 1980). Transformed plant cells are characterized by the following properties: the ability to grow in azenic culture without an exogenous supply of the plant hormones auxin and cytokinin (Braun, 1958) and the synthesis of unusual amino acids called opines (Petit et al., 1968; Menage and Morel, 1964; Goldman et al., 1968; Goldman et al., 1969; Fermin and Fenwick, 1978). The transferred plasmid DNA (T-DNA) is transcribed, (Drummond et al., 1978; Yang et al., 1979; Gelvin et al., 1981; Ledeboer, 1978; Gurley et al., 1979) influences the levels of plant hormones, and directs the synthesis opines (Bomhoff et al., 1976; Montoya et al., 1977; Kemp et al., 1979; Hack and Kemp, 1980; Guyon et al., 1980) in transformed plant cells. Thus, crown gall tumorigenesis is a model system for the study of the mechanism by which a bacterial plasmid transforms a eukaryotic cell causing a neoplastic disease.

While the T-DNA plays an essential role in crown gall induction and maintenance, it only comprises 8-20% of the Ti-plasmid. Koekman and coworkers (1979) found that only 40% of the Ti-plasmid could be deleted before the bacteria could no longer produce tumors. Thus, other areas of the plasmid must encode functions necessary for tumor formation. Avirulent mutants have been generated by insertion of the transposons Tn7 (Hernalsteens et al., 1978) and Tn904 or Tn1821 (Ooms et al., 1980) into the Ti-plasmid of Agrobacterium tumefaciens. These studies were only concerned with Ti-plasmid borne insertions, while gene products necessary for tumorigenesis might be encoded by the chromosome or by other plasmids present in some virulent strains. In this study we have utilized the transposon Tn5 to mutagenize the entire bacterial genome. We then selected mutants with altered virulence, host range and ability to catabolize opines; properties known to be coded by the plasmid (Bomhoff et al., 1976; Montoya et al., 1977; Guyon et al., 1980; Thomashow et al., 1980c). We have mapped these insertions to specific restriction fragments of the Ti-plasmid or to the chromosome. In addition we have also investigated the transcription of the Ti-plasmid during different growth regima and will correlate the information from the transcriptional studies with the mutant data.

RESULTS AND DISCUSSION

Isolation and Mapping of Transposon Induced Mutants. Berg (1973) has shown that mutations due to Tn5 insertion result from direct gene inactivation or polarity effects and usually result in complete loss of gene function. We used the vehicle pJB4J1 to deliver the Tn5 transposon to Agrobacterium. This plasmid has been shown to be unstable in Rhizobium (Beringer et al., 1978) and Agrobacterium (Garfinkel and Nester, 1980). The kanamycin resistant gentamycin sensitive transconjugants represent Tn5 transpositions into the Ti-plasmid, the chromosome or other cryptic plasmids. Insertions into loci that code for functions necessary for tumor induction or maintenance will yield strains that are avirulent. We screened 8,900 kanamycin resistant transconjugants for virulence by inoculating wounds on leaves of Kalanchoe diagremontiana and 40 mutants were identified with altered virulence properties. All transconjugants were also screened for the utilization of octopine as a sole source of nitrogen on bromthymol blue indicator plates (Hooykaas et al., 1979). Seven mutants were isolated which failed to utilize octopine.

Ti-plasmid was isolated from the 40 avirulent and 7 octopine non-utilizing mutnats. These preparations were cleaved with the restriction endonucleases KpnI, HpaI, and SmaI and subjected to electrophoresis on 0.7% horizontal agarose slab gels. The gels were then stained with ethidium bromide, visualized with a short wavelength ultra violet light, and photographed. The restriction endonuclease KpnI does not cut the Tn5 transposon, while SmaI cuts it once near the center and HpaI cuts it twice in the inverted repeats approximately 0.2 Md from the end of the transposon. Therefore, in KpnI digests of the plasmid the fragment in which the transposon is located will increase in molecular weight by 3.5 Md, the size of Tn5, and will exhibit an altered mobility upon electro-

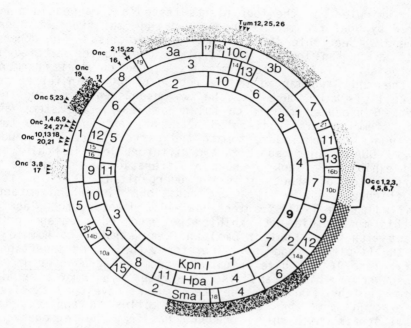

Fig. 1.   Restriction endonuclease map of the pTiB$_6$806 plasmid
(Chilton et al., 1978b; Ooms et al., 1980) showing locations of Tn5 transposition insertions and regions of transcription in the bacterium. ▨▨▨ Regions showing low
levels of homologous transcripts. ▨▨▨ Regions showing
high levels of homologous transcripts. ▨▨▨ Regions showing homologous transcripts inducible by octopine.▨▨▨
Regions showing homologous transcripts inducible by agropine.   Onc - mutants with altered virulence properties.
Tum - mutants which give rise to tumors with altered morphologies.   Occ - mutants which are unable to catabolize
octopine.

phoresis.   In SmaI digest the original fragment in which Tn5 has
transposed will disappear and two new fragments will appear.   Three
new fragments will appear in the HpaI digest.   Any ambiguities presented by multiple fragments of similar molecular weights in any
one digest can be resolved in this way and the Tn5 insertions can
be located on the map of the octopine plasmid established by
Chilton et al. (1978b) and extended by Ooms et al. (1980) (see
Figure 1).

Twenty-five of the 40 mutants affected in virulence had Tn5
located on the Ti-plasmid.   Twenty-one of these mutants were com-

pletely avirulent on the four plants tested and mapped in a region bordered by HpaI fragment 9 on one end and SmaI fragment 8 on the other end. (See Table 2 and Figure 1 for details.) The other four mutants which had Tn5 on the Ti-plasmid exhibited altered tumor morphologies. Two of these mutants mapped on HpaI fragment 6, while the other two mapped in the region of DNA transferred to the plant cell (T-DNA)(Figure 1). The two mutants which mapped in HpaI fragment 6 produced tumors on Kalanchöe leaves and stems and on tobacco stems which proliferated abundant roots from the tumors, while tumors on sunflower, tomato and carrot slices were normal. The two T-DNA mutants mapped in two different loci in HpaI fragment 14 and exhibited a lack of root proliferation on Kalanchoe stems and production of shoots from the unorganized callus on tobacco stems (Figure 1, Table 1). One additional insertion mutant was identified on the T-DNA fragment HpaI-14. However, the plasmid DNA from this mutant did not exhibit the expected cleavage patterns when cut with HpaI, KpnI or SmaI and demonstrated no homology between the Ti-plasmid and Tn5. Therefore, the 1.0 Md insertion into HpaI fragment 14 may have originated from an <u>Agrobacterium</u> insertion sequence. This mutant also gave rise to a tumor with altered tumor morphology. On Kalanchöe stems tumors developed massive root proliferation from the center of the callus in contrast to the parental strain which only produced roots from the periphery of the callus. In addition tumors produced on carrot slices and tobacco stems also developed a proliferation root from the callus, while the parental strain exhibited no root proliferation. All of the plasmids which gave rise to tumors with altered morphologies were transformed into a plasmidless strain. The transformants retained all of the characteristics of the original mutant.

Twelve of the avirulent mutants did not map on the Ti-plasmid when these plasmids were transformed into a plasmidless strain selecting for octopine catabolism, all twelve preparations gave transformants which were kanamycin sensitive and virulent. These data confirm that the Tn5 was not located on the plasmid. Plasmid DNA preparations were made from these strains by the procedure of Casse et al. (1978) and were then subjected to electrophoresis on 0.7% vertical agarose gels. Under these conditions the Ti-plasmid, cryptic plasmid and chromosomsal DNAs migrate to different locations in the gel. The DNAs were then transferred to nitrocellulose by the procedure of Southern (1975). The nitrocellulose transfers were then hybridized with a radiolabeled Tn5 probe, washed and autoradiographed. The resulting autoradiograph demonstrated homolgoy between the Tn5 probe and only the linear chromosomal DNA. No homology was detected to the cryptic or Ti-plasmids, even after extended periods of time for exposure of the autoradiograph. Thus, the insertions in these twelve strains must be in chromosomal genes that encode virulence functions. Seven of these mutants which were avirulent on Kalanchöe were virulent on sunflower, with two of the seven also being virulent on tomato. The other five chromosoaml

Table 1. Virulence of Agrobacterium tumefaciens strains harboring mutated Ti-plasmids

Strain	Position of insertion			Virulence						Octopine[a] production
	HpaI	KpnI	SmaI	Klanchoe Stems	Klanchoe Leaves	Carrot	Sun-flower	Tomato	Tobacco	
Controls										
A114	-	-	-	-[a]	-	-	-	-	-	Negative
A722	-	-	-	+[b]	+[c]	+[c]	+[c]	+[c]	+[c]	Positive
A723	-	-	-	+[b]	+[c]	+[c]	+[c]	+[c]	+[c]	Positive
A6NC	-	-	-	+	+[c]	+[c]	+[c]	+[c]	+[c]	Positive
Avirulent										
onc-3,8,17	9	11	1	-	-	-	-	-	NT	NT
onc-14	16	5	1	-	-	-	-	-	NT	NT
onc-10,13,18,20,21	15	5	1	-	-	-	-	-	NT	NT
onc-1,4,6,9,14,27	12	5	1	-	-	-	-	-	NT	NT
onc-5,23	6	5	1	-	-	-	-	-	NT	NT
onc-11	6	5	8	-	-	-	-	-	NT	NT
onc-2,15	3	2	8	-	-	-	-	-	NT	NT
onc-28	ND	ND	ND	-	-	-	-	-	NT	NT
onc-29	ND	ND	ND	-	-	-	-	-	NT	NT
Tumor morphology										
onc-16	6	2	8	+[e]	+[f]	+[c]	+[c]	+/-[h]	+[e]	Positive
onc-19	6	5	1	+[e]	+[f]	+[c]	+[c]	+/-	+[e]	Positive[j]
tum-12	14	10	10c	+[g]	+[g]	+/-[f]	+[c]	+/-	+[i]	Positive[j]
tum-25	14	10	10c	+[f]	-	+	+[c]	+/-	+[f]	Positive
tum-26	14	10	10c	+	+	+/-	+/-	+/-	+	Positive[j]

a Avirulent. b Unorganized callus overgrowth with roots proliferating from the callus periphery. c Unorganized callus overgrowth. d NT, not tested; ND, not determined. e Abnormal callus with roots proliferating from the entire callus. f Unorganized callus with roots proliferating from the callus overgrowth. g Necrotic callus overgrowth. h Unorganized callus overgrowth. i Unorganized callus with shoots proliferating from the entire callus. j Unorganized callus produced octopine, but shoots did not produce detectable levels of octopine.

mutants were avirulent on all plants tested. The parental strains
are virulent on the plants tested. Therefore we can conclude that
some chromosomal mutations may influence the host range of the bacterium.

Two additional mutants were isolated which were avirulent on
all plants tested. The restriction endonuclease patterns of these
plasmids appeared identical to the parental plasmid and the Tn5
probe hybridized to the linear DNA. Thus, the Tn5 insertion in
these strains is in the chromosome. However, when these plasmids
were transformed into a plasmidless strain selecting for octopine
catabolism the resulting transformants retained the avirulent characteristics of the mutant and were kanomycin sensitive. Thus,
there must be an alteration in the plasmid that cannot be detected
at the level of restriction endonuclease digestion pattern.

Seven mutants were isolated that could not utilize octopine as
a sole source of nitrogen. These Tn5 insertions were located in
HapI fragment 7 and KpnI fragment 4. This map position is consis-
tant with the location of the octopine catabolism genes which had
previously been roughly mapped by deletion mutants (Koekman et al.,
1979). These octopine non-utilizing mutants were plated on minimal
media with octopine a the sole carbon and nitrogen source.
Octopine-utilizing revertants arose at a frequency of 5×10^{-8}.
The revertants were kanomycin sensitive, indicating that the Tn5
excision repaired the gene function and that Tn5 was lost from the
cell. All of the octopine non-utilizing mutants were virulent on
all plants tested.

Transcriptional analysis of the Ti-plasmid. In order to gain
some insight into the pattern of gene expression of the Ti-plasmid,
the bacteria were analyzed for transcripts originating from various
regions of the Ti-plasmid. When the steady state population of
RNAs were examined by production of ^{32}P-labeled complementary
DNA and subsequent hybridization to nitrocellulose transfers of the
Ti-plasmid two areas are delineated which have abundant RNA populations present in cells grown both in minimal and rich medium. The
larger area extends from HpaI fragment 4 to SmaI fragment 6. To
date no genetic loci have been mapped in this region. The other
area homologous to abundant messanger RNAs is located within SmaI
fragment 1 and HpaI fragment 6. Garfinkel and Nester (1980) have
located insertion mutants within this region which are avirulent or
demonstrate an altered tumor morphology, suggesting that these
transcripts may have a function in the process of tumorigenicity.
Lower levels of RNAs were reproducibly detected that were homologous to three other regions of the Ti-plasmid. The first region is
SmaI fragment 11, to which no genetic loci have been mapped. The
second region is KpnI fragment 11 and HpaI fragment 9. Garfinkel
and Nester (1980) have isolated avirulent mutants which map in this
fragment. The final region of homology to low levels of RNAs ex-

tends from SmaI fragment 3a to SmaI fragment 3b. This region encompasses the DNA that is transferred to the plant upon initiation of a tumor and is found to be transcribed in the plant tumor. Insertion mutants within this region have given rise to tumors with altered morphologies (Ooms et al., 1980; Garfinkel and Nester, 1980). Additional studies are being carried out and it will be very interesting to see if the messenger RNA transcripts found in the bacterium are the same as those found in the tumor.

Klapwijk and Schilperoort (1979) have shown that three and possibly four genes are concerned with the conversion of octopine to pyruvic acid and arginine. Two other operons also appear to be under the coordinate control of octopine. These are the degradation of arginine for utilization as a carbon source (Ellis et al., 1979) and the transfer of the Ti-plasmid to other strains by conjugation (Klapwijk et al., 1978; Petit and Tempe, 1978). Thus, one would expect to see a difference in the messenger RNA populations isolated from cells grown on minimal medium in the presence and absence of octopine. Gelvin et al. (1981) have shown that the region from SmaI fragment 13 to SmaI fragment 10b is heavily transcribed both in cells grown in the presence of octopine and in constitutive octopine utilizing strains while this region has very low levels of transcription when the bacteria are grown in minimal media without octopine (Figure 1). This data also indirectly confirms the map position of the genes concerned with octopine degradation as mapped by deletion mutants (Koekman et al., 1979) and transposition insertions (Garfinkel and Nester, 1980).

Fermin and Fenwick (1978) have shown that octopine utilizing strains can also catabolize another tumor specific metabolite called agropine. Tempe and co-workers (1980) have suggested that this inducible degradation involves at least three genes. The first is a permease which permits agropine to be taken up by the cell and the other two would degrade the agropine by first opening the cyclic structure and then cleaving the noncyclic compound to metabolites that could be used as a carbon source by the bacteria. Thus, one would expect to detect the transcription of such an operon when the messenger RNA populations of induced and noninduced bacteria are compared. Gelvin and co-workers (1981) have shown that ^{32}P-labeled complementary DNA made to RNA isolated from agropine induced bacteria hybridized to a region extending from SmaI fragment 9 to SmaI fragment 14a (Figure 1). This area of the plasmid showed no detectable level of transcription in cells grown in the absence of agropine. Thus the genes concerned with agropine degradation most likely map within the region encompassed by SmaI fragments 9 and 14a and KpnI fragments 7 and 9.

Very low levels of transcripts were occasionally detected in the remaining areas of the plasmid. Thus, we cannot exclude the possibility that all regions of the plasmid are transcribed. Identification of messages and fine structure mapping would be required before silent regions of the plasmid might be identified. Identification of transcripts from regions where genetic loci have not yet been identified suggest that there is a great deal to be established before we have characterized the Ti-plasmid and understand the mechanisms of tumor induction and maintenance.

REFERENCES

Berg, D.E. 1977. Insertion and excision of the transposable kanamycin resistance determinant Tn5 p205-212 in DNA insertion elements, plasmids and episomes. A.I. Bukari, J.A. Shapiro, and S.L. Adhya (ed.) Cold Spring Harbor Laboratory, Cold Spring Harbor, N.Y.

Beringer, J.E., J.L. Beynon, A.V. Buchanan-Wolaston, and A.W.B. Johnson. 1978. Transfer of the drug-resistance transposon Tn5 to Rhizobium. Nature (London) 276: 633.

Bomhoff, G.H., P.M. Klapwijk, H.C.M. Kester, R.A. Schilperoort, J.P. Hernalsteens, and J. Schell. 1976. Octopine and nopaline synthesis and breakdown is genetically controlled by a plasmid of Agrobacterium tumefaciens. Mol. Gen. Genet. 145: 177.

Braun, A.C. 1958. A physiological basis for autonomous growth of the crown gall tumor cells. Proc. Natl. Acad. Sci. USA 44: 344.

Casse, F., C. Boucher, J.S. Jullito, M. Michal, and J. Denarie. 1978. Identification and characterization of large Plasmids in Rhizobium meliloti using gel electrophoresis. J. Gen. Microbiol. 13: 229.

Chilton, M.-D., M.H. Drummond, D.J. Merlo, D. Sciaky, A.L. Montoya, M.P. Gordon and E.W. Nester. 1978a. Stable incorporation of plasmid DNA into higher plant cells: the molecular basis for crown gall tumorigenesis. Cell 11: 263.

Chilton, M.-D., A.L. Montoya, D.J. Merlo, M.H. Drummond, R. Nutter, M.P. Gordon, and E.W. Nester. 1970b. Restriction endonuclease mapping of a plasmid that confers oncogenicity upon Agrobacterium tumefaciens strain B6-806. Plasmid 1: 254.

Chilton, M.-D., R. Saiki, N. Yadav, M.P. Gordon, and F. Quertier. 1980. T-DNA from Agrobacterium Ti-plasmid is in nuclear DNA fraction of crown gall tumor cells. Proc. Natl. Acad. Sci. USA 77: 4060.

Drummond, M.H., M.P. Grodon, E.W. Nester and M.-D. Chilton. 1977. Foreign DNA of bacterial plasmid origin is transcribed in crown gall tumors. Nature (London) 269: 535.

Ellis, J.G., A. Kerr, J. Tempe, and A. Petit. 1979. Arginine catabolism: a new function of both octopine and nopaline Ti-plasmids of Agrobacterium. Mol. Gen. Genet. 173: 263.

Firmin, J.L. an G.R. Fenwick. 1978. Agropine - a major new plasmid-determined metabolite in crown gall tumors. Nature (London) 276: 842.

Garfinkel, D.J. and E.W. Nester. 1980. Agrobacterium tumefaciens mutants affected in crown gall tumorigenesis and octopine catabolism. J. Bacteriol. 144: 732.

Gelvin, S.B., M.P. Gordon, E.W. Nester, and A.I. Aronson. 1981. transcription of Agrobacterium Ti-plasmid in the bacterium and crown gall tumors. Plasmid in press.

Goldman, A., J. Tempe, and G. Morel. 1968. Quelques particu- larites de diverses souches d'Agrobacterium tumefaciens. Comp. Rend. Acad. Sci. (Paris) 162: 630.

Goldman, A., D.W. Thomas, and G. Morel. 1969. Sur la structure de la nopaline metabolite abnormal de certaines tumeurs de crown gall. Comp. Rend. Acad. Sci. (Paris) 268: 852.

Gurley, W.B., J.D. Kemp, M.J. Albert, D.W. Sutton and J. Callis. 1979. Transcription of Ti-plasmid derived sequences in three octopine type crown gall tumor lines. Proc. Natl. Acad. Sci. USA 76: 2828.

Guyon, P., M.-D. Chilton, A. Petit, and J. Tempe. 1980. Agropine in "null-type" crown gall tumors: evidence for generality of the opine concept. Proc. Natl. Acad. Sci. USA 77: 2693.

Hack, E. and J.D. Kemp. 1908. Purification and characterization of the crown gall-specific enzyme, octopine synthase. Plant Physiol. 65: 949.

Hernalsteens, J.P., H. DeGreve, M. VanMontagu, and J. Schell. 1978. Mutagenesis by insertion of the drug resistance trans- poson Tn7 applied to the Ti-plasmid of Agrobacterium tume- faciens. Plasmid 1: 218.

Hooykaas, P.J.J., C. Roobol, and R.A. Schilperoort. 1979. Regula- tion of the transfer of Ti-plasmids of Agrobacterium tume- faciens. J. Gen. Microbiol. 110: 99.

Kemp, J.D., D.W. Sutton, and E. Hack. 1979. Purification and characterization of the crown gall specific enzyme nopaline synthase. Biochemistry 8: 3755.

Klapwijk, P.M., J. Scheuldermon, and R.A. Schilperoort. 1978. Coordinate regulation of octopine degradation and conjugative transfer of Ti-plasmids in Agrobacterium tumefaciens: evi- dence for a common regulator gene. J. Bacteriol. 136: 775.

Klapwijk, P.M. and R.A. Schilperoort. 1979. Negative control of octopine degradation and transfer genes of octopine Ti-plas- mids in Agrobacterium tumefaciens. J. Bacteriol. 139: 424.

Koekman, B.P., G. Ooms, P.M. Klapwijk, and R.A. Schilperoort. 1979. Genetic map of an octopine Ti-plasmid. Plasmid 2: 347.

Ledeboer, A.M. 1978. Large plasmids in Rhizobiaceae. I. Studies on the transcription of the tumor inducing plasmid from Agro- bacterium tumefaciens in sterile crown gall tumor cells. II. Studies on large plasmids in different Rhizobium species. Thesis, University of Leiden, The Netherlands.

Lemmers, M., M. De Beuckleer, M. Holsters, P. Zambryski, A. Depicker, J.P. Hernalsteens, M. Van Montagu and J. Schell. 1980. Internal organization, boundaries and integration of Ti-plasmid DNA in nopaline crown gall tumors. J. Mol. Biol. 144: 355.

Menage, A. and G. Morel. 1964. Sur la presence d'octopine dans les tissus de crown gall. Comp. Rend. Acad. Sci. 259: 4795.

Montoya, A.L., M.-D. Chilton, M.P. Gordon, D. Sciaky, and E.W. Nester. 1977. Octopine and nopaline metabolism in Agrobacterium tumefaciens and crown gall cells: role of plasmid genes. J. Bacteriol. 129: 101.

Ooms, G., P.M. Klapwijk, J.A. Poulis, and R.A. Schilperoort. 1980. Characterization of Tn904 Insertions in octopine Ti-plasmid mutants of Agrobacterium tumefaciens. J. Baceriol. 144: 82.

Petit, A., S. Delhaye, J. Tempe, and G. Morel. 1970. Recherches sur les guanidines des tissus de crown gall. Mise en evidence d'une relation biochemique specifique entre les souches d' Agrobacterium tumefaciens et les tumeurs qu'elles induisent. Physiol. Veg. 8: 205.

Petit, A. and J. Tempe. 1978. Isolation of Agrobacterium Ti-plasmid regulatory mutants. Mol. Gen. Genet. 167: 147.

Southern, E.M. 1975. Detection of specific sequences among DNA fragments separated by gel electrophoresis. J. Mol. Biol. 98: 503.

Tempe, J., P. Guyon, A. Petit, J.G. Ellis, M.E. Tate, and A. Kerr. 1980. Preparation et propertietes de nouveaux substrats catabolique pourdeux types de plasmides oncogenes d' Agrobacterium tumefaciens. Comp. Rend. Acad. Sci. Paris 290: 1173.

Thomashow, M.F., R. Nutter, A.L. Montoya, M.P. Gordon and E.W. Nester. 1980a. Integration and organization of Ti-plasmid sequences in crown gall tumors. Cell 19: 729.

Thomashow, M.F., R.C. Nutter, K. Postle, M.-D. Chilton, F.R. Blattner, A. Powell, M.P. Gordon, and E.W. Nester. 1980b. Recombination between higher plant DNA and the Ti-plasmid of Agrobacterium tumefaciens. Proc. Natl. Acad. Sci. USA 77: 6448.

Thomashow, M.F., C.G. Panagopoulos, M.P. Gordon, and E.W. Nester. 1980c. Host range of Agrobacterium tumefaciens is determined by the Ti-plasmid. Nature (London) 283: 794.

Yadav, N.S., K. Postle, R.K. Saiki, M.F. Thomashow, and M.-D. Chilton. 1980. T-DNA of a crown gall teratoma is covalently joined to host plant DNA. Nature (London) 287: 458.

Yang, F.-M., J.C. McPherson, M.P. Gordon, and E.W. Nester. 1980. Extensive transcription of foreign DNA in a crown gall teratoma. Biochem. Biophys. Res. Commun. 92: 1273.

Zaenen, I., N. Van Larebeke, H. Teuchy, M. Van Montagu, and J. Schell. 1974. Supercoiled circular DNA in crown gall inducing Agrobacterium strains. J. Mol. Biol. 86: 109.

TRANSFER, MAINTENANCE AND EXPRESSION OF GENES INTRODUCED INTO PLANT CELLS VIA THE TI PLASMID

M. Van Montagu[*+], J. Schell[o*], M. Holsters[*],
H. De Greve[+], J. Leemans[+], J.P. Hernalsteens[+],
L. Willmitzer[o], and L. Otten[o]

[*]Laboratory of Genetics, Rijksuniversiteit Gent, Belgium
[+]Laboratory GEVI, Vrije Universiteit Brussel, Belgium
[o]Max-Planck-Institut für Züchtungsforschung, Köln, FRG

K.L. Ledeganckstraat 35, B-9000 Gent (Belgium)

INTRODUCTION

The capacity of a microorganism to establish itself successfully in a particular ecological niche often seems to depend upon
the activities of a very small number of genes that are absent in
competing species. This additional DNA is frequently part of a
plasmid that allows its host to metabolize rarely exploited
carbon or nitrogen sources. Because of the presence of such
genes, these plasmids have been called degradative or catabolic
plasmids[1]. We believe that the Ti plasmids of Agrobacterium
tumefaciens form a special class of catabolic plasmids[2,3]. In
addition to encoding for proteins that catabolize several common
amino acids[4,5] and some polyphenols[5], these plasmids also carry
genes whose products catabolize compounds calles opines. Opines
are unusual amino acids, such as nopaline[6], octopine[6] or agropine[7] and phosphorylated sugars, such as the agrocinopines[8].
These opines have only been found in plant cells transformed by
Ti plasmids into crown gall tumor cells. By inducing crown gall
tumors, Agrobacterium tumefaciens forces a plant to synthesize
compounds which only the same virulent strains can use.

The Ti plasmids isolated from different strains can be
grouped into three major classes named after a characteristic
opine produced in the tumor cells. Consequently, these plasmids
are called nopaline, octopine or agropine Ti plasmids[9]. Agropine

is also synthesized in the hairy root tissue, a tumor induced by Agrobacterium rhizogenes[10]. The plasmids from the hairy root strains however, show only limited homology with the A. tumefaciens plasmids[11].

Upon tumor induction, a segment of the Ti plasmid becomes stably integrated in the plant chromosomes. This segment, called the T-DNA, encodes for the functions responsible for the biosynthesis of the opines and for the maintenance of the transformed phenotype of the tumor cells. The extent of the T-DNA has been determined by Southern blot analysis. The T-DNA of the nopaline plasmids was found reproducibly to be 23 Kb[12,13,14]. The octopine T-DNA, in contrast, was about 15 Kb long, although the extent of the right border of this T-DNA varied significantly in some cases[15,16]. Genomic cloning of crown gall DNA allowed the identification of the T-DNA border sequences and proved that this DNA was inserted into plant DNA[17,18]. The sum of available evidence suggests that the "ends" of the T-DNA are involved in the integration event. The exact number of T-DNA copies varied from tissue to tissue and in some tumors was five or more. Some of these copies were arranged as interspersed tandem repeats[17]. This amplification may have occurred after the initial integration event as a result of unequal crossing over between flanking sequences. The latter, indeed, were in all cases investigated, repetitive DNA. In simple terms, Agrobacterium changes its environment by selective gene transfer to plants. Perhaps feats of genetic engineering are not as infrequent as commonly thought.

The physical organization of both the octopine[19,20,21] and nopaline[21] plasmids has been established. This has allowed the construction of a genetic and functional map of these plasmids. Mutations have been isolated by transposon insertion mutagenesis [23,24,19,18] and by deletion formation[23,25].

The most important conclusion from this work was that the non-T-DNA part of the Ti plasmid contains extensive regions essential for tumor induction. These oncogenic (Onc) regions seem to be conserved among nopaline and octopine plasmids[26]. Some of the DNA segments possibly may encode for functions essential for the transfer of the T-DNA into the plant nucleus. Others might interfere with the balance of growth factors (plant hormones) of the infected tissue and therefore be essential to the initial stimulation of cell proliferation. We have indeed shown that exogenous auxin can restore the tumor-inducing capacity of some mutant strains, while exogenous cytokinins inhibit tumor formation[5].

A second conclusion was that no unconditional ONC⁻ mutations in the T-DNA were found which were not the result of extensive deletions. Small deletions or insertions have allowed identification of T-DNA regions responsible for opine synthesis and host specificity. Mutations in the latter regions permit tumors to form on some plant species (e.g. Kalanchoë) but not on others (e.g. tobacco). Remarkably, large portions of the T-DNA can be disrupted by insertion sequences or deletions without visibly affecting tumor formation or opine production. Recent efforts have concentrated on making a more detailed analysis of this area.

RESULTS

The transposon insertion mutagenesis of Ti plasmids allowed a rudimentary localization of some relevant loci[23,24]. Due to their rather high site or regional specificity, transposons cannot be expected to integrate in all the genes of the T-DNA. For this reason, we have begun an extensive program of site specific mutagenesis of cloned segments of the T-DNA.

Construction of a mutant Ti plasmid by in vitro mutagenesis of cloned T-DNA fragments

In an initial phase, well-defined insertions and deletions were constructed in cloned T-DNA fragments using identified restriction sites as endpoints. The alterations were then introduced in the corresponding Ti plasmid by in vivo recombination. To accomplish this, a cloning vector containing the mutated T-DNA fragment was transmitted from an E. coli host into an Agrobacterium harboring a transfer constitutive Ti plasmid. Two consecutive conjugations, the first one followed by selection for markers of the cloning vector and the second one followed by screening or selection for the loss of these markers, readily allowed the isolation of the required mutant Ti plasmid. The first conjugation gives rise to cells in which the vector plasmid has been inserted in the Ti plasmid by a single cross-over between the cloned T-DNA segment and the corresponding segment in the Ti plasmid. This event is easily selected since it occurs with a frequency between 10^{-3} and 10^{-6}, depending on the length of the fragments involved (respectively 16 Kb and 2 Kb). The resulting plasmids carrying a segment in duplicate are relatively unstable since the inserted vector DNA can be lost upon cross-over in the manipulated T-DNA segment. We found that this occurs with a frequency of 1 to 0.01 %, depending upon the length of the fragments (respectively 8 and 1 Kb). The second conjugation produces strains harboring the desired Ti plasmid recombinant. The definitive proof of the structure of the isolated plasmid is obtained by Southern blot analysis of digests of the total bac-

terial DNA, using a cloned segment of the mutated T-DNA as probe
[27].

In a first set of experiments, DNA segments isolated from
the antibiotic resistance determinants of R factors were introduced either as a simple insertion in a restriction site or as a
substitution insertion, replacing a restriction fragment. Once
this type of mutant Ti plasmid was obtained it could be used for
subsequent exchanges. When this exchange employed a T-DNA fragment containing an insert of a cloned eukaryotic gene, a Ti-plasmid was obtained which could transfer the new gene into plants.

Similarly, a well-defined T-DNA mutation could be introduced
by exchanging the insert for a homologous Ti fragment harboring a
deletion spanning the site of the insert. By using two cloned
fragments derived from the borders of the T-DNA, or from outside
the T-DNA, it is possible to construct Ti plasmids which lack
most or all of the T-DNA.

Construction of mutated Ti plasmids using in vivo mutagenesis of cloned T-DNA fragments

In vivo mutagenesis is basically analogous to the in vitro
technique, instead of using recombinant DNA technology to constructing an insertion, this second procedure inserts a copy of a
movable element into the cloned T-DNA fragment when the T-DNA
fragment is mobilized from one bacterium to another[28]. One practical advantage of the in vivo method is that many independent
insertions can be isolated through a single replica conjugation.
Following mutagenesis, the mutated T-DNA fragment is recombined
into the Ti plasmid by double cross-over, following the procedure
described in the previous section. Through this in vivo approach
to mutagenesis, Tn1 has been inserted into several different
sites in the T-DNA. As was previously demonstrated for the 15 Kb
long Tn7[29], the transposon can be co-transferred to a plant
without any apparent rearrangements as part of the T-DNA[29]. This
proves that the T-DNA can serve as a vector to introduce foreign
genes into plants.

Stability of the inserted T-DNA

The crown gall tissues induced by nopaline Ti-plasmids have
a tendency to redifferentiate into shoots. For this reason, this
kind of tumor is called teratoma tissue. These shoots can be
grafted to new plants where they grown into reasonably well
developed tobacco plants. Southern blot analysis has shown that
the T-DNA was conserved in the different tissues of the regenerated plants[14,30]. In marked contrast, in those rare cases where
fertile flowers formed, T-DNA was absent both from cultures

derived from anthers and from the F_1 generation.

This loss of the T-DNA after meiosis could seriously limit the use of the T-DNA as a cloning vector in plants. Studies of various mutants of the T-DNA have indicated a particularly attractive method of overcoming this difficulty. Some mutated T-DNAs induce tumors that proliferate into either roots or shoots. Frequently, these shoots do not contain any opines and in this way resemble shoots formed from some "genetic tumors". At the same time, shoots do arise which produce opines and therefore presumably contain intact portions of T-DNA. Therefore, by inserting foreign DNA into a suitable site, it should be possible to mutagenize the T-DNA in such a way as to ensure that the foreign DNA will become part of a new plant. One such example is particularly noteworthy. In this case, Tn7 was inserted into the EcoRI-32 fragment of the T-DNA of an octopine plasmid (pGV2100) [24]. The tumors of this mutant, unlike normal octopine tumors, gave rise to shoots which are able to form roots. Intact plantlets could be separated from this mass that grew well in isolation and were found to contain octopine. One shoot is particular developed into a fully grown, flowering plant. Both the pollen and ova of this tobacco plant were fertile and, after selfing, provided seeds for further analysis. These seeds germinated into normal-looking plants of which 75% contained octopine and 25% did not. In addition to this 3:1 segregation, we found the progeny of a cross between the regenerated plant and a wild type plant segregated 1:1. Finally, 50% of the haploid plantlets obtained from anther cultures derived from the mother plant contained octopine and 50% did not. The results indicate that the T-DNA segregates as a Mendelian trait and consequently, that the T-DNA is present as a single locus on one of the chromosomes.

Expression of the T-DNA

Several transcription studies of the T-DNA[32,33,34] have been published. Our results with both the octopine and the nopaline plasmids indicate that all of the T-DNA is transcribed but that some segments, particularly those situated at the ends of the T-DNA, are transcribed most actively[35,36]. Roughly, the same pattern was found when T-DNA was hybridized to nuclear or polysomal RNA. Interestingly, different regions of the T-DNA were transcribed in stationary phase tumor cells than in actively dividing ones. This may be the first evidence that some genes of the T-DNA are transcriptionally regulated in the plant host. In plants the transcription the T-DNA sequences is completely inhibited by 0.7 µg/ml α-amanitin as if it was dependent upon RNA polymerase II[36].

As expected from genetic studies[23,24], portions of the

Ti plasmid are transcribed in <u>Agrobacterium</u>. This was shown by
hybridizing total, <u>in</u> <u>vivo</u>-labelled RNA, isolated from bacteria,
to restriction fragments covering the whole Ti plasmid. The
portions of the plasmid coding for proteins which catabolize
opines are preferentially transcribed. On the other hand, the
T-DNA is expressed only very weakly. From these results, it
would appear that the Ti plasmid is organized into discrete
blocks of prokaryotic and eukaryotic genes.

Expression of a prokaryotic gene in a plant

One of the more important questions that must be answered
before the Ti plasmid is used to produce new kinds of plants, is
whether the DNA of one species is readily expressed in the cells
of another. With this in mind, several experiments were performed to determine whether the bacterial DNA of Tn<u>7</u> is expressed in
a eukaryotic host. In these experiments, RNA was extracted from
tumors induced by a Ti plasmid with Tn<u>7</u> inserted in the right
border of the T-DNA, in the nopaline synthase locus. Nuclear
transcripts were found which correspond to the entire Tn<u>7</u> genome
[29]. At least some of these transcripts were found also in the
polyA fraction of the polysomal RNA. Significantly, Tn<u>7</u> transcripts in polysomes lacked detectable poly A sequences. This may
indicate that the RNAs terminate within Tn<u>7</u>, perhaps at prokaryotic termination sequences, and not at the end of an adjacent
gene. Although it is still not certain that any Tn<u>7</u> gene is
translated in plants, these results indicate that plant enzymes
may be able to produce some messenger-like RNAs from foreign
genes, transport them out of the nucleus, and incorporate these
molecules into polysomes.

CONCLUSION

The Ti plasmids present some intriguing questions to plas-
midologists. For example, is the T-DNA segment derived from
eukaryotic DNA that became integrated into a prokaryotic host ?
This could account for the presence of an uninterrupted block of
genes that are transcribed only by polymerase II of plants and
that can control plant growth.

A second question is, how is the T-DNA transferred to the
nucleus ? Virtually nothing is known about early steps in the
infection of the plant. The Ti plasmid (or some portion of it)
may enter the cell as a naked molecule. In this event, infection
may be similar to bacterial conjugation, and may even employ the
same origin of transfer of the Ti plasmid. This model still
provides no explanation for how the DNA can reach the nucleus
safely. Perhaps it is worthwhile to reassess the evidence a-
gainst the uptake of whole <u>Agrobacterium</u> cells by plants.

Finally it is necessary to determine how the T-DNA integrates into the host chromosome. At this time, it is not possible to provide a specific model. The T-DNA may have the properties of a movable element. The T-DNA in nopaline-producing tumors, at least, appears to integrate quite precisely. However, no transposition of the whole T-DNA has been observed in a bacterial background. It should be possible to detect transposition of the T-DNA in plants by cloning from tumors the ends of T-DNAs that have been tagged with antibiotic resistance markers. Such markers provide a method of selecting clones containing the sites of T-DNA integration. Analysis of these sites might clarify how the T-DNA is incorporated into chromosomes and whether the integrated form can jump to a new location.

ACKNOWLEDGEMENT

We thank Dr. A. Caplan for his help with assembly of this manuscript. We thank all the members of the cooperating laboratories for their contributions. This research was supported by grants from the "A.S.L.K.-Kankerfonds", the "Instituut tot aanmoediging van het Wetenschappelijk Onderzoek in Nijverheid en Landbouw" (I.W.O.N.L., # 2481A), the "Fonds voor Geneeskundig Wetenschappelijk Onderzoek" (F.G.W.O., # 30052.78) and the "Onderling Overlegde Akties" (O.O.A., # 12052179) to J.S and M.V.M.

REFERENCES

1.   A.M. Chakrabarty, Plasmids in Pseudomonas. Ann. Rev. Genet.
         10: 7 (1976).
2.   J. Schell, M. Van Montagu, M. De Beuckeleer, M. De Block, A.
         Depicker, M. De Wilde, G. Engler, C. Genetello, J.P.
         Hernalsteens, M. Holsters, J. Seurinck, B. Silva, F.
         Van Vliet, and R. Villarroel, Interactions and DNA
         transfer between Agrobacterium tumefaciens, the Ti-plasmid and the plant host. Proc. R. Soc. Lond. B 204:251
         (1979).
3.   M. Van Montagu, M. Holsters, P. Zambryski, J.P. Hernalsteens,
         A. Depicker, M. De Beuckeleer, G. Engler, M. Lemmers,
         L. Willmitzer, and J. Schell, The interaction of Agrobacterium Ti-plasmid and plant cells. Proc. R. Soc. B,
         210:351 (1980).
4.   J. Ellis, A. Kerr, J. Tempé, and A. Petit, Arginine catabolism: a new function of both octopine and nopaline
         Ti-plasmids of Agrobacterium. Molec. gen. Genet. 173:
         263 (1979).
5.   Unpublished results from this laboratory.

6.   G. Bomhoff, P.M. Klapwijk, H.C.M. Kester, R.A. Schilperoort,
      J.P. Hernalsteens, and J. Schell, Octopine and nopaline
      synthesis and breakdown genetically controlled by a
      plasmid of Agrobacterium tumefaciens, Mol. gen. Genet.
      145:177 (1976).
7.   J. Tempé, P. Guyon, A. Petit, J.G. Ellis, M.E. Tate, and A.
      Kerr, Préparation et propriétés de nouveaux substrats
      cataboliques pour deux types de plasmides oncogènes d'
      Agrobacterium tumefaciens, C. R. Acad. Sci. Paris
      290:1173 (1980).
8.   J.D. Ellis and P.J. Murphy, Four new opines from crown gall
      tumours - their detection and properties, Molec. Gen.
      Genet. 181:36 (1981).
9.   P. Guyon, M.-D. Chilton, A. Petit and J. Tempé, Agropine in
      "null type" crown gall tumors: evidence for the genera-
      lity of the opine concept, Proc. Natl. Acad. Sci. USA
      77:2693 (1980).
10.   D.A. Tepfer and J. Tempé, Production d'agropine par des
      racines formées sous l'action d'Agrobacterium rhizo-
      genes, souche A4, C. R. Acad. Sc. Paris 292:153 (1981).
11.   F.F. White and E.W. Nester, Relationship of plasmids respon-
      sible for hairy root and crown gall tumorigenicity,
      J. Bacteriol. 144:710 (1980).
12.   M. De Beuckeleer, M. De Block, H. De Greve, A. Depicker, R.
      De Vos, G. De Vos, M. De Wilde, P. Dhaese, M.R.
      Dobbelaere, G. Engler, C. Genetello, J.P. Hernalsteens,
      M. Holsters, A. Jacobs, J. Schell, J. Seurinck, B.
      Silva, E. Van Haute, M. Van Montagu, F. Van Vliet, R.
      Villarroel and I. Zaenen, The use of the Ti-plasmid as
      a vector for the introduction of foreign DNA into
      plants. Proc. IVth Int. Conference on Plant Pathogenic
      Bacteria, INRA-Angers (1978).
13.   N.S. Yadav, K. Postle, R.K. Saiki, M.F. Thomashow and M.-D.
      Chilton, T-DNA of a crown gall teratoma is covalently
      joined to host plant DNA, Nature 287:458 (1980).
14.   M. Lemmers, M. De Beuckeleer, M. Holsters, P. Zambryski, A.
      Depicker, J.P. Hernalsteens, M. Van Montagu and J.
      Schell, Internal organization, boundaries and integra-
      tion of Ti-plasmid DNA in nopaline crown gall tumours,
      J. Mol Biol. 144:355 (1980).
15.   M.F. Thomashow, R. Nutter, A.L. Montoya, M.P. Gordon and E.W
      Nester, Integration and organisation of Ti-plasmid
      sequences in crown gall tumors, Cell 19:729 (1980).
16.   D.J. Merlo, R.C., Nutter, A.L. Montoya, D.J. Garfinkel, M.H.
      Drummond, M.-D. Chilton, M.P. Gordon and E.W. Nester,
      The boundaries and copy numbers of Ti plasmid T-DNA
      vary in crown gall tumors, Molec. Gen. Genet. 177:637
      (1980).

17. P. Zambryski, M. Holsters, K. Kruger, A. Depicker, J. Schell,
    M. Van Montagu and H.M. Goodman, Tumor DNA structure in
    plant cells transformed by A. tumefaciens, Science
    209:1385 (1980).
18. M.F. Thomashow, R. Nutter, K. Postle, M.-D. Chilton, F.R.
    Blattner, A. Powell, M.P. Gordon and E.W. Nester,
    Recombination between higher plant DNA and the Ti
    plasmid of Agrobacterium tumefaciens, Proc. Natl. Acad.
    Sci. USA 77:6448 (1980).
19. G. Ooms, P.M. Klapwijk, J.A. Poulis and R.A. Schilperoort,
    Characterization of Tn904 insertions in octopine Ti
    plasmid mutants of Agrobacterium tumefaciens, J.
    Bacteriol. 144:82 (1980).
20. D.J. Garfinkel and E.W. Nester, Agrobacterium tumefaciens
    mutants affected in crown gall tumorigenesis and octo-
    pine catabolism, J. Bacteriol. 144:732 (1980).
21. G. De Vos, M. De Beuckeleer, M. Van Montagu and J. Schell,
    Restriction endonuclease mapping of the octopine tumor
    inducing pTiAch5 of Agrobacterium tumefaciens, Plasmid
    (in press).
22. A. Depicker, M. De Wilde, G. De Vos, R. De Vos, M. Van
    Montagu and J. Schell, Molecular cloning of overlapping
    segments of the nopaline Ti-plasmid pTiC58 as a means
    to restriction endonuclease mapping, Plasmid, 3:193
    (1980).
23. M. Holsters, B. Silva, F. Van Vliet, C. Genetello, M. De
    Block, P. Dhaese, A. Depicker, D. Inzé, G. Engler, R.
    Villarroel, M. Van Montagu and J. Schell, The function-
    al organization of the nopaline A. tumefaciens plasmid
    pTiC58, Plasmid 3:212 (1980).
24. H. De Greve, H. Decraemer, J. Seurinck, M. Van Montagu and
    J. Schell, The functional organization of the octopine
    Agrobacterium tumefaciens plasmid pTiB6S3, Plasmid (in
    press).
25. B.T. Koekman, G. Ooms, P.M. Klapwijk and R.A. Schilperoort,
    Genetic map of an octopine Ti-plasmid, Plasmid 2:347
    (1979).
26. G. Engler, A. Depicker, R. Maenhaut, R. Villarroel-Mandiola,
    M. Van Montagu and J. Schell, Physical mapping of DNA
    base sequence homologies between an octopine and a
    nopaline Ti-plasmid of Agrobacterium tumefaciens,
    J. Mol. Biol. (in press).
27. P. Dhaese, H. De Greve, H. Decraemer, J. Schell and M. Van
    Montagu, Rapid mapping of transposon insertion and
    deletion mutations in the large Ti-plasmids of Agrobac-
    terium tumefaciens, Nucl. Acids Res. 7:1837 (1979).
28. J. Leemans, D. Inzé, R. Villarroel, G. Engler, J.P.
    Hernalsteens, M. De Block and M. Van Montagu, Plasmid
    mobilization as a tool for in vivo genetic engineering,

in:"Molecular Biology, Pathogenicity and Ecology of
Bacterial plasmids," S.B. Levy, ed., Plenum Press, New
York (1981).

29. J.P.Hernalsteens, F. Van Vliet, M. De Beuckeleer, A. Depicker,
G. Engler, M. Lemmers, M. Holsters, M. Van Montagu and
J. Schell, The Agrobacterium tumefaciens Ti plasmid as
a host vector system for introducing foreign DNA in
plant cells, Nature 287:654 (1980).

30. F. Yang, A.L. Montoya, D.J. Merlo, M.H. Drummond, M.-D.
Chilton, E.W. Nester and M.P. Gordon, Foreign DNA
sequences in crown gall teratomas and their fate during
the loss of the tumorous traits, Molec. Gen. Genet.
177:707 (1980).

31. A.C. Braun, Plant tumors, Biochim. Biophys. Acta 516:167
(1978).

32. W.B. Gurley, J.D. Kemp, M.J. Albert, D.W. Sutton and J.
Callis, Transcription of Ti plasmid-derived sequences
in three octopine-type crown gall tumor lines, Proc.
Natl. Acad. Sci. USA 76:2828 (1979).

33. F. Yang, J.C. McPherson, M.P. Gordon and E.W. Nester, Extensive transcription of foreign DNA in a crown gall
teratoma, Biochem. Biophys. Res. Comm. 92:1273 (1980).

34. J.C. McPherson, E.W. Nester and M.P. Gordon, Proteins encoded by Agrobacterium tumefaciens Ti plasmid DNA (T-DNA)
in crown gall tumors, Proc. Natl Acad. Sci. USA 77:2666
(1980).

35. L. Willmitzer, L. Otten, G. Simons, W. Schmalenbach, J.
Schröder, G. Schröder, M. Van Montagu, G. De Vos and J.
Schell, Nuclear and polysomal transcripts of T-DNA in
octopine crown gall suspension and callus cultures,
(submitted).

36. L. Willmitzer, W. Schmalenbach and J. Schell, Transcription
of T-DNA in octopine and nopaline crown gall tumours is
inhibited by low concentrations of α-aminitin, (submitted).

RHIZOBIUM PLASMIDS: THEIR ROLE IN THE NODULATION OF LEGUMES

A. W. B. Johnston, G. Hombrecher and N. J. Brewin

John Innes Institute
Colney Lane
Norwich NR4 7UH
England

Many important crop plants, such as soybeans, groundnuts, beans, peas, clover and alfalfa are legumes, and hence the symbiotic nitrogen fixing relationship between Rhizobium and the roots of legumes is of major agronomic importance. The cost of nitrogenous fertilizer is closely linked to the cost of oil, so it is not surprising that there is an increasing interest in a biological process that allows some crop plants to grow without the application of nitrogen fertilizer.

The symbiosis is also noteworthy purely as a problem in developmental biology because it involves biochemical and morphological differentiation in both partners. The infection process has been reviewed by Newcomb (1976). Typically, penetration by the bacteria begins at the tip of root hairs. An infection thread is formed within the root hair by invagination of the plant cell wall. The bacteria multiply inside this thread. As it grows into the cortex unknown signals induce localised plant cell proliferation ahead of the zone of infection. As the nodule develops the infection threads continue to penetrate the host cells and the bacteria near the tips are pinched off, surrounded by plant membrane and liberated into the cytoplasm. These forms are known as bacteroids; owing to the loss of much of the bacterial cell wall they are pleiomorphic and much larger than free-living Rhizobium. The bacteroids synthesise nitrogenase and the ammonia that is produced is exported to the plant cytoplasm where it is assimilated and from which it is transported to the rest of the plant.

Although the precise morphology of root nodules varies between different legumes, in all cases they are organised structures with a defined meristem and a well developed vascular system.

A feature of the symbiotic interaction is its specificity: different legume species are nodulated by different Rhizobium strains and the host-range of the bacteria is used to define Rhizobium species. Thus R. leguminosarum, R. phaseoli and R. trifolii nodulates peas, Phaseolus beans and clover respectively.

It is reasonable to suppose that during the course of nodule development a number of genes in both partners have to be expressed in a co-ordinate manner. Although we know little or nothing of the precise control and function of any 'symbiotic' genes, it is apparent that genes determining nodulation, nitrogen-fixing ability and host-range are plasmid-borne in at least some Rhizobium species. In this paper we shall describe the evidence that has led to this conclusion.

Isolation of Rhizobium Plasmids

Since Nuti et al. (1977) first demonstrated, in R. trifolii and R. leguminosarum, the presence of plasmids of > 100 Md it has become clear that such plasmids are widespread in other species also (Casse et al., 1979; Gross et al., 1979; Beynon et al., 1980). A single strain may contain several large plasmids of different molecular weights but the number and sizes may vary between strains of the same species. In a small survey of strains of R. leguminosarum the number of plasmid bands per strain seen on agarose gels ranged from two to seven but there was no plasmid of the same size present in all strains (Beringer et al., 1980). Thus there does not appear to be a 'pea nodulation plasmid' of uniform molecular weight. The situation may be different in strains of R. meliloti; in this species there is a plasmid of c. 350 Md in many strains of diverse geographical origin (J. Dénarié, personal communication). There is strong evidence that this plasmid determines nodulation and nitrogen-fixing functions (see below).

Transcription of Plasmids

A clear demonstration of the importance of plasmids in the

nodulation process comes from the observations by Krol et al. (1980) that RNA isolated from bacteroids of pea root nodules hybridised extensively to R. leguminosarum plasmid DNA whereas there was no detectable hybridisation between plasmids and RNA obtained from cells grown in vitro. Thus, between the free-living state and the bacteroid form, there appears to be a major shift in the pattern of transcription of plasmid-linked genes.

Location of nif genes

The genes that specify the components of the nitrogenase complex (nif genes) are normally expressed only within the root nodule bacteroids: hence the nif genes are an obvious example of what we describe as 'symbiotic genes'. In some Rhizobium species nif genes have now been shown to be plasmid-linked. The demonstration of this depends on the fact that two of the nif genes (nif D and nif H) which specify the structural components of nitrogenase are highly conserved among nitrogen-fixing bacteria so that cloned nif DNA from Klebsiella pneumoniae can hybridise with nif DNA from a wide variety of nitrogen-fixing bacteria (Ruvkun & Ausubel, 1980).

Nuti et al. (1979) found that the plasmid pSA30, which contained the nif K, D and H genes of K. pneumoniae, specifically hybridised to plasmid DNA of R. leguminosarum. By transferring plasmids which had been separated on agarose gels to nitrocellulose filters ("Southern blotting") and probing with labelled pSA30 we have identified specific 'nif' plasmids in several strains of R. leguminosarum and R. phaseoli (see below).

It is clear that this hybridisation with pSA30 is not due to some spurious homology. In some elegant studies (Ruvkun & Ausubel, 1981; Ditta et al. , 1981) it was found that non-fixing mutants of R. meliloti could be isolated by insertion of the transposon Tn5 into DNA that hybridised with pSA30.

Other plasmid determined symbiotic functions

Other symbiotic genes, less well defined than those specifying nitrogenase, have been shown to be plasmid-linked. In the discussion that follows we shall refer to 'Nod⁻' or 'Fix⁻' mutants, meaning respectively that the defective strains induce no detectable nodules or that nodules are formed which fail to fix nitrogen. Presumably these classes will become sub-divided as we know

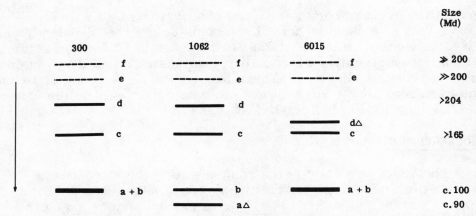

Fig. 1.   Representation of agarose gels of R. leguminosarum
          strain 300 and two derivative strains. Plasmids were
          isolated and the gels were run according to the method
          of Hirsch et al. (1980). The dotted lines indicate that
          these two bands were seen only in some preparations.

more of the biochemical and genetic detail of symbiosis but at
present such analyses are not available.

Most of the work to be described involves the study of
plasmids in strains of R. leguminosarum and R. phaseoli. In the
former species we have concentrated on the genetically well
characterised strain 300 (Beringer et al. , 1978b) and derivatives
of this strain into which plasmids were introduced from other
R. leguminosarum field isolates.

Strain 300 yields five plasmid bands following electrophoresis
on agarose gels (see Figure 1), the two largest being seen only in
some preparations (Hirsch et al. ; 1980). The fastest migrating
band (a + b in Figure 1) actually comprises two co-migrating
plasmids which in strain 1062 were resolved by a deletion of c.
10 Md in the a plasmid.

Of the six plasmids in strain 300, only the one corresponding
to band d in Figure 1 has been shown to be required for nodulation
and nitrogen fixation on peas (Hirsch et al. , 1980). Following UV
treatment, we have isolated a Nod⁻ derivative of strain 300 and it
can be seen that in this strain (6015) there has been a substantial
deletion of the d plasmid. This deletion appears not only to have
removed genes essential for pea nodulation; at least some of the

R. leguminosarum nif genes are also absent from this strain.
Following Southern blotting of gels containing the plasmids of
strains 300 and 6015, pSA30 (the plasmid containing the K. pneumoniae nif genes) hybridised to band d of strain 300 but there was
no detectable hybridisation to the d△⁻plasmid of strain 6015 (unpublished observations). Similarly, when pSA30 was used as a
probe against total DNA from strain 300 which had been digested
with endonuclease EcoRI, a 1.5 Md fragment was found to hybridise but there was no homology between pSA30 and any EcoRI fragment derived from strain 6015.

The plasmid d is apparently not self-transmissible. Derivatives of strain 300⁻ in which the transposon Tn5 has been inserted
into this plasmid fail to transfer kanamycin resistance (specified
by Tn5) to other strains of R. leguminosarum (frequency $< 10^{-9}$).

A. Kondorosi (personal communication) and J. Dénarié
(personal communication) have found that in R. meliloti a single
deletion in a large (c. 350 Md) plasmid can lead to the loss of nod
and nif genes. It is interesting that genes governing such different
steps as the early stages of nodule induction and of nitrogenase
synthesis should be closely linked on single plasmids in at least
two Rhizobium species.

Of the other plasmids in strain 300 we know very little: indeed
the plasmids corresponding to bands c, e and f determine no known
phenotype. We have inserted Tn5 into both the b and the a△
plasmids in derivatives of strain 1062 using the method of Tn5
mutagenesis described by Beringer et al. (1978a). These
plasmids are both transmissible at low frequencies (c. 10^{-6} and
10^{-7} respectively) to other R. leguminosarum strains. We have
isolated derivatives in which either the a△ or the b plasmid is
missing and in both cases the strain nodulates and fixes nitrogen
normally, indicating that neither is required for symbiotic proficiency.

Transmissible plasmids with symbiotic functions

In addition to the plasmids of R. leguminosarum strain 300
we have identified a number of plasmids originating in other R.
leguminosarum field isolates which can be transferred by conjugation into strain 300 and have shown in some cases that such
conjugative plasmids determine symbiotic functions.

pRL1JI.   This plasmid has a molecular weight of c. 130×10^6 (Hirsch et al., 1980) and was identified initially by the fact that the field isolate (strain 248) of R. leguminosarum in which it was detected made a bacteriocin whose production could be transferred at high frequencies (c. 10^{-2}) to non-producing strains such as strain 300 (Hirsch, 1979). Our interest in this plasmid was stimulated by the finding that when it, or a derivative containing Tn5, was transferred to the Nod⁻ Nif⁻ strain 6015 (see above) all the transconjugants induced nitrogen-fixing nodules on peas (Johnston et al., 1978). This plasmid can also suppress a number of chemically induced Fix⁻ mutants of R. leguminosarum strain 300 (Brewin et al., 1980a) and several Nod⁻ and Fix⁻ derivatives of pRL1JI have been isolated following Tn5 insertion into the plasmid (Buchanan-Wollaston et al., 1980; C-S. Ma, personal communication).

A Tn5-marked derivative of pRL1JI has also been transferred to strains of R. phaseoli and R. trifolii. The transconjugants gain the ability to nodulate and fix nitrogen on peas and they retain their ability to nodulate their normal hosts, although the nodulation both on peas and on clover or Phaseolus is later than when these hosts are inoculated with the normal homologous species (Johnston et al., 1978).

Some properties of the transconjugants of strain 1233 of R. phaseoli have been examined by Beynon et al. (1980). As will be seen, another plasmid-linked character relevant to the understanding of these interspecific transconjugants is the production of melanin. For reasons that are not understood, strains of R. phaseoli but not of R. leguminosarum or R. trifolii make melanin following prolonged growth on rich medium.

Following the transfer of pRL1JI to strain 1233 the transconjugants contained three plasmids, the smallest corresponding to pRL1JI plus the two larger plasmids of strain 1233 (see track 1 in Fig. 2). These transconjugants were stable in culture and could still make melanin. As mentioned above, peas inoculated with these transconjugants nodulated later (by about one week) than when R. leguminosarum strains were used. The great majority (c. 95%) of bacteria isolated from nodules induced by the strain 1233 pRL1JI transconjugants differed in three ways from the original transconjugants: (a) they could no longer make melanin; (b) they nodulated and fixed nitrogen on peas as well as did strains of R. leguminosarum but failed to nodulate Phaseolus beans;

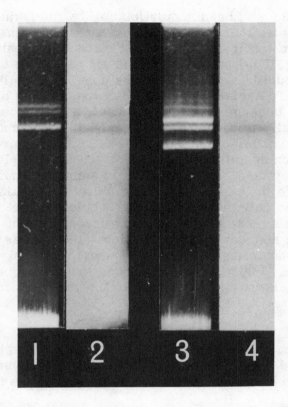

Fig. 2.   Isolation of plasmids from R. phaseoli containing pRL1JI
and demonstration of plasmid-linked nif genes.   Plasmids
were isolated according to the method of Hirsch et al.
(1980).   Transfer of DNA from gels to filters was essentially as described by Wahl et al. (1979).   Track 1.
Agarose gel of R. phaseoli strain 1233 containing pRL1JI.
The two larger plasmids are those of strain 1233 - the
fastest migrating band corresponds to pRL1JI.
Track 3.   Gel of R. leguminosarum strain 248.   The
second smallest plasmid corresponds to pRL1JI (Hirsch
et al, 1980).   Tracks 2 and 4.   Hybridisation of pSA30 to
plasmid DNA blotted from the gels in tracks 1 and 3
respectively.

(c) they had lost the smaller of the strain 1233 resident plasmids
(termed pRP1JI) but still retained pRL1JI and the larger of the two
plasmids of strain 1233.

The fact that following passage through pea nodules there was concomitant loss of bean nodulation ability, melanin production and pRP1JI indicates that both characters are determined by pRP1JI. This has been confirmed by the fact that some spontaneous deletions of pRP1JI in strain 1233 itself result in the loss of melanin production and of Phaseolus nodulation ability (Beynon et al., 1980). To explain why pRP1JI is lost at such high frequency following the passage through pea nodules, it has been proposed that the initially formed strain 1233 pRL1JI transconjugants are in fact unable to nodulate peas because of some uncharacterised inhibitory action specified by pRP1JI which acts on pRL1JI. Only when pRP1JI is lost, as it might be in some bacteria in the rhizosphere, would the pRL1JI-specified ability to nodulate peas be expressed and only these individuals would be able to induce nodules on this host. We know from reconstruction experiments that peas can nodulate if they are inoculated with as few as 10 Nod$^+$ R. leguminosarum cells even in the presence of 10^8 Nod$^-$ bacteria (Brewin et al., 1980a) so if pRP1JI was lost at frequencies as low as 10^{-6}, nodulation of peas by the transconjugants might still be detected.

In strain 1233, pRP1JI also carried nif genes; in Fig. 2, track 2, radioactively labelled pSA30 can be seen to hybridise both to pRL1JI and to pRP1JI so here is another case where at least some nod and nif genes are on the same Rhizobium plasmid.

pRL5JI.   There is some specificity even within 'classical' cross-inoculation groups. For example a primitive pea line called Afghanistan is resistant to nodulation by European strains of R. leguminosarum but can be nodulated by a strain of R. leguminosarum which was isolated in Turkey (Winarno & Lie, 1979). This strain, termed TOM, contains a 160 Md plasmid, pRL5JI, that is transferable at frequencies of c. 10^{-6} to other R. leguminosarum strains. Derivatives of the Nod$^-$ Nif$^-$ strain 6015 (see above) containing pRL5JI are Nod$^+$ Nif$^+$ both on Western pea cultivars and on the variety Afghanistan (Brewin et al., 1980b). Thus pRL5JI appears to carry the determinants that confer on strain TOM the ability to nodulate primitive pea lines.

Transfer of genes for an uptake hydrogenase (Hup)

Biological nitrogen fixation is energetically demanding with approximately 18 moles of ATP being consumed for the reduction of 1 mole of N_2. As much as 25% of this energy is not directly involved in the reduction of nitrogen but in a sense is wasted in the reduction by nitrogenase of protons to H_2 (see review by Robson & Postgate, 1980). Some strains of some species of nitrogen-fixing bacteria, including Rhizobium, possess an uptake hydrogen-ase which can oxidise the $\overline{H_2}$ that is liberated and in the process recycle some of the energy that would otherwise have been lost.

Albrecht et al. (1979) isolated Hup$^-$ derivatives from a Hup$^+$ field isolate of R. japonicum and found that soybeans inoculated with the mutants were smaller (by about 25%) than those inoculated by the Hup$^+$ parents, suggesting that Hup$^+$ bacteria are superior and that it would be desirable for any inoculant strain to be Hup$^+$.

In one Hup$^+$ field isolate of R. leguminosarum (strain 128C53) the hup genes appear to be on a plasmid termed pRL6JI which also carried nod and nif genes (Brewin et al., 1980c; unpublished observations). This plasmid is not self-transmissible but it can be transferred into Hup$^-$ field isolates of R. leguminosarum after recombination with a transmissible plasmid.

Hirsch (1979) identified two R. leguminosarum transmissible bacteriocinogenic plasmids termed pRL3JI and pRL4JI which were in the same incompatibility group as pRL1JI but which differed from pRL1JI in that they did not appear to carry genes for nod-ulation or nitrogen-fixing ability (Brewin et al., 1980a). However, they were shown to recombine with the 'symbiotic' plasmid of strain 300 (band d in Fig. 1) and such recombinants could then transfer Nod$^+$ and Fix$^+$ at high frequency (Brewin et al., 1980a).

When either pRL3JI or pRL4JI was transferred into the Hup$^+$ strain 128C53 they recombined with the smaller of the two resi-dent plasmids at high frequency. When this happened such recombinant plasmids could be transferred by conjugation to the Nod$^-$ Nif$^-$ strain 6015. Approximately 70% of the strain 6015 transconjugants could induce nitrogen-fixing nodules on peas and in all cases such nodules contained hydrogenase and liberated less H_2 than did the plants inoculated with Hup$^-$ control strain (Brewin et al., 1980c). We are presently investigating whether inocula-tion by these construction Hup$^+$ strains results in enhanced plant growth.

Conclusions

The importance of Rhizobium plasmids in determining several symbiotic functions is now clear. In some cases it is apparent that the genes concerned with rather different steps in the infection process are clustered on one plasmid. However we have virtually no knowledge of the proportion of plasmid DNA which is devoted to symbiotic functions nor do we have any real idea of the contributions of chromosomal genes in the infection process.

Methods are available both for chromosomal and plasmid mapping in Rhizobium (Beringer et al., 1980). As more symbiotically defective mutants are isolated, located, and analysed in detail for the basis of their defects it should be possible to use this information to dissect the various steps that are required for Rhizobium to induce a functioning nitrogen-fixing root nodule.

Armed with such information it may then become feasible to construct rationally strains of Rhizobium that would be of value as inoculants for legume crops.

References

Albrecht, S. L., Maier, R. J., Hanus, F. J., Russell, S. A. Emerich, D. W., and Evans, H J, 1979, Science, 203: 1255-1257.

Beringer, J. E., Beynon, J. L., Buchanan-Wollaston, A. V., and Johnston, A. W. B., 1978a, Nature 276:633-634.

Beringer, J. E., Brewin, N. J, and Johnston, A. W. B., 1980, Heredity 45:161-186.

Beringer, J. E., Hoggan, S. A., and Johnston, A. W. B., 1978b, J. gen. Microbiol., 98:339-343.

Beynon, J. L., Beringer, J. E., and Johnston, A. W. B., 1980, J. gen. Microbiol., 120:421-429.

Brewin, N J., Beringer, J. E., Buchanan-Wollaston, A. V., Johnston, A. W. B., and Hirsch, P. R., 1980a, J. gen. Microbiol., 116:261-270.

Brewin, N. J., Beringer, J. E., and Johnston, A. W. B., 1980b, J. gen. Microbiol., 120:413-420.

Brewin, N. J., De Jong, T. M., Phillips, D. A., and Johnston, A. W. B., 1980c, Nature 288:77-79.

Buchanan-Wollaston, A. V., Beringer, J. E., Brewin, N. J., Hirsch, P. R., and Johnston, A. W. B., 1980. Molec. gen. Genet., 178:185-190.

Casse, F., Boucher, C., Julliot, J. S., Michel, M., and Dénarié, J., 1979, J. gen. Microbiol., 113:229-242.

Ditta, G., Stanfield, S., Corbin, D., and Helinski, D. R., 1981, Proc. natl. Acad. Sci. U.S.A. (In press).

Gross, D. C., Vidaver, A. K., and Klucas, R. V., 1979, J. gen. Microbiol., 114:257-266.

Hirsch, P. R., 1979, J. gen. Microbiol., 113 219-228.

Hirsch, P. R., van Montagu, M., Johnston, A. W. B., Brewin, N. J., and Schell, J., 1980, J. gen. Microbiol. 120: 403-412.

Johnston, A. W. B., Beynon, J. L., Buchanan-Wollaston, A. V., Setchell, S. M., Hirsch, P. R., and Beringer, J. E., 1978, Nature 276:634-636.

Krol, A. J. M., Hontelez, J. G. J., Van den Bos, R. C., and van Kammen, A., 1980, Nucleic Acids Res., 8:4337-4347.

Newcomb, W., 1976, Can. J. Bot., 54:2163-2186.

Nuti, M. P., Ledeboer, A. M., Lepidi, A. A., and Schilperoort, R. A., 1977, J. gen. Microbiol., 100:241-248

Nuti, M. P., Lepidi, A. A., Prakash, R. K., Schilperoort, R. A., and Cannon, F. C., 1979, Nature 282:533-535.

Robson, R. L., and Postgate, J. R., 1980, Ann. Rev. Microbiol., 34:183-207.

Ruvkun, G. B., and Ausubel, F. M., 1980, Proc. natl. Acad. Sci. U.S.A., 77:191-195.

Ruvkun, G. B., and Ausubel, F. M., 1981, Nature 289:85-88.

Wahl, G. M., Stern, M., and Stark, G. R., 1979, Proc. natl. Acad. Sci. U.S.A., 76: 3683-3687.

Winarno, R., and Lie, T. A., 1979, Plant and Soil 51:135-142.

METABOLIC PLASMID ORGANIZATION AND DISTRIBUTION

I. C. Gunsalus, K-M. Yen

Biochemistry Department
University of Illinois
Urbana, Illinois 61801

SUMMARY

Pseudomonas strains carry plasmids under regulation of
natural and synthetic organic residues and bear primary roles in
mineralization. Aromatic compounds of known oxidation pathways
provide convenient models for genetic analyses and for plasmid
DNA isolation and structure determination. The alkane and terpene
catabolic systems, coded on larger self-fertile plasmids, have
provided primary data on gene organization and regulation, as
well as plasmid chromosome gene redundancy.

Two aromatic plasmids, NAH7 and SAL1, of about 80 to 90 kb
(kilobases), code respectively the conversion of naphthalene and
of salicylate to the anaplerotic intermediates, pyruvate and
acetaldehyde, plus CO_2 or formate, thus supporting cell growth.
The NAH plasmid codes for these two conversions on separate
operons, both controlled by salicylate or anthrinilate. Operon 1
codes the conversion of naphthalene to salicylate; operon 2, salicylate via catechol with "meta" (2,3 oxygenase) aromatic ring
cleavage. Plasmid DNA isolated from wild type and transposon Tn5
induced insertion mutants was scored for defective loci by enzyme
assays in the genomes subjected to gel electrophoresis after
restriction digestion. An EcoRl digest fragment A of 23 kilobases
carries the bulk of both operons; Smal yields 5 fragments, A of 42
kilobases and B of 18. The latter which lacks the left hand 5+
kilobases of EcoRl A reveals that the replicon in the *nah*A gene
are within this 5 kilobase region. The transcription is from left
to right in both operons; an 8 to 10 kilobase segment between the
operons carries at least one regulatory locus. The cell plasmid
in Smal digest yields 5 fragments identical in size to those of

NAH7, plus two smaller, about 3 kb, segments which constitute an insertion in naphthalene operon 1 in the gene AB region. The methods now available for plasmid isolation and DNA analyses, the genetic scoring and cloning, now appear capable of providing, in the near future, a complete structure, organization, and regulation model of the aromatic plasmids in fluorescent *Pseudomonas* species.

INTRODUCTION

The state of metabolic plasmid research in *Pseudomonas* strains can be presented most readily in the space available as examples of work in progress. The relevance of the "metabolic" - to the "resistance" plasmids - procaryote tolerance to therapeuti chemicals - requires additional discussion. Essential references and a suitable working background of *Pseudomonas* biology is provided by the Clarke-Richmond monograph (1) as updated by the rece mini-reviews of Chakrabarty (2) and of Williams (3).

Metabolic plasmid is offered as a more general term than degradative (2) or catabolic (3). It refers to reaction pathways presumed roles in nature, and methods of phenotypic scoring. It is now well documented that many plasmids coding resistance by antibiotics degrade or modify the active structures by forming less active or inactive derivatives (4).

Genetic exchange among gram negative procaryotes is now generally accepted. While subject to some expression barriers, fluo rescent pseudomonads are recognized as a single genetic group (1, The problems of plasmid compatibility (5), inhibition of expressi and the host range, are only partially documented (1-3). Number and variety of fertility factors among the fluorescent pseudomona whether scored by growth or as resistant phenotypes remain to be delineated. The total array of plasmids carrying markers for aro matic metabolism and their conformation, aggregate or cointegrate mode remain unexplored. For many aspects of the fundamental gene tics, even among the most studied group, the fluorescent pseudo-monads, the data are incomplete; for the nonfluorescent soil-wate forms (P. acidovorans-P. testosteroni) genetic problems are virtually undocumented. This, however, should not be difficult as Dagley, Evans, Gibson, and others have provided elegant chemical and enzymatic identities, and Stanier, Doudoroff, and Palleroni have provided taxonomic identity among many of the most-studied strains.

The fluorescent pseudomonad plasmid structure will be illustrated with a self-fertile aromatic plasmid coding naphthalene-salicylate oxidation, e.g., NAH7 and SAL1. The NIC1 plasmid, cod for nicotine-nicotinate oxidation, with or without the fertility factor "T", will be considered briefly. The plasmid isolation procedures, the preliminary maps of restriction and gene organization in some homology studies have been published (6, 7). Primary data are on the NAH/SAL and the TOL plasmids (8-10, 3). The transposon Tn5 has been employed in the study reported here for the elucidation of the gene order including polar effects. The gene loci, regulation and transcription, are presented; the relevance of these data to the aromatic metabolic processes in this genus is offered as a working hypothesis.

RESULTS

Table 1 indicates the principle metabolic plasmids studied so far in the fluorescent pseudomonads. The size of those coding growth phenotypes on alkane, terpene, and aromatic carbon sources range from 50 to > 200 megadaltons (75-300 kilobases, kb). The extent and precision of the data varies widely, primarily as a function of the more recent studies and the extent of commonality in methods used by the more active working groups. The growth data phenotypes are still incomplete in many key instances, pathway intermediates remain to be identified, and the scoring of enzyme lesions and activities are at best rudimentary. In certain cases, gene linkages have been established by transduction and, in others, plasmids accumulated within preferred hosts by transduction or conjugation to auxotrophic recipients. Plasmid DNA has been isolated from both wild type and derived strains in structures deduced from point or transposon-induced mutants with restriction enzyme digestion.

The aromatic plasmid data in Table 1 are perhaps, at this time, the more advanced. See, for example, Chakrabarty (2), Williams (3), Johnston (6), and Farrell (7). This paper provides additional fine structure of gene loci and organization in the NAH7 and SAL1 plasmids. Equivalent data are also included on the heterocyclic nicotine plasmid, NIC, for comparative purposes. The earlier data in Table 1 suffer from defects in 1) multiple bands in agarose gel electrophoresis due to the presence of supercoil, open circle and linear forms, and 2) errors in the size estimation of the larger fragments from restriction digests resulting from underestimates on flat bed agarose gel electrophoretic patterns. Multiple enzyme digests to yield smaller fragments, comparative measurements, among the laboratories working in this area, and elimination of contamination by chromosomal fragments remain to be optimized. The native plasmids are unusually large for optimum analysis by electron micrography although some confirmatory data are available.

Naphthalene oxidation via salicylate. The bicyclic aromatic hydrocarbon, naphthalene, is oxidized to salicylic acid with the generation of the three-carbon residue, pyruvate, as outlined in the first half of Scheme A. Enzymes and gene designations are indicated. These five genes are controlled as a single replicon. It appears likely that several of the enzymatic transformations require

Table 1.   Some *Pseudomonas* Catabolic Plasmids

Phenotype	DNA	Host No. wt	Host No. 277
	mD		*(trpB615)*
Alkane			
OCT	>̄100	6	972
CAM–OCT		1+6	970/977
Terpene			
CAMphor	>̄100	1	273
CAMphene	~70	93	
αPN, (pinene)	~70	93	
βPN, "	~70	93	
LINalool	~155	158	
PCYmene	"	"	
Aromatic			
NAH	42	7	1343
"	4,10,42	63	x000
"	–	90	
SAL	45	R1	2100
XYL	–	26,*xy*[†]	1525
XYL·K	90	AC142	1311
TOL	76	9,*mt2*	2116
TOL*	54	" AC804	1327*
TOLΔ	39	" AC803	1328*
TOL*K	108	" AC797	1318*
TOL·RP4	53	AC810	1329
Heterocyclic			
NIC	44	25,*pcl*	2501

[†]For strains, we thank P. K. Bhattacharyya, A. Chakrabarty, D. Gibson, and J. Shapiro.

*In *met-1*, PpG1 derivative.

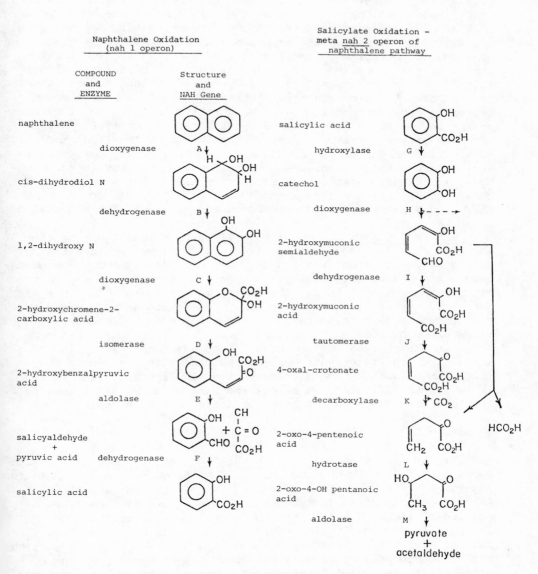

Scheme A. Naphthalene-salicylate oxidation pathway: Enzyme and gene designations

two or more proteins, thus, for example, *nah*A may turn out to be
two or three cistrons. Genetic distinction and locus identification
have not been completed. Salicylate oxidation to catechol aromatic
ring fission and the oxidation of the resulting aldehyde to hydroxy
mutanate are under control of a second operon, nah2. Catechol, a
first product of salicylate oxygenase, is a primary convergent point
of aromatic metabolism. The presence of the plasmid ring fission
occurs by the so-called "meta", 2,3 dioxygenase pathway in plasmid-
free *P. putida* chromosomal genes and regulation specify ring fission
by the "ortho" 1,2 oxygenase. Whether the regulation of these processes is dependent on inducer concentration or other chemical mechanisms in unclear. Catechol and substituted catechols are metabolized by enzymes relatively relaxed in tolerance to alkane and acidic
side chains on the aromatic nuclei. The loci, plasmid or chromosome,
in the late steps of conversion of salicylate to pyruvate acetaldehyde, i.e., the hydration and retrograde aldol reactions remain to
be identified. Present data suggests plasmid loci in operon 2, but
the possibility of plasmid chromosome redundancy is not eliminated.

The NAH7 plasmid. A Smal Type II restriction digest of the
isolated NAH7 DNA produces five fragments. Figure 1 indicates
diagrammatically their size, order, and the position of the naphthalene operons 1 and 2. Clearly, fragment B of nearly 18 kb, carries
most of the *nah* gene loci. The initiation of operon 1 and the *nah*A
loci over to the left in fragment A, ∿ 42 kb, is approximately half
of the entire plasmid. Operon 2, for which only three gene positions are shown, is near the right B fragment terminus. Later
steps in the pathway may be coded in the adjacent restriction fragment. The gene placements were established with transposon Tn5
insertion mutants by the data summarized in Figure 2. The Tn5,
about 5.7 kb (10), carries a Smal restriction site, 3.2 kilobases
from one terminus, and 2.5 from the other. With the polarity of
insertion unknown, an uncertainty of about 0.7 kb remains in determining the insertion locus.

Figure 2 indicates also an EcoRl fragment A, about 24 kb, with
overlap of 5.3 kb to the left of the Smal fragment B ∿ 0.5 kb to the
right. A BamHl site, also indicated in this region, also is useful
as will be indicated subsequently. The expanded diagram, lower
portion of Figure 2, indicates the *nah*A gene loci in the EcoRl
fragment A, presumably also including the replicon. Preliminary
data of Gibson (11) indicate for the naphthalene dioxygenase, three
protein components, thus multiple cistrons, presumably in the A
region. The region of 10 kilobases unmapped between operons 1 and
2, contains at least one regulatory locus.

Table 2 provides enzyme activity data on the wild type strain
and representative Tn5 insertion mutants. The levels induced by
salicylate, 2.5 mM, are compared to the noninduced levels, i.e.,
cells grown on sodium glutamate. The insertion mutants show

Table 2. Naphthalene Oxidation Enzyme of NAH7: :Tn5 Mutants

Gene & locus Enzyme	wt 1343	A1	B11	C24	D32	G66	I82
nah	n/i*	nkat -- n moles/min/mg protein					
A dioxygenase	0/2	0	0	.3	.5	1.5	1.5
B dehydrogenase	0/10	0	0	18	6	6	8
C oxygenase	.1/20	.1	.1	0	14	9	13
D isomerase	0/.4	0	0	0	0	<.1	.3
E aldolase	.3/5	.2	.3	.2	.01	3	9
F dehydrogenase	.7/4	.5	.2	.6	4	3	3
G hydroxylase	.06/2	5	2	4	2	0	3
H 2,3-dioxygenase	.2/11	27	8	19	8	.1	6
I dehydrogenase	.05/1	2	1.6	2	1	.04	.05

*n/i = Non or induced 2.5 mM salicylate; < sensitivity of assay

Table 3. NAH7 plasmid + Tn5 insertion mutant restriction
          pattern with SmaI

Gene loci Nah	SmaI fragments, kb						
	A	B	C	D	E	F	>Tn5 (5.7kb)
wt.1343	42.3	17.6	12.7	6.8	3.7	-	-
A1	42.7					5.19	+.21
A2	44.6					3.72	+.34
B11		20.0				3.93	+.63
C21		19.5				3.96	+.16
D31		14.8				8.84	+.34
G67		17.0				6.77	+.47
I81		20.2				3.44	+.34

blanks = fragments were wild type size.

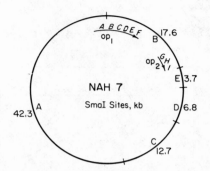

Figure 1. Plasmid NAH7 *nah* operons 1 and 2: <u>Sma</u>I digest

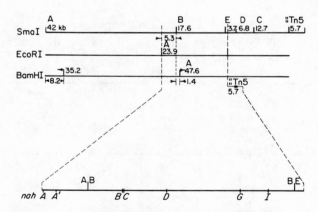

Plasmid Gene Organization--Napthalene Oxidation in NAH-7

Figure 2. The *nah* gene loci in plasmid NAH7: Restriction maps
          with <u>Sma</u>I, <u>EcoR</u>l, and <u>BamH</u>l

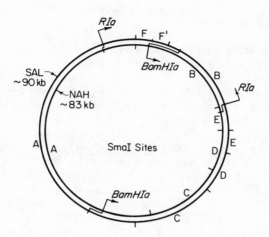

Figure 3.   NAH7 *vs* SALl plasmid restriction homologies. F and F'
            insertion segments in the *nah* operon 1 gene AB region

polarity in both operons 1 and 2. The anomolous value of "F" de-
hydrogenase in the *nah*D mutant remains to be explained. Additional
strains conform to the conclusions drawn from these examples. Since
the preparation of Table 2, we have synthesized the substrates for
later steps in the salicylate oxidation, and identified gene lesions
which map to the right of I in an adjacent restriction fragment.

     Table 3 presents the electrophoretic data for the Smal digest
of wild type and Tn5 insertion mutants upon which the gene positions
were assigned.

     NAH7 and SALl plasmid homology. The NAH7 and SALl plasmids
are of approximately equal size, 83 and 90 kilobases, respectively.
Figure 3 presents superimposed maps of their Smal digest and indicates the loci of EcoRl and BamHl cleavage which provides the
A, largest, fragment of each.

     The Smal digest of the SALl plasmid yields five fragments
identical in size to those from NAH7 plasmid, and in addition, two
smaller fragments, F and F', each of about three kilobases. These

arise from an insertion in the <u>Smal</u> fragment B segment, a position
which would coincide with NAH operon l. This insertion too, produces a polar mutation as occurs in Tn5 insertions. Thus, as one
would presume, the reaction pathway from naphthalene to salicylate
is inactive. The working hypothesis for homology analyses currently
is based on this assumption.

Heteroduplex analyses, by Southern Blot, of the NAH and SAL
fragments of <u>Smal</u> and <u>EcoRl</u> digests, indicate a high degree of
homology further supporting the working hypothesis. To date we
have been unable to delete the F-F' region from the SAL plasmid
nor do we have data indicating whether other insertions or deletions
have occurred in this region.

<u>Aromatic plasmids and oxidative pathways</u>. It would appear
from the data of Dagley and coworkers (12) and from the molecular
genetic data of Farrell (7) that a high degree of homology exists
among the TOL, XYL, NAH, and SAL plasmids of the fluorescent
pseudomonads. Taken with a relaxed specificity for aromatic
derivatives with ring substitutes, with activity in hydroxylation
and ring fission, one would seek further evidence of convergence
in structure and processes among the aromatic oxidation systems
as the molecular genetic studies are refined and the phenotypic
and genotypic scoring extended.

REFERENCES

1. P. H. Clarke and M. H. Richmond, Evolutionary Prospects
    for *Pseudomonas* species, in: "Genetics and Biochemistry
    of *Pseudomonas*," P. H. Clarke and M. H. Richmond, eds.,
    John Wiley & Sons, New York, 1975.
2. A. M. Chakrabarty, Plasmids in *Pseudomonas*, in: "Annual
    Reviews of Genetics," H. L. Roman, A. Campbell, and L. M.
    Sandler, eds., Vol. 10, Annual Reviews, Inc., Palo Alto,
    Ca., 1976.
3. P. A. Williams, Catabolic plasmids, TIBS, 6:23, 1981.
4. P. H. Clarke and M. H. Richmond, eds., "Resistance of
    Pseudomonas aeruginosa," John Wiley & Sons, New York, 1975.
5. G. A. Jacoby, Classification of Plasmids in *Pseudomonas
    aeruginosa*, Microbiology-1977, D. Schlessinger, ed.,
    American Society for Microbiology, 1977.
6. J. B. Johnston and I. C. Gunsalus, Isolation of Metabolic
    Plasmids DNA from *Pseudomonas putida*, Biochem. Biophys.
    Res. Commun., 75:13, 1977.
7. R. Farrell, Ph.D. Thesis, Biochemistry Department, Uni-
    versity of Illinois, Urbana, 1979.

8. R. Farrell, and A. M. Chakrabarty, Degradative Plasmids:
    Molecular Nature and Mode of Evolution, in: "Plasmids
    of Medical, Environmental and Commercial Importance,"
    K. N. Timmis and A. Pühler, eds., Elsevier/North Holland
    Biomedical Press, 1979.

9. N. J. Palleroni, General Properties and Taxonomy of the
    Genus *Pseudomonas*, in: "Genetics and Biochemistry of
    Pseudomonas," P. H. Clarke and M. H. Richmond, eds., John
    Wiley & Sons, New York, 1975.

10. R. A. Jorgensen, S. J. Rothstein, and W. S. Reznikoff,
    A Restriction Enzyme Cleavage Map of Tn5 and Location
    of a Region Encoding Neomycin Resistance, Molec. Gen.
    Genet., 177:65, 1979.

11. W. K. Yeh and D. T. Gibson, Resolution of toluene
    dioxygenase into three separate protein components,
    Bact. Proc., p. 166, 1974.

12. S. Dagley, Pathways for the Utilization of Organic Growth
    Substrates, in: "The Bacteria," Vol. VI, I. C. Gunsalus,
    ed., Academic Press, New York, 1978.

DEGRADATIVE PLASMIDS: TOL AND BEYOND

Paul Broda[1], Robert Downing[2], Philip Lehrbach[1], Ian McGregor[1] and Pierre Meulien

Department of Molecular Biology, University of Edinburgh
Edinburgh EH9 3JR, U.K.
(1) Present address: Biochemistry Department, UMIST, Manchester M60 1QD, U.K.
(2) Present address: CAMR, Public Health Laboratory Service, Porton Down, Salisbury, Wilts, SP4 0JG, U.K.

INTRODUCTION

The bacteria of soil and water have been presented with major challenges by the chemicals disseminated by man. Although many of these compounds are detoxified, degraded or mineralised, others are more or less recalcitrant. The activities and changes in bacterial populations in these circumstances are of great concern to micro-biologists interested in evolution and those seeking solutions to problems of pollution, utilisation of resources and recycling. The question relevant here is how plasmids contribute to these processes.

The degradative plasmids that have emerged (clearly the first of a very large number) are mainly in strains of Pseudomonas, a genus renowned for nutritional versatility. Work in a number of labora-tories has centred on the TOL plasmid, since it specifies a well-defined pathway and because it was possible to isolate its DNA. Such work has been facilitated by the cleavage map we have established (Downing et al, 1978; Downing and Broda, 1979). There is now evi-dence that translocatable elements, re-arrangements of genetic material and transfer between unrelated strains can all contribute to the variation upon which natural selection acts.

THE TOL PLASMID pWWO

The TOL plasmid pWWO (117 kb) encodes 12 enzymes responsible

511

for the degradation of toluene and the m and p xylenes by a pathway
that involves meta cleavage of the aromatic ring (Worsey and Williams,
1975). Cells lacking the meta pathway can be isolated after growth
on benzoate, which is an intermediate of this pathway and also of
the chromosomally-encoded ortho pathway. In cells carrying the
genes for both pathways only the meta pathway is expressed. However,
in variants that have lost the meta pathway the (more efficient)
ortho pathway functions; such cells then overgrow the others.
"Benzoate-cured" variants arise either by loss of the whole plasmid
or by excision of a specific contiguous 40 kb segment (Bayley et al,
1977). It is believed that the genes specifying the 12 enzymes are
organised within two regulons, and are contained within this 40 kb
segment (Worsey et al, 1978; Nakazawa et al, 1980; Inouye et al,
1981; Franklin et al, 1981).

THE EXCISION EVENT

        We have been studying the excision of the 40 kb segment, exemp-
lified by the formation of Tol plasmid pWWO-8 from pWWO (Table 1).
We find that it involves reciprocal recombination between two direct-
ly-repeated sequences at its boundaries. These repeats are within
the pWWO HindIII restriction fragments HD and HF; a novel fragment
present in pWWO-8 is termed Hd. Restriction mapping of cloned fragments of HD, HF and Hd showed that part of Hd is derived from HD and
the rest from HF. Heteroduplexes of HD and HF show that there is
a direct repeat of 1.4 kb at or near the ends of the excised region.
Comparison with the cleavage mapping data shows that the cross-over
must occur within this repeat. We are presently seeking to establish
whether this repeat is a translocatable element.

HYBRIDS OF pWWO AND RP4

        It has been proposed that the formation of hybrids between RP4
and TOL (RP4-Tol plasmids) involves transposition (Jacoby et al,
1978; Chakrabarty et al, 1978) perhaps of the 40 kb moiety. Although
the independence of this interaction from homologous recombination
has not been tested, some kind of illegitimate recombination is
likely since we have been unable to detect any homology between the
two parental plasmids. We have tested the transposition model using
six independently-isolated RP4-Tol plasmids by examining (1) what
RP4 and TOL DNA they carry and (2) the nature of the junction regions. Restriction digests show that all of the six hybrids contain
the whole of RP4 (to a level of resolution of 2 kb) as well as TOL
DNA. In each case the TOL segment includes the 40 kb segment and
extends beyond it in both directions. In four of the plasmids this
segment at this level of resolution was the same, as was the region
of RP4 that was interrupted (the tetracycline-resistance determi-

Table 1. HindIII restriction fragments of TOL and their fate in various derivatives. The top row gives the co-ordinates of the boundaries of the HindIII fragments given in the next row, according to the kilobase map of Downing and Broda (1979). Asterisks represent the positions and number of minor fragments. The remaining lines show which fragments are present wholly or in part in various derivative strains.

Map co-ordinate (kilobase)	111	15	35	35	39	44	53	62	67	90	99	103	106	111	
Fragment	HB	HC	*	HJ	HG	HE	HD	5*	HA	*	HF	HH	HK	HI	*	**Amount of TOL DNA (kb)**
Plasmid																
pWWO[a]	+	+	+	+	+	+	+	+	+	+	+	+	+	+	+	117
pWWO-8[a]	+	+	+	+	+	+	+	+	-	+	+	+	+	+	+	77
pWWO-339[b]	+	-	-	-	+	+	+	-	+	-	+	+	+	+	+	66
RP4-Tol[c]	+	-	-	-	-	+	+	+	+	+	+	+	+	+	+	59
pTN2[d]	-	-	-	-	-	-	+	+	+	-	+	-	+	-	+	56
pWWO-1211[e]	+	+	+	+	+	+	+	-	+	-	+	+	+	+	+	77
pWWO-1001[f]	+	+	+	+	+	+	+	-	+	-	+	+	+	+	+	117
pWWO-1216[g]	+	+	+	+	+	+	+	+	+	+	+	+	+	+	+	98

(a) Plasmid pWWO-8 is the archetypal plasmid lacking the 40 kb segment.
(b) From strain PAW339 (Williams, unpublished). The PR4 Tol plasmids from strains PAW153 (Williams, unpublished), PU21 (RP4-Tol) (Jacoby et al, 1978) and AC810 (Chakrabarty et al, 1978) are similar. The junction of RP4 and TOL DNA is at about 14' on the RP4 map.
(c) From strain AC836 (Chakrabarty, unpublished). The junction of RP4 and TOL DNA is at 16' on the RP4 map.
(d) Nakazawa et al, (1978, 1980). The junction of RP4 and TOL DNA is at about 32' on the RP4 map.
(e) And also the plasmid from strain PAM1 (Williams, personal communication).
(f) There is a 3 kb insert in fragment HD, near the excision site (Williams, personal communication).
(g) There are two 3 kb inserts, in HA and HC (Williams, personal communication).

nant). However, the plasmids from the other two strains had less TOL DNA and different insertion sites on RP4 (Table 1). We conclude that RP4-Tol plasmids do not arise through transposition involving an unique TOL segment.

A benzoate-cured derivative of the plasmid from strain PaW339 was used to study the boundaries of the RP4 and TOL moieties of the hybrid plasmids. A PstI fragment including one of the junctions was used as a ^{32}P-labelled probe against PstI digests of the hybrid plasmids in strains PU21 (RP4-Tol), PaW339 and PaW153, and of the parent plasmids RP4 and TOL. With each of the parent plasmids only one fragment hybridises with the probe DNA, as expected. However, with each of the RP4-Tol plasmids there was hybridisation with both junction fragments. This suggests that there is a sequence that is present at both junctions.

We have preliminary data that this sequence is not part of native TOL or RP4. When this same PstI fragment is hybridised against digests of chromosomal DNA from several plasmid-free strains of Pseudomonas putida (e.g. AC34) several fragments with homology are revealed. When RP4 or parts of TOL that are on this PstI fragment are used as probes no such homology is revealed. It is possible that there is an element resident on the chromosome that can translocate to TOL and/or RP4 as a preliminary to the formation of hybrids.

MOVEMENT OF TOL DNA TO THE CHROMOSOME

The DNA of some apparently plasmid-free benzoate-cured strains of P.putida mt2 showed homology with pWWO. We have been assessing the extent of this homology by hybridisation, using cloned pWWO fragments as probes. When fragments HD and HF were used against HindIII-restricted chromosomal DNA, a single band co-mobilising with HF showed homology with both probes. Further analysis with HindIII-XhoI double digests showed that this fragment was Hd, the novel fragment produced in the 40 kb excision event. The possibility therefore exists that an excision event similar to that yielding pWWO-8 occurred before, during or after integration.

Not all TOL DNA is present; thus no DNA homologous to the DNA contained in HA, HB, HC, HG, or HI was found. However, both HE and HK had homology with chromosomal HindIII fragments of different sizes.

OTHER DERIVATIVES OF pWWO

Reineke and Knackmuss (1979) have studied a strain of Pseudomonas, B13, that can utilise 3-chlorobenzoate (3CB) but not 4-chlorobenzoate (4CB). The reason for this inability to degrade 4CB was the specificity of the chlorobenzoate dioxygenase. Since pWWO specifies a benzoate dioxygenase with a wider substrate specificity, they introduced this plasmid into B13 to form B13/TOL strains (e.g. WR211). Such strains were still 4CB$^-$, but yielded 3CB$^+$4CB$^+$ derivatives with a frequency of 10^{-3} of the cells plated on selective medium. In such clones (e.g. WR216) expression of the <u>meta</u> pathway is lost. This loss is probably obligatory to avoid the synthesis by this pathway of non-metabolisable products. It is significant that 4CB$^+$ strains can be obtained so easily from B13/TOL clones, and also that strain WR216 yields Mtol$^+$ revertants, and that these revertants are always 4CB$^-$.

The structure of the plasmids of these strains (Williams and Jeenes, 1981) are interesting. That from strain WR211, pWWO-1211, is identical to pWWO-8. However, whereas the strain carrying pWWO-8 is irreversibily Mtol$^-$, strain WR211 is Mtol$^+$. One explanation is that the 40 kb moiety lacking in both carries all the degradative functions and that in strain WR211 it has become translocated to the chromosome.

Evidence to support this comes from matings of WR211 with the <u>P.putida</u> archetypal strain, which carries no known <u>meta</u> cleavage function or plasmid. A Mtol$^+$ transconjugant carried a plasmid (pWWO-1001) identical to the original TOL plasmid pWWO, except for a 3 kb insertion in HD (very close to the excision site). Its presence may account for the inability of this strain to grow on <u>m</u>-xylene.

The idea that the whole pathway is coded by this 40 kb segment is corroborated also by studies on strain PAM1, a clone of the original pWWO-carrying strain that had been maintained independently for 10 years. This too is Mtol$^+$Mxyl$^+$ but its plasmid is like pWWO-8. This strain remains Mtol$^+$Mxyl$^+$ even when the plasmid is eliminated by introducing the incompatible R plasmid pMG18, suggesting again that the 40 kb moiety is carried chromosomally and specifies these phenotypes.

The plasmid in strain WR216 (pWWO-1216) has regained some of the DNA excised in pWWO-1211. This confirms that at least part of this segment can be rescued. It was also noted that there are two novel inserts of 3 kb. A number of independently-isolated WR216-like derivatives of WR211 have similar structures. Whether the remaining TOL DNA is present chromosomally is not yet clear.

A further strain (WRB80) is a Mtol$^+$ derivative of WR216. Its plasmid differs from pWWO-1216 only in the loss of the 3 kb segment in HA, suggesting that this segment contains a structural or regulatory gene involved in the expression of the <u>meta</u> pathway.

The conclusion from the experiments is that there is movement
of plasmid material to and from the chromosome that is demonstrable
using the methods of molecular genetics and DNA-DNA hybridisation.
Indeed, such integration of specific functions in the past may have
been the basis of the accretion by Pseudomonas strains of their
range of degradative capacities.

FUTURE DIRECTIONS WITH DEGRADATIVE FUNCTIONS

Those working with degradative plasmids have a number of oppor-
tunities. These include: (1) pursuing more detailed studies on
plasmids that are already well studied, such as TOL and OCT (2) testing whether any of the plasmid/organism combinations that have been
devised can actually be developed as effective agents for environmental cleanup (3) establishing whether mutant strains can provide
aromatic or other compounds on a scale and with an efficiency that
would be attractive to industry (4) establishing the role of plasmids
in strains already involved in the degradation of natural and man-
made compounds.

An example of the last of these is the work of Salkinoja-Salonen
et al (1981) reported briefly in this volume. They implicate plasmids in the degradation by bacteria of soluble aromatic compounds
formed in the industrial breakdown of lignin, in the effluent of
pulp mills. Lignin is a major component of all plant material.
There would therefore be major benefits from developing biological
methods for delignification: these include energy saving and therefore cheaper production of cellulose from wood, reduction of pollution downstream from pulp mills, utilisation of straw residues for
paper and animal feed, and more efficient use of sugar cane for
ethanol production. The building blocks of lignin might also serve
as feedstocks for chemical industry.

We do not yet know what the importance of plasmids might be in
such systems, or even which are the organisms (e.g. bacteria or
fungi) of choice. Nevertheless it is clear that it is a test of
Molecular Biology how soon it can provide answers in terms of processes here as well as in the production of fine chemicals such as
hormones.

ACKNOWLEDGEMENTS

Work in our laboratory was supported by the Medical Research
Council and the Science Research Council. We thank P. Williams for
providing us with data before their publication.

REFERENCES

Bayley, S.A., C.J.Duggleby, M.J.Worsey, P.A.Williams, K.G.Hardy and
    P.Broda. 1977. Two modes of loss of the TOL function from
    Pseudomonas putida mt-2. Molec. Gen. Genet. 154 203-204.
Chakrabarty, A.M., D.A.Friello and L.H.Bopp. 1978. Transposition of
    plasmid DNA segments specifying hydrocarbon degradation and
    their expression in various microorganisms. Proc. Nat. Acad.
    Sci. U.S.A. 75 3109-3112.
Downing, R.G. and P.Broda. 1979. A cleavage map of the TOL plasmid
    of Pseudomonas putida mt2. Mol. Gen. Genet. 177 189-191.
Downing, R.G., C.J.Duggleby, R.Villems and P.Broda. 1979. An endonu-
    clease cleavage map of the plasmid pWWO-8, a derivative of the
    TOL plasmid of Pseudomonas putida mt2. Mol. Gen. Genet. 168
    97-99.
Franklin, F.C.H., M.Bagdasarian and K.N.Timmis. 1981. Genetic organi-
    sation of a TOL plasmid. This volume.
Inouye, S., A.Nakazawa and T.Nakazawa. 1981. Molecular cloning of
    TOL genes xylB and xylE in Escherichia coli. J. Bacteriol.
    145 (in press).
Jacoby, G.A., J.E.Rogers, A.E.Jacob and R.W.Hedges. 1978. Transpo-
    sition of Pseudomonas toluene-degrading genes and expression
    in Escherichia coli. Nature 274 179-180.
Nakazawa, T., E.Hayashi, T.Yokota, Y.Ebina and A.Nakazawa. 1978.
    Isolation of TOL and RP4 recombinants by integrative suppres-
    sion. J. Bacteriol. 134 270-277.
Nakazawa, T., S.Inouye and A.Nakazawa. 1980. Physical and functional
    mapping of RP4-TOL plasmid recombinants: analysis of insertion
    and deletion mutants. J. Bacteriol. 144 222-231.
Reineke, W. and H.J.Knackmuss. 1979. Construction of haloaromatics
    utilising bacteria. Nature 277 385-386.
Salkinoja-Salonen, M.S., A.Paterson and J.Buswell. 1981. Plasmid-
    coded degradation of salicylic acid and isovanillic acid in
    the soil bacterium K17. This volume.
Williams, P.A. and D.J.Jeenes. 1981. The origin of catabolic plasmids,
    in:"Microbiology 1981," D.Schlessinger ed. American Society for
    Microbiology.
Worsey, M.J., F.C.H.Franklin and P.A.Williams. 1978. Regulation of
    the degradative pathway enzymes coded for by the TOL plasmid
    (pWWO) from Pseudomonas putida mt2. J. Bacteriol. 134 757-764.
Worsey, M.J. and P.A.Williams. 1975. Metabolism of toluene and
    xylenes by Pseudomonas putida (arvilla)mt2: evidence for a
    new function of the TOL plasmid. J. Bacteriol. 124 7-13.

PLASMIDS IN THE BIODEGRADATION OF CHLORINATED

AROMATIC COMPOUNDS

D.K. Chatterjee, S.T. Kellogg, D.R. Watkins* and
A.M. Chakrabarty

Department of Microbiology and Immunology
University of Illinois Medical Center
Chicago, IL 60612
*Environmental Protection Agency
Cincinnati, OH 45268

Over the past several decades, man-made chlorinated aromatic compounds have been released into the environment in massive amounts in the form of herbicides, pesticides, refrigerants, lubricants or simply as industrial or hygienic household products. The presence of chlorine atoms on such molecules renders them toxic for microorganisms, insects and pests, and in some cases for human beings. The effectiveness of such compounds as insecticides or bacteriocidal agents prompted the chemical industry to manufacture varied types of the compounds and use them for enhanced agricultural productivity, various industrial processes and as health and beauty aids. The number of naturally-occurring compounds having carbon-chlorine bonds is very limited, so that microorganisms in nature have a limited capability to act upon all the complex chlorinated compounds synthesized by man[1]. This has resulted in the persistence of these compounds and because such compounds have been widely disseminated in nature, they have created enormous problems of toxic chemical pollution, as exemplified by the episodes in the Love Canal area, the pollution in the James River or the accidental release of extremely toxic dioxins in Seveso, Italy[2].
Although over the years, microorganisms have been reported to slowly biodegrade various chlorinated compounds by co-oxidative metabolism[3], there is still no evidence that pure cultures have acquired the ability to biodegrade highly chlorinated compounds. Reports of pure cultures capable of degrading simple mono- or dichloro compounds are now becoming available[4,5]. The purpose of this short article is to review the genetic

basis of the biodegradation of simple chlorinated aromatic compounds such as 4-chlorobiphenyl (pCB) or 3-, 4- or 3,5-dichloro-
benzoic acids by pure cultures, and examine the roleof plasmids
in extending the range of chlorinated substrates that can be
consumed by various bacterial genera.

Metabolism of Simple Chlorinated Aromatic Compounds by Pure Cultures

Although mixed cultures have long been known to slowly
biodegrade a variety of chlorinated compounds, there are
reports of pure cultures capable of dissimilating simple
chlorinated compounds. For example, pCB is known to be
metabolized by Alcaligenes, Acinetobacter, Klebsiella etc to
4-chlorobenzoic acid (4Cba)[6,7]. The Alcaligenes or the
Acinetobacter species can also convert di- or trichlorobi-
phenyls to the respective chlorobenzoic acids. In none of the
cases the pure cultures are known to further breakdown the
chlorobenzoic acids, which therefore accumulate in the medium.
The modes of biodegradation of other chlorinated compounds such
as 4-chloro-phenoxyacetic acid, 2,4-dichlorophenoxyacetic acid
and (2,4-D) 3-chlorobenzoate (3Cba) have been studied by a
number of workers[4,8,9]. Evans et al.[8] have described the
characterization of a pseudomonad that could degrade 4-chloro-
phenoxyacetic acid with the release of chloride ions in the
medium. Based on the accumulation of various intermediates and
their oxidation by resting cell suspensions, these workers
postulated a pathway for the oxidation of 4-chlorophenoxy-
acetate that involves 4-chlorocatechol, β-chloromuconic acid
and maleylacetic acid as intermediates. A similar pathway for
the degradation of chlorobenzoates by Pseudomonas B13 has been
postulated by Schmidt and Knackmuss[10]. In detailed studies
on the enzymes involved in the biodegradation of 3-chloroben-
zoate, Knackmuss and his co-workers[4,10] have defined the
strict specificities of many of these enzymes for chlorinated
substrates and have delineated the major parts of the dissimila-
tory pathways. We have recently demonstrated the ability of a
plasmid-containing 3-chlorobenzoate-positive Pseudomonas species
to utilize maleylacetic acid (Mac)[11]. Some of the mutants,
incapable of utilizing 3Cba were also rendered Mac⁻. Transductional repair of such mutations to 3Cba⁺ simultaneously
rendered them Mac⁺, suggesting that Mac is an intermediate of
3Cba degradation by this Pseudomonas species. Based on the
evidence presented by various workers, a plausible pathway for
the biodegradation of 3Cba is presented in Fig. 1.

Plasmids in the Biodegradation of Chlorinated Compounds

Plasmids specifying biodegradation of several chlorinated
compounds such as pCB, 2,4-D and 3Cba are now known (Table 1),

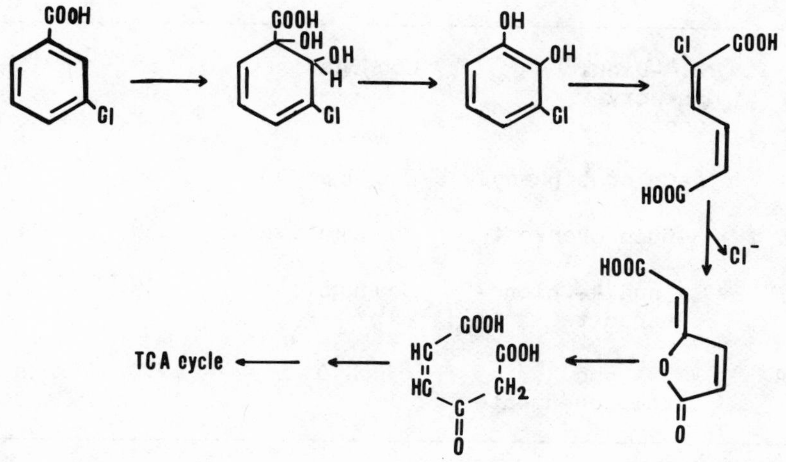

Fig. 1. Proposed pathway for the biodegradation of 3-chloro-benzoate by Pseudomonas species.

While plasmids such as pJP1 and pAC21 are known to encode a partial degradative pathway i.e., allowing conversion of 2,4-D to 2,4-dichlorophenol and 4-chlorobiphenyl to 4-chlorobenzoic acid (4Cba) respectively, pAC25 and pAC27 plasmids encode a complete degradative pathway for the biodegradation of chlorobenzoates with the release of chloride ions in the medium. We have previously reported that pAC25-positive P. putida or P. aeruginosa cells are incapable of utilizing 4Cba[11]. Growth of the pAC25-positive cells in presence of cells harboring the TOL plasmid in a chemostat enriched with 4Cba led to the emergence of cells that could also utilize 4Cba[5]. This observation is analogous to that previously reported by Hartmann et al.[4] that the benzoate oxidase complex induced by 3Cba in Pseudomonas B13 has a stringent substrate specificity so that it does not use 4Cba as a substrate. The presence of the TOL plasmid allows induction of a broad substrate specific benzoate oxidase which can also act on 4Cba with the formation of 4-chlorocatechol. The catechol oxygenase

Table 1. List of plasmids specifying dissimilation of chlorinated compounds

Plasmid	Degradative Pathway	Transmissibility	Size (Mdal)	Reference
pJP1	2,4-Dichloro-phenoxy-acetic acid	Conjugative	58	9
pAC21	4-Chlorobiphenyl	Conjugative	65	7
pAC25	3-Chlorobenzoate	Conjugative	68	11
pAC27	3- and 4-Chloro-benzoate	Conjugative	59	5
pAC29	3-,4- and 3,5-Dichlorobenzoate	N.D.	N.D.	This Manuscript

N.D. - not determined

and subsequent enzymes induced by 3Cba in Pseudomonas B13 can act upon 4-chlorocatechol, leading to its biodegradation. It was therefore anticipated that the pAC25-positive P. putida cells that also acquired the ability to utilize 4Cba due to chemostatic selection in presence of the TOL plasmid would either demonstrate the presence of the TOL plasmid or would have the benzoate oxidase gene(s) recombined with the pAC25 plasmid. Examination of the plasmid profiles of such 4Cba+ strains demonstrated the presence of a single chlorobenzoate plasmid with an average molecular size of 59 million daltons (Mdal). This plasmid is termed pAC27. It is also possible to transfer pAC25 and TOL to P. aeruginosa. These two plasmids are normally unstable in the same cell. Growth of the cells with 3Cba also induces the TOL-specified meta pathway, whereby 3-chlorocatechol derived from 3Cba is partly metabolized by the meta pathway. Metabolism of 3Cba by the meta pathway is believed to generate a chlorinated intermediate that is toxic for the cells. TOL and pAC25 are therefore incompatible due to metabolic reasons. It is, however, possible to isolate single colonies of P. aeruginosa capable of utilizing 4Cba from unstable TOL+ pAC25+ cells. Such 4Cba+ colonies are phenotypically Tol-, but can generate Tol+ revertants at a frequency of nearly 1 x 10^{-8}. Isolation of plasmid DNA from

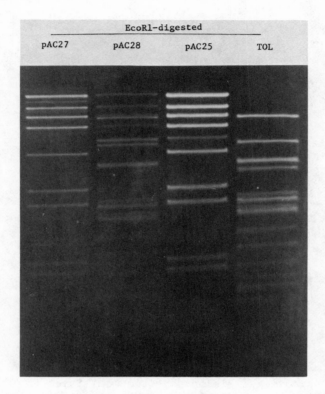

Fig. 2.   Agarose gel electrophoretic mobilities of fragments of
pAC27, pAC28, pAC25 and TOL plasmids on digestion with EcoRI.

such colonies and subsequent EcoRI digestion demonstrates that
both plasmids undergo deletions in order to become compatible in
the 4Cba$^+$ cells (Fig. 2).   The pAC25 plasmid has a 6.4 Mdal
band missing in the EcoRI digest.   This modified plasmid is
termed pAC28.   The fragment missing in pAC28 is different from
the fragment missing in pAC27 obtained by chemostatic selection
in presence of the TOL plasmid (Fig. 2).   The TOL plasmid
demonstrates the absence of a 5.6 Mdal fragment in the EcoRI
digest of the plasmids isolated from the 4Cba$^+$ P. aeruginosa
cells.   Since such 4Cba$^+$ cells are normally Tol$^-$ but can
revert to Tol$^+$ it is clear that the deletion does not span the
structural genes involved in toluate metabolism.

Hartmann et al.[4] have also demonstrated that it is possible
by continuous enrichment of 4-Cba$^+$ Pseudomonas B13 cells with
3,5-dichlorobenzoate to isolate cells that can utilize 3,5-di-

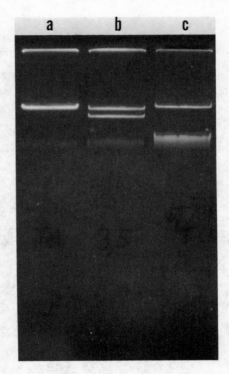

Fig. 3. Agarose gel electrophoretic mobilities of TOL (lane a)
plasmid DNA from 3,5-dichlorobenzoate positive cells (lane b)
and pAC28 (lane c).

chlorobenzoate. We have grown the 4-Cba$^+$ P. aeruginosa cells
in minimal media enriched with 3,5-dichlorobenzoate, and by
continuous subculturing in minimal dichlorobenzoate media have
isolated cells that can utilize this compound as a sole source
of carbon and energy. The profiles of TOL, pAC28 and the
plasmid DNA isolated from 3,5-dichlorobenzoate-positive cells
are shown in Fig. 3. It is interesting that during selection
for the 3,5-dichlorobenzoate character, both the plasmids
(pAC28, TOL) appear to undergo further structural rearrangements to generate the plasmid pAC29.

Genetic Homology Between the Chlorobenzoate (pAC25) and Other
Degradative Plasmids

In order to determine how much homology pAC25 may have with
other hydrocarbon degradative plasmids, we have nick-translated

pAC25 DNA and used it as a probe in hybridization experiments
with EcoRI restriction fragments of degradative plasmids such
as SAL and TOL, and an antibiotic resistance plasmid pAC30
which specifies resistance to tetracycline, carbenicillin and
streptomycin. Both SAL and TOL exhibited considerable homology,
while 3 out of 12 fragments of pAC30 demonstrated some degree

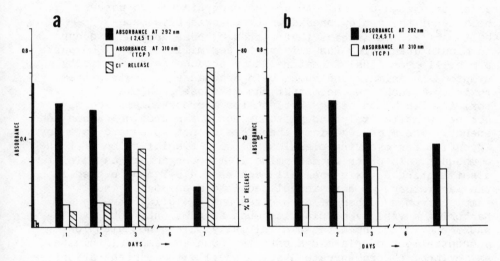

Fig. 4. (a) Growth of mixed cultures with 2,4,5-T as a sole
source of carbon with accumulation of 2,4,5-trichlorophenol
(TCP) and release of chloride; (b) demonstrates loss of 2,4,5-T
and accumulation of TCP during growth of a pure culture
isolated from the chemostat. No chloride release was
demonstrated in the latter case.

of homology. It is thus clear that a plasmid such as pAC25 may
have evolved by recombination of various genetic fragments from
plasmids such as TOL and SAL (and to some extent pAC30) specifying biodegradation of analogous non-chlorinated compounds.
The homology with pAC30 may be in the region of the replication,
maintenance or transfer genes of the plasmids.

Molecular Breeding of Strains for 2,4,5-T Dissimilation

The extensive homology of pAC25 with SAL and TOL, and to a lesser extent with an antibiotic resistance plasmid, appears to indicate that pAC25 may have evolved by recruitment of genes from various plasmids. If it is a general mode of evolution of plasmids, then perhaps it might be possible to allow evolution of degradative plasmids for various toxic chemicals in a continuous culture in the chemostat by supplying a variety of plasmids to microorganisms isolated from toxic waste dump sites. It is known that toxic chemicals such as 2,4,5-T (2,4,5-trichlorophenoxyacetic acid), TCDD (2,3, 7,8-tetrachlorodibenzo-p-dioxin) etc are very persistent in nature because of their slow breakdown by co-oxidative metabolism[12,13]. It appears that although these compounds occur in minute quantities (usually parts per million; for TCDD parts per billion or less) in nature, they produce severe toxicity symptoms in animals and human beings because of their extreme toxicity. Such low concentrations may pose problems of toxicity for human beings but not for microorganisms and may not be quantitatively enough to serve as a source of carbon and energy. The microorganisms therefore do not appear to have any incentive for evolving plasmids allowing dissimilation of these compounds. In order to determine if microorganisms capable of dissimilating a toxic chemical such as 2,4,5-T can be bred in the laboratory, we have inoculated into a chemostat, soil samples from a number of dump sites and P. putida strains harboring a variety of plasmids such as CAM, SAL, TOL, pAC21, pAC25 etc. The chemostat was initially maintained with low concentrations of plasmid substrates such as camphor, toluate, salicylate, chlorobenzoate etc. Gradually the concentrations of plasmid substrates were reduced while that of 2,4,5-T was increased. After about 6 months, the chemostat was run with 2,4,5-T alone (500 µg/ml) as a sole source of carbon. After several weeks with 2,4,5-T as sole carbon source, the medium in the chemostat gradually turned light brown, and an increase in turbidity was visible. Continuous monitoring of the medium demonstrated appreciable loss of 2,4,5-T and release of chloride ions in the reactor medium. This is more clearly seen from the results in Fig. 4a, where an aliquot from the chemostat vessel was inoculated into a minimal 2,4,5-T (500 µg/ml) medium and grown for 7 days. At different intervals, aliquots were taken, diluted and the levels of 2,4,5-T, 2,4,5-trichlorophenol (Tcp) and inorganic chloride were measured. In 7 days, about 72% of the 2,4,5-T was degraded with the release of an equivalent amount of chloride ions. Although initially the Tcp level increased steadily, the level of Tcp fell down considerably after 3 or 4 days. Streaking of the cell suspension on a nutrient agar plate demonstrated the presence of several types of colony morphologies suggesting the presence of a mixed

culture. On streaking on a minimal 2,4,5-T plate, single
colonies grew slowly within the first 3 days, but stopped
growing thereafter. On further examination, they were found to
be capable of converting 2,4,5-T to Tcp, but unable to attack
Tcp any further (Fig. 4b). No chloride release was observed
from 2,4,5-T or Tcp by such cells. The cells were also found
to be capable of producing Tcp from 2,4,5-T when grown with
glutamate.

Concluding Remarks

The need for the presence of the TOL plasmid in extending
the substrate range of the 3Cba degradative plasmid (pAC25) to
include 4Cba and 3,5-dichlorobenzoate, and consequent structural changes of the plasmids giving rise to pAC27, pAC28 and
pAC29 is an interesting example of the interactions of plasmids
in a natural environment for the degradation of novel xenobiotic
compounds. The biochemistry of this phenomenon has previously
been elucidated by Hartmann et al.[4], and the present study
simply delineates the role of plasmids involved in such a
process. The emergence of a mixed culture that can continu-
ously be cultivated indefinitely with 2,4,5-T as a sole source
of carbon reaffirms the utility of chemostats as a means of
selecting specific strains under defined growth conditions, and
additionally points out the important roles played by degradative plasmids in the evolution of new genetic functions. It
would be interesting to find out if continued growth of the
mixed culture with 2,4,5-T will ultimately lead to the emergence
of a single culture capable of total degradation of 2,4,5-T, and
if such a culture would harbor a 2,4,5-T degradative plasmid.
In the event of a positive response for both, plasmid-assisted
molecular breeding of strains under chemostatic selective conditions with specific toxic chemicals will become a powerful tool
in the application of such strains for practical removal of
toxic chemicals from the environment.

REFERENCES

1.   S. Dagley., Pathways for the utilization of organic growth
       substrates, in: "The Bacteria, Vol VI", L.N. Ornston
       and J.R. Sokatch, eds., Academic Press, N.Y. (1978).
2.   F. Cattabeni, A. Cavallaro and G. Galli, "Dioxin", SP
       Medical λ Scientific Books, New York (1978).
3.   M. Alexander, Biodegradation of chemicals of environmental
       concern, Science 211:132 (1981).
4.   J. Hartmann, W. Reineke and H.-J. Knackmuss, Metabolism of
       3-chloro, 4-chloro, and 3,5-dichlorobenzoate by a
       pseudomonad, Appl. Environ. Microbiol. 37:421 (1979).

5.   D.K. Chatterjee and A.M. Chakrabarty, Plasmids in the bio-
     degradation of pCBs and chlorobenzoates, in: "Microbial
     Degradation of Xenobiotics and Racalcitrant Compounds",
     T. Leisinger, A.M. Cook, J. Nuesch and R. Hutter, eds.,
     Academic Press, London (in press).

6.   K. Furakawa, N. Tomizuka and A. Kamibayashi, Effect of
     chlorine substitution on the bacterial metabolism of
     various poly-chlorinated biphenyls, Appl. Environ.
     Microbiol. 38:301 (1979).

7.   P.F. Kamp and A.M. Chakrabarty, Plasmids specifying p-
     chlorobiphenyl degradation in enteric bacteria, in:
     "Plasmids of Medical, Environmental and Commercial
     Importance", K.N. Timmis and A. Puhler, eds.,
     Elsevier/North-Holland Biomedical Press, Amsterdam
     (1979).

8.   W.C. Evans, B.S.W. Smith, P. Moss and H.N. Fernley,
     Bacterial metabolism of 4-chlorophenoxyacetate,
     Biochem. J. 122:509 (1971).

9.   P.R. Fisher, J. Appleton and J.M. Pemberton, Isolation and
     characterization of the pesticide-degrading plasmid
     pJP1 from Alcaligenes paradoxus, J. Bacteriol. 135:798
     (1978).

10. E. Schmidt and H.J. Knackmuss, Chemical structure and bio-
     degradability of halogenated aromatic compounds,
     Biochem J. 192:339 (1980).

11. D.K. Chatterjee, S.T. Kellogg, S. Hamada, and A.M.
     Chakrabarty, A plasmid specifying total degradation of
     3-chlorobenzoate by a modified ortho pathway, J.
     Bacteriol. (in press).

12. A. Rosenberg and M. Alexander, 2,4,5-Trichlorophenoxy-
     acetic acid (2,4,5-T) decomposition in tropical soil
     and its cometabolism by bacteria in vitro, J. Agric.
     Food Chem. 28:705 (1980).

13. P.C. Kearney, E.A. Woolson and C.P. Ellington, Jr., Per-
     sistence and metabolism of chlorodioxins in soils, Env.
     Science and Tech. 6:1017 (1972).

Acknowledgements

     This investigation was supported by grants from the
National Science Foundation (PCM79-17526 and PFR79-05499) and
under a contract with the Environmental Protection Agency
(68-03-2936).

ANTIBIOTIC RESISTANCE OF GRAM NEGATIVE BACTERIA IN MEXICO:

RELATIONSHIP TO DRUG CONSUMPTION

Yankel M. Kupersztoch-Portnoy

Departamento de Genética y Biologia Molecular, Centro
de Investigación y de Estudios Avanzados del I.P.N.
Apartado Postal 14-740, México 14, D.F. México

The selection of bacterial strains resistant to antibiotics
is closely linked to the usage of antimicrobial agents[1,2,3]. In
Japan during 1951, six years after the clinical introduction of
sulfanilamide, approximately 80% of the strains of Shigella
studied were found resistant to it, whereas in 1949 only 10% were
resistant. Similarly, increases in the incidence of drug resistant
microorganisms have been reported in Great Britain[4], the United
States[5], the Netherlands[6] and other countries[1,7]. In addition to
the increase in the percentage of strains resistant to individual
antibiotics, multiple resistant strains have been isolated with
greater frequency as the age of antibiotherapy grows older[4,7,8,9].
In Mexico, Olarte and co-workers[10,11] have reported the incidence
of resistance to antibiotics in strains of Shigella, Salmonella
and enteropathogenic E. coli and they have noted an increase in the
frequency of multiple resistant strains.

We present here the antibiotic resistance patterns of entero-
toxigentic E. coli strains (Ent ST+ and Ent LT+) isolated during
1976-1977 (H. Stieglitz, R. Fonseca, J. Olarte, and Y.M.
Kupersztoch-Portnoy, unpublished); the comparison of the antibiotic
resistance patterns of strains of Salmonella and Shigella isolated
during 1978-1979 (R. Fonseca, P. Mendoza, S. Garcia, V. Vázquez,
and Y.M. Kupersztoch-Portnoy, unpublished); and the antibiotic
resistance of Proteus mirabilis, indole positive Proteus, E. coli,
and Salmonella isolated in the city of Toluca (Mexico) and its
relationship to the consumption of antibiotics in Mexico (R. Lara,
J. Silva, and Y.M. Kupersztoch-Portnoy, unpublished).

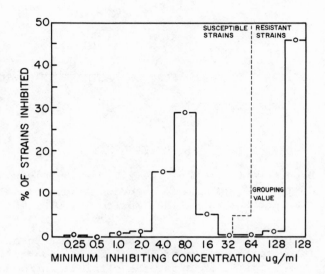

Fig. 1. Discrimination between drug sensitive and drug resistant
         bacteria. The lowest point between peaks is taken as the
         grouping value. In all the determinations(30 strains per
         test) E. coli ATCC10536 and Klebsiella pneumoniae ATCC10031
         were included. For Su, Tm, and Tm-X (sulfa-trimethoprim
         19:1) Wellcotest Sensitivity Test Agar was used. The data
         shown are from 252 strains of Salmonella tested for ampi-
         cillin susceptibility. As more strains were tested (1419
         in total), the most frequent value changed to 4µg/ml.

         The determination of the minimal inhibiting concentration
(mic) was done by the agar dilution method according to the recom-
mendation of the ICS Report[12]. The criterion we used to distinguish
drug sensitive from drug resistant microorganisms groups bacteria
from the same species according to the frequency distribution of
their mics[13](Fig. 1). It avoids the classification of a strain
as sensitive or resistant considering only preestablished values,
regardless of both the statistical fluctuation in a bacterial
population and the individual differences in implementation of the
same methodology. Table 1 shows a comparison of the values used by

Table 1. Antimicrobial drug resistance in Salmonella and Shigella

| | Grouping criterion | | | | | | ICS criterion | | |
| | Salmonella[1] | | | Shigella[2] | | | | | |
Drug	Mode of Sensitive Strains (µg/ml)	Grouping Value (µg/ml)	% Resistant Strains	Mode of Sensitive Strains	Grouping Value (µg/ml)	% Resistant Strains	Resistant Strains (µg/ml)	Resistant Strains Salmonella	Resistant Strains Shigella
Ap	4	32	47	4	32	20	32	47	20
Cb	4	128	46	2	64	18	32	46	20
Ce	4	32	40	8	64	2	32	40	5
Cm	8	64	34	8	64	16	25	35	18
Gm	1	16	26	2	16	0.34	6	27	1
Km	2	32	43	4	32	9.5	25	44	12
Nx	4	32	3	1	8	1	32	3	1
Fn	32	256	6	8	256	2	100	18	4
Rif	16	256	1	16	128	0			
Sm	8	64	45	8	32	60	15	67	69
Su	256	512	53	8	32	91	350	63	79
Tc	2	32	31	1	8	71	12	36	71
Tm	0.125	4	1.5	0.125	2	1.5			
Tm-X	2	64	0.35	2	32	0.6	200	0.35	0.5

[1] 1419 independently isolated strains were used for the calculations.
[2] 319 independently isolated strains were used for the calculations.

the grouping method and the ICS criterion to distinguish drug sensitive and drug resistant <u>Salmonella</u> and <u>Shigella</u>, and also the
percent of resistant strains with both methods. Even though the
values to differentiate drug resistant from drug susceptible
microorganisms show differences using the two criteria, the overall percent of resistant strains is similar in the majority of
cases. However if we were to take 15μg/ml for streptomycin in the
case of <u>Salmonella</u>, we would have had to split a clearly bimodal
curve (data not shown) artificially near the mode of the sensitive
population; for the clinical distinction of resistant bacteria,
the serum concentration of the drug is unquestionably of vital
importance, but it is not in the intrinsic properties of a genus or
species of bacteria. I feel that the grouping value should be used
in antibiotic resistance studies but not in the clinical ones.

Table 2 shows a remarkable difference in the percent of resistant strains isolated in hospitalized patients (no antibiotherapy
was given in the hospital before the sample was taken) and from
ambulatory patients. These data suggest that before the patient

Table 2. Comparison of the resistance to antimicrobial agents
between <u>Salmonella</u> strains isolated in hospitals and
in private laboratories.

Antimicrobial agent	Percent of resistant strains	
	Hospitals	Laboratories
Ap	73.95	11.42
Cb	70.86	9.49
Ce	60.98	8.08
Cm	34.25	8.78
Fn	1	0
Gm	42.2	2.63
Km	53.55	8.08
Nx	2	0
Rif	0	0
Sm	63.88	10.19
Su	89.44	95.26
Tc	42.32	16.13
Tm	2.28	2.63
Tm-X	0.38	2.63

50.2% and 26.8% of the <u>Salmonella</u> isolated from hospitals and
private laboratories respectively were serotyped as typhimurium.

was referred to the hospital he had had antibiotic treatment and/or that the strains were to begin with resistant (virulent) and the patient had to be hospitalized for proper treatment. The fact that 50.2% of the <u>Salmonella</u> isolated in hospitals were <u>S. typhimurium</u> as compared to 26.8% of the private laboratories favors the latter alternative but does not rule out the former. There is a notoriously high level of Su^r strains in both populations.

Table 3. Multiresistance in strains of <u>Salmonella</u> and <u>Shigella</u>

Type of resistance	Number of strains (%)		Most frequent pattern of resistance	Number of strains with the most frequent pattern (%)	
	Shigella	Salmonella		Shigella	Salmonella
11	0	5(0.72)	ApCbCeCm GmKmFnSm SuTcSi	0	5(100)
10	0	48(6.91)	ApCbCeCmGm KmSmSuTcSi	0	40(83)
9	0	59(8.49)	ApCbCeCmGmKm SmSuSi	0	27(46)
8	0	35(5.04)	ApCbCeCmGmKmSmSu	0	9(27.7)
7	·2(1.035)	45(6.43)	ApCbCmKmSmSuTc	0	13(28.9)
6	5(2.56)	34(4.89)	ApCbCeKmSmSu ApCbCmKmSmSi·	0 5(100)	10(29.4) 2(5.88)
5	11(5.64)	34(4.89)	CmKmSmSuTc ApCbKmSmSu	0 3(27.3)	13(38.24) 7(20.6)
4	16(8.2)	56(8.06)	CmSmSuTc ApCbSmSu	2(12.5) 6(37.5)	13(23.2) 4(7.1)
3	23(11.8)	43(6.2)	ApCbKm CmSmSu	0 13(56.5)	13(30) 0
2	71(36.4)	41(5.9)	SmSu	57(80.3)	8(19.5)
1	40(20.5)	83(11.9)	Su	29(72.5)	41(49.4)

Table 3 shows the multiple drug resistance of 697 strains of
Salmonella and 195 strains of Shigella (before the collection was
completed). It can be seen that 20.5% of the strains of Salmonella
were resistant to eight or more antibiotics while no Shigella was
found resistant to more than seven antibiotics; it is not clear as
to why this difference exists among the two genera. It also shows
that the two general do not share the most frequent pattern; i.e.
while 13 Salmonella strains were found resistant to ApCbKm (30%
of the 43 strains found resistant to three antibiotics), in Shigella,
the prevailing group of resistance to three drugs was CmSmSu (56.5%).
These results may be taken to indicate different evolutionary
patterns in the emergence of multiple drug resistance among the
two genera.

We have studied the antibiotic resistance of enterotoxigenic
LT^+ and ST^+ E. coli strains isolated during 1976-1977. As seen
in Table 4, not one of the 50 strains was susceptible to the 14
antimicrobial agents tested. 2% were resistant to one antibiotic
and the rest were multiple drug resistant. It is noticeable that
35 of the 50 enterotoxigenic strains were Tc^r; it is unlikely that
the prevention of travelers diarrhea due to enterotoxigenic E. coli
will be effective by deoxycycline[18] in a population of bacteria
that is 70% resistant to the drug. Thus, on top of the ecological
implications of the prophylactic use of antibiotics and the self-
limiting nature of diarrheal disease caused by enterotoxigenic
E. coli, the high percentage of resistant bacteria should dis-
courage the use of antibiotics in the prevention of the disease.

More detailed studies have been performed on the genetic and
physical linkage of antibiotic resistance and Ent ST^+. We have
shown that a naturally occurring single plasmid is responsible
for Ap^r and Ent ST^{+17} and that the same plasmid is widely distributed in the population studied (H. Stieglitz et al., this
volume).

An attempt to correlate the incidence of drug resistant
enterobacteria and the national consumption of antibiotics was
done in a study in the city of Toluca. From the cultures of each
case of diarrhea (500 in total) the prevailing microorganisms and/
or well-characterized bacterial pathogens were isolated; not more
than one of each genus was isolated from each case. The grouping
values were determined for each gera or species and the percentage
of resistant strains is shown in Table 5. The national consumption of these drugs[19] (Grunner, personal communication) is indicated in the same table; it includes the human, veterinary, and
agricultural consumption. It is clearly seen that the less
effective antibiotics are the most widely consumed. Thus, as
shown elsewhere[20,21], the appearance of antibiotic resistant
strains in bacteria is closely linked to the use of antimicrobial
agents.

Table 4. Resistance to antibiotics in enterotoxigenic Escherichia coli strains.

LT[+] Strains[1]	Antibiotic resistance	ST[+] Strains[2]	Antibiotic resistance
3IEC-1 and 2	ApCmKmSmSuTc	23IEC-4	ApCbSmSuTc
31IEC-5	ApCeCmKmSmSuTc	*40IEC-2	ApCbSmSuTc
*4IEC-1, 2 and 3	ApCmKmSmSuTc	*40IEC-3	CmSuTc
8IEC-5	CmSmSuTc	*40IEC-4	ApCbSuTc
10IEC-1	ApCbCmKmSmSuTc	*40IEC-5	ApSuTc
16IEC-2	ApCbCeCmKmSuTc	81IEC-3	ApCbSmSuTc
*18IEC-2	CmKmSuTc	*93IEC-3	ApCbSmSuTc
31IEC-5	ApCbCmSuTc	98IEC-1	Cm
67IEC-5	ApCbCmKmSuTc	101IEC-3 and 4	ApCmSmSuTc
78IEC-3	ApCbCmKmSuTc	102IEC-1 and 2	ApCbCmKm
*80IEC-1	ApCbCmKmSmSuTc	*108IEC-2	ApCbKmSmSu
*80IEC-2	ApCbCeSuTc	109IEC-3	SmSu
88IEC-4	ApCbCmKmSuTc	*111IEC-3	ApCbCmKmSu
*96IEC-2	ApCbCmKmSuTc	*113IEC-1	ApCbCmKmSmSuTc
*99IEC-3,4 and 5	ApCbSmSuTc		SuTc
101IEC-1	CmSuTc	*116IEC-2	SmTc
101IEC-2	CmSmSuTc	123IEC-2	ApCbCeTc
*104IEC-2	ApCbCeCmSuTc	123IEC-3	ApCbSmSuTc
104IEC-3	ApCbCeCmSu		
104IEC-4	ApCbCmTc		
110IEC-1	SuTc		
*113IEC-1 and 2	ApCbCeCmKmSmSuTc		
*113IEC-4	ApCbCeCmKmGmSmSuTc		
*113IEC-5	ApCbCmKmSmSuTc		
117IEC-4			

[1]
LT enterotoxin was determined initially by the adrenal cell assay as described by Sack[14], and confirmed in the rabbit ileum loop assay[15].

[2]
ST enterotoxin was determined initially by the suckling mice assay; positive cultures were then confirmed by the rabbit ileum loop assay[15].

*Patients that had medication before admission to the hospital.

Table 5.   Relation between antibiotic consumption and resistant
           strains

Antibiotic	Mexican consumption 1977 (tons)	Resistant strains (%)*
Tc	134	86.5
Su	111	70.8
Ap	101	63.7
Cb	0.3	55.0
Sm	133**	54.1
Ce	15	36.1
Km	133**	35.6
Cm	85	45.2
Fn	–	19.7
Nx	20	9.6
Rif	5	4.0
Tm	1.33	0.3
Gm	0.55	2.2

*Based on total number of strains studied: 295 E. coli, 198
Proteus mirabilis, 63 indole positive Proteus and 39 Salmonella

**Total consumption of Sm, Km, and neomycin.

References

1. Mitsuhashi, S. 1971. Epidemiology of Bacterial Drug Resistance
   in: "Transferable Drug Resistance Factor R," S. Mitsuhashi,
   ed., University Park Press. Baltimore
2. WHO Technical Report Series No. 624. 1978. Surveillance for
   the Prevention and Control of Health Hazards due to Antibiotic-resistant Enterobacteria. Report of a WHO Meeting,
   Geneva.
3. Swann, M. M. (Chairman). 1979. Report of the Joint Committee
   on the Use of Antibiotics in Animal Husbandry and Veterinary
   Medicine. H.M. Stationery Office. London.
4. Anderson, E. S. 1968. Ann. Rev. Microbiol. 22:131-180.
5. Finland, M. 1971. Ann. N. Y. Acad. Sci. 182:5-20.
6. Manten, A., P.A.M. Guinee, E.H. Kampelmacher and C.E. Voodg.
   1971. WHO Bulletin 45:8593.
7. Falkow, S. 1971. "Infectious Multiple Drug Resistance."
   Pion Limited. London.
8. Mitsuhashi, S. 1969. J. Infect. Dis. 199:89-100.
9. Dulaney, E.L. and A.L. Laskin (eds.). 1971. "The Problems
   of Durg Resistant Pathogenic Bacteria." Ann. N.Y. Acad.
   Sci. 182.
10. Olarte, J. and J.A. de la Torre. 1959. Amer. J. Trop. Med.
    Hyg. 8:324-326.

11. Olarte, J. and E. Galindo. 1973. Gaceta Médica México 105: 123-133.

12. Ericsson, H.M. and S.C. Sherris. 1971. Acta Pathol. Microbiol. Scand. Sect. B suppl. 217.

13. Otaya, H. 1974. J. Antibiotics 27:686-695.

14. Sack, D.A. and R. Bradley Sack. 1975. Infect. Immun. 11: 334-336.

15. Evans, D.G., D.J. Evans, Jr., and N.F. Pierce. 1973. Infect. Immun. 7:873-880.

16. Dean, A.G., Y.C. Ching, R.G. Williams and L.B. Harden. 1972. J. Infect. Dis. 125:405-411

17. Stieglitz, H., R. Fonseca, J. Olarte, and Y.M. Kupersztoch-Portnoy. 1980. Infect Immun. 30:617-620.

18. Sack, D.A., D.C. Kaminsky, R.B. Sack, J.M. Itotia, R.R. Arthur, A.Z. Kapikian, F. Ørskov, and I. Ørskov. 1978. N. Engl. J. Med. 298:758.

19. Fernández Viaña F. 1979. La Industria Farmacéutica en México. Seminario Regional Sobre Aplicaciones Industriales de la Microbiología en la Industria Farmacéutica. UMICO. La Habana (Cuba). Distribución limitada.

20. Ayliffe, G.A.J. 1976. In:"Current Antibiotic Therapy," A.M. Geddes and J.D. Williams, eds., Churchill/Livingstone, London. pp. 53-60.

21. Mouton, R.P., I.H.Glerum, and A.C. Van Loenen. 1976. J. Antimicrob. Chemother. 2:9-19.

Acknowledgements

Enterotoxin Studies were supported in part by grants 026, 1264,790154 from Programa Nacional Indicativo de Salud-Concejo Nacional de Ciencia Y Techologia.

Antibiotic Resistance Studies in Salmonella and Shigella by a donation of the following laboratories:
Burrows-Wellcome de Mexico, Cor S.A., Le Petit
Scheramex

The Studies in the City of Toluca by a grant of the government of the State of Mexico.

PLASMID MEDIATED AMPICILLIN RESISTANCE IN A STRAIN OF

HAEMOPHILUS PLEUROPNEUMONIAE ISOLATED FROM SWINE

Dwight C. Hirsh,[1] Lori M. Assaf,[1] and Melissa C. Libal[2]

[1]Deptartment of Veterinary Microbiology, School of
Veterinary Medicine, University of California, Davis, CA
95616/[2]Animal Disease Research and Diagnostic Laboratory
South Dakota State University, Brookings, SD 57007

INTRODUCTION

Haemophilus pleuropneumonia is a hemolytic, nicotinamide
adenine dinucleotide requiring member of the genus Haemophilus. H.
pleuropneumoniae produces lobar pneumonia with fibrinous pleuritis
in swine. The disease has high morbidity and, when introduced into
highly susceptible animals, high mortality. When the microorganism
becomes bacteremic, meningitis and arthritis may result. Young,
rapidly growing pigs seem to be the most susceptible, though any age
pig may contract the disease. The source of H. pleuropneumoniae in
the environment is the respiratory tracts of affected as well as
recovered asymptomatic pigs (1,2).

Disease produced by H. pleuropneumoniae was first recognized in
the 1960s following the independent isolation of the agent from
infected tissue in Great Britain, California, Argentina, and
Switzerland (1,3-6). Following these initial reports, the agent has
been shown to be responsible for diseases in swine herds in Europe,
Scandanavia, Australia, and Canada (7-11).

Though infrequently reported, the susceptibility of the
isolates obtained from outbreaks occurring through 1970, were found
to be susceptible to antimicrobial agents, including penicillin,
kanamycin, tetracycline, and chloramphenicol. There is disagreement
regarding streptomycin and the sulphonamides, some reports indicate
susceptibility others, resistance (4,6,9,10).

In 1980, most of the isolates of H. pleuropneumoniae possessed
resistance to streptomycin and the sulphonamides (Libal MC: Personal

communication). An isolate from one particular outbreak, involving
100 pound feeder pigs, demonstrated resistance not only to
streptomycin and the sulphonamides, but to ampicillin as well. This
report presents preliminary data concerning this isolate. For
comparative purposes, data concerning an ampicillin susceptible, but
streptomycin and sulphonamide resistant isolate obtained during this
period of time is also presented.

MATERIALS AND METHODS

Bacterial strains: Haemophilus pleuropneumoniae strain SD-1B
and SD-2A were isolated from the lungs of swine that had died from
porcine pleuropneumonia. Haemophilus pleuropneumoniae strain M26
was a plasmid-less strain of serovar 4 obtained from E. L.
Biberstein, University of California, Davis, California.

Media and growth conditions: Haemophilus cultures were grown
in brain heart infusion broth or agar supplimented with 1 µg NAD/ml.
All incubations were performed at 37°C in an atmosphere of 10% CO_2
and air.

Susceptibility testing: An agar dilution method was used for
all isolates (12).

Preparation of DNA: Bacteria were grown to late logarithmic
phase in NAD supplemented brain heart infusion broth. The cells
were harvested by centrifugation and lysed by Triton X-100 (13).
Covalently closed circular plasmid DNA was purified by isopycnic
centrifugation in a cesium chloride-ethidium bromide gradient (14).
The final density was adjusted to 1.6199 g/cm^3 (refractive index,
1.3920), and the solution was centrifuged for 48 hours at 15°C and
34,000 rpm in a Beckman type 40 rotor.

DNA bands in the gradients were located with a black-light lamp
(UVS-11, Ultraviolet Products, Inc., San Gabriel, CA). Plasmid DNA
was removed by puncturing the side of the gradient tube with a 18-
gauge needle attached to a syringe.

Transformation: The transformation method was that described
by Cohen et al (15). Following transformation, the mixture of cells
and DNA was diluted 1:10 in NAD supplemented L-broth and incubated
for 6h. When ampicillin resistant transformants were desired, 15 µg
of ampicillin per ml were added prior to overnight incubation.
Following overnight incubation, transformants were selected by
plating on chocholate agar containing ampicillin (15 µg/ml) or
streptomycin (25 µg/ml).

Agarose gel electrophoresis: Vertical gel electrophoresis was
performed using the method of Meyers et al (16).

Beta-lactamase measurement: Three 100 X 15 mm petri plates
containing chocolate agar were flooded with an overnight broth
culture of H. pleuropneumoniae. Thirty minutes later, excess
culture fluid was removed, and the plates incubated for 18-24h at
37°C under an atmosphere of 10% CO_2 and air. The growth of the
organisms on the surface of these plates was removed by gentle
washing with 25 mM phosphate buffer, pH 7.0 (3 mls per plate). The
cells were pelleted by centrifugation (approximately 10,000 xg, 15
min, 2°C). The pellets were resuspended in 5 ml of 25 mM phosphate
buffer, pH 7.0. The cells were sonicated (setting 35 using a
microprobe, Biosonik III, Bronwill Scientific, Rochester, NY) three
times. The suspension was cooled in ice for 2 min between each
sonication. Following sonication, the suspension was spun (20,000
xg, 15 min, 2°C) and the supernatant saved and assayed for
β-lactamase activity.

The method used for the determination of β-lactamase activity
was the hydroxylamine assay (17). Activity (decrease in substrate
in μ moles/min) of the sonicate supernatants against penicillin G
was taken as 100.

RESULTS

The susceptibility of the isolates is shown in Table 1.

Agarose gel electrophoresis of DNA isolated following
CsCl-ethidium bromide centrifugation is shown in Figure 1, lanes A
and B. Two plasmids are seen, one of molecular mass 3.5 MDal, the
other 2.3.

Transformation of H. pleuropneumoniae M62 with purified plasmid
DNA gave transformants resistant to SmSu and to ApSu (Table 2).
Agarose gel electrophoresis of DNA obtained from transformed H.
pleuropneumoniae M62 (Figure 1, lanes C through E) shows that the
plasmid (pVM105) of molecular mass 3.5 MDal codes for resistance to
ApSu, whereas the other of mass 2.3 Mdal (pVM104, pVM106) code for
resistance to SmSu.

Table 1 Susceptibility of Haemophilus pleuropneumoniae
        isolated from swine.

Isolate	Minimal inhibitory concn (μg/ml)								
	Ap	Pc	Tc	Su	Sm	Km	Gm	Cp	Cm
SD-1	32	32	16	256	128	2	0.5	1	0.5
SD-2	<0.25	0.5	8	2048	>128	16	8	<0.25	0.5

Ap = ampicillin; Pc = penicillin G; Tc = tetracycline;
Su = sulfadiazine; Sm = streptomycin; Km = kanamycin;
Gm = gentamicin; Cp = cephalothin; Cm = chloramphenicol

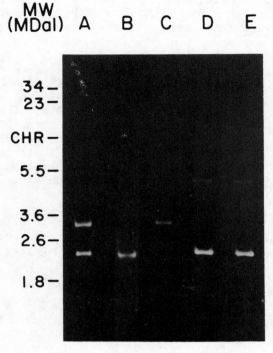

Figure 1. Agarose gel electrophoresis of plasmid DNA obtained from
Haemophilus pleuropneumoniae. Lane A: SD-1 (ApSmSu), B:
SD-2 (SmSu), C: M62 (pVM105, ApSu), D: M62 (pVM 104;
SmSu), E: M62 (pVM 106; SmSu).

Table 2.   Susceptibility of transformed _Haemophilus pleuropneumoniae_
strain M62.

Strain of _H. pleuropneumoniae_	Minimal inhibitory concentration (µg/ml)		
	Ap	Sm	Su
SD-1	32	128	256
SD-2	<0.25	>128	2048
M62(pVM105)	>128	16	>2048
M62(pVM104)	<0.25	>128	>2048
M62(pVM106)	<0.25	>128	>2048
M62	<0.25	8	<100

The activity of sonicate supernatants against various
penicillins used as substrates is shown in Table 3.   The substrate
profile is consistent with a TEM type β-lactamase.

Table 3. Relative rates of hydrolysis of various penicillin substrates by sonicates of Haemophilus pleuropneumoniae

Strain of H. pleuropneumoniae	Substrate				
	Penicillin G	Ampicillin	Oxacillin	Cephalothin	
M62(pVM105)	100*	149	0	0–27	
M62(pVM104)	0	–	–	–	

*Activity, μ moles/minute, against penicillin G arbitrarily set at 100

DISCUSSION

We have presented evidence that indicates that the genes responsible for resistance to ampicillin, streptomycin, and the sulphonamides in H. pleuropneumoniae strain SD-1 are located on two small molecular weight plasmids, pVM105 (3.5 MDal) coding for ApSu resistance and pVM104 (2.3 MDal) coding for SmSu. The genes responsible for SmSu resistance in H. pleuropneumoniae strain SD-2 appear to be located on the small molecular weight plasmid pVM106 (2.3 MDal).

The somewhat sudden acquisition of these resistance determinants is not surprising. Almost all swine in the midwestern United States are fed feed supplemented with antimicrobials. The most common additive contains a mixture of chlortetracycline (100 gms/ton), sulphonamides (100) and penicillin (50).

The genetic basis for the acquisition of resistance determinants is purely speculative. We hypothesize, as was done in the case of resistance in Neisseria gonorrhoeae and H. influenzae, that SmSu resistance genes were acquired from without, possibly from members of the family Enterobacteriaceae (13,18). These genes became associated with a small resident plasmid already possessed by H. pleuropneumoniae. On the other hand, the plasmid with SmSu resistance markers may have already been in an occasional strain of H. pleuropneumoniae. At first rare, these SmSu resistant strains were selected gradually by the antimicrobics used in animal husbandry.

Ampicillin resistance genes were shown to code for a TEM type β-lactamase. This type of β-lactamase is the most common in members of the family Enterobacteriaceae and is the type seen in H. influenzae and Neisseria gonorrhoeae (13,18,19). The data suggest that Ap resistance may have occurred because of the acquisition of an Ap transposon by a SmSu resistant H. pleuropneumoniae. This element could have inserted into the Sm resistant genes found on the 2.3 MDal plasmid yielding an ApSu phenotype with a higher molecular weight (20,21). An explanation for the disparity of the molecular weight between TnA (3 MDal) and the increase in molecular weight of pVM105 relative to pVM104 is not readily apparent.

REFERENCES

1. Biberstein, EL, Cameron HS. Annu. Rev. Microbiol. 15: 93-118, 1961.
2. Kilan M, Nicolet J, Biberstein EL. Int. J. Syst. Bacteriol. 28: 20-26, 1978.
3. Matthews PRJ, Pattison IH. J. Comp. Pathol. 71: 44-52, 1961.
4. Olander HJ. Ph.D. Thesis, University of California, Davis, 1963.
5. Shope RE. J. Exp. Med. 119: 357-368, 1964.

6. Nicolet J. Pathol. Microbiol. 31: 215–225, 1968.
7. Radostits OM, Ruhnke HL, Losos GJ. Can. Vet. J. 4: 265–270, 1963.
8. Nielsen R. Nord. Veterinaermed. 22: 240–245, 1970.
9. Schiefer B, Moffatt RE, Greenfield J, Agar JL, Majka JA. Can. J. Comp. Med. 38: 99–104, 1974.
10. Schiefer B, Greenfield J. Can. J. Comp. Med. 38: 105–110, 1974.
11. Mylrea PJ, Fraser G, MacQueen P, Lambourne DA. Aust. Vet. J. 70: 255–259, 1974.
12. Washington JA, Barry AL. "Manual of Clinical Microbiology", EH Lennette, EH Spaulding, JP Truant, eds., American Society for Microbiology, Washington, DC (1974) pp. 410–417, 1974.
13. Elwell LP, DeGraaff J, Seibert D, Falkow S. Infect. Immun. 12: 404–410, 1975.
14. Guerry PJ, vanEmbden J, Falkow S. J. Bacteriol. 117: 619–630, 1974
15. Cohen SN, Chang ACY, Hsu L. Proc. Natl. Acad. Sci. 69: 2110–2114, 1972.
16. Meyers J, Sanchez D, Elwell LP, Falkow S. J. Bacteriol. 127: 1529–1537, 1976.
17. Sykes RB, Matthew M. "Beta Lactamases", JMT Hamilton-Miller, JT Smith, eds., Academic Press, New York (1979) pp. 17–49.
18. Elwell LP, Roberts M, Mayer LW, Falkow S. Antimicrob. Agents Chemother. 11: 528–533, 1977.
19. Laufs R, Kaulfers PM. J. Gen. Microbiol. 103-277–286, 1977.
20. Heffron F, Rubers C, Falkow S. Proc. Nat. Acad. Sci. 72: 3623–3627, 1975.
21. Heffron F, Rubens C, Falkow S. "DNA: Insertion Elements, Plasmids, and Episomes", AI Bukhari, JA Shapiro, SL Adhya, eds., Cold Spring Harbor Laboratory, New York (1977) pp. 151–160.

R PLASMIDS IN PATHOGENIC ENTEROBACTERIACEAE FROM CALVES

John F. Timoney

Department of Microbiology
N.Y. State College of Veterinary Medicine
Cornell University, Ithaca, N.Y.   14853

INTRODUCTION

Pressure for selection of antibiotic resistant bacteria is greater in intensive calf raising than in any other livestock raising operation. The newborn calf is particularly vulnerable to enteric infections because it is often colostrum deprived, transported long distances without food, mixed with calves from other sources and therefore simultaneously stressed and exposed to a variety of pathogenic strains to which it may have no immunity. The crowded nature of the intensive rearing environment further facilitates spread of infection and favors accelerated feco-oral transfer of enteric pathogens in the group.

Antibiotics are administered in great quantity to minimize the effects of these infections and not surprisingly, have resulted in the emergence of resistant populations of Salmonella typhimurium and Escherichia coli (1, 2, 3). In at least two instances, clones of S. typhimurium selected in this way have spread into the human population (4, 5). Heavy antibiotic usage as described also increases the probability of novel recombinant plasmids. One instance of this was an unusually large inc Hl plasmid carrying a lac gene as well as resistance to antibiotics including chloramphenicol that occurred in a S. typhimurium strain from calves. This strain caused a mortality of 50% in a group of 320 calves in a veal unit (6). The ability to utilize lactose in the milk replacer apparently allowed the salmonella strain to rapidly attain lethal numbers. The combination of lactose positivity and multiresistance was obviously a formidable problem in respect of therapy, diagnosis and pathogenicity.

Intensive calf raising is therefore a useful model for study of untoward effects of excessive use of antibiotics. In this contribution I shall examine antibiotic resistance in S. typhimurium and enteropathogenic E. coli from calves in N.Y. State in an attempt to elucidate some of the factors that underlie the responses of these two populations of enteric pathogens to heavy antibiotic selection pressure.

Antibiotic Resistance in S. typhimurium from Calves

Since the early 1970's, strains of S. typhimurium from calves in the N. E. United States have exhibited a frequency of resistance to tetracycline, streptomycin and kanamycin that is virtually 100% (Table 1). Only 5% of strains were sensitive to the commonly used antibiotics. Since 1973, when ampicillin was approved for use in food producing animals, resistance to this antibiotic has also increased greatly in frequency (Fig. 1), a situation similar to that observed earlier in strains of S. typhimurium from calves in England in the 1960's (4). In the latter instance spread of resistant strains into the human population was noted. A similar spread has not apparently occurred in N.Y. (2). Although chloramphenicol is not approved for use in food-producing animals in the United States, circumstantial evidence for its use in calves is evident from Table 1 where 5% of calf strains were resistant.

When the frequency of antibiotic resistance in S. typhimurium strains from calves is compared with that of strains from other animals the effect of the greater selection pressure in calves is clearly seen (Table 1). About one third of strains from other animals were antibiotic sensitive and the frequency of resistance to kanamycin, streptomycin and tetracycline, although high, was less than half that present in calves. The high frequency of resistance to ampicillin in horses, dogs and cats probably reflects heavy therapeutic use.

Table 1. Antibiotic Resistances of S. typhimurium and Enteropathogenic E. coli from Calves Compared with the Resistances of S. typhimurium from Other Domestic Animals (N.Y. 1973-78).

	% Resistant		
	Calves		Other Domestic Animals
	S. typhimurium	E. coli	S. typhimurium
Antibiotic	(146)	(115)	(153)
Ampicillin	39	80	33
Chloramphenicol	5	31	3
Kanamycin	88	94	41
Streptomycin	97	98	47
Tetracycline	93	97	39
Sensitive	4	0	33

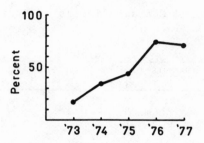

Fig. 1 Increase in frequency of ampicillin resistance in strains
of S. typhimurium from N.Y. calves from 1973-77.

Antibiotic Resistance in Enteropathogenic E. coli from Calves

Enteropathogenic E. coli exhibit an even worse situation in
respect of the extent of multiple antibiotic resistance than is the
case with S. typhimurium. The extent of resistance clearly indicates
that antibiotic therapy of colibacillosis in calves in N.Y. is now
strongly contraindicated as it can serve only to increase the reservoir of virulent strains without exerting any beneficial effect what-
soever.

The existence of clonal effects is underlined by the finding
that 70% of the E. coli studied belonged to O groups 8, 9, 20 and
101. In contrast to the situation in enteropathogenic strains the
frequency of resistance in nonpathogenic E. coli strains from healthy
calves has been shown to be less (7), a reflection of less severe
selective pressure from sub-therapeutic use of antibiotics for prophylaxis and growth promotion.

Characteristics of R Plasmids in S. typhimurium and Enteropathogenic
E. coli

Conjugation experiments at 28° and 37° revealed that resistance
in S. typhimurium and E. coli in this study were transferable in 91%
and 70% of strains respectively. The reason for the larger proportion of nontransferable plasmids in E. coli is not known. In 74% of
strains of S. typhimurium that transferred, the plasmids involved were
shown to be inc H2 (8). Only one inc H2 plasmid was found in the
collection of E. coli strains. Other major differences in distribution of plasmid incompatibility groups between the 2 enteric species
were also detected (Table 2). Most of the antibiotic resistance in
E. coli was carried on inc Iα or FII plasmids in contrast to S. typhimurium where similar resistance patterns were carried on inc H2 or,
to a lesser degree on a nontypeable 73 Md plasmid (10% of strains).
A 5.5 Md plasmid carrying ampicillin resistance was present in 19% of
S. typhimurium strains but in only 2% of E. coli strains. This

Table 2. Occurrence and Characteristics of Resistance Plasmids from
         Calves (N.Y. 1973-78).

| Inc Group | Source | | Enteropathogenic E. coli[+] (115) | |
| or Size | S. typhimurium (140) | | | |
	%	R Type(s)	%	R type(s)
H2	74	ApKmSmTc KmSmTc	1	KmSmTc
Iα	0		32	ApKmSmTc KmSmTc
FII	7	Tc ApKmTc	47	ApKmSmTc KmSmTc
5.5 Md	19	Ap	2	Ap
73.0 Md[++]	10	KmSmTc	Not known	–

[+] 84 strains belonged to "O" groups 8, 9, 20 and 101.

[++] Compatible with inc FI, FII, FIV, Iα, M and N plasmids.

plasmid is similar to the prototype ampicillin plasmid described by
Anderson in S. typhimurium from English calves in the 1960's (9) and
later observed in other enteric bacteria elsewhere (10). The transfer factor of this plasmid has been shown to be inc Iα (9). Although
not identified in this study, it is probable that its presence would
have increased the actual number of inc Iα plasmids shown in Table 2
for S. typhimurium.

The results outlined above clearly indicate that the two enteric
pathogens in the calf harbour rather different sets of R factor
plasmids. This is surprising since the calves from which the isolates were obtained were from the same general area of N.Y. and were
collected over the same time period (1973-78). Antibiotic selection
pressures must also have been similar because colibacillosis and
salmonellosis are diseases seen early in the calf's life.

It seems clear that the host bacterium is a critical factor in
the epidemiology of R factor plasmids in the calf and that the relationship of each pathogenic enteric species with the normal background enteric flora of the intestine and of the animals' environment
must be of considerable importance in the eventual dominance of
certain R plasmids in enteric pathogens. This seems to be the case
in respect of inc H2 plasmids whose thermosensitivity of transfer
(Figure 2) implies transfer outside the host. In vitro experiments
with feces from 2 four week old calves revealed that a typical inc
H2 plasmid (pJT4) did not transfer at 37° but was transferred between
E. coli strains at a frequency of 10^{-3} at 30°. S. typhimurium
strains must therefore acquire their inc H2 plasmids in the calf's
environment. The original source of these plasmids for this transfe
is unknown. They have been observed in Serratia (11), Citrobacter

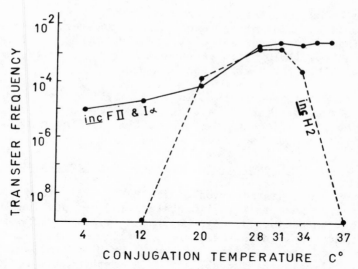

Fig. 2.   Effect of temperature of mating mixture on transfer of inc
          H2, FII and Iα plasmids.

and Klebsiella sp.but are uncommon in E. coli (12) with the possible
exception of E. coli strains isolated from calves recently infected
with S. typhimurium that already possessed inc H2 plasmids (13).

Non-Transfer of inc H2 Plasmids in the Intestine of the Calf

     The failure of typical inc H2 plasmids to transfer at 37° in
calf feces suggested that they did not transfer in the intestine.
Some recent work (Timoney and Linton, 1980 Unpublished Data) has
provided direct experimental confirmation of this.   Three attempts
to demonstrate in vivo transfer in groups of 4 calves were made using
E. coli strains of O groups 21, 45 and 69 as donors of inc H2 plasmids.   These plasmids were obtained from E. coli isolated from
calves that survived an outbreak of S. typhimurium (Phage type 193)
infection in S. W. England and were similar to the epidemic inc H2
plasmid in calves in Britain that has been recently described by
Threlfall et al. (5) and by Rowe in this volume.   Recipient E. coli
used in the in vivo transfer attempt were smooth Nal^R mutants of the
donor E. coli.   Both donor and recipient E. coli were excellent
colonizers of the calf intestine and were selected because of their
dominance in the intestine of the calves from which they were originally isolated.   Transfer of the inc H2 plasmids was not detected
following oral (stomach tube) administration when calves were
muzzled and denied oral contact with their environment.   This was the
case even when tetracycline or chloramphenicol was administered to
exert selection pressure for transconjugants the day after donor and
recipient E. coli were given.   Evidence of transfer of non-thermosen-
sitive R factors was obtained under these conditions and suggested

that conditions permissive of R factor transfer did exist in the
intestine at the time of the experiment. However, transfer of the
inc H2 plasmids to a variety of E. coli "0" types was detected at
a low frequency (1×10^{-6}) in experiments when the calves were not
muzzled or after the muzzles had been removed.

An attempt to demonstrate in vivo mobilization of an inc H2
plasmid in the intestine by a coexisting Class 2 complex consisting
of a 5.5 Md plasmid coding for ampicillin resistance and an inc Iα
transfer factor was also unsuccessful.

Effects of inc H2 Plasmids on Virulence and Colonization

The epidemic distribution of inc H2 plasmids in S. typhimurium
from calves as seen in N.Y., in Britain (5) and previously in man
in the Iberian Peninsula suggests that they may confer advantages
additional to antibiotic resistance. Williams Smith et al. (12)
were unable to show an effect of inc H1 or H2 plasmids on virulence
or intestinal colonization ability of S. typhimurium for chickens.
Similar experiments comparing mouse virulence of twenty inc H2 +
and eleven inc H2 - strains of S. typhimurium from N.Y. calves have
failed to show that inc H2 plasmids increase virulence (Figure 3).
This result was perhaps to be expected because the effects of inc H2
plasmids are more likely to be expressed in the intestine than elsewhere in the body. Accordingly, three experiments to compare the
colonization or persistence in the calf intestine of E. coli strains
(021, 045 and 069) with and without inc H2 plasmids were run. The
results of 2 of these experiments are shown in Figure 4. Both inc
H2 +   E. coli and its Nal^R counterpart cured of the plasmid by incubation at 43° (14) were administered by stomach tube in equal quantities (3×10^{11} CFU) and counts of both strains compared in the calf's
feces for the following 3 weeks. A consistent finding in respect of
all three E. coli serotypes was that the E. coli with the inc H2
plasmid persisted to a progressively greater extent than its cured
counterpart. The difference became most apparent at between 7 to 10
days. By 20 days the inc H2 + organisms were still present in substantial numbers ($\simeq 10^7$ CFU/g feces) whereas counts of the identical

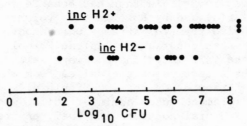

Fig. 3.   Comparison of the virulence for mice (i/P LD_{50}) of strains
of S. typhimurium with and without inc H2 plasmids. Three
strains carrying inc H2 plasmids were avirulent.

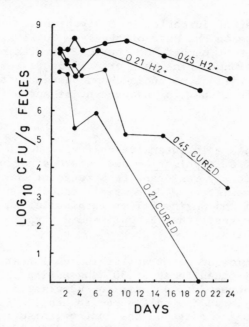

Fig. 4. Effect of the presence of an inc H2 plasmid on the persistence of E. coli strains (021 and 045) in the intestine of
the calf. Each point represents the mean of counts from
four calves.

but cured organisms were zero to 3 x 10^3/g feces. Thus a marked
effect on persistence was evident. This appears to be quite different to the colonization effect of the K88 antigen of E. coli where
differences of up to 1000 X in counts of K88$^+$ and K88$^-$ strains in pig
intestinal contents occur 24 hours after oral administration. The
relatively accelerated disappearance of the cured strains was not
caused by antibiotics because the calves were not receiving antibiotics of any kind. As well, antibiotic sensitive E. coli were detected at a frequency of 10^7 CFU/g feces throughout the experiments.

These results indicate that inc H2 plasmids carry genes which
augment the host bacterium's ability to maintain itself in the calf
intestine. The accelerated decrease of the cured strains at 7 to 10
days suggests the possibility that the intestinal immune response may
be involved and that inc H2$^+$ strains are in some way able to counter-
act host antibody or are not initially as antigenic because of differences in cell surface chemistry or structure. In any event,
increased persistence in the intestine could be contributing to the

epidemic character of infection by S. typhimurium strains carrying inc H2 plasmids as in the case of the Type 204/193 epidemic in Britain. The greater numbers of inc H2 + strains produced in the intestine over a longer time span greatly increases the probability that such clones will be maintained and passed on to other suscepti- ble hosts, an effect that is independent of antibiotic usage.

SUMMARY

Antibiotic usage in intensive calf raising in N.Y. has resulted in populations of S. typhimurium and enteropathogenic E. coli that were almost completely resistant to a range of commonly used anti- biotics. These resistances were mainly encoded on inc H2 plasmids in S. typhimurium and on inc FII or Iα plasmids in enteropathogenic E. coli. This suggests that E. coli and S. typhimurium share different reservoirs.

Inc H2 plasmids do not transfer in the intestine of the calf but transfer well in voided feces at 30° suggesting that multiresistant S. typhimurium clones derive their inc H2 plasmids by conjugation with other bacteria in the calf's environment. The presence of these plasmids in E. coli confers on the host organism an enhanced ability to persist in the calf's intestine beyond 7 to 10 days, a property which could be an important factor in the clonal character of inc H2 positive S. typhimurium infections in the calf.

Acknowledgement

Part of the work described in this paper was performed during the tenure of a Senior International Fellowship of the Fogarty International Center at the Department of Bacteriology, University of Bristol. I am also grateful to Dr. Alan Linton for his help and advice.

REFERENCES

1. J. F. Timoney. The epidemiology and genetics of Salmonella typhimurium isolated from diseased animals in New York. J. Infec. Dis. 137:67 (1978).
2. C. E. Cherubin, J. F. Timoney, M. F. Sierra, P. Ma, J. Marr, and S. Shin. A sudden decline in ampicillin resistance in Salmon- ella typhimurium. J. Am. Med. Assoc. 243:439 (1980).
3. D. P. Aden, N. D. Reed, N. R. Underdahl, and C. A. Mebus. Trans- ferable drug resistance among Enterobacteriaceae isolated from cases of neonatal diarrhea in calves and piglets. Appl. Microbiol. 18:961 (1969).
4. E. S. Anderson. The ecology of transferable drug resistance in the enterobacteria. Annual Review of Microbiology 22:131 (1968).

5. R. V. Threlfall, L. R. Ward, and B. Rowe. Epidemic spread of a chloramphenicol resistant strain of Salmonella typhimurium phage type 204 in bovine animals in Britain. Vet. Rec. 130: 438 (1978).

6. J. F. Timoney, D. E. Taylor, S. Shin, and P. McDonough. pJT2: Unusual H1 plasmid in a highly virulent lactose positive and chloramphenicol-resistant Salmonella typhimurium strain from calves. Antimicrob. Agents Chemother. 18:480 (1980).

7. K. Howe and A. H. Linton. The distribution of O-antigen types of Escherichia coli in normal calves, compared with man and their R plasmid carriage. J. Appl. Bact. 40:317 (1976).

8. D. E. Taylor and R. B. Grant. Inhibition of bacteriophage lambda, T1, and T7 development by R plasmids of the H incompatibility group. Antimicrob. Agents Chemother. 10:762 (1977).

9. E. S. Anderson and L. S. Lewis. Characterization of a transfer factor associated with drug resistance in Salmonella typhimurium. Nature. 208:843 (1965).

10. J. H. Crosa, J. Olarte, L. S. Mata, C. K. Lattrop, and M. E. Penarenda. Characterization of an R plasmid associated with ampicillin resistance in Shigella dysenteriae type 1 strains isolated in epidemics. Antimicrob. Agents Chemother. 11:553 (1977).

11. D. E. Taylor and R. B. Grant. R plasmids of the S incompatibility group belong to the H2 incompatibility group. Antimicrob. Agents Chemother. 12:431 (1977).

12. H. W. Smith, Z. Parsell, and P. Green. Thermosensitive antibiotic resistance plasmids in enterobacteria. J. Gen. Microbiol. 109:37 (1978).

13. A. H. Linton, J. F. Timoney, and M. Hinton. The ecology of chloramphenicol resistance in Salmonella typhimurium and Escherichia coli in calves. J. Appl. Bact. In Press. (1981).

14. D. E. Taylor and J. G. Levine. Studies of temperature-sensitive transfer and maintenance of H Incompatibility group plasmids. J. Gen. Microbiol. 116:475 (1980).

15. H. W. Smith and M. A. Linggood. Observations on the pathogenic properties of the K88, HCY and ENT plasmids of Escherichia coli with particular reference to porcine diarrhoea. J. Med. Microbiol. 4:467 (1971).

EFFECTS OF ANTIBIOTICS IN ANIMAL FEED ON THE ANTIBIOTIC RESISTANCE OF THE GRAM POSITIVE BACTERIAL FLORA OF ANIMALS AND MAN

Gary M. Dunny[1], Peter J. Christie[1], Jean C. Adsit[1], Ellen S. Baron[2], and Richard P. Novick[2]

[1]New York State College of Veterinary Medicine
 Cornell University
 Ithaca, N.Y. 14853
[2]The Public Health Research Institute of New York
 455 1st Avenue
 New York, N.Y. 10016

INTRODUCTION

The use of antibiotics in the raising of farm animals has become an area of considerable controversy in recent years. There have been numerous allegations that this practice, particularly the incorporation of subtherapeutic levels of antibiotics into feed for purposes of growth promotion, is contributing to the increasing incidence of drug resistance in bacterial pathogens that infect man. It has been suggested that the selective pressure exerted upon the bacterial flora of animals by these antibiotics gives rise to large populations of resistant microorganisms. The organisms are then postulated to enter the human population, either through agricultural and meat processing workers, or via the food chain, as a result of contamination of meat products. Once in contact with man, the resistant bacteria could presumably cause disease directly, or transfer their resistance to organisms more pathogenic for humans. Although there is documentation of specific instances of human disease caused by resistant organisms from the farm, the extent to which this occurs has been difficult to assess. Representatives of the drug and animal raising industries have argued that therapeutic use of antibiotics in the treatment of human diseases has a much larger effect on the human resistance problem than agricultural use of antimicrobials. In fact, proponents of both points of view have used the same experimental data to support their particular position on several occasions. Virtually all of the research done in this area has been focused on the gram negative bacteria, particularly the members of the Enterobacteriaceae.

557

Our laboratories are engaged in studies of the plasmids of gram
positive bacteria, especially staphylococci and streptococci. Although there has been considerable interest in plasmid-determined
drug resistance in human isolates of these genera, there is a surprising dearth of knowledge about the resistance and plasmid properties of the gram positive bacteria found in animals. Examples of
several basic questions to be considered in assessing the effects of
antibiotic use in animals on human drug resistance include the following:

    1) Are antibiotic resistance plasmids prevalent in the bacterial
    flora of normal animals on the farm and/or animals being treated
    for diseases, and if so, are these plasmids similar to those
    found in bacteria isolated from human infections?

    2) Does the feeding of an antibiotic to farm animals affect the
    resistance of the bacterial flora of the animals, their care-
    takers, and the environment?

    3) Do resistant and/or pathogenic microorganisms from animals
    enter the human food chain in significant numbers?

While numerous studies on gram negative bacteria have been
directed toward these questions, virtually no data on gram positive
organisms is available in this regard. In this communication, we
will summarize the results to date, of studies begun in our laboratories during the past year. We feel that these initial findings
suggest that the effects of antibiotics in animal feed on gram
positive drug resistance are very relevant to these questions and
should be strongly considered in making decisions regarding future
use of these substances.

RESULTS AND DISCUSSION

The U. S. Food and Drug Administration has been collecting
representative bacterial isolates from farm animals throughout the
country. We have examined 100 isolates each of staphylococci and
fecal streptococci for plasmid content and antibiotic resistance
profiles. We have found that virtually all of these strains are
resistant to at least one antibiotic, and the vast majority carry
multiple resistance. Table 1 shows the resistance and plasmid
profiles of 20 animal streptococci which are typical of what was
found with the streptococcal isolates. Multiple resistance and
multiple plasmid species were commonly observed, including a number
of fairly large plasmids. Similar findings were obtained when human
strains isolated from infections of New York Hospital patients were
examined (data not shown here). We are presently attempting to
identify specific macrolide resistance plasmids from the two groups
of strains, so that their sequence homology may be determined. When
a similar analysis was carried out on staphylococci from human

Table 1. Properties and Plasmids of Animal Streptococci

Strain Number	Resistances	Plasmid Sizes (Mdal)
1	Tc, Pn, Km	4.7; 1.6
2	-	47.8; 2.0
3	Tc, Em, Ne, Km, Sm	35.4; 2.6; 1.0; .8; .4
4	Tc, Em, Sm	22.9
5	Tc, Em, Sm	22.3; 17.3; 9.5; 6.7; 3.2; 1.0; .5
6	Tc, Em	-
7	-	27.5
8	Tc, Ne	53.7; 41.6; 33.4; 25.1; 9.3; 8.3; 5.7; 5.0; 2.4; 2.2
9	Tc	35.0
10	Tc	-
11	Tc	4.3
12	Tc, Km	16.9
13	Tc, Em, Km, Sm	2.1
14	Tc, Km	-
15	Tc	37.1; 29.5
16	Tc, Em, Sm	39.8; 1.3; .95
17	Tc, Km, Sm	-
18	Em, Km, Sm	45.7; 35.4; 2.5; 2.4
19	Tc, Em	.8
20	Tc, Km, Sm	-

Antibiotic resistance was determined by disc diffusion method and plasmid content was determined by agarose gel electrophoresis.

infections and farm animals, multiple resistances and multiple plasmids were also observed, but most of the plasmids were relatively small in size, many having a molecular weight less than 5×10^6. In the case of the staphylococci, several macrolide resistance plasmids have been identified (Table 2) and the restriction enzyme digests of a few of these isolates have been compared. In Table 3, it can be seen that there is considerable similarity in the banding pattern of human and animal plasmids, suggesting a common evolutionary origin. As shown in Table 4, multiresistant streptococci are also readily isolated from animals in a veterinary hospital and many of these isolates transfer their resistance to a recipient strain of human origin. Taken together, the data obtained from examination of gram positive bacteria from humans and animals reveal that drug resistance and plasmids are prevalent in both populations. Although the comparison of the sequence homology of specific plasmids from these isolates has not been completed, there is already evidence for common evolutionary origins of animal and human macrolide resistance plasmids.

Table 2. Molecular Weight of Macrolide Resistance Determinants
          in Staphylococci

Strain or Plasmid Number	Source	Location of Determinant	M.W.x10^{-6}	Transposon
RN1550	Human	Chromosome	5000	Tn554 (4.3 Mdal)
pr258	Human	Plasmid	18.4	Tn551 (3.4 Mdal)
pe194	Human	Plasmid	2.4	-
pSA1104	Human	Plasmid	1.45	-
pSA1105	Human	Plasmid	1.40	-
pEB111	Human	Plasmid	1.58	-
EB116	Human	Plasmid	*1.75,0.85	-
pEB201	Animal	Plasmid	2.4	-
pEB102	Animal	Plasmid	2.7	-
pEB100	Animal	Plasmid	2.7	-
pEB203	Animal	Plasmid	2.8	-
pEB97	Animal	Plasmid	2.8	-
pEB88	Animal	Plasmid	2.8	-
pEB90	Animal	Plasmid	2.9	-
pEB214	Animal	Plasmid	3.15	-

*Plasmid screening of Em^r transductants always revealed two
plasmid DNA species - = uncharacterized

Table 3. Molecular Sizes of Restriction
          Fragments of MLS Plasmids from
          Humans and Animal Staphylococci

HincII Fragments	pE194	pEB97	pEB102
A	1.0	1.35	1.15
B	0.83	1.0	1.08
C	0.7	0.74	0.74
D	0.62	0.635	0.615
E	0.38	0.39	0.395
F	0.245	0.25	0.25
G	0.205	0.205	0.205
	3.98Kb	4.58Kb	4.43Kb

Table 4. Multi-Resistant Fecal Streptococci from Animals at
the Cornell Veterinary Hospital

Species	Strain Number	Resistances
Canine	1	Pen, Amp, Tet, Kan, Str$_*$
"	2	Tet, Neo, Str. Chl, Kan
Bovine (Adult)	3	Amp, Chl, Kan, Pen, Str, Tet, Neo*
"	4	Chl, Tet, Neo*
Bovine (Calf)	5	Tet, Chl, Str, Kan*
Equine	6	Tet, Chl, Str, Kan, Neo$_*$
"	7	Tet, Chl, Str, Kan, Neo*
Porcine	8	Str, Kan, Tet, Amp
Avian	9	Pen, Amp, Chl, Kan, Tet
"	10	Kan, Str, Tet, Neo

*Indicates that strain could transfer Tet resistance to a
human recipient strain, JH2-2.

A second problem which we have addressed in our research is
the effect of incorporation of the antibiotic tylosin, in the feed
of pigs on the macrolide resistance of their gram positive microflora. A major obstacle in this work was the lack of availability of
animals carrying low levels of indigenous drug-resistant bacteria.
After an extensive search, we succeeded in obtaining 16 piglets
having less than 20% macrolide resistant staphylococci and streptococci in their normal flora. We constructed pens on open land which
had not been previously used for raising animals, and carried out the
study outlined in Table 5. As can be seen in Figure 1, the resistance of the tylosin-fed pigs' gram positive flora was relatively
low during the baseline period. The fecal streptococci in these
animals became almost 100% macrolide-resistant within a few days of
the addition of tylosin to their feed, whereas the staphylococcal
populations appeared to be reduced initially, followed by establishment of a resistant population within a few weeks. In contract,
there was considerable fluctuation in the percentage of resistant
organisms in the control group. During the baseline sampling period,
there was a steady rise in the percentage of resistant fecal streptococci in these pigs at a time when both groups were being fed the
same, non-tylosin containing ration. We feel that this rise may have
been due to the presence, in the herd, of a fortuitously resistant
strain which was very proficient at colonizing the pigs' intestinal
tracts. This strain may have become predominant during this time and
was eventually displaced by sensitive strains, resulting in the
decrease in resistance seen during the middle portions of the experiment. Near the end of the study, there was a second rise in

Table 5. Pig Raising Studies

2 groups of piglets (8 per group)
   Group A - fed 100 g/ton tylosin in feed
   Group B - no tylosin

Culture biweekly - rectal swabs —— CNA-horse blood agar
              skin and nasal swabs —— mannitol-salts agar

Culturing procedure:
   1) Suspend material from swab in 10 ml of sterile
      saline + 0.05 µg/ml Em. Incubate at 37°.
   2) Make serial dilutions and plate on media
      described above + 10 µg/ml Em.

Caretakers and environmental samples are also periodically
cultured and feed is tested for antibiotic residues. We
tested erythromycin resistance and preincubated our samples
as described above because the most common macrolide resistance phenotype in gram positive bacteria is the so-called
"MLS" phenotype.[1] CNA agar selects for gram positive bacteria,
whereas mannitol-salts agar selects for staphylococci.

----

[1] Weisblum, et al. J. Bacteriol. 138:990-998 (1979).

resistance of the streptococci and staphylococci. Based on the
results of assays for tylosin residues (carried out in the laboratory
of Dr. S. Katz, Rutgers University) in the various batches of feed
used in the study, we believe that this increase in resistance was
due to inadvertant contamination of two batches of feed (see Figure
1) with approximately 20 g/ton of tylosin. This unfortunate incident
actually illustrates a very serious problem which we encountered in
this work. Namely, that it is surprisingly difficult to obtain
"clean" feed (and animals) to do this sort of project, even in university experimental animal raising facilities, due to the prevalence
of antibiotics in the environment. In spite of these problems, the
percentages of resistant organisms in the control group never
reached the levels observed in the tylosin-fed pigs, nor did we see
the abrupt rise in resistance in the controls that was evident in
the tylosin group. It is our feeling that these data do show that
tylosin feeding does cause an increase in macrolide resistance of the
gram positive bacteria of pigs. Analysis of resistance and plasmid
profiles of strains isolated from the pigs during the experiment
(which is currently being carried out) should reveal effects on
multiple resistance and plasmid content of the bacterial flora. Even
though tylosin is not used in human medicine, its agricultural use
would appear to result in an increase in resistance to drugs useful
in human medicine, such as erythromycin.

We also cultured the caretakers of the two groups of pigs, and

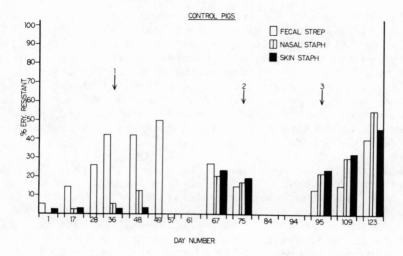

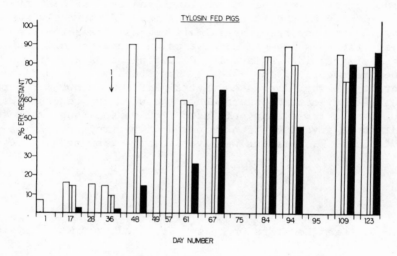

Fig. 1   The percentages of resistant organisms at various samplings
         are plotted in this figure. Arrow #1 indicates the time
         tylosin feeding was initiated. Arrows 2 and 3 indicate the
         time period when inadvertantly (tylosin) contaminated feed
         was given to the control group. The numbers are cumulative
         averages of all the pigs in the two groups. The data for
         each pig is based on the average of four plates.

we found that the fecal streptococci of the control and experimental
caretakers both increased from less than 5% erythromycin resistant
to about 15%. The resistance of the nasal staphylococci of the
control caretaker increased from 2% to 9%, whereas the percentage of
resistant organisms of the tylosin group's caretaker increased from

less than 1% to 20% at the end of the study. Plasmid analysis of
erythromycin resistant strains from the caretaker revealed that so
staphylococci from the tylosin-fed pigs had similar plasmid profil
to organisms isolated from their caretaker. While these data are
suggestive of some colonization of the caretaker by organisms from
the animals, we feel that more frequent sampling of the caretakers
as well as using larger numbers of experimental animals (to increa
the exposure of the caretakers to the animals and feed) would be
necessary to conclusively determine the extent to which this color
zation actually occurs.

While the evidence discussed above indicates that there is a
production of resistant organisms in farm animals, the next questi
that arises is whether these organisms reach the human population
via the food chain in significant numbers to facilitate a direct
interaction with man and his bacterial flora. We have recently be
to culture the gram positive bacteria present on cuts of meat whic
might reach the consumer. Table 6 shows that fairly large numbers
staphylococci and streptococci contaminated cuts of meat from our
tylosin fed pigs at the time of processing. We strongly suspect t
these organisms were from the animals because the butchering was
under very rigorous hygenic conditions, and the bacteria isolated
were mostly macrolide-resistant. Culturing of pork portions which
have been refrigerated for several days, to simulate conditions on
meat market shelves, indicates that significant growth of streptococci and staphylococci occurs under these circumstances. We have
also cultured chicken meat purchased from various supermarkets and
found it to be invariably contaminated with streptococci, as illu
trated in Table 7. Strains we have isolated from this source

Table 6. Gram Positive Organisms Isolated from Meat Samples

Cut	Total staph	Em-resistant staph	Total strep	Em-resis stre
Chops (pig 4)	6.1×10^3	4.4×10^3	1.1×10^3	1.0×1
Ham (pig 4)	1.5×10^3	3.0×10^3	1.0×10^3	1.0×1
Chops (pig 1)	1.6×10^4	7.0×10^3	1.0×10^2	1.0×1
Sausage (pig 1)	4.1×10^4	5.0×10^4	1.5×10^3	1.0×1

Meat samples from tylosin fed pigs at the time of packaging. The
numbers represent the number of organisms isolated (on Erythromyc
containing, and drug-free plates) from swabs rubbed vigorously on
cuts of meat.

Table 7. Drug-Resistant Streptococci from Supermarket
          Chickens

	Drug-free plates	Tet plates	Ery plates
cfu/mlon:			
Chicken 5	4.2×10^4	6.1×10^3	5.3×10^3
Chicken 6	3.2×10^5	2.6×10^5	2.5×10^2

Fluid was aseptically removed from a package containing
a whole fryer or roasting chicken and plated on CNA agar
plus the antibiotics indicated above. Under these
conditions about 60-80% of the colonies which grew
were streptococci.

included β-hemolytic group L streptococci (whose identity was confirmed by Dr. R. Facklam of the Center for Disease Control) and group
D streptococci which transferred drug resistance to a human recipient
strain.   There is certainly indication from these results that gram
positive bacteria from farm animals do reach the human food chain
in significant numbers, representing a significant reservoir of
pathogens and resistance genes.

    Although much of our data is preliminary, we feel that the use
of antibiotics in animal raising does markedly effect the gram
positive bacteria of animals, and there appears to be considerable
potential for these organisms to interact with humans and their bacterial flora. We hope to confirm and extend these observations in
the near future, and it is our belief that the effects we have
observed with the gram positive bacteria should be taken into account
in considering any future changes in the use of antibiotics in animal
raising.

    Acknowledgements. This work was supported by contract #RFP-223-
79-7050 from the U.S. Food and Drug Administration to the Public
Health Research Institute and a subcontract to Cornell University.

Commissioned Reports Summarizing Studies on Antibiotic Use in Animal Raising

Penicillin. Use in Animal Feed. Federal Register 42 #168. August
30, 1977.

Tetracycline in Animal Feeds and Tetracycline-Containing Premixes.
Federal Register 42 #204. October 21, 1977.

Joint Committee on the Use of Antibiotics in Animal Husbandry and
Veterinary Medicine. Report. 1969. Her Majesty's Stationery
Office. London.

MULTIPLY-RESISTANT CLONES OF <u>SALMONELLA TYPHIMURIUM</u> IN BRITAIN:

EPIDEMIOLOGICAL AND LABORATORY ASPECTS

B. Rowe and E. J. Threlfall

Division of Enteric Pathogens
Public Health Laboratory Service
Colindale Avenue, London, NW9 5HT

In Britain, salmonellosis is the most important cause of food-poisoning and <u>Salmonella typhimurium</u> causes about 25 per cent of all human salmonella infections each year. Poultry and cattle are the main sources of human infections with this serotype and phage typing studies have demonstrated that in general the poultry-associated phage types are almost exclusively drug-sensitive whereas the majority of cattle-associated types are resistant to antimicrobial drugs. This reflects the use of antibiotics in the different animal species.

Salmonellosis in cattle can be a severe disease, particularly amongst calves and is an important economic factor in the cattle-rearing industry. Antibiotics are used extensively for therapy and prophylaxis in cattle although their use for growth promotion has been prohibited since 1971. In contrast, salmonellosis is not an economically important disease in poultry and the use of antibiotics is comparatively insignificant.

The effects of the legislation resulting from the recommendations of the Swann Committee[1] are difficult to quantify. Prior to 1963, about three per cent of S.typhimurium from cattle were drug-resistant but the incidence of resistance increased dramatically between 1963 and 1969 following the appearance and epidemic spread of a multiresistant clone of phage type 29 in calves. The peak was reached in 1965 when 73 per cent of all isolations of <u>S.typhimurium</u> from cattle were caused by this strain[2]. By the time the Swann recommendations were implemented, isolations of type 29 were at a low level and the strain has subsequently disappeared from bovine animals in Britain. Thus although the appearance and spread of this particular clone contributed to the enactment of the Swann

567

legislation, its disappearance was related to other factors.

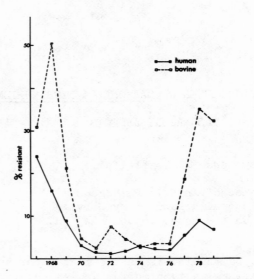

Fig. 1. Multiple drug resistance in S.typhimurium in Britain

Fig. 1 shows the percentage of multiresistant S.typhimurium
from cattle and humans in Britain from 1968 to 1979. The early
peak corresponds to the period when type 29 was predominant. It
is tempting to speculate that the low proportion of multiresistant
strains between 1971 and 1976 (about eight per cent of bovine and
two per cent of human isolations) was a direct result of the Swann
legislation, but this cannot be proved and there was little
diminution in the overall use of antibiotics in animal husbandry
during this period.

The increase in the proportions of multiresistant S.typhimuriu
in cattle and humans since 1977 has followed the sequential
acquisition of resistance plasmids in the bovine host by one strain
of S.typhimurium, type 204 and the resultant epidemic dissemination
of resistant clones (Table 1). Because of the influence of the
drug-sensitive poultry types, the overall increase in multiresistance in S.typhimurium from humans has been not as pronounced
as may be expected from that observed in cattle.

Type 204 resistant to sulphonamides and tetracyclines (R-type
SuT) was identified in calves in Britain in 1974. The strain sprea
in cattle and entered the human food chain. Sulphonamides and
tetracycline resistance were encoded by independent plasmids and
the tetracyclines resistance plasmid was found to be type-
determining. Thus the probable progenitor of type 204 was a strai
of phage type 49, a phage type common in cattle before 1974.

Table 1. Appearance of type 204 and related strains

Strain	R-type	Date
Type 204	SuT	1974 January
	CSSuT	1977 June
Type 193	ACKSSuT	1977 December
Type 204c	CSSuTTm	1979 March
	ACKSSuTTm	1979 October
	SSuTTm	1980 July

In June 1977 a strain of type 204 resistant to chloramphenicol, streptomycin, sulphonamides and tetracyclines (R-type CSSuT) appeared in calves and spread epidemically. Genetic studies showed that a type 204 strain of R-type SuT had acquired a compatibility group H_2 plasmid coding for the complete resistance spectrum. Human infections were subsequently identified[3].

In December 1977 a new strain appeared spread epidemically in calves in Britain. This strain was assigned to phage type 193, and was resistant to ampicillin, chloramphenicol, kanamycin, streptomycin, sulphonamides and tetracyclines (R-type ACKSSuT). Genetic and molecular investigations demonstrated that this strain had been derived from type 204, R-type CSSuT, following the acquisition of a group I_1 plasmid specifying resistance to ampicillin, kanamycin and streptomycin. This plasmid also coded for restriction of S.typhimurium typing phages and thereby converted type 204 R-type CSSuT to type 193, R-type ACKSSuT[4,5]. During 1978 and 1979 these multiresistant strains of types 204 and 193 spread to Europe following the export of infected calves from Britain[6].

In March 1979 a strain of S.typhimurium resistant to chloramphenicol, streptomycin, sulphonamides, tetracyclines and trimethoprim (CSSuTTm) was identified in calves. This strain was designated type 204c because of its derivation from type 204 of R-type CSSuT by a complex process involving loss of typing phage restriction from the type-determining tetracycline resistance plasmid present in all type 204 strains, acquisition of a trimethoprim transposon by the H_2 resistance factor and acquisition of a temperate bacteriophage, the presence of which converted type 49 to the new type, type 204c[7]. This strain became established in calves during 1979 and in due course acquired further resistance plasmids coding for ampicillin and kanamycin resistance. By

December 1979 the predominant R-type in type 204c isolations was
that of ACKSSuTTm. All type 204c isolations have been resistant to
trimethoprim and the appearance of type 204c coincided with an
intensive promotional campaign in Britain to encourage the use of
trimethoprim for the treatment and prophylaxis of bovine
salmonellosis.

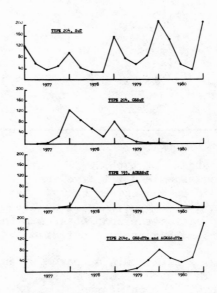

Fig. 2. *S.typhimurium* types 204, 193 and 204c in cattle, 1977-1980

    The clone of type 204 of R-type CSSuT had become the predominant
strain in cattle by late 1977 and has subsequently disappeared.
Type 193 peaked in 1978/1979 but the frequency of isolations of
this clone was reduced in 1980. Type 204c, which appeared in 1979,
became the predominant multiresistant clone in cattle during 1980
(Fig. 2). In contrast, strains of type 204 of R-type SuT have
been regularly isolated throughout this period. The initial rise in
prevalence of these multiresistant clones, followed by their
subsequent decline may be related to changes in selective pressure
brought about by the successive use of different antimicrobials in
animal husbandry in attempts to combat the increasing spectrum of
resistance in these strains.

    As with all strains of S.typhimurium, there was a range of
symptoms in calves infected with the multiresistant strains.
However the disease appeared unusually virulent; many reports
mentioned severe scouring frequently accompanied by septicaemia and
mortality was high - up to 50 per cent in some calf herds. The
proportion of infections in cattle caused by these multiresistant

clones has increased from 14.7 per cent in 1977 to 27.4 per cent
and 24.2 per cent in 1979 and 1980 (Table 2) and economic losses
have been considerable. In terms of the actual number of animals
infected, it is important to realise that the strains referred to
this laboratory represent only a proportion of infections in cattle
since in many instances only representative strains are referred
from an outbreak.

Table 2.   <u>S.typhimurium</u> types 204, 193 and 204c from
            cattle, 1977-1980

Year	Strains received	Per cent type 204		Per cent type 193	Per cent type 204c
		SuT	CSSuT		
1977	1194	20.0	14.1	0.6	0
1978	1790	14.2	13.6	15.8	0
1979	1732	26.4	2.3	16.4	8.7
1980	1585*	28.8	0	3.4	20.9

*Provisional figures

<u>Source</u>: Strains referred to DEP

     Since 1977, 457 human infections with the multiresistant clones
of types 204, 193 and 204c have been recognised. In addition a
further 48 patients have been infected with a related multiresistant
strain of type 204a, R-type CKSSuT which appeared in 1980 (Table 3).
In the majority of instances the symptoms were those of mild to
moderate enteritis but severe diarrhoea which persisted for several
weeks was reported. Enteritis was reported as the cause of death of
two patients. The strain spread extra-intestinally in ten patients
and one child died of septicaemia in a family outbreak of type 193
of R-type ACKSSuT. When these multiresistant clones spread extra-
intestinally, the clinicians choice of drug for therapy is obviously
extremely limited.

     The therapeutic and prophylactic use of antibiotics in cattle
has directly contributed to the appearance of these multiresistant
clones but the importance of drug resistance in their epidemic spread
cannot be quantified. However there is no doubt that the
prophylactic use of antibiotics in animal husbandry has provided
selective pressure which has allowed the strain to persist and
become disseminated in calf herds. It is noteworthy that epidemic
spread occurred subsequent to the acquisition of resistance plasmids.

Table 3. Human infections with multiresistant S.typhimurium
types 204, 193, 204c and 204a

Year	Type 204 CSSuT	Type 193 ACKSSuT	Type 204c CSSuTTm and ACKSSuTTm	Type 204a CKSSuT	Total
1977	37	4	0	0	41
1978	51	89	0	0	140
1979	15	94	20	0	129
1980	0	29	118	48	195
	103	216	138	48	505

Source: Strains referred to DEP

Although reports indicated that infections in calves were
unusually severe, as yet there is no evidence that the multiresistant strains have increased virulence. However the use of
antibiotics to which the strains were resistant may have
aggravated the disease by suppressing competition by sensitive
bacteria in the bowel and certainly infected animals have not
responded to treatment.

The dissemination of these clones was facilitated by the
extensive movements of young animals due to the distribution
practices of the calf-dealing trade and cross-infection in dealers'
premises was undoubtedly a major contributory factor. In Britain,
existing legislation - the Zoonoses Order[8] - permits movement contro
restrictions on infected animals and effective use of this
legislation would help limit the spread of infection. However it
is essential that any measures to prevent cross-infection and the
dissemination of infected stock be combined with a more judicious
use of antibiotics for therapy and prophylaxis in cattle.

REFERENCES

1. Joint Committee on the use of antibiotics in Animal Husbandry
   and Veterinary Medicine. Report. 1969. Her Majesty's
   Stationery Office, London.
2. E. S. Anderson. Drug resistance in Salmonella typhimurium and
   its implications. Br.Med.J. 3:333 (1968).
3. E. J. Threlfall, L. R. Ward and B. Rowe. Epidemic spread of a
   chloramphenicol-resistant strain of Salmonella typhimurium
   phage type 204 in bovine animals in Britain. Vet.Rec.
   103:438 (1978).

4. E. J. Threlfall, L. R. Ward and B. Rowe. Spread of multi-resistant strains of Salmonella typhimurium phage types 204 and 193 in Britain. Br.Med.J. 2:997 (1978).

5. G. A. Willshaw, E. J. Threlfall, L. R. Ward, A. S. Ashley and B. Rowe. Plasmid studies of drug-resistant epidemic strains of Salmonella typhimurium belonging to phage types 204 and 193. J.Antimicrob.Chem. 6:763 (1980).

6. B. Rowe, E. J. Threlfall, L. R. Ward and A. S. Ashley. International spread of multiresistant strains of Salmonella typhimurium phage types 204 and 193 from Britain to Europe. Vet.Rec. 105:468 (1979).

7. E. J. Threlfall, L. R. Ward, A. S. Ashley and B. Rowe. Plasmid-encoded trimethoprim resistance in multiresistant epidemic Salmonella typhimurium phage types 204 and 193 in Britain. Br.Med.J. 1:1210 (1980).

8. Statutory Instruments 1975. No. 1030. Animals. Diseases of Animals. The Zoonoses Order 1975.

R PLASMIDS FROM S. typhi AND S. typhimurium

STRAINS ISOLATED IN MEXICO CITY HOSPITALS

Guillermo Alfaro

Departamento de Biotecnología
Instituto de Investigaciones Biomédicas
Universidad Nacional Autónoma de México
Apartado Postal 70228
México 20, D.F., México

S. typhi strains harboring R plasmids are a common finding in Mexico City hospitals. The predominant R plasmids share the following properties: they belong to the same incompatibility group (H_1), have a molecular weight of 135 Mdal, carry a temperature sensitive transfer system, and code for the resistance to Cm, Sm, Su, Hg and Tc. The general organization of the resistance genes resembles that of R100, since homogenic derivatives which have lost the r-determinants, Tn10 or all the resistance genes can be isolated in vitro by several methods. Furthermore, naturally occurring R plasmids deleted for the r-determinants or Tn10 have been found, although at low frequency. Complementation experiments indicated that the ts transfer system of the mexican plasmids is not related to that of Flac, R1-19 or Col Ibdrd.

Although the resistance patterns of S. typhimurium are more complex than those of S. typhi, it has been possible to isolate R plasmids which are indistinguishable from those described above. This is epidemiologically important since S. typhimurium strains may be one of the sources of R plasmids in Mexico. The use of antibiotics in animal feedening programs and the lack of appropiate sanitary conditions may play an important role in the distribution of R plasmids.

Furthermore, most of the S. typhimurium strains are resistant to Ap, the second antibiotic of choice in the treatment of typhoid in Mexico. The resistance to this antibiotic is encoded by a small conjugative plasmid of 17 Mdal.

A PLASMID-MEDIATED SURFACE ANTIGEN OF THE CLINICALLY ISOLATED *ESCHERICHIA COLI* STRAINS

Toshihiko Arai, Takao Ando, Sadao Komatsu and Yoko Komatsu

Department of Microbiology, Keio University School of
Medicine, Tokyo, Japan

A plasmid-mediated surface antigen of naturally occurring
Escherichia coli strains were detected. This antigen was classified into L type (heat-labile K) antigens but suggested not to be
pilus antigen, because we found no pilus on the surface of common
pili-free *E. coli* C strains carrying these plasmids, and because
these strains did not hemagglutinate any red blood cells. Incidences of this antigen-forming strains were high in the strains isolated from feces and respiratory tract secretions. Plasmid DNAs
from these strains were different in their molecular sizes, but
they had a common size band after digestion by EcoRI endonuclease,
suggesting that they had the similar or same origen(s).

Distributions of the strains which had the surface antigen
common to the *Klebsiella* strain

| Strains | No. of strains isolated from   (%) | | | | | |
	feces	urine	pus	resp.sec#	others	total
examined*	271	268	141	88	58	826
K*	20(7)	3(1)	2(1)	5(6)	1(1)	31(4)
plasmid*	4	1	0	1	0	6

\# resp.sec.; respiratory tract secretion.
* examined ; Numbers of strains examined.
  K   ; Numbers of strains which had the surface antigen
            common to *Klebsiella pneumoniae*.
  plasmid ; Numbers of strains which had plasmid mediating this
            antigen. Transfer of these plasmids to *E. coli* C
            which is agglutinated by all commercially available
            anti-sera against K antigens of *Vibrio parahemolyti-
            cus* but not agglutinated by any of the commercially
            available anti-sera against OK antigens of entero-
            pathogenic *E. coli* removes or covers antigens for
            V. parahemolyticus groups I, II, III, VII and VIII
            and adds antigens agglutinated by anti-sera against
            enteropathogenic *E. coli* K60, K62, K69, K74 and Kxl.

RESISTANT AND BIOACTIVE *ESCHERICHIA COLI* STRAINS FROM CLINICAL MATERIALS AND THEIR PLASMIDS

Toshihiko Arai, Sadao Komatsu, Yoko Komatsu and
Akio Kobayashi*

Department of Microbiology, Keio University School of
Medicine, Tokyo, Japan *Cnetral Clinical Laboratories
Chiba University Hospital, Chiba, Japan

We surveyed tha antibiotic resistant, adhesive, enterotoxigenic, hemolytic, colicin producing, cell invasive, capsule forming, special surface antigen producing and actively iron incorporating strains in the *Escherichia coli* strains from various clinical materials of five general hospitals in different districts in
Tokyo area. Some of the bioactive strains were isolated in different frequencies from various organs but in similar frequencies
from every hospitals. The differences of distributions of the
strains carrying these various activities suggesting that human
cell specific adhesins and hemolysins gave advantages to the strains to reside in respiratory tract, that capsules helped the
strains to survive in pustular foci, and that the surface antigens
common to enteropathogenic bacteria helped the strains to grow in
intestine and respiratory tract. Antibiotic resistances, colicin
productions and active incorporations of iron could give advantages to grow over other bacteria but gave no preferences to the
special organs. Enterotoxigenic and cell invasive strains were
found to be very rare in the clinically isolated strains in general hospitals. Conjogative R plasmids were detected in average
40% of the resistant strains by direct drug selection. Conjugative plasmids mediating all other bioactive characters were examined by their mobilizations of a non-conjugative R plasmid. But,
we detected only a few colicinogenic plasmids and plasmids which
mediated a surface antigen common to *Klebsiella* by the mobilization test.

577

GENETICAL BASES OF MICROCIN CLASSIFICATION

F.Baquero, F.Sanchez, V.Rubio and A.Tenorio

Servicio de Microbiología
Centro Especial Ramón y Cajal
Carr. Colmenar km 9.1. Madrid-34. Spain

Microcins are low molecular weight antibiotic substances produced and excreted by Enterobacteriaceae. About 25% of hospitalized patients harbour microcinogenic strains in the intestinal tract.

With the purpose to study the biological diversity of microcins, 26 wild type E.coli microcinogenic strains have been classified by cross-activity spectra into four groups. Microcin producing E.coli transconjugants were obtained from several strains of each group in order to applie cross-immunity criteria excluding tolerance or resistance of wild strains.

E. coli transconjugants of each group II,III or IV showed internal cross-immunity and are susceptible to the activities of the other groups. Group I contains two different microcin activities which can be separated by conjugation or transformation, one of them presenting cross-immunity with group IV.

Groups I and IV activities are associated with the presence of a 3.7 Md plasmid. Transconjugants with group II activity-immunity group presents a single 48 Md plasmid of very similar restriction pattern in all the studied strains. A physical map of this plasmid including the location of the microcin immunity region by cloning is presented.

GENETIC, MOLECULAR, AND BIOCHEMICAL CHARACTERIZATION OF PLASMID-MEDIATED ATYPICAL UTILIZATION OF CITRATE BY ESCHERICHIA COLI

L.S. Baron, D.J. Kopecko, W.C. Reid, and S.M. McCowen*

Walter Reed Army Institute of Research, Wash., D.C.
and *Virginia Commonwealth Univ., Richmond, VA.

Although Escherichia coli strains normally do not utilize citrate, citrate utilizing (Cit$^+$) variants of otherwise normal E. coli strains have been detected at a low frequency in animal and human isolates. We have examined citrate utilization in the atypical E. coli variant strain V414 isolated from a diseased human. Plasmid-mediated citrate assimilation was suspected because citrate-nonutilizing derivatives of the Cit$^+$ strain appeared spontaneously at a high frequency. In conjugation experiments with plasmid-free E. coli K12 recipients, we found the atypical Cit$^+$ character to be part of a self-transmissible plasmid which also conferred resistance to tetracycline and chloramphenical. Purified plasmid DNAs from the original Cit$^+$ host or K12 Cit$^+$ transconjugants were examined by agarose gel electrophoresis and electron microscopy. Both strain V414 and the transconjugants contained a 130 megadalton conjugative plasmid which is transferable upon selection for citrate utilization or the antibiotic resistances. The cit$^+$ determinant was cloned from the 130 megadalton plasmid into the PstI site of pBR325. Several independent Cit$^+$ recombinant plasmids were examined and found to contain essentially identical cloned PstI fragments of approximately 9 kilobases in size. Although E. coli cells are normally unable to transport exogenous citrate, they do possess the enzymes necessary to catabolize it intracellularly. Metabolic studies of cells containing the Cit$^+$ plasmid indicate, however, that intact citrate is not incorporated directly into whole cells, but is metabolized at the cell surface before uptake and assimilation by the cell. Further studies show that this plasmid does not enhance the ability of an enterochelin-deficient E. coli Cit$^+$ transconjugant to grow in the absence of iron, thus demonstrating that citrate utilization does not involve iron uptake.

ANTIBIOTIC RESISTANCE IN *VIBRIO CHOLERAE* 01 AND ITS PUBLIC HEALTH SIGNIFICANCE

D. Barua

Diarrheal Diseases Control Programme

World Health Organization, Geneva, Switzerland

Clinical studies have firmly established the value of tetracycline and of a number of other antimicrobial drugs as adjuncts to rehydration therapy in the treatment of cholera; they have also been shown to be effective in reducing the transmission of infection, provided their use is limited to close contacts of patients. Sporadic isolations of drug-resistant strains have been reported from time to time in different areas since the early sixties, but the resistance has generally been found to be unstable. Although in a few strains it was found to be stable and encoded by a group C plasmid, it is only in the recent years that such strains have become a cause of concern to public health authorities. Since 1977, outbreaks of cholera caused by resistant strains have been reported from Tanzania and Bangladesh. In the former, the incidence of tetracycline-resistant organisms increased from 0% in November 1977 to 76% in March 1978, during which period about 1788 kg of tetracycline were reported to have been used for mass prophylaxis and treatment of cases. During 1977/78, 67% of the isolates were resistant to tetracycline when 4436 kg of tetracycline were consumed. Thereafter, use of tetracycline for mass prophylaxis was restricted and during 1979/80 only 4.8% of strains were tetracycline resistant when 1028 kg of tetracycline were used.

In Bangladesh, isolation of resistant strains increased from 5% in the first month of the epidemic to 13%, 28%, and 36% in subsequent months and then gradually declined. This increase and decrease in drug-resistance could not be ascribed to any unusual increase or decrease in the drug consumption. The R-types in Bangladesh (ApKmSmSpTcSuTm, ApKmTcSuTm, ApTcSuTm) differed from those in Tanzania (ApKmSmTcCmSu, ApKmSu) in that they did not include resistance to chloramphenicol, but in both countries the plasmid responsible belonged to incompatibility group C. An understanding of the factors involved in the acquisition and loss of resistance in <u>V. cholerae</u> is important for ensuring a rational use of antimicrobials.

CHARACTERISATION OF THE TETRACYCLINE RESISTANCE REGION OF THE INCP PLASMID RP1.

P.M. Bennett and S.W. Shales

Department of Bacteriology
University of Bristol
Bristol, U.K.

Preliminary investigations (1,2) indicated that the tetracycline resistance gene(s) carried on RP1 are located approximately 14 kb from the EcoR1 site of the plasmid. Plasmid pUB307 is a deletion derivative of RP1 which has lost the resident TnA of RP1 but carries the tet-gene(s) intact. Tn802 (TnA) and Tn501 (TnM) insertion mutants of pUB307 have been used to map more precisely the tet region of RP1. The structural gene(s) comprise a nucleotide sequence of about 1.3 kb. Adjacent to this and proximal to the EcoR1 site of the plasmid is a region of about 500 bp which encodes a repressor. A fragment of about 2.2 kb which carries the entire 1.8 - 1.9 kb tet region of RP1 has been cloned into pSF2124. The new plasmid, pUB1246, confers inducible tetracycline resistance at a level approximately twice that conferred by RP1. The tet resistance determinant of RP1 (which is indistinguishable from RP4) is homologous with the prototype tetA of pIP7, a finding consistent with that of Mendez et al (3).

1. Barth, P.T. and Grinter, N.J. Map of plasmid RP4
        derived by insertion of transposon C.
        J. molec. Biol. 113, 455-474 (1977).
2. Grinsted, J., Bennett, P.M., Higginson, S. and
        Richmond, M.H. Regional preference of insertion
        of Tn501 and Tn802 into RP1 and its derivatives.
        Molec. gen. Genet. 166, 313-320 (1978).
3. Mendez, B., Tachibana, C. and Levy, S.B.
        Heterogeneity of tetracycline resistance
        determinants. Plasmid, 3, 99-108 (1980).

REGULATION OF TRANSPOSON Tn10 TETRACYCLINE RESISTANCE

K. Bertrand, K. Postle, L. Wray* and W. Reznikoff*
Department of Microbilogy
University of Californis, Irvine CA 92717
*Department of Biochemistry
University of Wisconsin
Madison, WI 53706

The maximal expression of Tn10 tetracycline resistance is induced by exposure to low concentrations of the drug itself. Induction appears to involve inactivation of a Tn10 encoded repressor protein that acts negatively to control the rate of transcription of the resistance function(s). We have analyzed the genetic organization of the resistance region by constructing in vitro recombinant plasmids that carry different segments of Tn10 DNA. The structural gene for the repressor is within a 695 base pair Hind II restriction fragment situated adjacent to the promoter for the resistance function(s). The DNA sequence of this region, in conjunction with mutational analyses, predicts the amino acid sequence of a 23,500 dalton repressor protein. Several lines of evidence indicate that the structural genes for the repressor and the resistance function(s) are transcribed in opposite directions from functionally overlapping promoters. Fusion of either the repressor promoter or the resistance promoter to an otherwise promoterless lacZ gene places lacZ under the control of the tet repressor in vivo. Repression of lacZ in these gene fusion strains is overcome by low concentrations of tetracycline. Plasmids that car the repressor gene direct the synthesis of a 23,000 dalton protein in minicells, and the synthesis of this protein is induced by tetracycli We conclude that the repressor is autogenously regulated--it negative regulates transcription of its own structural gene as well as regulat ing transcription of the resistance gene(s). In vitro studies employ ing purified RNA polymerase and various restriction fragments as DNA templates indicate that the transcription initiation sites for the repressor and resistance promoters are only 15-20 base pairs apart. The DNA sequence of the regulatory region suggests a model in which transcription of the repressor and the resistance function(s) is controlled simultaneously by repressor binding to a common operator sites.

PLASMIDS AND PHAGES AND COMPLEMENT RESISTANCE

M.M. Binns, F.P.A. Carr and R.P. Levine

James S. McDonnell Department of Genetics
Washington University School of Medicine
St. Louis, Missouri   63110

Plasmid-specified resistance to complement is well documented; R100, R6-5 and ColV.I-K94 have been studied extensively (see article by Dr. K. Timmis in this volume). Resistance conferred by temperate phages is less well understood.

Results using "Southern blots" and specific antibody against the traT protein of R100 indicate that the iss gene of ColV.I-K94 and the traT gene of R100 are distinct. However the levels of resistance conferred to a range of serums by each gene, cloned into the plasmid vector pBR322, are remarkably similar. Resistance in both cases is to the classical and the alternative pathway of complement action.

The consumption of C8 by cells with and without the plasmid genes which had been treated with R8 (complement from which C8 had been removed using a C8 specific antibody column) were identical. This result indicates that the gene products which confer resistance do so at the level of C8 action or C9 binding or action, i.e. the gene products inpair the formation and/or structure of the terminal complex.

traT-containing cells remain resistant to complement after pretreatment with antibody to either traT or to E. coli, indicating that the traT protein may have a "passive" structural role rather than an "active" function in complement resistance.

E. coli J6-2 lysogenic for λ is approximately four-fold more resistant to a range of serums than the non-lysogenic strain. Two major genes, cI and rex are expressed in prophage λ. Complement resistance conferred by the prophage does not involve the rex gene as demonstrated by studies with rex⁻ mutants. The role of the cI gene is unclear. A cI clone producing high levels of cI .repressor confers increased sensitivity to complement. Further studies to determine the genetic basis of the complement resistance by λ are in progress.

POSSIBLE VIRULENCE DETERMINANTS IN YERSINIA PSEUDOTUBERCULOSIS

Ingrid Bölin, Birgitta Engberg and Hans Wolf-Watz

Department of Microbiology
National Defence Research Institute
S-901 82 Umeå, Sweden

It is known that certain strains of Yersinia pseudotuber-
culosis (Y.p.) are highly virulent for birds, rodents and other
animals. When given orally these strains cause lethal infection in
Swiss albino mice (1). It was found that one of these virulent
strains of Y.p. (strain III) carried a plasmid showing a molecular
weight of about 60 Kb. A plasmid free derivative of this strain
was incapable to cause a lethal infection in mice when given
orally. These results clearly indicate that the virulence of Y.p.
is associated with a plasmid. This is also confirmed by results
obtained by others (1). Several temperature effects of Y.p. may
also be correlated to the presence of a plasmid. When a growing
plasmid containing strain (Y.p. III), was shifted from growth at
$26^{o}C$ to $37^{o}C$ a number of differences in the protein profile of the
sarcosyl insoluble membrane fraction was found. At least one
protein showing a molecular weight of about 100 000 Mdal was
induced by this temperature shift. This protein was correlated
with the presence of plasmid, as a plasmid free derivative of Y.p.
III lacked this protein in the corresponding membrane fraction.
In addition we were unable to detect any differences in the rate
of synthesis of this 100 K protein correlated to the presence of
either Ca^{2+} or Mg^{2+} ions in the growth medium after the temperature shift. We have shown that strains of Y.p. are virlent for
guinea pigs when injected intraperitionally and that this virulence
is correlated to the capability of these strains of adhere to HeLa
cells. However, this HeLa cell attachment is not associated with a
plasmid, as we found strains of Y.p. lacking plasmid but still
maintaining the capacity to adhere to HeLa cells. This HeLa cell
adherence of Y.p. was found to be mannose insensitive but temperature dependent. When strains of Y.p. was grown at $26^{o}C$ they adhered
in a high degree to HeLa cells in sharp contrast to cells grown at
$37^{o}C$ which showed a very low capacity to bind to HeLa cells. We
were unable to detect pili on the bacterial cell surface, indicating
that the Y.p. adherance to HeLa cells is not mediated by pili. By
allowing a total cell extract of sonicated Y.p. to react with HeLa
cells prior to the addition of intact Y.p. we were able to block
the specific attachment between the bacteria and HeLa cells. The
adherance was markedly decresed after addition of sonicated cell
extract. Furthermore, by using the same strategy it was shown that
the sarcosyl insoluble membrane fraction contained maximum blocking
capacity. These results indicate that the ligand mediating the adherance between Y.p. and HeLa cells can be recovered in the sarcosyl
insoluble membrane fraction.

1. P. Gemski, J. R. Lazere, T. Casey, and J. A. Wohlhieter,
   Infect. Immun. 28:1044-1047 (1980).

INFLUENCE OF HOST CELL METABOLISM ON EXPRESSION OF FERTILITY OF F-LIKE R PLASMIDS

Lars G. Burman and Solveig Lindh
Department of Clinical Microbiology
University of Umeå
S-90185 Umeå, Sweden

INTRODUCTION:

The natural habitat of enteric bacteria is largely anaerobic. Anaerobic growth of an E. coli K12 host did not affect replication or drug resistance of 45 R plasmids studied, whereas transfer was strongly reduced (by 10^2 to 10^4-fold) for F-like plasmids but not for I or N plasmids. The conjugative process per se was not impaired by anaerobiosis. Instead, this condition appeared to increase repression of the tra operon of F-like plasmids and augmented their inhibition of F factor fertility (fin). Thus, anaerobic "superrepression" of plasmid fertility was active also in trans. (L.G.Burman; J.Bacteriol. 123:265, 1975 and 131:69, 1977.)

RESULTS:

The response of the F-like R plasmid R1 to anaerobiosis can be mimicked by aerobic growth of the host in the presence of high concentrations of glucose (0.5-2%), which is known to induce a metabolic state similar to anaerobiosis, i.e. increased glycolysis and repression of TCA cycle enzymes. This glucose effect occurred only in yeast extract based media, was not alleviated by cyclic AMP and was seen in all Enterobacteriaceae spp. investigated. Other sugars, glycolytic intermediates and end products tested had no effect on tra control except for pyruvate which decreased R1 fertility by 100-fold. A possible clue to the effect of host cell metabolism on tra control was suggested by experiments with NaF. This glycolysis inhibitor alleviated the glucose effect but augmented that of pyruvate. However, the intermediate implicated, phosphoenol pyruvate (PEP, see Fig.), could not be assessed in vivo since it was not taken up by E. coli cells.

DISCUSSION:

It seems unlikely that O_2 tension per se influences the control of fertility of F-like plasmids. In situations when the PEP pool is large (anaerobiosis, high glucose, pyruvate + NaF) repression of tra is much stronger than during low PEP (aerobiosis, high glucose + NaF). Therefore, one hypothetical interpretation of the findings is that phosphorylation of a soluble control element using PEP as donor is involved in the expression of the tra operon of F-like plasmids.

Fig. Glycolysis. Glucose .. <$\xleftrightarrow{\text{enolase}}$> PEP <——> pyruvate -- TCA cycle

↑
NaF

TRANSFERABLE DRUG RESISTANCE IN BACTEROIDES FRAGILIS:

IN VITRO AND IN VIVO OBSERVATIONS

T. Butler, M.D.[1], K. Joiner, M.D.[1], F. Tally, M.D.[1],
S. L. Gorbach, M.D.[1,2], J. Bartlett, M.D.[3],
M. Malamy, PhD[2].
Departments of Medicine[1], Microbiology and Molecular
Biology[2], Tufts-New England Medical Center and The
Boston Veterans Administration Hospital[3], Boston, Mass.

Plasmid-mediated transferable drug resistance (tetracycline,
clindamycin) has been described among strains of Bacteroides
fragilis. As beta-lactamase production by bacteroides is known
to be common, we sought to determine if transferable resistance to
beta-lactam drugs occured among strains and if it could be ascribed
to transfer of extrachromosomal elements. Transfer of drug resistance among these strains of bacteroides was also examined in an
experimental subcutaneous abscess model, to ascertain if resistance transfer occurs at infected sites.

The findings indicate that transferable beta-lactam (penicillin, ampicillin, cephalothin, cephamandole) resistance occurs
between strain TMP 16 and a suitable recipient. Localization of
the beta-lactam resistance determinant has not been established.
In addition, we have detected, in the experimental abscess model,
transferable clindamycin and tetracycline resistance between TMP
10 and TM 4500. A 10 megadalton plasmid encoding clindamycin
resistance and originating in TMP 10 is seen in clindamycin
resistant progeny.

E. COLI K1 PATHOGENICITY

F.C. Cabello and M.E. Aguero
New York Medical College, Valhall, NY 10595

The work of the Cooperative Neonatal Meningitis Study demonstrated that 81% of the E. coli strains isolated from the spinal fluid of sick neonates have the K1 capsular antigen. Animal studies showed that E. coli K1 strains were more virulent than non K1 E. coli and that antibodies against K1 antigen were protective, confirming the role of K1 antigen as a virulence factor. The fact that not all the neonates colonized with E. coli K1 develop disease, that the rates of colonization among neonates fluctuates widely and that there are variations in the LD50 of different E. coli K1 strains for the mice led us to think that these strains are not a homogeneous population and that other bacterial factors may be involved in their ability to colonize and produced disease. These factors could be the same ones that have been associated with the ability of E. coli to invade, i.e. harboring of ColV plasmids, hemolysin production and the capacity to hemagglutinate.

To investigate the heterogeneity of E. coli K1 strains regarding these properties we tested several E. coli K1 strains isolated from stools, blood and spinal fluid for production of colicin V, hemolysin and ability to agglutinate human red blood cells. We found that E. coli K1 isolates carry these traits with high frequency regardless of the site of isolation. To further prove the relevance of these characters and K1 antigen to E. coli K1 pathogenicity isogenic strains were isolated and their LD50 for mice were determined. The results showed that the K1 antigen is essential for pathogenicity and that this basal pathogenicity can be increased by the presence of the ColV and hemolysin plasmids. Additional experiments indicated that the presence of K1 antigen but not that of ColV protect the bacteria from the action of complement and phagocytosis. The isolation, by transposition, of colicin negative ColV plasmids allowed us to demonstrate that the increase of pathogenicity is not mediated by colicin production. Preliminary results suggest that the ColV plasmid confers a selective advantage to E. coli K1 in an iron poor environment (see P. Williams this volume).

The newborn rat model is now being used to test the importance of these factors in colonization and ability to invade (see Clancy and Savage, this volume). The cloning of the K1 antigen genes and the ColV plasmid DNA has been achieved and will facilitate progress in further understanding of their biology and their relationship to disease formation.

This work is supported by N.I.H. Grant R01 AI 116078-01 and funds from Smith, Kline and French.

ANTIBIOTIC RESISTANCE IN STAPHYLOCCI ISOLATED IN DUBLIN HOSPITALS

M Cafferkey, G Dowd, C Keane, R Hone, H Pomeroy, G Dougan

Departments of Clinical Microbiology and Microbiology

University of Dublin, Dublin 2. Ireland

A large number of isolates of Staphylococcus aureus from nosocomial infections and the hospital environment were characterised by phage typing and plasmid analysis. The strains were isolated in a group of eight hospitals over a four year period. Isolates which were resistant to gentamicin and several other antibiotics including penicillin, tetracycline, erythromycin and methicillin belonged to four main 'phage types'. The gentamicin resistant strains (GMRSA) were widespread in the hospitals and were responsible for cases of serious infection including 34 cases of septicaemia. The Table shows the periods when the different 'phage types' were present in the hospitals.

Plasmid screening of more than 200 out of a total of some 2,000 GMRSA isolates revealed a conserved plasmid profile. Restriction analysis, transformation and transduction studies allowed antibiotic resistance markers to be assigned to particular plasmids. All strains harboured a 21Md penicillinase plasmid. Type 85 and 77 strains harboured a 3.0Md tetracycline resistance plasmid whereas type 90 and 6/47/54/84/85 strains harboured a 24Md tetracycline resistance plasmid. GMRSA contained acetyl and phosphotransferase aminoglycoside inactivating activity. However gentamicin, amikacin, erythromycin and methicillin resistance seemed to be encoded on the host chromosome. Thus a small number of related strains were responsible for a large number of nosocomial infections.

TABLE

Phage type	Period of Isolation of Strains
77	1977 - 1979
85	1978 - 1979
6/47/54/84/85	1980 - present day
90	1979 - present day

PLASMIDS AND DELTA-ENDOTOXIN PRODUCTION IN BACILLUS THURINGIENSIS

Bruce C. Carlton and José M. González, Jr.

Department of Molecular and Population Genetics
University of Georgia
Athens, Georgia 30602 USA

Five strains of Bacillus thuringiensis that produce crystalline δ-endotoxin were used as parental strains to isolate acrystalliferous (Cry⁻) mutants: HD-2 (B. thuringiensis var. thuringiensis, flagellar serotype 1); HD-1 and HD-73 (both var. kurstaki, serotype 3ab); HD-4 (var. alesti, serotype 3a), and HD-8 (var. galleriae, serotype 5ab). The parental strains contain complex plasmid arrays ranging from 4 to 11 plasmids per strain, with sizes from 1.4 to 150 Md. The plasmid patterns of both Cry⁻ and Cry⁺ variants were analyzed and compared to the parental strains using a modified Eckhardt lysate-electrophoresis method.

Most Cry⁻ mutants derived from strain HD-2 exhibited a distinctive colony morphology which facilitated their isolation. Loss of crystal production was associated with loss of a 75-Md plasmid. A 50-Md plasmid of strain HD-73 was lost in the Cry⁻ mutants. Crystal production in strain HD-4 appeared to be associated with a plasmid about 105 Md in size; in strain HD-1, a smaller plasmid (29 Md in size) seemed to be involved. In strain HD-8, a large plasmid (∼130 Md in size) was implicated in crystal production. Direct bioassay of several mutant strains confirmed the loss of δ-endotoxin activity in the acrystalliferous isolates.

The evidence supports the notion of a relationship between specific extrachromosomal DNA elements and δ-endotoxin production in B. thuringiensis, and suggests that in each strain only a single plasmid is involved, although the size of the implicated plasmid varies from one strain to another.

CONJUGAL TRANSFER OF PLASMID-ASSOCIATED LACTOSE METABOLISM IN LACTOBACILLUS CASEI subsp. CASEI.

Bruce Chassy and Enid Rokaw
NIDR-NIH
Bethesda, Maryland   20205   U.S.A.

Many strains of *Lactobacillus casei* subsp. *casei* lose the ability to ferment lactose when cultured in the presence of plasmid curing agents such as acriflavin. The curing is accompanied by the loss of distinct plasmids ranging in size from 17.5 to 36 Mdalton (Mdal) depending on the strain studied. Analysis of these lactose plasmids with several restriction endonucleases revealed no fragments of identical size, however, the possible presence of a homologous sequence of DNA associated with lactose metabolism has not been evaluated. In order to assess possible mechanisms for the widespread distribution of lactose plasmids in *L. casei*, a number of Lac^+ and Lac^- strains were crossed by a filter pad mating technique. For example:

DONOR: *L. casei* 4646 Lac^+, Rif^s, $Ribitol^-$, white smooth colonial morphology

RECIPIENT: *L. casei* 64H Lac^- (cured of 23 Mdal lactose plasmid) Rif^r, $Ribitol^+$, glassy mucoid colonial morphology

Cells (10^8 of donor and recipient) were mixed onto a Millipore filter pad, incubated for 18 hr at 37° on glucose-LCM-agar and then transferred to lactose-rifampin-LCM-agar for 3-5 days at 37°. Typically, 100-200 glassy mucoid, Lac^+, $Ribitol^+$, Rif^r transconjugant colonies were observed. Spontaneous reversion to Lac^+ has not been observed in *L. casei* 64H Lac^-, nor has spontaneous acquisition of $Ribitol^+$ been observed with *L. casei* ATCC 4646. The latter strain spontaneously becomes Rif^r at a frequency of $<1/10^7$ cells, but colonies resulting from this mutation were easily distinguished from *L. casei* 64H. Plasmid isolation, followed by agarose gel electrophoresis, revealed that transconjugants always contained a plasmid which was identical in size to that found in the donor (36 Mdal). Some isolates also contained one, or both, of the small cryptic plasmids found in the donor; perhaps indicative of a conjugal "mobilization". While purified plasmid DNA from ATCC 4646 would not transform 64H Lac^- under these conditions; experiments incorporating DNAse into the agar were not performed. These results indicate that the plasmid-determined ability to ferment lactose is transmissible among *L. casei* strains by a "conjugation-like" process. To our knowledge, no naturally occuring system of conjugation, transformation or transduction has been described previously in the genus *Lactobacillus*.

DIFFERENCES IN RECOMBINATION BETWEEN TWO TRANSPOSON SEQUENCES

ORIENTED AS DIRECT OR INDIRECT REPEATS IN recA OR recA+ HOSTS

S. J. Chiang and R. C. Clowes

Programs in Biology, The Univ. of Texas at Dallas

P.O. Box 688, Richardson, Texas 75080

When intramolecular transposition occurs to produce a second copy of the transposon, Tn3 or Tn2660, this copy is invariably oriented inversely to the resident transposon, and in some cases, the plasmid DNA sequence between the two transposons has undergone an inversion. We have recently determined that the orientation of the DNA sequence between these two inverse repeat transposons is stable (less than 2% change after 60 generations of growth), irrespective of whether inversion of the plasmid DNA occurred during transposition, and irrespective of whether growth is observed in a recA or recA+ host. This stability has been observed in two plasmids differing in their replication control.

In contrast, the DNA sequence between two direct repeats of the same transposon (in the one host tested) appears to be highly unstable. We draw this conclusion from experiments attempting to couple two plasmids in vitro, each with a Tn2660 transposon, each with a mutually-compatible replication control and with different antibiotic resistance markers, followed by selection of transformants in a recA⁻ host. Whereas, these two plasmids can be coupled with the Tn2660 sequences as an inverse repeat, no composite plasmids with the transposons as a direct repeat can be isolated, but two recombinant plasmids, consistent with recombination between the two transposons are isolated with a high frequency. There thus appears to be a marked difference in the frequency of recombination in recA or recA+ cells between two transposons in a plasmid, depending upon whether they are oriented as a direct or an indirect repeat.

Tn 10 ENCODED PROTEINS THAT MEDIATE TETRACYCLINE RESISTANCE IN E. COLI

I. Chopra, P.R. Ball, S.J. Eccles and S.W. Shales
Department of Bacteriology
University of Bristol. U.K.

Other workers have shown that transposon 10 probably codes for 3 proteins (of molecular weights 36K, 25K and 13-15K) which are involved in tetracycline resistance. The function of these proteins is unknown but studies on their location in whole cells may clarify their roles. Immuno-precipitation demonstrated the 25K protein in the outer membrane. Expression of Tn10-mediated resistance was defective in certain outer membrane mutants suggesting that the 25K protein is involved in resistance. The 36K protein (p I about 6.4) was resolved by two dimensional electrophoresis and its content in the inner membrane was corre-lated with reduced drug uptake. The 25K protein was not resolved by standard 2D-electrophoresis suggesting that it is basic (pI>7). The 25K and 36K envelope associated proteins probably contribute to decreased antibiotic uptake. The location of the third polypeptide (13-15K) is presently unknown, but might be ribosomal.

ANOTHER COLICIN V PHENOTYPE: ADHESION IN VITRO OF ESCHERICHIA

COLI TO MOUSE INTESTINAL EPITHELIUM

Joanna Clancy and Dwayne C. Savage*

Department of Microbiology
University of Illinois
Urbana, Illinois 61801

ABSTRACT

Two assays were designed with which isogenic laboratory
strains of E. coli K12 with and without ColV plasmids were compared for their ability to adhere in vitro to mouse intestinal
epithelium. In both assays discs of intestinal tissue were exposed
to bacteria. In the first, discs were homogenized and the numbers
of viable bacteria adherent to them were estimated from colony
counts of plates inoculated with dilutions of the homogenates. In
the second, bacteria were labeled with ^{14}C-aspartic acid; the
number of adherent cells per disc was estimated by liquid scintil-
lation spectrometry. Data from each assay were compared by analysis of variance. In both assays, strains bearing the ColV plasmid
adhered in two to three-fold greater numbers than isogenic strains
without the plasmid. These differences were highly significant
statistically. A non-colicinogenic strain free of the ColV plasmid
was selected by treatment of a ColV strain with Sodium Dodecyl
Sulfate (SDS). In the radioisotopic assay, the ColV strain associated with the epithelium in significantly greater numbers than the
cured derivative. A ColV strain was created by conjugation; in the
radioisotopic assay this strain bound to epithelium in significantly
greater numbers than the recipient strain without the plasmid. The
original ColV strain, when negatively-stained and examined by
electron microscopy, had pili that adsorbed male-specific bacteriophage while its isogenic variant without ColV did not. Some such
properties, coded by the plasmid, may increase the virulence of
the bacteria.

*Infect. Immun. (1981) 31: in press.

EXPRESSION OF TN10 ENCODED TETRACYCLINE

RESISTANCE IS REDUCED IN MULTIPLE COPIES

D.C.Coleman and T.J.Foster

Microbiology Department

Trinity College, Dublin 2

Plasmid pNK133 carries the tet genes of Tn10 inserted in a multicopy vector derived from pBR322. The Tc^r level was 10-fold lower than determined by a chromosomal element. Minicells harbouring pNK133 failed to synthesize the 36K tet protein. Most deletions and Tn5 in tet on pNK133 caused Tc^s mutations which also prevented expression of high level Tc^r from chromosomal Tn10 present in the same cell. Only those insertions in the promoter-proximal 90-130bp of a 1275bp HindII fragment known to carry the tet structural genes did not reduce the single copy Tc^r level.

A gene-fusion system resulting in constitutive expression of β-galactosidase from a tet promoter was used to assay tet repressor. Multicopy plasmids encoding tet repressor reduced the basal (uninduced) level of β-galactosidase by 17-fold, whereas single copy tet repression was 2-fold. The tet::Tn5 mutants defective in the trans-dominant multicopy effect still made normal amounts of repressor. This shows that overproduction of repressor was not responsible for the multicopy effect.

In conclusion, the trans-acting multicopy tet effect was inactivated only by Tn5 insertions located in the first 90-130bp of the tet structural gene, possibly in the coding region for the amino-terminus of a tet protein. We postulate that a regulatory mechanism in addition to repressor control of induction exists which prevents attempts to overproduce the tet protein.

NATIONAL INSTITUTES OF HEALTH PROGRAMS IN ANTIBIOTIC RESISTANCE AND RECOMBINANT DNA

Irving P. Delappe
Microbiology and Infectious Diseases Program, NIAID
National Institutes of Health, Bethesda, Maryland

These two programs are supported by the Molecular Microbiology and Parasitology Branch in the Microbiology and Infectious Diseases Program of the National Institute of Allergy and Infectious Diseases.

The first of these is Mechanisms of Resistance to Antimicrobial Agents whose principal goal is to elucidate fundamental biological mechanisms involved in the development of microbial drug resistance and to increase our basic understanding of this phenomenon. More specific goals involve investigations of the origin, development, evolution, expression and mechanisms of drug resistance in a variety of specific microorganisms. Of particular interest to the program are the Enterobacteriaceae, Pseudomonas, Neisseria, staphylococci, streptococci, mycobacteria, mycoplasmas, and pathogenic fungi.

Research of special interest to this program is included in one or more of the following categories: (1) genetic and structural studies of R factors and related plasmids; (2) origin, development, and evolution of drug resistance in microorganisms; (3) replication and conjugal transfer of plasmids; (4) biochemistry and genetics of plasmid-determined functions, especially resistance to antimicrobial agents; (5) correlated epidemiological and microbiological studies of naturally-occurring plasmids with special reference to R factors. The branch currently has approximately 3.7 million dollars invested in this program.

The branch has also supported the Stanford Plasmid Reference Center for 4 years. This serves as the sole collection and coordination center of its type in the United States, and, as such, is an important establishment that is very useful to workers in this rapidly expanding area of research.

The second program, Recombinant DNA, had its origins in the first. Our most important goal in this program is the utilization of the recombinant DNA technology to provide us with a greater knowledge of the molecular basis of pathogenicity. This information may lead to improved prevention, diagnosis, and treatment of infectious diseases.

Another goal is the production of a variety of biologically useful substances through the construction of bacterial cells containing functional DNA of animal origin. Currently, Institute-supported scientists are working to clone the interferon gene.

An equally important goal is the identification, assessment, and elimination of any and all potential biohazards encountered in the exploitation of this technology. Currently the branch invests 3.3 million dollars in this program.

DNA SEQUENCE OF THE ST_{A2} ENTEROTOXIN GENE FROM AN E. COLI STRAIN OF HUMAN ORIGIN

Michel De Wilde[1], Marc Ysebaert[2], and Nigel Harford[1]

Genetics Group[1], Smith Kline - RIT, Rixensart, and
Department of Molecular Biology[2], University of Ghent,
BELGIUM

The DNA sequence of the ST_{A2} gene from CRL25090 (see Harford et al : this meeting) is presented and compared to the DNA sequence derived by So and McCarthy (PNAS 1980 ; 77 : 4011) for the ST_{A1} gene from Tn1681. The genes are similar in having a conserved promoter region and an open reading frame of 72 amino acids including a 19 amino acid putative signal sequence. However there are 27 % base mismatch and 38 % amino acid differences between the two coding sequences. This explains the lack of homology between the two genes in stringent DNA-DNA hybridizations. The C-terminal region is highly conserved in the two genes including 6 half cysteine residues. In the case of ST_{A1} this region corresponds exactly to the amino acid composition found by Staples et al (J. Biol. Chem. 1980 ; 225 : 4716) for a purified ST_A toxin from a human E. coli isolate. It appears that the primary gene product undergoes extensive processing during the release of mature toxin from the cell.

GENETIC ANALYSIS OF CONJUGATION IN <u>STREPTOCOCCUS</u> <u>FAECALIS</u>

G. Dunny, C. Funk, and E. Ehrenfeld

N.Y.S. College of Veterinary Medicine
Cornell University
Ithaca, N.Y. 14853

pCF-10 is a 35 megadalton plasmid which was identified in a human clinical isolate of <u>S. faecalis</u>. A series of conjugation and curing experiments has revealed that this conjugative plasmid determines tetracycline resistance and also carries genes which enable its host cell to elicit a clumping response and high frequency of transfer when exposed to bacterial sex pheromones (CIAs). This plasmid is the first naturally occurring R-factor identified which carries genes for CIA response. We have been using pCF-10 to begin genetic analysis of streptococcal conjugation. In the course of attempting to cure pCF-10, we obtained tetracycline sensitive variants which still carried pCF-10. Some of these plasmids appear to carry small deletions and are also affected in their CIA response. These plasmids may be very useful in physical analysis of the transfer region of the plasmid. A second type of variant of pCF-10 has been identified by looking at rare transconjugants obtained after short matings in the absence of CIA. This variant plasmid transfers at higher frequencies than wild-type pCF-10 in the absence of CIA, and cells carrying it spontaneously clump in liquid culture. Further genetic and physical characterization of these plasmids should help to better define the conjugal transfer process.

TANDEM DUPLICATIONS OF THE ampC GENE OF ESCHERICHIA COLI K-12

Thomas Edlund and Staffan Normark

Department of Microbiology
University of Umeå
S-901 87 Umeå, Sweden

The ampC gene at 93.8 min on the E. coli K-12 linkage map codes for a β-lactamase. By selection for ampicillin resistance mutants have been isolated that carry multiple tandem ampC repeats[1]. The size and end points for ten independent amp duplications were determined by direct cleavage of chromosomal DNA with relevant restriction endonucleases. The amp duplications were all between 9 and 18 kilobasepairs in size. The end points for seven of these duplications were accurately determined and found to be essentially randomly distributed. By reciprocal recombination between a ColE1-ampC hybrid plasmid and the chromosome of an amp amplified mutant, a plasmid derivative was isolated carrying multiple copies of a 9.8 kb amp repeat. The nucleotide sequence of the novel joint created by the duplication was compared to the sequences of the two DNA segments that participated in the formation of this novel joint. The fusion had occurred within a 12 bp perfect homology with the sequence 5'-CAACACCACGCG-3'. It is suggested that tandem ampC duplications are the result of unequal recA dependent crossing overs between short homologous sequences of any composition. E. coli strains carrying about 10 tandem ampC repeats were virtually stable in a recA background. In contrast, a plasmid carrying five 9.5 kb repeats was found to segregate these repeats as covalently closed circular (ccc) DNA molecules in a recA background. This provides evidence for intramolecular recA independent recombinations in plasmids carrying repetitive DNA.

REFERENCE

1. Edlund, T., Grundström, T., and Normark, S. 1979. Isolation and characterization of DNA repetitions carrying the chromosomal β-lactamase gene of Escherichia coli K-12. Molec.Gen.Genet. 173: 115-125.

R67: A NATURALLY OCCURRING R PLASMID ENCODING TWO DISTINCT TRIMETHOPRIM-RESISTANT DIHYDROFOLATE REDUCTASES

Lynn P. Elwell, Mary E. Fling and Leslie Walton

Wellcome Research Laboratories
North Carolina 27709

The mechanism of plasmid-associated trimethoprim (Tp) resistance involves the synthesis of novel dihydrofolate reductases (DHFRs) which are highly resistant to Tp. R plasmid-encoded DHFRs can be arbitrarily divided into two broad classes (type I and II) based on different levels of sensitivity to Tp and related antifolate compounds. Hence, type I DHFRs have 50% inhibitory concentrations in the micromolar range whereas type II enzymes are inhibited by millimolar amounts of trimethoprim. Representative enzymes of each class appear to differ antigenically as well as in subunit structure. Plasmid R67 is a multiply antibiotic resistant plasmid originally isolated from a citrobacter sp. We previously cloned a DNA segment encoding a type II DHFR from R67 and characterized this enzyme in E. coli minicells. This R67 reductase was shown to consist of 4 identical 8,444 molecular weight subunits and to be antigenically unrelated to the type I DHFR harbored by transposon 7 (Tn7). In cloning experiments using purified R67 DNA and pSC101 DNA a small number of transformants (4% of the total) had an ampicillin-resistant, trimethoprim-resistant, tetracycline-sensitive phenotype. These transformants harbored plasmids 2-5 X 10^6 daltons in mass. Unexpectedly, these chimeric plasmids directed the synthesis of an 18,000 molecular weight polypeptide in E. coli minicells (the type I DHFR harbored by Tn7 has a subunit molecular weight of 18,000). Furthermore, the reductases harbored by three independently isolated derivative plasmids appeared to be type I - like on the basis of inhibition kinetics, pH activity profile, stability studies and lack of antigenic reactivity with anti-type II (R67) antibody. Chimeric plasmids of this description were never isolated when pBR322 DNA was substituted for pSC101 DNA or when either cloning vehicle was omitted from the reaction mixture. EcoRl-digested R67 was probed, using the Southern blotting technique, with ^{32}P-labeled DNA segments containing a type I or a type II gene sequence. Different EcoRl digestion fragments showed homology with either the type I or the type II probe. Therefore, both gene sequences appear to be present in this plasmid. Hence, plasmid R67 appears to harbor the genes for two distinct trimethoprim-resistant dihydrofolate reductases. The evolutionary implications of this finding are intriguing but, as yet, are unclear.

BEHAVIOR OF ANTIBIOTIC RESISTANT PLASMIDS OF Staphylococcus Aureus STRAINS.

Espinosa-Lara, A. and Martínez.

Depto. de Microbiología. Escuela Nacional de Ciencias Biológicas. IPN. Apartado Postal 4-870. México 17, D.F.

Thirteen multirresistant strains of S.aureus coagulase positive, isolated from different lesions were used. The strains were maintained at 4°on slants of soja-tripticaseine agar added with antibiotics. The propagation, segregation and curing experiments were carried out in soja-tripticaseine agar and broth.

The strains have different patterns of resistance to aminoglycosides They were resistant, to five, four and two antibiotics. The strains were considered resistant if they grew on medium with concentration of antibiotics higher than the maximal concentration found in blood after a therapeutic dose.

In order to determine if the aminoglycoside resistance markers were in chromosomal or in plasmid DNA, the genetic material of the resistant strains was isolated and separated by agarose gel electrophoresis. The data showed that strains have at least one and some of them more than one plasmid.

Experiments of spontaneous lost of these markers were conducted by incubation of the strains 4 h and 18 h in TSA without selective pressure. The markers are lost together in a characteristic frequency for each strain, except in R13, R14 and R5 in which the percentage of lost for amikacin marker was higher than that of - the other markers, indicating the location of this marker in a different plasmid.

Ethidium bromide (EtBr) and sodium dodecyl sulphate (SDS) effect on the resistance patterns was the last parameter analized. Six strains were treated and only two were cured. With strain R13 the curing of the amikacin marker was less than that of the other markers, suggesting again its location in a different plasmid.

Strain	Resistance pattern	% segregation		% curing		No Electro-
		3h	18 h	EtBr	SDS	phoretic bands
R1	K,G,T,S,A	63	78	–	–	2
R2	K,G,T,S	–	–	18	–	–
R5	K,G,T,S,A	5	97	–	–	1
R8	T,S	45	19	0	0	–
R10	T,S	4	15	–	–	–
R11	K,G,T,S,A	0	28	0	0	3
R12	K,G,T,S,A	5	84	0	0	3
R13	K,G,T,S,A	0	68	28	18	3
R14	K,G,T,S	–	–	–	–	1

K=Kanamycin,G=Gentamicin,T=Tobramycin,S=Sisomycin, A=Amikacin

MULTIPLE KIL GENES OF THE BROAD HOST RANGE PLASMID RK2

D. Figurski, R. Pohlman, D. Bechhofer, A. Prince,
C. Kelton

Department of Microbiology, College of Physicians &
Surgeons Columbia University, New York, New York 10032

The broad host range capability of IncP plasmids very likely involves plasmid-specified functions. We are examining the IncP plasmid RK2[1] for genes involved in host-plasmid interactions. Our results show that three separate regions of RK2 contain genes whose expression can apparently kill an E. coli host cell. Each "kil" gene (kil I, II, III) has a corresponding "kor" ("kil-override") gene (korI, II, III) to prevent cell death.

The three kor genes have been cloned. Since the kor functions act in trans, the Kor+ strains allowed cloning of the kil genes. None of the kor genes is close to the kil gene it controls. KorI and korII map together in the 50-56.4 kb region of the plasmid, but deletions of korII suggest that these are separate genes. Kil I and kil III map in regions known to be non-essential for RK2 replication in E. coli. Kil II is near a replication gene, trfA,[2] but mutations of kil II show that these are different genes.

The kor genes are also non-essential, unless kil genes are present. Previous work[2] indicates that at least two separate genes (trfA and trfB) code for the trans-acting functions[3] essential for RK2 in E. coli. Our studies show that trfA alone is sufficient for replication at ori. The trfB region is only needed to control a non-essential kil-like gene (possibly kil II) that maps next to trfA.

Four different IncP plasmids (R906, R995, pUZ8, R751) were tested for korI- and korII-like genes, and all four were found to have both. This predicts that kil I and kil II are also present on these plasmids. If the kil and kor genes are truly conserved among IncP plasmids, they are likely to have a significant role in the proliferation of these plasmids, perhaps in hosts other than E. coli.

The existence of kil genes on promiscuous plasmids rich in antibiotic resistance genes suggests a novel approach for the control of organisms carrying these plasmids. An understanding of the regulation of kil genes may lead to antibiotics that will induce suicide by these bacteria specifically.

1. Ingram L, Richmond M, Sykes R, 1973, Antimicrob. Ag. & Che. 3:279.
2. Thomas CM, Meyer RJ, Helinski DR, 1980, J. Bacteriol. 141:213.
3. Figurski DH and Helinski DR, 1979, Proc. Natl. Acad. Sci. USA, 76:1648.

ISOLATION AND IDENTIFICATION OF A DNA FRAGMENT OF Rts1 PLASMID

RESPONSIBLE FOR TEMPERATURE SENSITIVE GROWTH OF HOST BACTERIA

S. Finver, T. Yamamoto, J. Bricker and A. Kaji

University of Pennsylvania
Philadelphia, Pennsylvania 19104

A kanamycin (KM) resistance factor, Rts1, causes inhibition of growth of host bacteria if grown from high density (10^6/ml) at 42° C (temperature sensitive growth effect, tsg$^+$), and replicates without forming covalently closed circular (ccc) DNA. On the other hand, at this temperature, this plasmid is eliminated from cultures if cells were grown overnight from low density inoculum (10^3/ml). To isolate the genetic region responsible for tsg$^+$, we utilized digests of pAK8, a spontaneous smaller derivative of Rts1 which retains all the characteristics of Rts1 except for the phenotype of T4 phage growth restriction. Electrophoresis of restriction enzyme digests of Rts1 and pAK8 DNA demonstrated overall sequence homology between these two plasmids. pAK8 DNA provided a better source of tsg$^+$ regions because the molecular weight of pAK8 is 83 Mdal, while that of Rts1 is 126 Mdal. Digests of pAK8 were rejoined with T4 ligase and used to transform E. coli 20S0. Transformants selected for KM resistance were found to contain Rts1 mini-plasmids expressing tsg$^+$ or the instability phenotype. In a second experiment, digests of pAK8 were inserted into the cloning vehicle pBR322. Restriction enzyme analysis of these pBR322 derivatives and Rts1 mini-plasmids allowed the identification of BAM HI fragments essential for replication (18.6 Mdal), KM resistance (14.1 Mdal), and the tsg$^+$ phenotype (8.0 Mdal). Alkaline sucrose gradient analysis of tsg$^+$ and tsg$^-$ mini-plasmids demonstrated that the presence of the 8 Mdal Bam HI fragment also correlated with thermosensitive inhibition of ccc DNA formation. It was observed that many pBR322 derivatives with Rts1 inserts became unstable and were rapidly eliminated from host cells, suggesting that Rts1 contains elements which adversely affect plasmid stability. This effect works only in cis since a co-existing second plasmid replicated normally. One mini-plasmid synthesized by ligation of Sal I digests of pAK8 was KM^r and tsg$^+$; since the total molecular weight of this plasmid was around 5 Mdal, the region(s) influencing tsg would be relatively small and therefore may not consist of multiple genes. Most Rts1 mini-plasmids expressed T group incompatibility, identical to Rts1, except for the Sal I mini-plasmid. This may suggest that one Rts1 replication region is separate from the T-incompatibility gene. Analysis of the phenotypes of various mini-plasmids led us to conclude that the elimination gene (the Rts1 gene causing instability) is distinct from tsg$^+$. These studies suggested that regions influencing tsg$^+$ instability, and replication appear to be independently controlled genes. (U.S.P.H.S. GM-12053).

MOLECULAR AND FUNCTIONAL ANALYSIS OF

THE TOL PLASMID pWWO

F.C.H. Franklin, M. Bagdasarian,
M.M. Bagdasarian and K.N. Timmis

Max-Planck-Institut für Molekulare Genetik
Ihnestrasse 63-73
D-1000 Berlin 33

Soil bacteria are able to utilize or transform an enormous range of natural and synthetic organic molecules. They are therefore of great value as vehicles for environmental protection and have virtually unlimited potential for recycling and regenerating valuable aromatic compounds.

Many of these pathways are known to be plasmid coded. We have made a detailed molecular analysis of one such plasmid, the TOL plasmid pWWO from Pseudomonas putida mt-2. This plasmid codes for the utilization of the hydrocarbons toluene, m- and p-xylene together with their alcohol, aldehyde and carboxylic acid derivatives via a meta-ring cleavage pathway. The analysis was made by Tn5 transposon mutagenesis and gene cloning in a system specially developed for soil bacteria. The gene cloning system consists of a number of vectors derived from the broad host range plasmid RSF1010 and strains of Pseudomonas aeruginosa and P.putida which are restriction deficient and can be transformed at high frequency.

The Tn5 insertions in pWWO were mapped by restriction endonuclease analysis and characterized phenotypically by studying their substrate utilization patterns. XhoI, SstI and HindIII generated fragments of pWWO were cloned and characterized by enzyme assay and complementation analysis. Based on this we have constructed a functional map of the TOL plasmid pWWO (Figure 1).

This reveals that the genes encoding the degradative enzymes map in two separate regions of the plasmid. One of the groups consists of the genes encoding the meta-ring fission enzymes, this is probably of evolutionary significance as the same enzymes are found in quite different degradative pathways. This suggests that there is a high degree of conservation of this DNA sequence. The cloned fragments encoding these enzymes are of great value in further investigation of the degradative pathway regulation and provide a basis for construction of novel degradative pathways with relaxed substrate specificity.

FIGURE 1

Functional map of pWWO. Filled triangles indicate Tn5 insertions that inactivate all or part of the xylene/toluene pathway, whereas open triangles indicate insertions that have no influence on the catabolic functions.

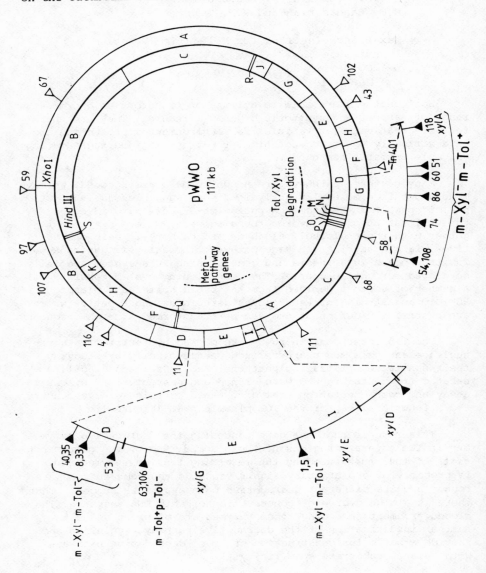

BIOCHEMICAL STUDIES ON THE ANTIGENIC DETERMINANTS OF CFA/I PILI

Laura Frost, Kerry Siminoski, Tania Watts, Betty Worobec and William Paranchych

Department of Biochemistry, University of Alberta, Edmonton, Alberta, Canada T6G 2H7

Enterotoxigenic E. coli H10407 (078:H11) produces CFA/I, a colonization factor antigen found on a plasmid (60 megadaltons) which also encodes the heat stable (ST) toxin and is mobilized by a second smaller plasmid encoding the heat labile (LT) toxin[1]. The CFA/I virulence factor was demonstrated to be pili which mediate adherence to human epithelial tissue of the upper small intestine as well as mannose-resistant hemagglutination of erythrocytes.

The CFA/I pilus is composed of a repeating protein subunit of molecular weight 14,200 which contains no sugar or phosphate. The amino acid composition (43% hydrophobic amino acids) and N-terminal valine residue agree with the findings of P. Klemm[2]. The circular dichroism spectrum for CFA/I pili shows that the amount of helix in the protein is 11% while there is approximately twice as much β-form. Preliminary fiber diffraction patterns indicate a 70 Å periodicity along the axis of the pilus filament/fiber. No values for the number of subunits/turn nor radial density distribution have been determined.

The pilin subunit was purified by gel filtration on a Sephadex G200 column in the presence of 1% SDS, followed by precipitation with acetone. The CFA/I monomer was digested with trypsin (E/S = 1/50) to yield 10 peptides (11 peptides expected). Four of these peptides were fairly large (15 - 47 amino acids) while the other 6 peptides were small (<3 amino acids). Using a competitive ELISA assay whereby a given amount of antibody was pretreated with a known amount of protein or peptide for 0.5 h at 37°C followed by 12-16 h at 4°C, the relative antigenicity of the pilin monomer and tryptic peptides relative to whole pili was determined. While tryptic digestion of the pilin monomer completely destroyed its antigenicity, digestion of whole pili decreased its antigenicity only slightly (21%). No conformational or compositional change in the pili could be detected by electron microscopy, circular dichroism or peptide mapping. The N-terminal peptide (MW4550) and the C-terminal peptide (MW1646) were found to compete with whole pili in the ELISA assay indicating the presence of antigenic determinants in these two peptides.

1. L.P. Elwell and P. Shipley (1980) Ann. Rev. Microbiol. 34:465-496.
2. P. Klemm (1979) FEBS Letters 108:107-110.

THE NATURE OF THE FOSFOMYCIN RESISTANCE DETERMINANT FOUND IN PLASMIDS

Juan M. Garcia-Lobo, Javier León and Jose M. Ortiz

Departamento de Bioquimica, Facultad de Medicina

Santander, SPAIN.

Fosfomycin (1,2,epoxy propyl phosphonic acid) is a cell-wall active antibiotic produced by some *Streptomyces* strains. Chromosomal mutants resistant to fosfomycin are easily found in nature, and this resistance is due to the lack of transport of the drug into the cell.

Recently we have described the finding of plasmids coding for resistance to fosfomycin in clinical isolates of *Serratia marcescens*. The fosfomycin resistance determinant from one of these plasmids, pOU 900, could be mobilized into the plasmid ColE1. The resultant plasmid was designated pSU912. It codes for colicin E1 production and immunity in adition to fosfomycin resistance. The size of the plasmid pSU912 was found to be 11.8 Mdal. This result implied the adition of a 7.6 Mdal fragment of DNA to the plasmid ColE1.

Using the plasmid pSU912 as donor we could observe the traslocation of the fosfomycin resistance determinant into the plasmid RP4 using a system composed of an *E.coli* recA containing both plasmids (pSU912 and RP4) as the donor and an *E.coli* polAts strain as recipient at the restrictive temperature.

On this way we isolated the plasmids pSU920 and pSU923 which showed a size of 43 Mdal. and carried the resistance to fosfomycin in adition to the other markers of the plasmid RP4. Restriction analysis of these two plasmids showed that they carried a 7.6 Mdal. DNA insertion, located at different sites. This result confirmed the existance of a DNA fragment of 7.6 Mdal. in size, capable to move from replicon to replicon independently of the recA host function. It was designated Tn2921.

In order to locate more precisely the DNA region responsible of the fosfomycin resistance we attempted the cloning of this region into the plasmid vector pBR322. Plasmids pSU912 and pBR322 were cleaved with the restriction enzyme PstI and ligated. The ligation mix was used to transform competent *E.coli* C600 cells. Several plasmids conferring to the host the Ap^s, Tc^r, Fo^r phenotype were analised and all of them showed the presence of a 3.45 Mdal. DNA fragment generated by the enzyme PstI.

MIC determination showed that the fosfomycin resistance level was not affected by the plasmid copy number.

TN916: A CONJUGATIVE TRANSPOSON IN STREPTOCOCCUS FAECALIS?

C. Gawron-Burke, A. Franke, and D. B. Clewell
The University of Michigan, Ann Arbor

Streptococcus faecalis strain DS16 harbors a hemolysin-determining conjugative plasmid pAD1 (35 Mdal) and a non-conjugative multiple drug resistance plasmid pAD2 (15 Mdal). A chromosome-borne tetracycline resistance determinant is located on a 10 Mdal transposon designated Tn916. Transposition to pAD1 occurs at a frequency of $\sim 10^{-6}$. A derivative of DS16 cured of both pAD1 and pAD2 (i.e., strain DS16C3) is capable of transferring Tn916 at low frequency ($\sim 10^{-8}$) to plasmid-free recipients (JH2-2) in "filter-matings" by a Rec-independent, DNase-resistant process resembling conjugation [J. Bacteriol. Vol. 145: 494 (1981)]. When examined using the Southern hybridization method, Tn916 was found to be inserted into different sites in different transconjugants. This was demonstrated by probing HindIII-digested chromosomal DNA with a ^{32}P-labeled EcoR1 restriction fragment of pAD1::Tn916 containing the entire transposon. Insofar as Tn916 has a single HindIII site, two transposon-host junction fragments are easily resolved. The size of these two fragments varied greatly in different transconjugants.

Certain Tc-resistant transconjugants of JH2-2, such as CG110, are able to donate Tc-resistance at 100-fold elevated frequencies ($\sim 10^{-6}$). Experiments which measure the frequency of Tn916 transposition from the chromosome to a newly introduced pAD1 indicate that for CG110, an increased (~ 100-fold) frequency of transposition is also exhibited. Southern hybridization experiments that probed host-transposon junction fragments in HindIII-digested chromosomal DNA isolated from successive cultures of CG110 that had originated from a single colony revealed that Tn916 readily moves from one site to another during growth.

It would appear then that a common step is involved in both transposition and conjugal transfer of Tn916. The conjugal transfer of Tn916 may, thus, represent a complex transposition event in which the transposon is excised from the donor chromosome, transferred by a conjugation-like event, and inserted into the recipient chromosome.

607

EFFECT OF NALIDIXIC ACID AND NOVOBIOCIN ON pBR322

GENETIC EXPRESSION IN Escherichia coli MINICELLS

M. Carmen Gómez-Eichelmann

Departamento de Biología Molecular
Instituto de Investigaciones Biomédicas
Universidad Nacional Autónoma de México
México 20, D. F., MEXICO

The E. coli enzyme DNA gyrase catalyzes the introduction of superhelical turns into closed, circular, double-stranded DNA in an ATP-dependent reaction. Gyrase has been shown to be involved in a number of cellular processes such as supercoiling of the chromosome; DNA replication, transcription, and repair; λ integrative recombination; and general recombination. Gyrase has also been involved in the selectivity of gene expression.

The purpose of this work was to determine and to compare the effects of two different gyrase inhibitors (nalidixic acid and novobiocin) on gene expression of the well-studied small plasmid pBR322 in E. coli minicells.

Quantitative estimates of the synthesis of pBR322-coded polypeptides in novobiocin-treated minicells showed that, compared to control levels, the synthesis of a polypeptide of molecular weight of 34,000 (the tetracycline resistance protein) was reduced to 10-16% while that of a polypeptide of 30,800 (the β-lactamase precursor) was increased to as much as 200%. Nalidixic acid affected the synthesis of pBR322-coded polypeptides in a manner similar to that of novobiocin, although to a lesser extent.

The results suggest that the gyrase inhibitors modifie the interaction of RNA polymerase with some promoters either by decreasing the supercoiling density of plasmid DNA or by changing the gyrase association constant at some specific DNA sites.

STRUCTURAL AND GENETIC ANALYSIS OF PLASMIDS OF
AMINOGLYCOSIDE RESISTANT <u>STAPHYLOCOCCUS AUREUS</u>

Gary S. Gray, Department of Biochemistry, University of
Wisconsin, Madison, Wisconsin 53706

Staphylococci resistant to aminoglycoside antibiotics were
first reported in 1975. Resistant strains usually contain
plasmids and frequently express multiple aminoglycoside modifying
enzymes in addition to other antibiotic resistances.

United States and Canadian clinical isolates of <u>Staphylococcus
aureus</u>, resistant to the aminoglycoside antibiotic amikacin, were
studied with respect to antibiotic resistances and plasmid
content. All isolates contained large ($\sim$ 30,000bp) plasmids and
express multiple aminoglycoside modifying enzymes including
phosphotransferase (3') and/or (2"), adenylyltransferase (4')
and/or (2") and acetyltransferase (6'). These enzymes mediate
resistance to high levels of amikacin, gentamicin, kanamycin,
tobramycin and sisomycin. In addition, all isolates studied were
resistant to penicillin and the inorganic ions cadmium +2, lead+2,
arsenate and mercury+2. The strains could be divided into two
groups on the basis of their sensitivity to ertyhromycin and
trimethoprim/sulfamethoxazole.

Restriction endonuclease analysis of isolated plasmid DNA
revealed that the erythromycin resistant strains possess a series
of similar plasmids which are related to the <u>S. aureus</u> penicillinase plasmid I524_p; a different interrelated series of plasmids
is present in the erythromycin sensitive strains. The variation
between plasmids in each related series is apparently due to the
insertion/deletion of specific DNA sequences. The location and
size of each insertion was confirmed by electron microscopic
examination of heteroduplex pairs of linearized plasmids from
each plasmid group. One insertion which occured in the erythromycin
resistant proup of plasmids appears as a stem-and-loop structure
in electromicrographs. Analysis of deleted and recombinant
plasmids suggests that this insertion encodes the kanamycin
modifying enzyme adenylyltransferase (4') and that this gene is
present in all plasmids studied and in the small <u>S. aureus</u>
kanamycin resistance plasmid UB110_p.

The stem-and-loop structure, similar to the one reported here,
is a common feature of the antibiotic resistance determinants
which have been observed to transpose. The data presented here
suggests that the kanamycin resistance determinant may transpose
and could be involved in the recent spread of aminoglycoside
resistant <u>Staphylococcus aureus</u>.

CHROMOSOMAL LOCATION OF CONJUGATIVE R DETERMINANTS

IN STRAIN BM4200 OF <u>STREPTOCOCCUS</u> <u>PNEUMONIAE</u>

Walter R. Guild, Shulamith Hazum, and Michael D. Smith

Biochemistry Department, Duke University
Durham, North Carolina 27710

BM4200 is a multiply resistant pneumococcus that transfers a
<u>cat tet erm aphA</u> block by conjugation.[1,2] No plasmid can be detected
in either BM4200 or the transconjugants. However, because conjugative transfer of chromosomal elements in gram positive eubacteria was
unprecedented when found by Shoemaker et al.,[3] it is essential to have
other evidence that the genes are in the chromosome. Our approach was
to use transformation to examine the physical nature of the DNA particles carrying the genes and to ask whether the results resembled
plasmid or chromosomal transformation. For BM6001 (<u>cat</u> <u>tet</u>) and derivatives, <u>cat</u> cosedimented with chromosomal DNA and was linked to
<u>tet</u> and a chromosomal gene. The genes in BM4200 will transform lab-
oratory strains; <u>cat</u> goes into wild type readily and all the genes
transform a strain that carries <u>tet</u> from BM6001 in its chromosome.

In lysates of BM4200 each transforming activity cosedimented
with the chromosomal DNA both when the lysate contained very large
DNA and after it had been sheared to a mean size near 6 Md. The shear
had only a small effect on the level of activity but shifted its
velocity distribution greatly. These results imply that the genes
were carried initially on very large DNA particles but could transform almost as well from much smaller fragments. Because they differ
strongly from those for plasmid transformation or phage DNA transfection, these results exclude the hypothesis that the transformants
arose by formation of new replicons in the recipients.

An alternative might be that the R determinants were on a very
large plasmid in the donor but transformed by inserting into the
normal genome of the recipient. <u>If</u> <u>so</u>, <u>the</u> <u>result</u> <u>is</u> that the determinants are inserted into the normal genome of the transformants,
which also transfer them by either conjugation or transformation
with properties not distinguishable from those of the original donor.
One is forced to the conclusion that inserted R determinants can
transfer from one chromosome to another by a process that looks like
conjugation. The absence of detectable plasmid DNA is consistent
with the chromosomal location but is not the basis for reaching this
conclusion. The conjugative plasmid pIP501 has no influence on the
transfers when it is deliberately added to the cells.

1. Buu-Hoi, A., and T. Horodniceanu. 1980. J. Bact. 143:313-320.
2. Smith, M.D., S. Hazum, and W.R. Guild 1981. (ms. in preparation).
3. Shoemaker, N., M.D. Smith, and W.R. Guild. 1980. Plasmid 3:80-87.

CLONING OF TWO DISTINCT BUT RELATED ST ENTEROTOXIN GENES FROM PORCINE AND HUMAN STRAINS OF E. COLI

Nigel Harford, Michel De Wilde, and Teresa Cabezon

Genetics Group, Smith Kline - RIT

1330 Rixensart, BELGIUM

Many strains of enterotoxigenic E. coli excrete a low molecular weight, heat stable toxin ($\overline{ST_A}$) into the culture medium. We have cloned an ST_A gene from a human enteropathogenic strain, CRL25090, as a 1.0×10^6 d PstI fragment inserted on pBR322. Evidence from restriction endonuclease mapping, DNA-DNA hybridization under stringent conditions and absence of IS1 sequence homology shows that the gene differs from the Tn1681 ST transposon described by So et al (Nature 1979 ; 277 : 453). Nevertheless the gene products are similar since both toxins are active in the baby mouse test and antisera directed against porcine ST_A neutralize the CRL25090 toxin. We propose to name the Tn1681 ST gene product ST_{A1} and the CRL25090 gene product ST_{A2}.

RELATION OF ENTEROTOXIN PLASMIDS TO KINDS OF ENTEROTOXIN PRODUCED AND THE PATHOGENICITY OF ST-PRODUCING ESCHERICHIA COLI FROM PIGS AND CATTLE

N. M. Harnett and C. L. Gyles

Department of Veterinary Microbiology and Immunology
University of Guelph
Guelph, Ontario, Canada N1G 2W1

Bovine enterotoxigenic Escherichia coli (ETEC) have several features in common with those porcine ETEC referred to as "porcine class 2 ETEC". These similarities include production of heat-stable enterotoxin (ST) and possession of the O antigens 8, 9, 20 or 101 as well as the K99 antigen. This study compared these two groups of ETEC for their toxin production and for their plasmid content with particular emphasis on the enterotoxin plasmids. Four strains behaved differently with respect to their ability to cause fluid secretion in suckling mice, 1-week-old piglets and 6-week-old piglets; one was assayable in the 1-week-old piglet and suckling mice, the second in 1-week and 6-week-old piglets and suckling mice, the third in 1-week and 6-week-old piglets but not in suckling mice and the fourth assayable only in the 1-week-old piglet. Two of the strains under investigation appear to carry plasmid-linked genes for antibiotic resistance and heat-stable enterotoxin activity. A total of 12 strains from 5 serogroups were examined for the presence of extrachromosomal genetic elements by a modified cleared lysate procedure and agarose gel electrophoresis.

[*]EFFECTS OF PORCINE CLASS 2 ENTEROTOXIGENIC E. COLI ON SUCKLING MICE AND LIGATED ILEAL LOOPS OF 1-WEEK-OLD AND 6-WEEK-OLD PIGLETS

| Strain | Serogroup | PIGLETS | | SUCKLING MICE |
		1 Week (V/L)	6 Weeks (V/L)	3 Days (GW/BW)
0329-A	09:K103	0.9 ± 0.4 (+)	0 ± 0 (-)	0.137 ± 0.015(+)
P16	09:K103	1.0 ± 0.1 (+)	0 ± 0 (-)	0.062 ± 0.001(-)
P16M	09:K103	1.8 ± 0.4 (+)	2.7 ± 0.6 (+)	0.129 ± 0.009(+)
G53	020:K?	0.9 ± 0.2 (+)	2.0 ± 0.4 (+)	0.062 ± 0.003(-)

V/L   Ratio of volume to length. The mean $\pm$ standard error of the mean for four trials.

GW/BW Ratio of Gut Weight to Body Weight. The mean $\pm$ standard error of the mean for four trials.

In parentheses: + = positive; - = negative.

GENETICS OF F PLASMID SEGREGATION INTO E. COLI MINICELLS

J. Hogan[1], B. Kline[2], and S.B. Levy[1]
Department of Microbiology and Molecular Biology
Tufts University School of Medicine[1], Boston, MA and
Department of Cell Biology, Mayo Clinic[2], Rochester, MN

F plasmid segregates poorly, if at all, into Escherichia coli minicells. Studies using mini-F plasmids constructed from the 40.3 - 49.3F (F kilobase coordinates) EcoRl fragment of F plasmid--which includes three inc loci: incB, 45.0 - 45.8F; incC, 45.8 - 46.4F; and incD, 47.5 - 49.3F--have shown that these F loci affect segregation of the plasmids into minicells.

The minimum amount of F DNA required for autonomous plasmid replication reported to date is 44.0 - 45.8F, which includes incB. Four such incB$^+$ plasmids segregated into minicells. Addition of incC$^+$ or incD$^+$ loci, or both, to these plasmids resulted in little, or no, segregation. Thus either incC or incD present with incB$^+$ inhibited segregation. Some understanding of this interaction emerged from studies of two plasmids which had retained the incB$^+$ incC$^+$ incD$^+$ phenotype but had copy number mutations (Cop$^-$) mapping in incB. One plasmid segregated, the other did not. This result demonstrated that a site in incB, apart from incompatibility, was involved in minicell segregation. Eleven of thirteen mini-F plasmids studied are Cop$^-$ with copy numbers increased up to fourteen-fold over the wild-type copy number of 1-2. Seven Cop$^-$ plasmids segregated into minicells. Thus there appears to be no direct relationship between copy number and the ability to segregate into minicells.

We have proposed that the ability of a plasmid to segregate into minicells reflects an association of the plasmid with a septation site, e.g., polar sites in the minicell strain (1). This would be one means of assuring proper partitioning into daughter cells at cell division. Another means, proposed for F (2), would be by association of the plasmid with the chromosome. These plasmids would not be expected to segregate into minicells, where chromosomal DNA is not found. There was no detectable difference in inheritance during cell growth of segregating and non-segregating mini-F plasmids after > 100 cell divisions. This result showed that segregation of the mini-F plasmids into minicells did not affect stable inheritance; however, the mechanism of partitioning could affect the ability of a plasmid to segregate into minicells.

1. Levy, S.B. 1971. Ann. N.Y. Acad. Sci. 182:217-225.
2. Jacob, F., Brenner, S., and Cuzin, F. 1963. Cold Spring Harbor Symp. Quant. Biol. 28:329-348.

STABLE RNA MOLECULES ENCODED BY THE RESISTANCE PLASMID R1

G. Högenauer, F. Kricek, and E. Ostermann

Sandoz Forschungsinstitut
Brunner Strasse 59
A-1235 Vienna, Austria

Some resistance plasmids code for stable RNAs of various size classes.[1,2] The biological role of these RNA molecules is unknown.

Genes coding for stable RNA species could be identified on a 7.7 kb (5.1 Mdal) EcoRI fragment and on a 3.6 kb DNA piece (situated on the edge of a 17.7 kb (11.7 Mdal) EcoRI fragment), belonging to the RTF-region of the resistance plasmid R1. The 7.7 kb piece, when analyzed by the Southern-hybridization technique, bound exclusively a 4S RNA while the second fragment proved to be complementary to 5S, 9S and still larger RNA molecules. Northern blots showed that the most prominent RNA species encoded by R1 belong to a large size class, measuring about 335 nucleotides. From this we conclude that the primary gene product is a large RNA which subsequently is cleaved to give the small RNA species mentioned above.

An increased amount of the 335 nucleotide long RNA and, in addition, still larger RNA molecules were found to be present in E. coli cells harboring the derepressed plasmid R1drd19. RNA of plasmid-less bacteria showed no hybridization to R1-DNA.

Map location and difference in RNA composition in the derepressed state indicate an involvement of the R-factor specific RNAs in the conjugational transfer process.

1. F. Kricek, G. Hartmann and G. Högenauer, Coding of Stable 4S RNA Molecules by the Resistance Factor R1, Molec. gen. Genet., 161:231 (1978).
2. M. De Wilde, J.E. Davies, and F.J. Schmidt, Low Molecular Weight RNA Species Encoded by a Multiple Drug Resistance Plasmid, Proc. Natl. Acad. Sci. USA, 75:3673 (1978).

HIGH-LEVEL, PLASMID-BORNE RESISTANCE TO AMINOGLYCOSIDE ANTIBIOTICS IN GROUP D STREPTOCOCCI

Thea Horodniceanu[1], Chantal Le Bouguenec[1] and
Annie Buu-Hoï[2]

Institut Pasteur[1] and CHU Broussais-Hôtel Dieu[2]
Paris, France

Group D streptococci are etiological agents of bacterial endocarditis. Four S. faecalis, 10 S. faecium and 7 S. bovis strains isolated from blood and urine cultures carried genetic markers for high-level resistance to aminoglycosides (streptomycin: Sm, kanamycin: Km, gentamicin: Gm) and tetracycline (Tc), chloramphenicol (Cm) and macrolides (MLS-type resistance). Mating experiments were carried out on membrane filters. Recipient strains were JH2-2 (S. faecalis) and BM132 (group B Streptococcus). Molecular weight (MW) of plasmid DNAs (isolated by dye-buoyant centrifugation) was calculated by agarose gel electrophoresis.

All S. faecalis strains transferred by conjugation their resistance to aminoglycosides into JH2-2 at a high (10^{-2}) or low (10^{-5}) frequency. Resistance to Gm and Km was carried by R plasmids of 44×10^6. Six S. faecium strains transferred their resistance markers into JH2-2 at a low frequency (10^{-8}). Resistance to Sm and Km alone was carried by R plasmids of 15×10^6 or 16×10^6. Resistance to Sm and Km linked to MLS, Cm and Tc was carried by R plasmids of 20×10^6, 24×10^6 or 25×10^6. Each of these plasmids had identical MW with one of the plasmids found in the donor strain. Two S. bovis strains transferred their resistance markers en bloc (Tc,MLS,Sm,Km) at a low frequency (10^{-7}) into BM132 or at a high frequency (10^{-4}) into JH2-2 and BM132 . When low, no plasmid DNA was found in both wild-type and transconjugant strains, suggesting that resistance markers are chromosome-borne. When high, plasmid DNA of 38×10^6 was found in transconjugants.

High-level aminoglycoside resistance is plasmid-borne in group D streptococci and the MW of the plasmids varied from 15×10^6 to 44×10^6. The relationships between all these plasmids are under study in our laboratory.

THE MER OPERON: POLYPEPTIDES AND A PROMOTER

W.J. Jackson, F. A. Bohlander, and A. O. Summers

University of Georgia
Department of Microbiology
Athens, Ga. 30602

Four polypeptides are synthesized in response to $HgCl_2$ induction of minicells carrying the cloned mer operon of the plasmid NR1. The molecular weights of these polypeptides are: 69,000 daltons, 15,000 daltons, 14,000 daltons, and 10,000 daltons. Antibody to the purified mercuric ion reductase reacts with the largest polypeptide. An additional inducible polypeptide of 65,000 daltons can occasionally be seen. Since this polypeptide also reacts with antibody to purified reductase, we believe it is the proteolytically degraded form of the enzyme observed by Schottel. Data on polypeptides synthesized by cloned sub-fragments of the operon suggest that the bulk of the reductase resides in the EcoRI-H fragment of NR1.

Hydroxylamine-generated mutants of the operon demonstrate sensitive, super-sensitive, and temperature-sensitive phenotypes. There are two classes of sensitive mutant: one class has no reductase activity and no inducible polypeptides; the other class has very high levels (both uninduced and induced) of the enzyme and all four polypeptides. The supersensitive mutants have no detectable reductase activity; only one can be seen to form an altered reductase polypeptide but all have pleiotropic alterations in the smaller polypeptides. All temperature sensitive mutations isolated are altered in regulation rather than in reductase activity.

Using EcoRI* we have cloned into the "promoter-cloning" vehicle pHB1, a $HgCl_2$-responsive promoter from the purified EcoRI-H fragment of NR1. This promoter requires a functional mer regulatory element in trans and the level of tetracycline resistance provided is directly proportional to the $HgCl_2$ concentration (at sub-toxic levels). The single HincII site in the 200 bp fragment carrying this putative mer promoter corresponds to a site in the EcoRI-H fragment approximately 380 bp from the "right" end of IS1b. Since this distance would be sufficient to determine a polypeptide of 14,000 daltons, and since genetic evidence suggests that the operon immediately abuts the end of IS1b, we believe that this is the promoter for one of the smaller, inducible mer polypeptides.

PROVIDENCIA PLASMIDS

J.F. John, C.M. Newton, and J.A. Twitty
V.A. Medical Center
Medical University of South Carolina
Charleston, South Carolina 29403

Providencia commonly cause nosocomial infections, usually of the urinary tract. Both P. stuartii and P. rettgeri readily become resistant to multiple antibiotics. At our medical center over the past four years, Providencia have often been amino-glycoside resistant. Aminoglycoside-resistant (Gm^r or Tm^r) P. rettgeri and P. stuartii (56 strains from 53 patients) were speciated by API biotype: 29 were from the Charleston VAMC, 11 from Columbia, S.C. V.A., 9 from Medical University Hospital (MUH), 1 from Walter Reed Army Medical Center, and 7 from the Center for Disease Control, Atlanta, Georgia. All strains were tested by Bauer-Kirby disc methods to 13 antimicrobials. Cleared lysates were subjected to agarose gel electrophoresis for detection of plasmid DNA. Conjugal transfer of plasmid containing strains was attempted using as recipients P. mirabilis F-67 (Rif^r) and E. coli C (Rif^r). Transformation of purified plasmid DNA from one strain of P. rettgeri was performed into E. coli C (Rif^r). Bristol Laboratories, Syracuse, New York, performed determination of aminoglycoside modifying enzymes for one strain. Of 56 different strains 18 were P. rettgeri, 38 P. stuartii (14 urease$^+$). The percent of susceptibility to various antimicrobial agents was as follows: Tet (0%), Col (2%), Tm (2%), Gm (5%), Cr (5%), Ch (11%), Tmp-Smz (14%), Su (17%), Ap (20%), Km (43%), Cb (46%), Nal (54%), and An (54%). Of the 56 strains, 43% contained one or more plasmids. The most common plasmid pattern was a 29-3.1 Md pair seen in 16 strains which were obtained from Charleston (VAMC and MUH) Columbia VA. Other plasmid sizes ranged from 2.9 to 115 Md. Conjugation of 13 different strains resulted in transfer of at least 1 marker in 9 strains. Ap^r and Cb^r were the most commonly transferred. Gm^r, Tm^r, Km^r transfer was seen only once, then associated with a 105 Md plasmid. Ap^r and Cb^r transconjugants contained the 29 Md plasmid and in one case also coded for urease. Transformation of purified plasmid containing the 29 and 3.1 Md plasmids demonstrated that the 29 Md plasmid coded for Ap^r and Cb^r and that the 3.1 Md plasmid coded for Cr^r. Aminoglycoside 2'-N-acetyltransferase (AAC-2') was elaborated by one organism containing the 29-3.1 Md pair, suggesting a chromosomal locus for production of this enzyme. We conclude that various size plasmids in multi-resistant Providencia were present in South Carolina and other geographic locations. Amikacin and carbenicillin were the most active agents in this group of Providencia. In these strains, aminoglycoside resistance was usually non-plasmid mediated; moreover, the presence of AAC-2' in Providencia may be chromosomally mediated. In addition, in some Providencia, we found urease$^+$ to be plasmid mediated and this may explain the variability of urease production within the genus Providencia.

A RAPID MINI-SCREEN PROCEDURE FOR THE DETECTION

AND ISOLATION OF SMALL AND LARGE PLASMIDS

C. I. Kado* and S.-T. Liu

Department of Plant Pathology
University of California
Davis, California 95616

High molecular weight plasmids of various gram-negative bacteri
can be resolved within 3 hr. Cells from a single colony or from 3
ml broth cultures are suspended in E buffer (40 mM Tris-acetate, pH
7.9, 2 mM Na_2EDTA) and lysed by adding 2 volumes of 3% Na dodecyl
sulfate (SDS in 50 mM Tris-OH, pH 12.6). The mixture is incubated
for 20 min at 50-95°C (depending on the bacterium) and then briefly
emulsified with an equal volume of a distilled unbuffered phenol/
chloroform mixture (1:1, vol/vol). The mixture is centrifuged for
10 min, 8000 g. A 20-50 µl sample of the aqueous phase is used
directly for electrophoresis in 0.7% agarose gel (in E buffer), 1.5
hr at 12 V/cm with water cooling. The plasmid DNA is visualized
by soaking the gel in a solution of ethidium bromide (0.5 µg EB/ml)
for 30 min and then placed over a short wave ultraviolet light
source. For preparative isolation, the phenol/choroform is removed
by dialysis. The plasmid preparation can then be used directly for
transformation, nick translated as probes, ligated and restricted.
Plasmids with molecular masses ranging from 2.2 to 350 mdal have
been clearly resolved and readily isolated. The procedure is
particularly useful for rapid screening of E. coli harboring recombinant plasmids. Single colonies can be analyzed for recombinant
plasmids as follows: A single colony is resuspended in 100 µl of
3% SDS in 0.05 M Tris-OH, pH 12.6. The suspension is thoroughly
mixed and heated at 50°C for 20 min. The lysate is then extracted
(briefly by shaking) with an equal volume of unbuffered phenol/
chloroform (1:1; vol/vol) and centrifuged at 10,000 rpm for 5 min.
A 25 µl sample of the upper aqueous phase is directly placed in
sample wells containing electrophoresis buffer in 1% agarose gel in
E buffer. Electrophoresis is carried out at 12-15 volts/cm for 1.5
hr with water cooling. Plasmid can be isolated from the aqueous
phase by first extracting the phenol/chloroform residue with ether
and then precipitating the plasmid with two volumes of -20°C ethanc
The precipitate is dried with nitrogen and is redisolved in distilled water.

This work was supported by NIH Research Grant CA-11526 and a grant
from the Science and Education Administration.

A MODEL FOR THE MECHANISM OF RESISTANCE TO AMINOCYCLITOLS

Sarah A. Kagan

Department of Biochemistry
University of Wisconsin
Madison, Wisconsin 53706

A clinically isolated plasmid, pJR89, confers resistance to aminocyclitol antibiotics. It encodes an enzyme, aminocyclitol acetyltransferase (3)-I, which both modifies the aminocyclitol molecules and diminishes the amount of drug accumulated by the bacteria. Both functions are important for the expression of the resistance phenotype.

This study addresses the mechanism by which the enzyme, (AAC 3-I,) diminishes cellular accumulation of drug. One possible mechanism invokes a stable enzyme-substrate complex, which blocks uptake of additional drug molecules. If this mechanism were correct, one would expect a good substrate for the enzyme to protect cells against the effects of poor substrates. However, this appears not to be the case. This was shown in two ways: 1) gentamicin (a good substrate) did not lessen the inhibition of protein synthesis, in vivo, by tobramycin (a poor substrate); 2) sisomycin, (a good substrate) did not diminish the amount or rate of netilmicin (a poor substrate) accumulation. Good substrates did not merely fail to protect cells against poorer substrates; in fact, when both were present in the growth media together, they exerted a synergistic antibiotic effect. Poor substrates also enabled the better substrates to overcome the block to transport.

The mechanism of enzyme-mediated resistance could have involved either modification of all intracellular drug or just of a critical portion thereof. Therefore, the complement of intracellular drug was assayed radioenzymatically to determine the ratio of modified to non-modified forms. One hundred percent of the intracellular aminocyclitol was found to be modified in resistant cells.

On the basis of these data the following model was proposed. Initially, there is a slow, energy-dependent phase of uptake. This corresponds to the drug crossing the cell membrane. Intracellular drug then binds to ribosomes. Ribosome-binding triggers the second, faster phase of uptake. In resistant bacteria, the first, slow phase of uptake occurs. However, the AAC 3-I modification rate is sufficient to modify all drug that gains access to the cytoplasm. Therefore, active drug cannot bind to ribosomes, and the faster phase of uptake does not occur.

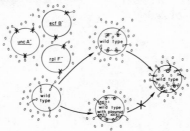

MOLECULAR CHARACTERISATION OF THE K88 MEDIATED ADHESION SYSTEM OF PORCINE ENTEROTOXIGENIC ESCHERICHIA COLI (ETEC)

M. Kehoe, R. Sellwood and G. Dougan

Department of Microbiology

Trinity College, Dublin 2. Ireland

By using DNA cloning techniques, Tn5 transposon mutagenesis and the E. coli minicell system we have identified and mapped four cistrons and their corresponding polypeptides which are involved in expression and assembly of the K88 fimbriae of procine ETEC. The cistrons are arranged in at least two operons which are located adjacent to each other and are transcribed in the same direction. The operons have been cloned separately onto different plasmids. Operon I encodes 70,000d, 29,000d and 17,000d polypeptides in that order. Operon II encodes the 23,500d K88 fimbriae subunit and is normally expressed at high levels. Cells harbouring Operon II alone do not express levels of the 23,000d polypeptide which can be detected using our assay systems whereas cells harbouring Operon I and Operon II on separate plasmids express near normal levels of the 23,000d K88 subunit.

Tn5 insertions in adhA (70,000d) express reduced levels of the 23,000d K88 subunit which is found in culture supernatents and not on the cell surface. Inserts in adhB (29,000d) produce reduced levels of the 23,500d K88 subunit, are phenotypically Adh$^+$ (bind in vitro to pig intestinal epithial cells) but are MRHA$^-$ (failed to agglutinate red blood cells in the presence of D-mannose). Inserts in adhC (17,000d) do not express detectable levels of the 23,500d K88 antigen from Operon II. Inserts in adhD (23,500d) are K88$^-$, Adh$^-$, MRHA$^-$. The adhD product is the K88 fimbrial subunit. The results suggest that the adhA product is part of a basal structure attaching the K88 fimbriae to the cell membrane. The adhC product may be a positive regulator controlling expression of adhD.

MULTIPLE ANTIBIOTIC RESISTANCE AMONG GRAM-NEGATIVE BACTERIA ISOLATED IN KARACHI

Hajra Khatoon, S. Amir Ali and S. M. Najeeb

Department of Microbiology, University of
Karachi, Pakistan

The incidence and extent of multiple antibiotic resistance among gram-negative bacteria, isolated from various sources in Karachi, was investigated. The bacterial strains were isolated from clinical specimens, food, milk, water and sewage and were screened against the commonly-used antibiotics: ampicillin (Ap), chloramphenicol (Cm), kanamycin (Km), neomycin (Nm), streptomycin (Sm) and tetracycline (Tc). Of the total 518 bacterial strains screened, 446 (86%) were resistant to one or more antibiotics. Among the clinical bacteria, the incidence was particularly high (93%), reflecting an indiscriminate use of antibiotics in chemotherapy. The most common resistance pattern among Escherichia coli was ApCmSmTc, followed by CmSmTc and ApCmKmNmSmTc. Pseudomonads were found to exhibit resistance to all or most of the antibiotics. Other gram-negative bacteria, including Salmonella, Shigella, Aerobacter and Proteus showed resistance to one or more antibiotics in different combinations. Seven R plasmids, R62, R63, R64, R65, R66, R67 and R68 isolated from resistant bacteria, were studied for their genetic behaviour.

EPIDEMIC SPREAD OF AN R PLASMID TO VARIOUS BACTERIA IN A HOSPITAL

Akio Kobayashi, Shinji Takahashi and Toshihiko Arai*

Central Clinical Laboratories, Chiba University
Chiba, Japan
*Department of Microbiology, Keio University School of
Medicine, Tokyo, Japan

Incidences of gentamicin resistant strains were very high in
the enteric bacteria isolated in the urology wards in our hospital.
Because of their antibiotic resistance patterns, we studied for
their R plasmids. Majority of these strains were found to have
conjugative R plasmids. Because of the similar resistance patterns of these R plasmids, we tried to classified these R plasmids
into incompatibility groups. We have two independent wards in the
urology department. Almost all R plasmids detected in the strains
in one ward were found to be A-C group and most of the R plasmids
in the other ward were not identified despite of the similar resistance markers, although detailed study for aminiglycoside antibiotic inactivating enzymes of these R plasmids suggested some differences of these two groups. Thus, it was found that only a certain R plasmid had been disseminated in various enteric bacteria in
the different patients and that this dissemination had been limited in a certain ward.

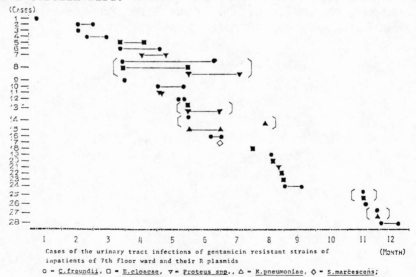

Cases of the urinary tract infections of gentamicin resistant strains of
inpatients of 7th floor ward and their R plasmids

○ = C.freundii, □ = E.cloacae, ▽ = Proteus spp., △ = K.pneumoniae, ◇ = S.marcescens;
Black symbols = A-C complex group; White symbols = other than I_2, A-C, H, W, M_1.

MODULAR CONSTRUCTION OF R PLASMIDS IN VIVO : TRANSLOCATION EVENTS IN SALMONELLA ORDONEZ.

A. Labigne-Roussel, G. Gerbaud, P. Courvalin

L.A. CNRS 271. Unité de Bactériologie Médicale
Institut Pasteur
25, Rue du Docteur Roux. F75724 Paris Cedex (France)

Salmonella ordonez strain BM2000 encodes ApCmKmSpSuTc resistances
and production of colicin Ib (Cib). The Km and Cib characters are
carried by a 97 kb IncI1 plasmid (pIP565). In addition to the Km
and Cib traits all or part of the other resistances (ApCmSpSuTc)
can be transferred by conjugation from S. ordonez to E. coli where
all the acquired characters are borne by an IncI1 plasmid designated complete or partial composite plasmid respectively. This suggests that in BM2000 the ApCmSpSuTc R determinants are encoded by
a DNA sequence able to translocate, en bloc or in part, from a donor replicon to pIP565. DNA from pIP565 and composite plasmids,
and total DNA from S. ordonez BM2000 have been studied by agarose
and polyacrylamide gel electrophoresis following digestion with
EcoRI, BamHI, or SalI, and by Southern hybridization.These comparative analyses enable us : a) to show that, in each case, acquisition by pIP565 of all or part of the resistances is due to the
insertion of a single DNA fragment into the receptor plasmid ;
b) to detect two types of composite plasmids with regard to the
specificity of insertion into pIP565 and the mapping of the inserts ; c) to demonstrate that the ApCmSpSuTc R determinants are
integrated into S. ordonez chromosomal DNA ; d) to map the endo-
nuclease-generated DNA fragments of the translocatable sequence
whether integrated into BM2000 chromosome or into pIP565.

The results obtained are compatible with the existence of two
distinct molecular mechanisms : a site specific recombination between two of the four directly repeated IS-like sequences present
in S. ordonez chromosome leading to the circularisation of all or
part of the ApCmSpSuTc R determinants followed by 1) either a second site specific recombination with the copy of the IS-like sequence of pIP565 (Type I composite plasmids), 2) or transposition
of precise groups of characters in various sites of pIP565 (Type II).

RELATIVE COLONIZATION POTENTIALS OF E. COLI K-12 AND HUMAN FECAL STRAINS IN STREPTOMYCIN-TREATED MICE

David C. Laux, M. Lynn Myhal, and Paul S. Cohen

Department of Microbiology
University of Rhode Island
Kingston, R.I.   02881

Relative colonization potentials of E. coli K-12 strains and human fecal isolates were assessed in a competitive streptomycin-treated mouse system. Mice pretreated and subsequently maintained on streptomycin were simultaneously fed two strains of streptomycin-resistant E. coli and the level of each strain was monitored for 10-14 days. Neither E. coli K-12 nor human fecal isolates were able to colonize mice which had not been treated with streptomycin. When a single strain of E. coli K-12 or a fecal isolate was fed to streptomycin-treated mice, all strains colonized at approximately equal levels (10^8 organisms/g feces). Experiments involving the competition of one fecal strain against another fecal strain also resulted in approximately equal levels of colonization (10^8 organisms of each strain/g feces). When a fecal strain was competed with any E. coli K-12 strain, both strains colonized the large intestine, however, the level of E. coli K-12 was always 100-1000 fold less than that of the human fecal strain.

In two instances genetic alterations were demonstrated to have an affect on colonization potential. In the first instance, two fecal isolates (F-18 & F-56), each cured of a single plasmid, demonstrated decreased colonization potential relative to the plasmid containing parent strain. In the second instance, a number of rifampicin-resistant mutants of both K-12 and fecal strains were isolated and assayed for colonizing ability relative to the parent strain. Interestingly, each rifampicin-resistant mutant which contained one or no plasmids demonstrated a decreased colonizing capacity, while those strains containing multiple plasmids failed to show a decreased colonizing capacity relative to the rifampicin-sensitive parent strain. Together these data indicate that both chromosomal and plasmid genes can influence the colonization potential of E. coli. Further characterization of these genes and the products they code for should contribute to our basic understanding of the colonization process.
Supported by NIH Grant AI 16370.

THE PLASMID REFERENCE CENTER (PRC)

E.M. Lederberg
Department of Medical Microbiology
Stanford University Stanford, California

The PRC serves as a central research resource facility for the acquisition, maintenance, and distribution of important, prototype plasmid cultures, and has been in operation for just over three years. The collection comprises plasmids carried by enteric bacteria, especially *Staphylococcus aureus* prototype plasmids, reflecting historically earlier research developments. New plasmids in other species have since been discovered and will gradually be added to the collection. In addition, some plasmids reported since the CSH compilation, including useful cloning vectors from the laboratories of S.N. Cohen and H. Boyer, have been deposited and are available.

The collection currently consists of over 800 members, but a catalog is not available. The CSH compilation serves as a basic catalog. If any plasmid listed or donated to the collection is requested, it will be shipped; if not available, it will be sought for the collection and sent when received. Certain plasmid bearing strains are assembled for distribution as kits. Those currently available include:

(1) an *E coli Inc* tester kit.
(2) Size Standards kit for agarose gel determinations.
(3) A kit of representative colicinogenic strains.
(4) Metabolic representatives: (β-lactamase-coding plasmids
and *Tc* subtypes).
(5) *Tn*1 to *Tn*10 standards kit.

Investigators are encouraged to deposit prototype plasmid strains, representatives of new *Inc* classes, new plasmid derivatives and mutants. The PRC will then assign a PRC catalog number, maintain, store, and distribute these cultures. Requestors of plasmid strains are encouraged to report to the PRC new information from their investigations of the plasmids provided.

The proposal for the uniform nomenclature for bacterial plasmids will be used. Symbols for newly discovered plasmid attributes may be registered with the PRC for inclusion in future compilation. To avoid duplications of plasmid names, a registry of plasmid prefix designations is maintained at the PRC. Over 200 permutations of the proposed code, pXY prefix, are still available. A registry of *Tn* allocations (*Plasmid* 2: 466, 1979) is also maintained.

Funded by Contract No1-A1-72531, National Institutes of Health.

UNDERSTANDING THE INVIRONMENTAL EFFECTS OF APPLIED GENETICS

Morris A. Levin
U.S. ENVIRONMENTAL PROTECTION AGENCY
WASHINGTON, D.C.

The Applied Genetics program evolving at EPA is an effort to prepare a
foundation for understanding the impact of increased production and
application of Applied Genetics products. To this end, we have insti-
tuted a contractual effort to survey the industry, an in-house research effort to estimate the probability of genetic exchange in
sewage, and an extramural grant effort to consider the probability of
escape from containment and to develop a model which will permit
estimation of the probability of survival and persistence of novel
genomes under a variety of environmental conditions. In addition, we
are examining the regulatory and legal bases under which EPA operates
to determine appropriateness as a basis for action. It must be
stressed that there have been no adverse effects or any real evidence
of significant potential hazards. However, questions relating to
large scale (factors of 10,000) processes and deliberate or accidental
release have simply not been encountered nor adequately explored.

Specifically, the program will attempt to:
(1) Scope The Industry: Estimate the types and quantities of products
anticipated as well as production methods involved. (Contract effort,
Battelle (Columbus) and Teknekron to be completed by April, 1981).
Battelle will concentrate on Agricultural aspects of Applied Genetics
research while Teknekron will survey the potential industrial applications and impacts;
(2) Assess Potential Effects: Develop a model which will permit the
evaluation of the potential effects of application and accidental
escape of these products on public health, welfare and environmental
problems (Grant Program, University of Rhode Island/Tufts University,
Carnegie Mellon/Naval Bioscience Laboratory, Cornell University). The
URI/Tufts study involves construction of a plasmid which can be traced
after it has been introduced to a model sewage plant to simulate accidental release. Evidence of transfer to sewage microflora and percent survival during treatment will be sought. The Carnegie Mellon/
Naval Bioscience Laboratory study will estimate the probability of
escape of organisms from large scale equipment. A model will be developed (using fault tree analyses) and verified both in laboratory
trials using large scale equipment and on site. The Cornell Study
will attempt to define and quantitate parameters in colonization of a
new niche by microorganisms. An attempt will be made to develop a
model relating colonization to physiological or biochemical characteristics of microorganisms.
(3) Evaluate Existing Regulations: Explore the regulatory and legal
mechanisms available to achieve the desired result (in-house); and
(4) Investigate Beneficial Components of the Applied Genetics Industry
(e.g., reduction in hazardous wastes, enhancement of clean-up capability) which should be encouraged (University of Illinois). This
study will attempt to categorize needs in terms of susceptibility to
techniques developed as a result of research in this area.

A MINI-Ti PLASMID OF AGROBACTERIUM TUMEFACIENS AS A VECTOR FOR THE INSERTION OF FOREIGN GENES INTO HIGHER PLANT CELLS

S.-T. Liu, M. Hagiya, J.C. Kao, K.L. Perry, and C.I. Kado[*]
Department of Plant Pathology
University of California, Davis, California

It has been long thought that oncogenic and virulence properties are conferred by large Ti plasmids in Agrobacterium strains. However, we predicted that Ti plasmids of much smaller sizes might exist in nature because only small segments of these Ti plasmids carry the genetic information necessary for crown gall oncogenesis. We report here the confirmation of this prediction by the discovery of an Agrobacterium strain that harbors a Ti plasmid one-fifth the size of its larger 120 mdal counterpart. The mini-plasmid, pTi1422, has a molecular mass of 28.7 mdal and is harbored in strain 1D1422 that was originally isolated from a tumor on a grapevine. Unlike many Agrobacterium strains, strain 1D1422 does not harbor any cryptic plasmids. It is oncogenic on a number of different hosts. Crown gall tumor formation is best expressed on carrot discs and is markedly delayed on woody hosts. Strain 1D1422 best fits the biotype-1 group of Agrobacterium strains similar to octopine and nopaline strains. However, strain 1D1422 is unable to utilize or produce octopine or nopaline and preliminary tests indicate that it produces two unidentified acidic opines. A small deletion of 2-3 kilobases in the mini-Ti plasmid is sufficient to cause complete loss of oncogenicity.

Unlike the usual large Ti plasmids, pTi1422 possesses single sites for restriction endonuclease BamHI and HpaI (Fig. 1). Thus, the whole intact mini-Ti plasmid has been cloned in E. coli HB101. Also proteins coded by cloned fragments of pTi1422 DNA were synthesized in P678-54 mini-cells except in the region designated in Figure 1. This region and the rest of the mini-Ti plasmid DNA have no apparent sequence homologies with large Ti plasmids such as in strains 15955 and C58 as judged by reciprocal Southern blot hybridizations. This is supported by the fact that the mini-Ti plasmid is compatible with the Ti plasmids of 15955 and C58 when they were either inserted in strain 1D1422 or when pTi1422 was transferred with pTiACH5 or pTiC58 into Ti plasmid-free avirulent strain NT1 by cotransformation.

These studies, therefore, clearly show that Ti plasmids substantially smaller than 120 mdal exist in nature. Although the mini-Ti plasmid has no detectable sequence homologies with large octopine and nopaline Ti plasmids, it nevertheless confers oncogenic properties on Agrobacterium. This suggests that T-DNA sequences can be quite distinct and argues against the notion of a common DNA among all Ti plasmids. Of primary significance is the presence of single sites for two restriction enzymes, which

permits the insertion of foreign DNA such as the β-lactamase gene
into these sites. Hybrid plasmids carrying this gene have already
been propagated and expressed in E. coli and such hybrid plasmids
can be readily transferred into plants. pTi1422 therefore has a
number of advantages over its larger counterparts: a) the
essential genes necessary for oncogenesis and virulence make up a
considerable portion of the mini-Ti plasmid; b) with fewer
restriction endonuclease sites, genes conferring functional
properties can be easily located on a physical map and therefore
isolated as cloned fragments; c) the whole plasmid can be
genetically manipulated in E. coli; d) single and double
restriction sites already exist on the mini-Ti plasmid. This will
permit us to reconstruct the plasmid into an useful vector that
can be used directly (direct insertion into plant protoplasts)
and indirectly (insertion mediated by Agrobacterium).

This work was supported in part by CA-11526.

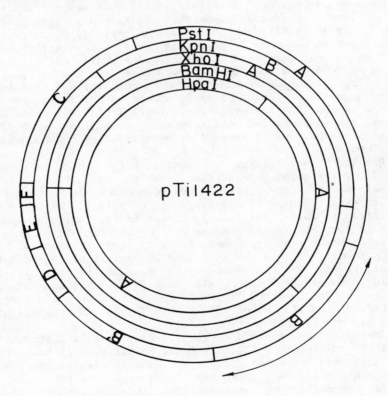

RECOMBINANT DNA SYSTEM IN STREPTOCOCCUS SANGUIS

F.L. Macrina, R.P. Evans, K.R. Jones and J.Ash Tobian
Virginia Commonwealth University
Richmond, Virginia 23298

We have previously described the construction of plasmids that may be used as vehicles in a streptococcal molecular cloning system (Macrina, et al. J. Bacteriol 143, 1425-1435 [1980]). Extended characterization of two such plasmids has revealed additional useful information. pVA380-1 is a 2.8 Mdal, multicopy plasmid originally isolated in S. ferus. It is a phenotypically silent plasmid but may be used to clone directly selectable markers (e.g., resistance determinants) using Eco RI, Ava I, Hind III or Hpa II. The Eco RI, Ava I and Hind III sites may be used in any paired combination to insert DNA into this vector. A derivative (designated pVA736; 5 Mdal) of pVA380-1 bearing an erythromycin-resistance (Em^r) determinant has been constructed for cloning non-selectable DNA sequences. Passenger DNA may be inserted into pVA736 using Hind III, Eco RI, Kpn I, Ava I or Hpa II restriction enzymes. The pVA380-1 plasmid has been used to study the organization of a 20 Mdal conjugative R plasmid, pIP501, originally isolated in S. agalactiae. Using molecular cloning methods, the chloramphenicol resistance (Cm^r) determinant of pIP501 was found to reside on the 4.1 Mdal Hind III A fragment while the Em^r determinant was located on the 3.0 Mdal Hind III B fragment. The Hind III A and B fragments were contiguous on pIP501. A 2.3 Mdal Hpa II - Ava I fragment bearing the Em^r determinant of pIP501 was replaced with a 2.3 Mdal Hpa II - Ava I fragment derived from pVA380-1. Unlike pIP501, the resultant 20 Mdal plasmid, pVA797, (bearing only Cm^r), did not display segregation from cells grown at 42°C, indicating that the pVA380-1 portion of pVA797 was governing its replication. In addition, pVA797 was unable to promote its own conjugative transfer suggesting that a structural or regulatory gene(s) for transfer proficiency resides near the Em^r determinant.

The use of pVA736 to clone chromosomal gene sequences from cariogenic S. mutans into S. sanguis is being assessed. Transformation of S. sanguis with purified monomeric pVA736 forms was found to be a second order process, whereas multimeric plasmid forms have been inferred to transform with one-hit kinetics. "Shotgun" cloning of S. mutans chromosomal fragments into S. sanguis resulted in the recovery of chimeras that had suffered deletions. We attributed this to the negligible amounts of monomeric or perfect oligomeric chimeras formed during ligation which are presumably needed for effective transformation. We are currently attempting to solve this problem by adapting the "helper plasmid" method of Gryczan, et al. (Molec. Gen. Genetics 177, 459-467 [1980]) to the S. sanguis cloning system. (Supported by USPHS Grant DE 04224).

ECOLOGY OF ANTIBIOTIC AND HEAVY METAL RESISTANCE IN NATURE

B. Marshall, S. Schluederberg, D. Rowse-Eagle,
A.O. Summers and S.B. Levy
Department of Molecular Biology and Microbiology
Tufts University School of Medicine, Boston, MA and
Department of Microbiology, University of Georgia,
Athens, GA*

We have studied the frequency of antibiotic and heavy metal
resistance in the fecal flora of approximately 1300 samples from
populations of patients, laboratory workers, urban and rural dwellers and farm animals. Computerization of the data base has produced statistics on the prevalence of antibiotic and metal sensitivity, and single, multiple and linked antibiotic resistances. Flora
was designated resistant if it contained $\geq$ 10% resistant coliforms
to any of eight antibiotics: tetracycline (tet), gentamicin (gm),
kanamycin (kan), ampicillin (amp), streptomycin (sm), keflin (kef),
chloramphenicol and naladixic acid. By this criterion, only 25% of
all samples were sensitive to all drugs. High level resistance was
defined as flora having $\geq$ 50% resistant coliforms.

In all populations studied, resistance to amp, tet, sm, kef
and kan was most common. 25-40% of samples from the hospitalized
population were resistant to one or more of these drugs. The frequency of resistance in lab workers was similar, except for a 33-
50% decrease in high level resistance to tet and amp. The urban
dwellers showed a lower frequency of resistance notably to kan
($\approx$15%) however, tet, amp and sm resistance levels were $\approx$30-35%.
High level resistance was also notably less in rural dwellers.
These findings indicated an unexpectedly high frequency of resistant fecal organisms in the general population, particularly among
those not taking antibiotics. A group of patients on one or more
antibiotics showed that multiple resistance to 4-7 drugs was significantly more common than among noningestors.

In 560 fecal samples examined, 15.6% had lead resistance in $\geq$
10% of the lactose fermenting populations. Other resistance frequencies were mercury (Hg) 14.3%, tellurite (Te) 13.9%, cadmium
(Cd) 6.6%, arsenate (As) 5.0%, metaborate (MBO) 3.0%, chromate (Cr)
2.6%, phenylmercuric acetate (PMA) 1.4% and silver 0%. Resistance
was unequally distributed in the fecal samples: e.g., many samples
were either sensitive (<10%), or showed large numbers ($\geq$ 90%) of
resistant organisms. This was particularly true for Hg, Pb, Cr
and MBO. Lactose nonfermenters were equally or less resistant to
all metals. The kinds of high frequency metal resistance (50%
resistance) differed in the various populations: in the hospital,
19.5% had high level Hg resistance; Te and Pb were at 12.6% and
Cd and MOB at 8.7%. In lab workers, 12.6% of samples were highly
resistant to Hg, whereas in rural dwellers the frequency was 6.4%.
In this latter group, Pb resistance was at 28.7 compared to 1.5%
in the lab group.

UNUSUAL CONJUGAL TRANSFER OF ANTIBIOTIC RESISTANCE IN BACTEROIDES: NON-INVOLVEMENT OF PLASMIDS

T.D. Mays, F.L. Macrina, R.A. Welch, and C.J. Smith

Virginia Commonwealth University
Richmond, Virginia 23298

Resistance to tetracycline (Tc^r) and lincosamide antibiotics (clindamycin resistance, Cc^r; erythryomycin resistance, Em^r) was transferred from a strain of <u>Bacteroides</u> <u>fragilis</u> (V503) to a plasmidless strain of B. uniformis (V528) during <u>in</u> <u>vitro</u> filter matings. Resistance transfer was detected at frequencies of 10^{-5} to 10^{-6} drug resistant progeny/input donor cell and was dependent on cell-to-cell contact of donors and recipients. Transfer was insensitive to DNase and was not mediated by chloroform or filter-sterilized donor broth cultures. The Tc^r and Cc^r markers did not segregate away from one another at readily detectable frequencies. Both markers were stable in the V503 donor and in resistant progeny and treatment of V503 cultures with coumermycin or ethidium bromide failed to yield drug-sensitive variants. By standard physical analyses, V503 was found to contain a 3.7 Mdal plasmid (pVA503). Attempts to isolate unusually large plasmids from V503 using the method of Hansen and Olsen (J. Bacteriol <u>135</u>, 227-238 [1978]) were unsuccessful. Drug resistant transconjugants of V503 x V528 matings usually contained pVA503, but up to 20% of the total transconjugants of such crosses were plasmid free. Filter blot DNA hybridization studies (Southern method) confirmed that V503 was not integrated into the host chromosome of the plasmidless transconjugants. Transconjugants from V503 x V528 matings (with or without pVA503) acted as donors for Cc^r. Tc^r transfer could not be monitored in such secondary crosses due to inherent Tc^r in the recipient strain. Chromosomal determinants for resistance to cefoxitin and rifampicin were not transferred in this system.

To further explore this seemingly plasmidless transfer we exploited a previously characterized conjugative R plasmid (pBF4) from <u>B</u>. <u>fragilis</u>. (Welch, et al. Plasmid <u>2</u>, 261-268 1979 , and Welch and Macrina, J. Bacteriol <u>145</u>, <u>in</u> <u>press</u> [1981]). pBF4 is 27 Mdal in size and confers constitutively-expressed Cc^r. ^{32}P labelled pBF4 was used as a probe in hybridizations against filter blotted <u>Hind</u> III cleaved V503 (donor), V528 (recipient) and selected Cc^r/ Tc^r progeny from V503 x V528 matings. A single ~4.2 <u>Hind</u> III fragment present in the V503 digest showed homology to pBF4. There was no pBF4-hybridizing material in the V528 recipient. Interestingly, all Cc^r/Tc^r progeny from V503 x V528 matings contained a 4.2 Mdal <u>Hind</u> III fragment that hybridized to pBF4. Our current hypothesis is that the Cc^r, Tc^r and conjugal transfer genes are on a discrete segment of DNA which resides on the host genome rather than a plasmid. (Supported by NSF grant 77-00858)

LAMBDA TRANSDUCING PHAGES CARRYING PLASMID R100 <u>tra</u> GENES

Sarah A. McIntire and Walter B. Dempsey

VA Med. Ctr. and
Univ. of Tx. Health Sci. Ctr.
Dallas, Texas

From the R100::λ cointegrate pEDR101, we have isolated a series of λ<u>tra</u> transducing phages which carry R100 <u>tra</u> DNA substituted into the left arm of λ. Five phages have been completely analyzed. The <u>tra</u> genes carried by each phage were assayed in complementation tests with known F'<u>lac tra</u>$_{am}$ plasmids, and this genetic analysis was then correlated with the amount of R100 DNA present in each phage (Fig. 1).

The proteins synthesized from each phage were determined [1] from infections of irradiated λ⁻ host cells so that all promoters on the phage (both λ and R100) were expressed. Similar infections of irradiated λ-lysogenic cells lead to repression of λ promoters and thus allow detection of any proteins synthesized from R100 promoters. Such experiments led to the unexpected observation that each phage directed the synthesis of one R100 protein (25,800 M.W.), even though the <u>tra</u> promoter located before <u>traY</u> was missing in all but one phage. By analogy with the reported molecular weight of plasmid F <u>traT</u> protein as 25,000, and since one phage encodes only <u>traS</u> and <u>traT</u>, we believe this protein represents R100 <u>traT</u> product. These experiments using the λ lysogen mean that either: (1) <u>traT</u> has its own promoter; or (2) a few λP$_R$, mRNA transcripts are made and <u>traT</u> has a much more efficient translation initiation mechanism than any other gene on these transcripts.

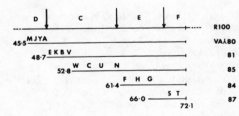

Figure 1. R100 DNA carried by the five λ<u>tra</u> phages. Arrows indicate EcoR1 sites. Numbers on the left are kb coordinates for the R100 DNA carried by each phage.

References:
1. Dempsey, W.B., S. McIntire, N. Willetts, J. Schottel, T. Kinscherf, S. Silver and W. Shannon. 1978. Properties of lambda transducing bacteriophages carrying R100 plasmid DNA: mercury resistance genes. J. Bacteriol. 136:1084-1093.

ACTIVE UPTAKE OF TETRACYCLINE IN MEMBRANE VESICLES OF SENSITIVE ESCHERICHIA COLI.

L. McMurry, J. Cullinane, R. Petrucci, Jr.& S. Levy
Department of Molecular Biology and Microbiology
Tufts University Medical School, Boston, MA 02111

Tetracycline inhibits protein synthesis in susceptible microbial organisms by interfering with binding of amino-acyl-tRNA to the A site on the ribosome. Since plasmid-borne resistance to this drug involves a decrease in drug uptake, we have studied tetracycline transport in resistant and sensitive E. coli cells. Sensitive E. coli cells have both an energy-dependent uptake and an energy-independent uptake (1).

There are 3 kinds of active transport in E. coli: that requiring ATP; that during which the substrate is modified (e.g. phosphorylated by PEP) and that which depends only upon proton motive force (pmf; an electrochemical gradient of hydrogen ions across the membrane formed by electron transport and/or by ATP hydrolysis specifically by the membrane ATPase).

Because tetracycline uptake in cells was inhibited to the same extent by agents which a) block respiration (cyanide, anaerobiosis), b) inhibit ATP synthesis (arsenate) and c) destroy the proton motive force (2,4-dinitrophenol) (1), it was not clear to which category active tetracycline uptake belonged. Membrane vesicles prepared by osmotic lysis of spheroplasts according to the method of Kaback (2) are free of cytoplasm and endogenous energy sources and serve to distinguish among these possibilities. With such vesicles, addition of electron transport substrates forms a pmf only, so that transport stimulated by such substrates must be pmf-dependent. We have found that such vesicles made from sensitive E. coli cells were indeed stimulated by electron transport substrates (D-lactate and phenazine methosulfate plus ascorbate) to concentrate tetracycline 3-5-fold above the level of the drug in the medium. Therefore at least part of the energy-dependent uptake of tetracycline in sensitive cells depends only upon pmf. The pH and Mg^{++} optima were pH 6.9 and 1 mM respectively.

The various inhibitors mentioned above (arsenate, cyanide, dinitrophenol, etc.) presumably all lower pmf to some extent in vivo. That they all inhibit tetracycline uptake completely might be explained if this uptake required a relatively high pmf below which no active transport of tetracycline could occur.

(1) McMurry, L. and S.B. Levy, 1978. Antimicrob. Agents & Chemotherapy 14, 201-209.
(2) Kaback, H.R. 1971. Methods Enzymol. 22, 99-120.

DISTRIBUTION OF PLASMID TYPE β-LACTAMASES IN AMPICILLIN-RESISTANT SALMONELLAE FROM HUMANS AND ANIMALS IN THE UNITED STATES

A.A. Medeiros, E.S. Gilleece and T.F. O'Brien

The Miriam Hospital, Brown University
Providence, RI &
Brigham and Women's Hospital,
Harvard Medical School, Boston, MA

The types of β-lactamase produced by 261 non-typhoidal ampicillin-resistant salmonellae, 114 human and 146 animal isolates, was determined by isoelectric focusing of crude sonic extracts. All isolates produced at least one of the types of beta-lactamase known to be plasmid-mediated. The most prevalent type was TEM-1 (n=203), followed by OXA-2 (n=50), OXA-1 (n=3) and PSE-1 (n=2). Three isolates each produced two plasmid-type beta-lactamases, i.e., TEM-1 + PSE-1 and TEM-1 + OXA-1. The PSE-1 β-lactamase, thought previously to be pseudomonas specific, was found in strains of S. typhimurium, S. newport, and S. heidelberg. None of the other 7 known types of plasmid-mediated beta-lactamase were found.

The OXA-2 β-lactamase was far more prevalent in Salmonella than has been reported for any other genera. It was found in 16 (31%) of 52 animal isolates but in only 4 (11%) of 38 human isolates of S. typhimurium. In contrast, the prevalence of OXA-2 was high in both animal (60%) and human (79%) isolates of S. typhimurium, var. copenhagen (n=29) but low in animal (9%) and human (5%) isolates of other serotypes (n=142).

OXA-2 was found rarely in human isolates of S. typhimurium, var. copenhagen from Massachusetts prior to February 1980. It occurred, however, in 8 isolates from different parts of the state over a 2 month period in February and March, suggesting that a previously undetected common source outbreak had occurred. These isolates had an unusual antibiotype to non β-lactam antibiotic characterized by intermediate level tetracycline resistant (mean diameter of zone of inhibition around 30 µg tetracycline disk = 10.5 ± 3.5mm) linked to high level resistance to streptomycin, kanamycin, and sulfonamides. Most animal isolates of OXA-2 containing S. typhimurium, var. copenhagen had the same anti-biotype indicating that this human outbreak may have been related to an animal source.

MOLECULAR STUDIES OF A COINTEGRATE PLASMID FORMED FROM PLASMID Flac AND PM10$_{LT2}$ IN Salmonella typhimurium LT2

Alexis Mendoza, José L. Ramírez & Vidal Rodriguez Lemoine
Departamento de Biologia Celular, Facultad de Ciencias
Universidad Central de Venezuela
Apartado 21201
Caracas 1020, Venezuela

Salmonella typhimurium LT2 strains has been shown to carry a large plasmid of molecular weight 53.5-60 Mdal (1). The plasmid PM10$_{LT2}$, previously named pLT2, appears to be highly stable and compatible with plasmids of F-like incompatibility groups (2).

In S.typhimurium dnaC strains plasmid Flac is highly unstable in presence of PM10$_{LT2}$ (3). Stable Lac$^+$ derivatives of these strains were shown, by alkaline sucrose gradients, to posses a large plasmid (130 Md) which appears to be a cointegrate of Flac and the PM10$_{LT2}$ plasmid (4).

We have further studied the formation of this plasmid (pSD-1) which have shown to be dissociable, in order to understand the mechanism of association/dissociation of the E.coli Flac plasmid with the stable resident PM10$_{LT2}$ of S.typhimurium.

Using a modified method for high MW extrachromosomal DNA separation we have confirmed the presence of PM10$_{LT2}$ in S.typhimurium strains(5)

Analysis of DNA extracts of S.typhimurium dnaC pM10$_{LT2}$ Flac strains carrying Lac$^+$ character relatively stable have shown the presence of a plasmid (pSD-1) of 137 Md Agarose gel diggestion patterns of plasmids pSD-1,PM10$_{LT2}$ and Flac/PM10$_{LT2}$ with restriction enzyme Sal I provide a strong evidence in support of the hypothesis that pSD-1 contains part or all of plasmid PM10$_{LT2}$ and Flac. Digestion of these plasmids using endo nucleases EcoRI or Bam HI also suggest that pSD-1 contains a substantial part of both plasmids.

References

1. Spratt, Rowbury & Meynel, 1973. M.G.G. 121, 341-353
2. Rodríguez Lemoine & Rowbury, 1975a. Rev. Lat. Microb.17, 79-85
3. Rodríguez Lemoine & Rowbury, 1975b. J.G. Microb. 90; 360-364
4. Rodríguez Lemoine & Rowbury, 1976. J.G. Microb. 96; 109-116
5. Mendoza, Ramírez & Rodríguez Lemoine, 1980. Acta Cient. Venez. 31 (s1)

ANALYSIS OF F SPECIFIC MEMBRANE PROTEINS

Deanna Moore, Blair Sowa and Karin Ippen-Ihler

Department of Medical Microbiology
Texas A&M University, College Station, TX   77843

Elucidation of the pathway which leads to the biosynthesis of F-pili has been complicated by the failure of previous analytical procedures to detect a pool of F-pilin in an unassembled state in the cell. Thus, gene products associated with synthesis of the polypeptide subunit have not been distinguishable from those which participate in its assembly into a pilus structure. We have analyzed 35-S methionine labelled membrane preparations from male and female cells by polyacrylamide gel electrophoresis using slab gels formed in an exponential gradient of 10-16% acrylamide. Under our conditions, an F specific band which co-migrates with purified F-pilin is resolved at an apparent molecular weight of 7,000 daltons. The F-pilin membrane band appears to represent a substantial pool of protein, and contains 4-5% of the total radioactive label in our whole membrane preparations. The polypeptide could be extracted from these preparations with Triton X-100, and was found in the inner membrane fraction of membranes separated on the basis of density. It would appear, therefore, that F-pili are assembled from the inner membrane. traJ mutations, which affect F tra operon transcription, and mutations in traA, the structural gene for F-pilin, resulted·in the absence of the F-pilin membrane polypeptide. The F-pilin band was still present, however, in membrane preparations from strains carrying mutations in traL, traE, traB, traV traW, traC, traU, traF, traH or traG, despite the inability of these mutants to elaborate F-pili filaments. This suggests that the products of these genes are concerned with F-pilus assembly and outgrowth rather than F-pilin biosynthesis. Analysis of Hfr deletion mutants, however, indicated that a previously unidentified tra operon activity, located between traF and traH is essential for the appearance of the F-pilin membrane polypeptide. We have named this locus traQ, and suggest that the traQ product is required for processing of the traA product to F-pilin.

Several other F specific polypeptides could also be detected in our membrane preparations. These included a 100,000 dalton polypeptide, identified as a product of traG, a 23,500 dalton polypeptide which co-migrated with traJ product, and a 12,000 dalton polypeptide. Presence of the 12,000 dalton protein is affected by amber mutations in traD.

DETECTION OF ENTEROTOXIGENIC ESCHERICHIA COLI

BY DNA COLONY HYBRIDIZATION

Steve L. Moseley, Imdadul Huq and Stanley Falkow

Department of Microbiology and Immunology
University of Washington, Seattle, Washington 98195

International Centre for Diarrhoeal Disease Research
Dacca, Bangladesh

Current methods for the identification of enterotoxigenic E. coli involve immunologic or biologic assays for the presence of enterotoxins, and are not entirely suitable for screening large numbers of strains. The object of this study was to test an alternative technique based on the detection of the genes encoding the enterotoxins rather than the toxins themselves.

Genes encoding the heat labile (LT) and heat stable (ST) toxins of E. coli have been isolated and characterized by recombinant DNA techniques (1,2,3). Portions of these isolated toxin genes were used as hybridization probes for homologous sequences in strains of E. coli isolated from patients with diarrheal disease. Isolated strains of diarrheal stools were inoculated onto nitrocellulose paper (NC) which had been placed on the surface of MacConkey's agar. After incubation at 37°C, the NC was removed from the agar and the resulting colonies lysed in situ. The DNA was fixed to the NC and hybridized with radiolabeled gene probes by a modification of the colony hybridization technique of Grunstein and Hogness (4). The strains were also tested for ST and LT production by the infant mouse assay and the CHO cell assay, respectively.

All of 31 strains producing ST+LT or LT-only were detected by the LT probe. The ST probe detected 12 of 17 ST-only strains (70%) and 3 of the 26 ST+LT strains (12%). These results suggest that while LTs produced by different strains of E. coli are homologous, there are at least two heterologous STs that are detectable in the infant mouse assay.

This method is suitable for screening very large numbers of strains and detects LT producing strains with complete accuracy. Preliminary data suggest that a probe prepared from one of the ST genes not detected by the ST probe in this study may allow more complete detection of ST-only strains. Isolation and characterization of other genes encoding virulence factors from a variety of organisms will allow a more general application of analagous genetic hybridization techniques to the study of infectious diseases.

1. Dallas, W.S. et al. J. Bacteriol. 139:850-858, 1979.
2. Lathe, R. et al. Nature 284:473-474, 1980.
3. So, M. and B.J. McCarthy. PNAS 77:4011-4015, 1980.
4. Grunstein, M. and D.S. Hogness. PNAS 72:3961-3965, 1975.

STRUCTURE, REARRANGEMENTS AND MODIFICATION IN THE SMALL

UBIQUITOUS PLASMID OF NEISSERIA GONORRHOEAE

Staffan Normark, John K. Davies, Per Hagblom, Mari
Norgren, Lena Norlander, and Christopher Korch
Department of Microbiology
University of Umeå
S-901 87 Umeå, Sweden

About 95% of clinical Neisseria gonorrhoeae isolates possess a
small 4.2 kilobasepair plasmid. A small unique DNA segment can be
deleted from a specific place on this plasmid molecule. The specific deletion was accurately mapped on the plasmid and the DNA
spanning the deletion site was sequenced. The DNA sequence of the
wild type and of two deletion bearing plasmids revealed that the
exact same 54 bp had been lost in the deletion plasmids. One end
point of the deletion was flanked by two blocks of 20 bp long sequences that was nearly homologous to two sequence blocks flanking the other end point. The two respective blocks were separated
by the sequence -A T C A- and -A G C A-, respectively. In the
deleted plasmids one sequence block from each end point was retained. However, unexpectedly the sequence separating these blocks
was -G T C G-. A nonequal crossover event between nearly homologous
sequence blocks associated with specific base alterations could
explain the deletion event. Gonococcal DNA is difficult to cleave
by a number of restriction enzymes. We have evidence for that the
partial or complete resistance to the restriction endonucleases
HaeII (NgoI), HaeIII (NgoII), SacII (NgoIII) and BamHI is due to
modification. During the sequencing of the 4.2 kbp gonococcal
plasmid we found a HaeIII/NgoII (-G G C C-) site where the internal cytosines are modified. Interestingly, this site is part of
both a BglII and a HpaII/MspI site. BglII and MspI will not cleave
at this site whereas HpaII will. The results show that: i) HpaII
but not MspI can cleave if one of the external cytosines is methylated, ii) BglII cannot cleave if the cytosine at the 3' end of its
recognition sequence is modified. Other recognition sequences were
also difficult to cleave without any evidence for DNA modification.
In some cases these sites on the plasmid were associated with short
DNA repeats.

PLASMIDS IN EPIDERMOLYTIC STRAINS OF STAPHYLOCOCCUS AUREUS

M. O'Reilly, J.P.Arbuthnott & T.J.Foster

Microbiology Department,

Trinity College, Dublin 2, Ireland

Some strains of S. aureus cause blistering conditions of the skin called the Scalded Skin Syndrome. A diffusible exotoxin, epidermolytic toxin (ET) caused the epidermal splitting. Two serological types of ET (types i and ii) have been characterized. Some strains produce type i and ii ET alone, while others produce both serotypes.

We have examined 34 ET-producing strains of S. aureus for presence of plasmid DNA. All serotype ii producers carried a 42kb plasmid. Elimination of this plasmid caused simultaneous loss of toxin and bacteriocin production (Bac+). This suggested that the serotype ii ET genes were linked to Bac+ on this plasmid. Type i ET was never eliminated and was presumably chromosomally determined. Some serotype i strains also contained a 42kb plasmid but its elimination only resulted in the loss of bacteriocin production. In some strains cadmium resistance was also linked to the 42kb plasmid.

The 42kb plasmids from seven strains expressing different phenotypes were analysed with restriction endonucleases EcoR1 and HindIII. The plasmids shared 19 of 22 HindIII fragments indicating that they are closely related to each other.

REPLICATION, INCOMPATIBILITY AND ACRIDINE ORANGE CURING OF F IN

E. COLI K12

Sunil Palchaudhuri and Gopa Mitra

Department of Immunology & Microbiology

Wayne State University, School of Medicine
540 E. Canfield Ave. Detroit, Michigan 48201

In recent years, several investigators reported the conflicting incompatibility behavior of the composite plasmids (Cabello et al., 1976; Ida, 1980; Katz and Palchaudhuri, 1980). In most cases, the multicopy replicon was joined to replicon with low copy number. We studied the incompatibility characteristics of a composite plasmid, pWS1 (the pSC101 plasmid-fragment 5 of F) which can use the replication of either of the two functionally distinct replicons. We aimed to determine the functional replicon of pWS1 by testing the sensitivity to acridine orange (AO). At subinhibitory concentration of AO, the 30% of cells had lost pWS1 even though only one component (f5) was AO sensitive. Presumably, the cells (70%) which escaped the inhibitory effect of AO, were using the pSC101 replicon of pWS1. Under these in vivo conditions, we compared the incompatibility of pWS1 against a number of well characterized F' plasmids in E. coli K12 hosts (recA$^+$, recA$^-$). The presence of genetically stable transconjugants carrying both plasmids was further confirmed by gel electrophoresis and electron microscopy. These results indicated the weak incompatibility behavior of pWS1 compared to the incompatibility of mini F. In recA background, the incompatibility of pWS1 against F's is little reduced. Hence it can be concluded that functional F-replicons show stronger incompatibility properties. As a corollary it was found that the plasmid ColVtrp$^+$ showed partial incompatilbility with F's and was highly compatible with pWS1. Our present data suggest that ColVtrp$^+$ is a double replicon and one of them is F replicon. (See Table on page 2). Incompatibility of pWS1 was further tested by mating the pWS1 containing recipients with Hfr donor. In this case the incompatibility was measured by comparing the number of recombinants from Hfr x MA140 (pWS1) and Hfr x MA140 (pSC138) matings. A few recombinants were formed by the recipients carrying miniF, pSC138,

Infecting Plasmid	Resident Plasmid	Selection for Markers	% of Daughter Colonies Containing		
			Incoming Only	Resident Only	Both
F'Trp+	pWS1(Tc)	Trp+	5	0	95
		Trp+,Tc	1	1	98
F'His+	pWS1(Tc)	His+	48	0	52
		His+,Tc	6	4	90
ColVTrp+	pWS1(Tc)	Trp+	0	0	100
F'His+	Mini F	His+	95	0	5
	(pSC138)	His+,Amp	65	35	0

whereas the F⁻ or pWS1 carrying recipient cells showed much higher number of recombinants.

The F prime plasmid superinfected into the male recipients (F⁺) was converted to the covalently closed, circular duplex form as in the F⁻ recipients but the subsequent replication of circular duplex of superinfected F was blocked due to incompatibility (Saitoh and Hiraga, 1975). The Hfr donor cells transferred the genes determining inc, rep and pif functions of the integrated F into recipients (male or female) along with early chromosomal markers (Palchaudhuri Ms in prep.). It is conceivable that the mechanism of incompatibility is primarily related to the initiation of replication of the circular duplex F-DNA subsequently followed by its proper distribution into daughter cells. This early step seems to be controlled by proteins, synthesized by the host in limited amount. Our data suggests that the pWS1 which can use pSC101 replicon does not recognize these proteins as efficiently as mini F and thus the F-specific incompatibility is relaxed.

References

Cabello, F., Timmis K. and Cohen S.N., 1976, Replication Control in a composite plasmid constructed by in vitro linkage of two distinct replicons, Nature, 259: 285-290.

Ida, S., 1980, A cointegrate of the bacteriophage P1 genome and the conjuative R plasmid R100, Plasmid, 3: 278-290.

Katz, I. and Palchaudhuri, S., 1980, Consequences of interaction between F plasmid and a drug resistance plasmid belonging to incompatibility group F1., Can. J. Microbiology, 26: 94-101.

Saitoh, T. and Hiraga, S., 1975, F-DNA Superinfected into pheno-copies of donor strains 121: 1007-1013.

VIRULENCE FOR MICE OF PLASMID-BEARING EPIDEMIC STRAINS OF

SALMONELLA TYPHIMURIUM

Ciro A. Peluffo and Kinue Irino.

Instituto de Higiene, Montevideo, Uruguay and
Instituto Adolfo Lutz, Sao Paulo, Brasil
Hidalgos 532, Montevideo, Uruguay

From a sample of 84 multi-resistant strains of Salmonella typhimurium obtained from outbreaks in children's hospitals of nine cities of five South American countries we selected at random two to four strains from each outbreak, 30 strains in all. The strains, with transferable drug-resistance, were of high virulence for children as judged by their transmissibility, systemic spread and high fatality rate. The epidemic strains and 18 normal, sensitive strains were tested by i.p. challenge in mice.

The arithmetic mean of the LD_{50} is 1.37×10^7, compared with a mean LD_{50} of 2.65×10^5 for the sensitive strains (P < 0.0005). Thirteen of the epidemic strains, highly virulent for children, have an LD_{50} over 10^7 and on the average they are 80 times less virulent than strain CDC 9 kept in the laboratory for over 40 years.

The unexpected results show that apparently the factor(s) which determine virulence for children are not the same as those for mice. It is suggested that the outbreaks are the consequence of the sudden emergence of a strain endowed with high virulence for children and that the genetic material carried by the transfer factor together with the resistance determinants might be held responsible for the increased virulence for children and low virulence for mice. Bacterial virulence depends on a delicate adjustment between the biological characteristics of the pathogen and those of the host. It is not a biological heresy to admit that the loss or acquisition of a metabolic function or structural character may change the pathogenicity in opposite direction for different hosts.

A RAPID METHOD FOR DETERMINING PLASMID INCOMPATIBILITY GROUP

E.J. Perea and J.C. Palomares
Department of Microbiology
School of Medicine
Seville-9, Spain

A rapid method for determining plasmid incompatibility group by determining plasmid size by agarose gel electrophoresis is described.

The method involves checking one plasmid against another to see if they are incompatible. One plasmid is transferred to a strain carrying the other plasmid, selecting only for the incoming plasmid. Transcipients are then checked by agarose gel electrophoresis to see if both plasmids are still present; if the resident plasmid is missing, the two plasmids are clearly incompatible. If both plasmids are still present independently, transcipients are grown up overnight in non-selective medium. Clones are then checked for their plasmid complement: if a plasmid has been lost, the pair of plasmids are incompatible, while if both are present, they are compatible.

To demonstrate the method, two naturally-occurring plasmids (pSE 6 and pSE 16), originally isolated from Salmonella typhimurium, were checked against the plasmid R386 that belong to the incompatibility group FI.

The data indicate that pSE 16 and R386 are incompatible, whereas pSE 6 is compatible with R386. Thus pSE 16 belongs to the incompatibility group FI.

Since this method involves examination of the plasmids themselves, it is much faster that the classical method of incompatibility testing and takesfewer working hours. Futhermore, since no changes in the plasmid DNA need be induced to give unique markers on each plasmid, there is no chance of incorrect classification due to alterations in the inc genes,

643

GENTAMICIN RESISTANCE IN CLINICAL ISOLATES,

"PICKING-UP" OF R-DETERMINANTS ON PHAGE P1

Wolfgang Piepersberg
Department of Biochemistry
University of Wisconsin
Madison, WI 53706

As a first step towards epidemiological studies on plasmid-encoded gentamicin resistance (gen^r) in gram-negative bacteria from human and animal sources the ability of transposition of the respective r-determinants was investigated. None of the gen^r genes from 48 different R-factors (RF) could be moved onto λ b515 b519 cI857 s7. However, out of 17 tested RF 10 gave rise to high-frequency-transducing (hft) gen^r derivatives of phage P1 cm0 clts100.

In the cases studied gen^r was always accompanied by other RF derived antibiotic resistances when "picked-up" by P1. First step (generalized) transduction frequencies of the gen^r phenotype varied between about 10^{-3} and below 10^{-7} per chloramphenicol resistant lysogens formed. Among those hft P1 gen^r derivatives were found within a range from below 5% up to 100% of the heat-inducible gen^r primary transductants.

The analysis of the DNA segments inserted into P1 prophage plasmids revealed the following: (i) their lengths varied within about 15 to 60 kb, but (ii) were constant in independent isolates from a given RF with the same phenotype transduced; (iii) the sites of the insertion into the genome of P1 cm0 varied from isolate to isolate, but (iv) were found to be always within either one of the BglII-2 or BglII-5 fragments (within map units 3 through 35). Further investigation will involve an analysis of their structure and mechanism of movement, and of possible homologies between them.

In conclusion, if the gen^r genes stably integrated into the DNA of phage P1 are within true transposons (which has to be proven), they seem to be mostly part of larger r-determinants together with other resistance genes. Since gentamicin was comparatively late intoduced into clinical use, the resistance conferring genetic material might have been preferentially incorporated into preexsisting selftransmissible elements. Also, the ease with which phage P1 accepts and transduces large fragments of RF's and its broad host range could suggest that this kind of phages might be potent vehicles for the distribution of r-determinants in natural environments.

GENETIC CHARACTERIZATION OF RESISTANCE PLASMID CONTENT IN THREE SALMONELLA SEROTYPE WHICH PRODUCED EPIDEMIC NOSO-COMIAL INFECTIONS.

Gustavo Prieto, Ada Martínez, Jeannette Vargas and Carmen Marín
Centro Regional de Referencia Bacteriológica. Hospital Universitario. Fac. de Medicina. Universidad del Zulia. Maracaibo Venezuela

Strains of Salmonella (S. enteritidis bioser Java, ser Saintpaul and ser Havana) which showing complex phenotype resistance produced impor tant epidemic nosocomial infections, involving one or more hospitals, we re analyzed in regard to their resistance plasmid content. Except for the resistance for nalidixic acid and nitrofurantoin present in some strains, which is a chromosomal type, any other resistance found, was an extra-chromosomal type, originated in a polyplasmid state, by the presence of autotransferable and non-autotransferable plasmids. In bioser Java are characterized the autotransferable plasmid H_2 R (Te-Cm) and a new plasmid F-like R (Kn-Nm-Am-Cb-Cr) which is able to propagate the phage fd but not u_2, it does not show incompatibility with any known plasmid F-like but it is incompatible with F-like plasmids that showing similar characteristics have been isolated locally from S. sonnei and S. anteriti dis ser Typhimurium. There are others two non-autotransferable plasmids r (Am-Cb) and r (Su-St). In ser Saintpaul coexist two autotransferable plasmid R (Su-Te-Cm-Kn-Nm-Am-Cb-Cr) and R (Am-Cb-Cr) incompatibility groups H_1 and $I_{1,k}$ respectively and r (St) determinant. Ser Havana has an autotransferable plasmid R (Te-Cm-Kn-Nm-Am-Cb-Cr) incompatibility group H_2 and two non-autotransferable plasmids r (Kn-Am-Cb-Cr-Gm) and r (Su-St). In the first two serotypes the polyplasmid state provi des for a double mechanism of resistance for ampicillin, carbenicillin and cephalosporins. The whole analysis of the plasmid content allows to deny or to assert the epidemiologic relationship that exists between resistance plasmids, which determine a similar complex phenotypic resistance, and appear in epidemics that happen during certain period of time in a some hospital or different hospitals.

EPIDEMIOLOGY OF ANTIBIOTIC RESISTANCE IN THE BACTEROIDES FRAGILIS GROUP

Gaetano Privitera[+],Françoise Fayolle and Madeleine Sebald

Institut Pasteur, Paris, France and Infectious Diseases
Clinic, Milan, Italy [+]

Bacteroides fragilis is the most frequently isolated anaerobic organism in human infections. In this species tetracycline (Tc)
and macrolide-lincosamide-streptogramins (MLS) resistances have been
recently demonstrated to be plasmid-mediated and transferable. In
the strains which initially came to our observation, the Tc resistan
ce appeared to be inducible; the transfer ability (tra) of Tc resistance was contemporaneously induced when the bacteria were grown
in the presence of subinhibitory concentrations of Tc before mating[1].

In the order to assess the epidemiology of transferable antibio
tic resistance in the B. fragilis group, we examined 63 clinical iso
lates sent for identification to the Anaerobe Reference Center in Pa
ris. The prevalence of Tc and MLS resistant strains was 82,5% and 2%
respectively. All Tc resistant strains were studied for inducibility
(i) vs. constitutivity(c) for expression and transfer ability of the
resistance. 60% of the strains were transfer proficient after induction (tra_i) or constitutively (tra_c); of these, about two thirds
were Tc_i tra_i, but Tc^r_c tra_c and dissociated phenotypes were also
found. Among the strains wich did not transfer the resistance both
Tc^r_i and Tc^r_c phenotypes were observed. MLS resistance is almost
constantly associated with Tc resistance. Except one strain which is
able to transfer MLS^r independently, this character is either not-
transferable or co-transferred with the Tc resistance. In the tra_c
strains, the number of all transcipients was increased by Tc induction, but for a given strain the percentage of MLS cotransfer was
remarkably stable.

Although different lysis and preparative techniques were employed, we failed to demonstrate any plasmid DNA in most wild-type
resistant strains and in their transconjugants.

Experiments performed in gnotoxenic mice colonized with B. fragilis strain 92 Tc^r_i tra_i showed that the Tc resistance and transfer
ability could be induced in vivo by sub-inhibitory concentrations
of the antibiotic. These properties appeared to be quickly lost once
the antibiotic was withdrawn; the prolonged administration of higher
doses lead however to the isolation of strains constitutive for Tc
resistance and transfer ability. The transfer of MLS resistance was
observed in vivo in the absence of antibiotic selective pressure.

1 - Privitera, G., Sebald, M., and Fayolle, F. 1979. Nature (London)
278: 657-659

IDENTIFICATION OF A BACTERIAL PATHOGENICITY DETERMINANT MODULATED BY PROPHAGE GENES.

C.Pruzzo, S.Valisena, E. Debbia and G. Satta.

Institute of Microbiology University of Genova and

Institute of Microbiology University of Cagliari ITALY

We have previously shown in <u>Klebsiella pneumoniae</u> a special case of lysogenic conversion which seems to be regulated by the expression of immunity to superinfection[1]. We have now studied if the conversion phenomenon, where the prophages FR2 and AP3 cause repression (or masking) of the receptors for the phages Pl and T3-T7 respectively also changed other properties of the converted cells. A possible influence on adherence to human epithelial cells (EC) was studied first. We have found that the non-converted Klebsiellae adhere to EC from intestine (75 bact./EC), oral cavity (180 bact./EC) and urinary tract (75 bact./EC), while the derivatives lysogenic for FR2 did not. Strains cured from AP3 showed the same adherence capability as the non-lysogenic parental strain[2]. The influence of lysogenization by AP3 and FR2 on resistance to phagocytosis by human neutrophils was then studied. It was found that the strains lysogenic for AP3, but not those lysogenic for FR2, were more sensitive to uptake (5 fold) and intracellular killing (8 fold) than the non-lysogneic parental strain. LD_{50} in mice of the non-lysogenic strain sensitive to T3 and T7 was 150 fold lower than that of the strian converted by AP3 to coliphage resistance. The AP3 lysogenic recombinants in which loss of immunity gene was transferred[3] showed the same adherence capability, resistance to phagocytosis and LD_{50} values as the non-lysogenic parental strain. Spontaneous mutants resistant to T3 and T7 showed adherence capability, sensitivity to phagocytosis and pathogenicity for mice similar to those of the AP3 lysogens. AP3-like phages, induced from two non-adhesive Klebsiellae isolated from clinical specimens, were able to convert bacteria to T3-T7 resistance. These lysogens were non-adhesive. Their sensitivity to phagocytosis and pathogenicity for mice were similar to those of the strains lysogenic for AP3.

1. Satta G.,C.Pruzzo,E.Debbia and L.Calegari 1978 J. Virol. <u>28</u>:786.
2. Pruzzo C.,E.Debbia and G.Satta 1980 Infect.Immun. <u>30</u>:562.
3.Satta G.,C.Pruzzo,E.Debbia and R.Fontana 1978. J. Virol. <u>28</u>:772.

SIMULTANEOUS EXPRESSION OF CFA/I AND ST IN 0128 ac SEROTYPES OF

E. COLI ISOLATED IN SÃO PAULO

M.H.L. Reis , T.A.T. Gomes, M.H.T. Affonso and
L.R. Trabulsi
Department of Micro, Immuno and Parasitology
Escola Paulista de Medicine
São Paulo, SP, Brazil

Escherichia coli strains of serotypes 0128 ac: H12 and 0128ac:H7 producing the heat-stable enterotoxin (ST) and the colonization factor CFA/I were isolated from children with diarrhea in São Paulo.

Genetic studies and analysis of plasmids by agarose gel electrophoresis and/or electron microscopy revealed that: 1) In 3 strains of serotype 0128ac:H12 (strains TR438/1, TR14/1 and TR99/1) and in 1 strain of serotype 0128ac:H7 (TR780) the expression of CFA/I and ST is coded for by genes from a single plasmid; 2) The CFA/I-ST coding plasmids of these strains are not self-transmissible and need for transfer a conjugative plasmid (plasmid B) which was isolated from strain TR438/1; 3) The CFA/I-ST coding plasmid of strain TR780 differs from plasmids of the other strains, being incompatible with the conjugative plasmid B; 4) The CFA/I-ST plasmid isolated from strain TR438/1 is 97 kilobases long and plasmid B has a length of 64 kilobases as determined by electron microscopy; 5) The molecular weight of the CFA/I-ST plasmids of strains TR14/1 and TR99/1 is about 49×10^6 daltons while that of the CFA/I-ST plasmid of strain TR780 is 59×10^6 daltons, as determined by agarose gel electrophoresis.

ON THE TRANSFER SYSTEM DETERMINED BY PLASMIDS BELONGING TO INCOMPATIBILITY GROUP S

Vidal Rodríguez Lemoine and María E. Cavazza
Departamento de Biología Celular, Facultad de Ciencias
Universidad Central de Venezuela
Apartado 21201
Caracas 1020, Venezuela

All plasmids belonging to an incompatibility group appear to deter mine the sinthesis of a particular transfer system.

Plasmids isolated from Serratia marcescens that were originally classified as incompatibility group S (1) determine a transfer system which is optimum when host strains are grown at 22°C (2). This transfer system typified by plasmid R477, appears to be different from plasmids of all other incompatibility groups so far studied.

Plasmids isolated from other genera of bacteria ie. S.typhimurium, K.pneumoniae, S.flexneri, S.anatum, C.freundii, E.cloacae and S.typhi and classified into incompatibility group H2 also appear to produce a transfer system that is most efficient at low temperature.

Incompatibility relationship between plasmids belonging to inc. groups S or H2 have been studied in order to demostrate our hypothe sis that they share a unique transfer system (3). Inc S plasmids are indeed incompatible with plasmids Mip235, R1022 and pSD114 (inc H2).

We have studied further the transfer system of inc S/H2 plasmids. Our results support those of Rodríguez Lemoine et al (2) that the growth temperature of the donor affect significantly transfer of all those plasmids grouped previously into inc. group S. The incubation temperature of recipient cells has little effect on transfer effi- ciency. Temperature of mating appears to has not effect on transfer efficiency of any of the S/H2 inc. plasmids studied. We have used different conditions that Taylor et al (4) but we found no apprecia ble differences using temperatures of 24°C or 37°C during 1 h or 10 min of mating in liquid medium.

We have found that temperature of growth of cells (24°C-37°C) carryng plasmids pSD114, Mip235 and R1022 but not N-1 appears to have little or not effect on their transfer.

The growth temperature of the donor cells appears to effect one to the early stages related to the union formation of pairs or aggrega te of donor and recipient cells. When donor cells grown at 37°are mixed with recipient cells and forced to bring together (i.e by con jugation on solid surfaces or using filters) the frequency of trans fer is increased to close the efficiency of donor grown at 24°C.

Presence of common fimbriae in donor cells but not in recipient cells appears to play an important role in transfer of S/H2 plasmids.

R e f e r e n c e s
1. Hedges, Rodríguez Lemoine & Datta, 1975 J.G.Microb. 86; 88-92
2. Rodríguez Lemoine, Jacob, Hedges and Datta, 1975.J.G.Microb.86 111-114
3. Cavazza & Rodríguez Lemoine,1980. Acta Cient. Ven. 31; (Supl.1)
4. Taylor & Levine, 1980. J.G.Microb. 116; 475-484

A SIMPLE PROCEDURE FOR THE DETECTION OF "CRYPTIC" CONJUGATIVE PLASMIDS OF THE INCOMPATIBILITY GROUP N

M. Rodriguez and V.N. Iyer

Department of Biology
Carleton University
Ottawa, Canada

Conjugative plasmids of the incompatibility group N are widely distributed and frequently isolated from natural populations of bacteria – often, but not exclusively, from Enterobacteriaceae. Sometimes, such plasmids, although conjugative, have been found to be otherwise cryptic. Their isolation supports the concept that in natural environments their exist pools of such plasmids that specify only functions related to bacterial conjugation and that they acquire other genes by recombination events such as those mediated by transposons. The detection of such "cryptic" conjugative plasmids is usually by indirect methods which involve their ability to mobilize genes from non-conjugative plasmids. Although bacteriophages specific for this group of plasmids exist, phage sensitivity tests frequently require first the transfer of the plasmid to a suitable standard host. We describe a relatively simpler procedure for detecting such plasmids. This procedure should facilitate and encourage the determination of the proportion of such "cryptic" conjugative plasmids in collections of N group plasmids from particular environments and provide information that could be useful in epidemiological or evolutionary studies.

The test is based on the observation that a variety of species of gram negative bacteria harbouring conjugative N group plasmids whether "cryptic" or "non-cryptic" kill Klebsiella pneumoniae strain M5a1. Plasmids of the groups P and W but not other groups also mediate killing of the K. pneumoniae strain but to a degree that is less than with the N group plasmids. The mechanism of killing is being investigated.

Procedure – Grow the test culture and strain M5a1 to late exponential phase in Penassay Broth at 37 C with aeration. Spread 0.1 ml of M5a1 (10^7-10^8 cells) on Penassay Agar. After the surface has dried, place a drop of the test culture on the M5a1-seeded surface. Incubate the plate for 24 hours at 37°C and observe for the inhibition of M5a1 at the area inoculated with the test culture. The procedure lends itself well to the use of multipoint inoculating devices enabling the simultaneous screening of large numbers of cultures. (We are grateful to M. Arroyo and H. Tschape for some of the test strains.)

650

INDICATOR PLATES FOR CHLORAMPHENICOL RESISTANCE IN
ENTEROBACTERIACEAE MEDIATED BY CHLORAMPHENICOL ACETYLTRANSFERASE

G. Neal Proctor and Robert H. Rownd

Laboratory of Molecular Biology and
Department of Biochemistry
University of Wisconsin
Madison, Wisconsin 53706

Rosanilin dyes such as crystal violet and basic fuchsin can be used as indicator dyes in agar plates to distinguish betwee chloramphenicol sensitive colonies and chloramphenicol resistant colonies containing the inactivating enzyme chloramphenicol acetyltransferase (CAT). On certain media containing rosanilins, enterobacterial colonies containing CAT are more darkly colored than colonies not containing this enzyme. This permits the direct detection of chloramphenicol sensitive cells in a population of chloramphenicol resistant cells by plating on agar medium containing rosanilin dyes but lacking chloramphenicol. This method should be valuable in cloning experiments using insertional inactivation of the CAT resistance gene. Enterobacteriaceae harboring unstable plasmids conferring chloramphenicol resistance form sectored colonies on rosanilin dye indicator plates. The color difference between chloramphenicol sensitive and resistance colonies is less dramatic than the color difference between Lac$^+$ and Lac$^-$ colonies on MacConkey lactose medium, but is sufficient for unambiguous distinction.

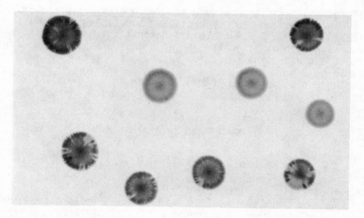

Figure Legend: Sectored colonies of <u>Salmonella typhimurium</u> harboring the R plasmid NR1 on broth plates containing 2 μg/ml crystal violet. The spontaneous loss of the r-determinants component of NR1 in <u>S</u>. <u>typhimurium</u> during colony formation results in the lighter colored sectors within individual colonies which contain chloramphenicol-sensitive cells. Non-sectored, light-colored colonies are colonies which do not contain the r-determinants component.

PLASMID-CODED DEGRADATION OF SALICYLIC AND ISOVANILLIC ACIDS IN THE SOIL BACTERIUM K17

M. S. Salkinoja-Salonen[*], A. Paterson[*] and J. Buswell[#]

[*]Dept. of General Microbiology, University of Helsinki
Mannerheimintie 172, 00280 Finland
[#]Dept. of Biology, Paisley College of Technology, Paisley
Renfrewshire, PA1 2BE Scotland UK

The soil bacterium K17[1] is able to degrade the lignan alpha-conidendrin via the intermediate isovanillic acid (4-methoxy,3-hydroxy benzoic acid) and grows on a number of aromatic carboxylic acids and lower aliphatic alcohols[2,3]. In K17, as in a great number of bacteria isolated by us from lignin-containing wastes[3], a number of phenotypes were found to be unstable and were irreversibly lost at high frequency with growth on nutrient media[4]. The frequency of loss was increased by introduction of the IncP plasmids RP4 and R68.44 into the strain.

K17 strain degrades salicylic acid via gentisic acid[2] after 5-hydroxylation of the aromatic ring. Isovanillic acid is degraded via protocatechuic acid. K17 easily lost the ability for growth on salicylic and isovanillic acids, but such "cured" mutants still grow on gentisic and protocatechuic acids.

The sal and the isovan phenotypes could be reintroduced into the cured mutants by conjugation with the parent strain, and also to heterologous recipients such as Pseudomonas putida PAW85, and with a lower frequency to Agrobacterium tumefaciens LBA202, provided that a conjugative P-plasmid was first introduced into the donor strain. The sal and the isovan phenotypes hitch-hiked into the recipient also when selection was made for the transfer of the R-plasmid only.

A large plasmid (over 100Md) was transferred from the K17 donor into the Agrobacterium recipient along with the sal phenotype.

We conclude that the degradation of salicylic acid and isovanillic acid is in K17 coded for by a plasmid.

References
1. V. Sundman, J. Gen. Microbiol. 36: 171 (1964)
2. J. A. Buswell, A. Paterson, and M.S. Salkinoja-Salonen, FEMS Microbiol. Lett. 8: 135 (1980)
3. M.S. Salkinoja-Salonen and V. Sundman, in "Lignin biodegradation : microbiology, chemistry and potential applications" T.Kent Kirk, T. Higuchi and H.-M. Chang eds., CRC Press, Boca Raton Fl. Vol.2: 179 (1980)
4. M. S. Salkinoja-Salonen, E. Vaisanen, and A. Paterson, in "Plasmids of Medical, Environmental and Commercial Importance", K.N. Timmis and A. Puhler, eds., Elsevier/North Holland Biomedical Press, p. 301 (1979)

MANIPULATION OF THE GENES CODING FOR THE HEAT-LABILE

ENTEROTOXIN OF ESCHERICHIA COLI

J. Sanchez, P.M. Bennett and M.H. Richmond

Department of Bacteriology
University of Bristol
Bristol, U.K.

Plasmid P307, isolated from a porcine strain of E. coli (1) carries genes (eltA and eltB) (2) which specify the synthesis of a heat-labile enterotoxin. These genes have been cloned into pBR313 to produce plasmid EWD299 (3).

Plasmid pUB1841 was generated in vitro from EWD299 by deleting the small EcoRI fragment carrying most of the eltB gene. An intact and functional eltA gene is left (3). Plasmids pUB1844 and pUB1845 were constructed by cloning the small HindIII fragment of EWD299, which carries eltB, into pACYC184 (4) in the two possible orientations. When whole cell lysates (WCL) (or cell free supernatants CFS) of UB5201 (pUB1841) were mixed with WCL (or CFS) of UB5201 (pUB1844 or pUB1845) no toxin activity was detected using the Y-1 tissue culture cell assay. In contrast, when pUB1841 and pUB1844 were both carried by UB5201, toxin activity comparable to that found in UB5201 (EWD 299) was observed. When pUB1845 replaced pUB1844 toxin activity was decreased to about 1%. The host strain is a recA strain of E. coli and tests confirmed that no recombination between pUB1841 and pUB1844 or pUB1845 had occurred to any detectable extent. The results indicate that either eltA and eltB have separate promoters or, when cloned into pACYC184 eltB is under the control of an external promoter.

1. Gyles, C., So, M. and Falkow, S. J. Infect. Dis. 130, 40
        (1974).
2. Dallas, W.S. and Falkow, S. Nature 288, 499 (1980).
3. Dallas, W.S., Gill, D.M. and Falkow, S. J. Bact. 139, 850
        (1979).
4. Chang, A.C.Y. and Cohen, S. J. Bact. 134, 1141 (1978).

GENETIC AND PHYSICAL CHARACTERISTICS OF ENTEROTOXIN PLASMIDS FROM HUMAN STRAINS OF ESCHERICHIA COLI

D.S. Santos, I.I. Tanaka and L.R. Trabulsi

Department of Micro,Imuno and Parasitology
Escola Paulista de Medicina
São Paulo,SP,Brazil

Enterotoxigenic strains of E.coli isolated from several sources were shown by genetic and physical analysis to possess plasmid DNA encoding the heat-labile enterotoxin genes. A study was conducted to investigate the relationship among six enterotoxin plasmids transferred into an E. coli K12 in the basis of incompatibility,repression and restriction analysis. The study have shown that all of them belongs to the incompatibility group L, and represses the tra genes of F-like plasmids. Analysis of plasmid DNA fragments on 1% agarose gel,revealed common genetic sequences. In two of them an identical cutting pattern was observed, indicating that they are a unique plasmid in different strains of clinical isolates. (This research was supported by grant 2222/15 81/77 - CNPq)

BINDING AND UPTAKE OF PLASMID DNA DURING TRANSFORMATION OF

$CaCl_2$-TREATED ESCHERICHIA COLI

J.R. Saunders and G.O. Humphreys
Department of Microbiology
University of Liverpool L69 3BX, U.K

Little is known of the mechanisms involved in uptake of plasmid DNA during transformation of $CaCl_2$-treated E.coli. Cells harvested in early exponential phase produce about 200 times more transformants at saturating DNA concentrations than cells in lag or stationary phases[1]. The efficiency of transformation (transformants/µg DNA at non-saturating concentrations), the amount of DNA required to saturate the transformation capacity of a fixed number of cells, and the total number of transformants at saturation increased to a maximum in early exponential phase (A_{660} = 0.1 - 0.2) and then declined progressively. Transformation was most efficient at a time when the modal volume of cells in the culture was greatest and when the size distribution was skewed towards cells of large volume. However, there cannot be a simple relationship between cell volume and transformability since during growth in batch culture the former varies over a two fold range whereas the latter varies about 200 fold.

About 10% of ^{3}H-NTP16 DNA in a transformation mixture remained tightly bound to the outside of cells in the presence of Ca^{2+}. <10% of such tightly bound DNA subsequently became DNase-resistant after a $42^{o}C$ heat-pulse. When the system was just saturating, 1-2 molecule equivalents of NTP16 DNA (Mol. wt. 5.7×10^6)/viable cell became DNase-resistant, but <1% of viable cells became transformed. This suggests that a large proportion of DNase-resistant DNA may be located in the periplasm after the heat pulse. Separation of membrane fractions (in the absence of DNase) after transformation showed that > 90% of bound DNA remained attached to the outer membrane. If cells were treated with DNase after the heat-pulse then most of the small amount of labelled DNA remaining was associated with inner membranes. Plasmid DNA bound equally well in vitro to isolated inner or outer membranes. The efficiencies of divalent cations in promoting binding to membranes or whole cells ($Ca^{2+} \gg Ba^{2+} > Sr^{2+} > Mg^{2+}$) paralleled their ability to induce transformability. DNA binding was greatly reduced if outer membranes were treated with trypsin. Proteolytic enzymes also reduced transformation frequencies in intact $CaCl_2$-treated cells, suggesting that protein components of the cell envelope are required for binding and/or transport of DNA during transformation.

1. M.G.M. Brown, A. Weston, J.R. Saunders and G.O. Humphreys. FEMS Microbiol. Lett. 5, 219-222, (1979).

INTERGENERIC MOBILIZATION OF NONCONJUGATIVE R PLASMIDS BY 24.5

MEGADALTON CONJUGATIVE PLASMID OF NEISSERIA GONORRHOEAE

J.R. Saunders, Fiona Flett and G.O. Humphreys

Department of Microbiology
University of Liverpool
Liverpool, L69 3BX, U.K.

Some strains of N.gonorrhoeae carry conjugative plasmids of 24.5 Mdal that are capable of mobilizing gonococcal β-lactamase plasmids[3]. We investigated the ability of one such plasmid, pLE2451[2], to mobilize nonconjugative plasmids in intergeneric triparental matings. Strains of N.gonorrhoeae carrying pLE2451 could mobilize plasmids residing in an intermediate donor $hsdR_k^- M_k^+$ strain of E.coli to an $hsdR_k^- M_k^+$ recipient. However, pLE2451 itself could not be detected physically in either strain of E.coli. This indicated that pLE2451 was unstable in E.coli but could survive sufficiently long to express mobilization functions. 3.2 Mdal and 4.4 Mdal gonococcal β-lactamase plasmids, plasmids originally isolated from enteric bacteria (ColEl and NTP5), from H.parainfluenzae (RSF0885) and from H.ducreyi (pJB1) were mobilized between strains of E.coli by pLE2451 at frequencies of 10^{-5} to 10^{-4} per initial donor. In contrast, the enteric plasmids NTP1 and NTP16, unlike other plasmids also encoding TEM β-lactamase, were not mobilized, presumably because appropriate mobility functions were not provided. However, transfer events involving transient survival of conjugative plasmids might play a general role in the dissemination of nonconjugative plasmids between bacterial species.

The molecular relatedness between β-lactamase plasmids found in N.gonorrhoeae and Haemophilus species has prompted speculation that the gonococcus may have acquired such plasmids from Haemophilus. None of the β-lactamase plasmids tested in our experiments could be mobilized from E.coli by pLE2451 if the final recipients were strains of N.gonorrhoeae or Haemophilus influenzae. This suggests that a substantial restriction barrier operates against passage of plasmids from E.coli to these organisms. Furthermore intergeneric mobilization experiments indicated that transfer of β-lactamase plasmids mediated by pLE2451 occurs much more readily out of the gonococcus to Haemophilus than in the reverse direction. In addition, the conjugative plasmids pUB701, pFR16017 and pRI234, isolated originally in H.influenzae, were incapable of mobilizing either gonococcal or Haemophilus β-lactamase plasmids, even in intraspecies crosses. Thus conjugative transfer from Haemophilus to Neisseria species as an origin of gonococcal β-lactamase plasmids would seem to be an infrequent event in vivo.

1. M. Roberts, L.P. Elwell and S. Falkow. J. Bacteriol. 131, 557-563, (1977).
2. M. Roberts, P. Piot and S. Falkow. J. Gen. Microbiol. 114, 491-494, (1979).
3. T.E. Sox, W. Mohammed, E. Blackman, G. Biswas and P.F. Sparling. J. Bacteriol 134, 278-286, (1978).

INTRASTRAND BASE PAIRING IN SINGLE-STRANDED DNA FROM pCR1 AND ITS POSSIBLE RELATIONSHIP TO ROLLING CIRCLE TRANSFER REPLICATION

Thomas D. Edlind and Garret M. Ihler, Texas A&M Collge of Medicine, College Station, TX

Numerous studies have indicated the existence of important short range intrastrand base pairing in DNA and RNA. The presence of such pairing can be inferred by inspection of the base sequence or by computer analysis. Long range interactions have not been as extensively studied and interacting regions at present cannot be readily predicted even by computer analysis. Our approach to this problem has been by electron microscopy to locate the interacting regions relative to an origin such as a transposon insertion site or unique ends created by a restriction enzyme. Standard formamide-cytochrome $\underline{c}$ spreading conditions modified by the addition of ammonium acetate are used to visualize reproducible stem and loop structures resulting from long range base pairing. The nucleotides responsible are then identified from the base sequence of the DNA.

Rolling circle DNA replication begins when a single strand nick is introduced at the origin of DNA synthesis, creating a 5' and a 3' end. The DNA strand displaced during synthesis may remain single-stranded. Transfer DNA replication probably proceeds by a rolling circle mechanism (Rupp, W.D. and Ihler, G. (1968) Cold Spring Harbor Symp. Quant. Biol 33, 647-650). Previous results with φX174 DNA (Edlind, T. and Ihler, G., (1980) J. Mol. Biol., 142, 131-144) demonstrated that base paired sequences bring the 5' and 3' ends of linear φX174 DNA, cleaved at the origin of viral strand replication, close together, which may facilitate their rejoining by φX174 gene $\underline{A}$ protein following DNA replication by the rolling circle mechanism. We have examined a small (13.7 kb) transferable plasmid, pCR1 carrying the transposon Tn903 for similar pairing. Unique ends were introduced with EcoRI. A 1.5 kb stem and loop often containing an internal hairpin was observed near the left end of the molecule and nucleotides likely to be responsible for this pairing have been located in the base sequence. Both the origins of vegetative and transfer DNA replication are located in this loop. Formation of the stem by long range base pairing would draw the 5' and 3' ends, created by cleavage at the origin of replication, closer together. Several molecules were observed in which the loop appeared completed paired, suggesting the existence of further, weaker base pairing which could hold the 5' and 3' ends much closer together and facilitate recircularization of the single-stranded DNA after transfer.

We have also found in pCR1 that Tn903 was inserted into a region already containing inverted repeat sequences and suggest that transposition may be facilitated by the presence of inverted repeats or potential long range base pairing.

This research was supported in part by NIH research grants GM24432 and GM27727.

CELL-TO-CELL TRANSFER OF R-PLASMIDS FROM <u>STREPTOCOCCUS</u> <u>FAECALIS</u> TO <u>STAPHYLOCOCCUS</u> <u>AUREUS</u>

D. R. Schaberg, D. B. Clewell, and L. Glatzer
The University of Michigan, Ann Arbor
University of Toledo, Toledo, Ohio

Erythromycin and clindamycin have proved useful as alternative therapies for S. aureus infections, especially in the penicillin-allergic patient as well as in some infections due to methicillin-resistant strains. Between 1978 and 1980, clinical isolates obtained at the University of Michigan Medical Center have exhibited an increase in resistance to these compounds with 5% of S. aureus strains showing resistance in 1978, while 40% of isolates are resistant in 1980. Resistance to these agents is frequently plasmid-mediated and thought to develop in S. aureus via transduction. However, a recent report by vanEmbden and coworkers [J. Bacteriol. 142:407 (1980)] suggested to us that transfer of macrolide-lincosamide-streptogramin (MLS) resistance plasmids from streptococci to S. aureus could contribute to the evolution of resistance in S. aureus. Mating experiments on filter membranes (overnight) using S. aureus 879 R-4 as a recipient and S. faecalis strain JH2-2 containing various known MLS R-plasmids as donors, we detected transfer as shown below:

Plasmid	Original Source of Plasmid	Transfer Frequency per Recipient
pAMβ1	S. faecalis	1×10^{-5}
pAM15346	S. pyogenes	5×10^{-5}
pAC1	S. pyogenes	7×10^{-6}
pIP501	S. agalactiae	1×10^{-6}

We also demonstrated transfer of pAMβ1 to three different clinical isolates of S. aureus at frequencies from 1×10^{-7} to 5×10^{-8}. When 25 clinical isolates of S. faecalis were examined, three could be shown to transfer MLS resistance to 879 R-4 at frequencies similar to pAMβ1. Matings were performed with S. faecalis carrying pAM∝1 (a small non-conjugative tetracycline-resistance plasmid) in addition to pAMβ1 and mobilization of tetracycline resistance could be demonstrated at frequencies of 1×10^{-8}. These studies suggest that intergeneric R-plasmid transfer is a potential factor in the evolution of resistant strains of S. aureus.

PLASMID-CODED LOW-MOLECULAR WEIGHT RNA SPECIES

Francis J. Schmidt and Virginia E. Peterson

Department of Biochemistry
University of Missouri-Columbia
Columbia, Missouri 65211

I. The evolution of antibiotic resistance transposons has selected
two separate functions: antibiotic resistance and the ability to
transpose between replicons. In some cases, it is possible to argue
that antibiotic resistance can be "picked up" by a mobile DNA element
to the mutual benefit of both. Such a model would explain, for
example, the ability of the Tn5 inverted repeats (IS50 sequences) to
transpose without the companionship of the neomycin phosphotransferase genes (see Berg, et al., this volume). On the other hand, the
transposition and resistance functions may be functionally linked
either de novo or by subsequent evolution of the Tn element
(Reznikoff, et al., this volume). We (F. Schmidt, R. Jorgensen, M.
De Wilde, and J. Davies) have recently identified a low molecular
weight RNA species which is encoded by the inverted repeat of Tn10.
By itself, this is not surprising; but this RNA (which when isolated
contains two molecular species) is induced by tetracycline. Figure
1 shows the results of Southern hybridization of this RNA mixture to
Tn10. Note particularly that the RNA hybridized to the outside 400
bp of Tn10 DNA. One can speculate that this RNA is in some way
involved in transposition. Although we have not demonstrated such
a connection, it is interesting that transposition of erythromycin
resistance in S. aureus is induced by subinhibitory concentrations
of drug (1).

II. We have also investigated in preliminary fashion, the tRNA-
like RNA coded by the tra region of R100 (NR1 or R222). We showed
earlier (2) that this RNA had a 3' C-C-A sequence and other characteristics (although not modified bases) of a tRNA. Furthermore,
this RNA cross-hybridized to the cloned f6 fragment of the F plasmid
which is contained in pRS5 (2). More recently, we have prepared and
characterized an RNA similar to that from R100 which is coded by
cloned F plasmid. The fingerprint analysis of this RNA shows that
it is not identical to that of R100, but it is similar in size and,
presumably, in sequence since R100 RNA hybridizes to the DNA from
which it is derived. Supported in part by funds from the University
of Missouri Medical School Research Council and NIH grant GM26756.

1. P.K. Tomich, F.Y. An, D.B. Clewell. J. Bacteriol. 124:1366-1374
     (1980).
2. M. De Wilde, J.E. Davies, F.J. Schmidt. Proc. Natl. Acad.
     Sci. USA 75:3673-3677 (1978).

CHARACTERIZATION OF MUTANTS OF A PLASMID ColE1 DERIVATIVE WHICH AFFECT PLASMID COPY NUMBER

L. Schmidt and J. Inselburg, Department of Microbiology
Dartmouth Medical School, Hanover, NH

pDMS6642 (Fig. 1), which exhibits an increased copy number, was mutagenized, and plasmids conferring increased resistance to ampicillin were selected. One mutant plasmid, pLS103, showed an increase in β-lactamase proportional to the plasmid copy number (Table 1b). Two plasmids, pLS54 and pLS57, exhibited an enhanced β-lactamase production that was 3 to 8 times greater than that expected for the increased copy number found (see Table 1b). Ligation of the promoter of the β-lactamase gene of pDMS6642 or the mutants to the promoterless tetracycline resistance gene carried by plasmid pGA46 (2) indicated that pLS54 and pLS57 promoters exhibit a 3-fold greater transcriptional activity as measured by conferred drug resistance (Table 1d) than does the promoter carried by pDMS6642. In an in vitro linked translation system pLS54 and pLS57 DNA was found to be about 2.5 - 3-fold more effective as templates for the synthesis of β-lactamase than pDMS6642. The insertion of either plasmid pGA46 or a nucleotide sequence containing a chloramphenicol resistance gene derived from the transposon Tn9 (Table 1c,d) into the Pst site of pDMS 6642, pLS54 and pLS57 reduced the plasmid copy number to between 20-30 per chromosome while failing to reduce the copy number of pLS103 significantly (Table 1c and e). The results suggest that the copy number of pDMS6642, pLS54 and pLS57 are all higher than ColE1 (which is about 15 - 20/chromosome) because of a trans-criptional-read-through from the β-lactamase promoter into the RNA-primer transcript (see Fig. 1) that normally governs replication initiation of ColE1. While the potential for copy number control exists in pDMS6642, a strong promoter upstream from the normal RNA primer of replication can apparently override the expression of that control as can mutants affecting the structure of RNA of ColE1 (1). Copy number therefore appears to be controllable at the transcriptional level in ColE1.

Table 1. Properties of plasmids.

	a) Copy #	b) β-lac/10^8 plasmids	c) Copy #	d) Tc^R μg/ml	e) X-Cm^R copy#
pDMS6642	57	0.05	22	5	23
pLS54	109	0.43	36	15	32
pLS57	84	0.15	24	15	21
pLS103	140	0.08	-	-	127

Fig. 1. pDMS6642 and its mutants. Origin of ColE1 replication. region of β-lactamase of Tn3. P. location of the β-lacta-mase promoter and its direction of transcription. Pst = site sensitive to endonuclease Pst1 into which pGA46 and a fragment of Tn9 was cloned.

INCOMPATIBILITY AMONG GROUP Y PLASMIDS

by June R. Scott and Jack A. Cowan
Department of Microbiology,
Emory University School of Medicine
Atlanta, Georgia 30322, USA

Incompatibility expressed by the group Y plasmid prophages P1 and P7 was investigated by analysis of the behavior on non-selective medium of heteroplasmid cells immediately after introduction of the second plasmid by infection. Since a marker effect biased the segregation results when both plasmids were selected on solid medium, we followed plasmid segregation on nonselective medium. P1 and P7 derivatives fall into two sub-classes based on the rapidity of expression of incompatibility: homologous plasmids (P1-P1 or P7-P7) express incompatibility more rapidly than heterologous (P1-P7) plasmids. The determinant of this difference is genetically separable from the immunity determinant of the prophage.

After homologous superinfection, no colonies with both plasmids are recovered. We call this rapid expression of incompatibility. It apparently results because neither plasmid can replicate in cells containing two plasmids, possibly because of a plasmid specific inhibitor that controls copy number. At cell division, the two unreplicated plasmids segregate into different daughters. This interpretation is supported by kinetic data.

Following heterologous superinfection there is no increase in the number of cells with the marker of the incoming plasmid; the number of heteroplasmid cells remains constant. We call this slow expression of incompatibility and suggest that the resident plasmid has a very much greater probability of replication than the newly introduced one. The replicated plasmid is then partitioned between the daughter cells while the one that does not replicate is inherited essentially unilinearly. This suggest a physical relation between plasmid replication and partition, possibly by way of a membrane site.

CLONING OF FOREIGN GENES IN B.subtilis, NATURE OF BLOCKS TO THE EXPRESSION OF E.coli hisG GENE

V.Sgaramella, G.De Fazio, L.Ferretti, G.Grandi, M.Mottes and E.Palla
Istituto di Genetica Biochimica ed
Evoluzionistica del CNR, Pavia, Italy

Several genes derived from E.coli have been cloned into B.subtilis, but for only two of them (thymidylate synthetase[1] and tetracyline resistance[2]) phenotypic expression of the traits has been demonstrated.

We have studied the ability of the E.coli hisG gene to complement a corresponding mutation in B.subtilis. The relevant gene, together with its E.coli vector pBR313, was inserted into a S.aureus/B.subtilis plasmid pCS194, a natural recombinant between two smaller S.aureus plasmids, pC194 and pS194. The resulting inter specific plasmid, pPV28, was found to be stable in E.coli, but highly unstable in B.subtilis, where the most frequent rearrangements involved the loss of the entire E.coli DNA sequence, plus the surrounding pS194 moiety, following a nearly precise excision process[3].

It has been possible to clone the E.coli hisG gene in B.subtilis via the interspecific E.coli-B.subtilis vector pHV14. The resulting plasmid, pPV48, could be faithfully replicated in B.subtilis but failed to complement the corresponding B.subtilis mutation in spite of the presence of a functional hisG gene.

Southern hybridization of mRNA produced in vivo by B.subtilis CU403 minicells, harboring pPV48, with restriction segments of this plasmid, as well as E.M. comparison of R-loops obtained through in vitro transcription of pPV48 with E.coli and B.subtilis RNA poly merases, suggest that B.subtilis RNA polymerase transcribes the E.coli hisG gene. Lack of his[+] phenotype could be due either to a wrong initiation of transcrip tion or to a post-transcriptional event occurring on a functional mRNA.

References
1. E.M.Rubin, G.A.Wilson and F.E.Young.Gene,10:227,1980
2. J.Kreft,K.J.Burger and W.Goebel. M.G.G., in press
3. G.Grandi,M.Mottes and V.Sgaramella. Plasmid,in press

THE DETECTION OF TRANSPOSABLE RESISTANCE ELEMENT

Tn5 IN A PORCINE DIARRHEAL ISOLATE

E. Scott Stibits

Department of Biochemistry
University of Wisconsin
Madison, Wisconsin 53706

A transposable kanamycin resistance element was isolated from an enterotoxigenic (ST) E. coli strain isolated as the cause of diarrhea in pigs (strain 1710). The transposon was detected as insertions in phage λ b515 b519 (λkan's) that were detected as kan^R transducing phage in an induced lysated from a kan^R exconjugant of 1710 and a lysogenic E. coli recipient. These insertions were shown to be indistinguishable from Tn5 by:
1) HindIII digestion patterns of λkan DNA's.
2) Hybridization patterns of PstI and HincII cleaved λkan and λ::Tn5 DNA's probed with ^{32}P-ColEl::Tn5.
3) HaeIII digestion patterns of pVH51 transposition derivatives.
4) In vivo resistance pattern and in vitro substrate range of aminoglycoside-phosphotransferase activity.

Plasmid DNA prepared from a kan^R exconjugant of 1710 (R1710 DNA) was compared to R-plasmid JR67 DNA. JR67 was the original source of Tn5 and was found in Klebsiella strains causing urinary tract infections in humans. From restriction analysis and Southern hybridizations using as probes JR67, ColEl::Tn5, and restriction fragments of Tn5's inverted repeats or resistance gene, it was shown that:
1) The EcoRl digestion patterns of the two plasmid preparations have no similarity.
2) R1710 DNA has more homology to JR67 than is attributable to Tn5. This may be explained in part by the fact that both plasmids code for resistance to streptomycin and to sulfisoxazole.
3) R1710 DNA contains an extra copy of sequences homologous to the inverted repeats of Tn5 (IS50), but not homologous to the resistance gene.
It was also shown by incompatibility testing that R1710 is not of the same incompatibility group as JR67 (Iα).

WIDESPREAD OCCURRENCE OF AN Ap^{r}ST$^+$ E. COLI PLASMID OF HUMAN ORIGIN

Heather Stieglitz,[*] Jorge Olarte,[†] and Yankel M. Kupersztoch-Portnoy[*]

Departamento de Genetica y Biologia Molecular, Centro de Investigacion y de Estudios Avanzados del I.P.N., Mexico 14,[*] and Laboratorio de Enterobacterias, Hospital Infantil de Mexico, Mexico 7,[†] D.F. Mexico

From 144 children admitted to the Hospital Infantil de Mexico with acute watery diarrhea during 1976-1977, five isolates of E. coli were tested for heat-stable(ST) and heat-labile(LT) toxin and for resistance to 14 antibiotics. Antibiotic resistance was determined by the agar dilution method.[12] ST$^+$ production was determined by the suckling mice assay [16] and LT toxin was determined by the adrenal cell assay.[14] Positive strains for either toxin were subsequently assayed in the rabbit ilium loop model.[15] The 31 LT$^+$ producing isolates came from 18 patients; 93.5% were resistant to between four and nine antibiotics. The 19 ST$^+$ producing strains came from 13 patients; 89.5% were resistant to as many as five antibiotics and 5% were resistant to seven antibiotics.

The linkage of antibiotic resistance and ST$^+$ enterotoxin activity was studied in six high level ST$^+$ isolates from five patients by conjugation to E. coli K-12 J54(Nal^r). The resistance markers used were ampicillin(Ap) and tetracycline(Tc)(three cases) and Ap, Tc, and streptomycin(Sm)(three cases). Transconjugants were selected for one antibiotic and then tested for resistance to the unselected antibiotics and for ST$^+$ production. In all cases Ap^r and ST$^+$ were tightly linked. In some instances we also found linkage of ST$^+$ with Tc^r and Sm^r.

Plasmid DNA was isolated from various ST$^+$ transconjugants representing the different patterns of antibiotic resistance; the partially purified DNA was analyzed on agarose gels. The only transconjugants that showed a single plasmid band(approximately 80 md)[17] were Ap^{r}ST$^+$. All others exhibited at least two extrachromosomal bands, one of which was 80 md. Four Ap^{r}ST$^+$ transconjugants, each derived from a separate clinical strain(different patients) and shown to have only one plasmid band, were further studied by EcoR1 restriction endonuclease analysis. Purified restricted plasmid DNAs from each were coelectrophoresed in a 1% agarose slab gel. The restriction pattern was identical in all cases: 11 fragments giving a total molecular weight of 81.5 md.[17] The four patients from whom these transconjugants were derived live in different section of Mexico City and had been hospitalized at different times of the year.

References

12,16,14,15,17: listed in Kupersztoch-Portnoy Y. M. this volume.

TRANSFER OF CHROMOSOMALLY INTEGRATED PLASMIDS IN

Haemophilus influenzae

Johan H. Stuy and Ronald B. Walter

Department of Biological Science
Florida State University
Tallahassee, Florida 32306

Chromosomally integrated conjugative R plasmids transfer with an efficiency of 0.001 to 0.01 in standard isogenic genetic transformation crosses of Haemophilus influenzae Rd (relative to a high-efficiency point mutation). There is no transfer at all to rec⁻ or $CaCl_2$-treated recipients while free plasmids in such donor DNA lysates transfer infrequently (0.000001) to all these recipients. We have constructed strains with long nonhomologous plasmid-derived DNA inserts (from 6 to 14 megadaltons) at a given site in the chromosome. These inserts are transferred with efficiencies which vary inversely with size (0.3 to 0.03). Transforming out these inserts is independent of size; the efficiency is close to one. Replacing one insert by another is about as efficient as adding alone. A closely linked point mutation in the recipient reduces all transfer phenomena by 3 to 100 times while the same mutation in the donor DNA gave a much smaller effect. Thus the transfer of integrated plasmids from hospital isolates to strain Rd is infrequent because of large plasmid size and because of imperfect homology in the plasmid-flanking DNA regions. Spreading of integrated plasmids between heterologous populations should thus be limited.

pLEB1 DNA added to 2 different insert strains was integrated within the insert (Campbell model?). This was accompanied by loss of plasmid-controled ampicillin resistance. The integrated plasmids could be transferred by transformation. In one strain the plasmid was not excised spontaneously. In the other strain excision appeared to be recA-independent.

TRANSFER OF N PLASMIDS TO PSEUDOMONAS AERUGINOSA

Ginette Tardif and Robert B. Grant

Research Institute and Department of Bacteriology
The Hospital for Sick Children
555 University Ave., Toronto, Canada   M5G 1X8

Our previous research, and the work of other investigators, has determined that the N plasmids transferred at very low frequencies to Pseudomonas aeruginosa, and that the retransfer of these plasmids from P. aeruginosa to either E. coli or P. aeruginosa was not detected. We have obtained P. aeruginosa mutants which show an increase in their recipient ability for N plasmids (Ren mutants). The N plasmids do not transfer at the same frequency to the Ren mutants; for example, the transfer of N3 is hardly affected by the mutations but there is a significant increase (10,000fold in some cases) in the transfer frequency of R46. Plasmid pCF290 is able to transfer from two Ren mutants to E. coli, but the retransfer of the other N plasmids is not detected. Differences among the N plasmids are also noted in their stability patterns: pCF290 is stable in each mutant but N3, R45 and R46 are lost at various frequencies depending on the host strain.

The mutations seem to be specific for N plasmid transfer since the transfer frequencies of several plasmids from other incompatibility groups (FII, Iα, C, W, P) are not affected. The antibiotic resistances mediated by the N plasmids are generally expressed by the Ren mutants, but the sensitivities to phages IKe and PRD1 could not be detected. In contrast, sensitivity to PRD1 was observed when the Ren mutants harboured RP1. The Ren mutations might possibly involve a membrane component as evidenced by a pyocin sensitivity test. One mutant is resistant to a particular pyocin, while two of the other mutants are more sensitive than the parental strain. Whether or not there is a direct correlation between N plasmid transfer and sensitivity to this pyocin remains to be determined.

COINTEGRATE FORMATION BETWEEN PLASMIDS CARRYING VIRULENCE FACTOR AND ANTIBIOTIC RESISTANCE GENES IN E. COLI

P.L. Shipley, A.D. Allen, and T.N. Swanson
Virginia Commonwealth University
Richmond, Virginia

Enterotoxigenic _Escherichia_ _coli_ (ETEC) strains which cause diarrhea in young pigs often possess the proteinaceous fimbrial surface antigen, K88, which enables the bacterium to adhere to the mucosal epithelium of the anterior small intestine of the pig. The genetic determinants for production of K88 fimbriae and utilization of the trisaccharide raffinose (Raf) are located on a 52 megadalton nonconjugative plasmid. The K88/Raf plasmid can be mobilized by a variety of conjugative plasmids in the ETEC strains Selection for Raf transfer frequently results in the isolation of cointegrate plasmids containing both the K88/Raf and mobilizing plasmid genomes. We have examined some parameters of cointegrate formation between a K88/Raf plasmid, pPS900, and pPS030, a conjugative R factor carrying the determinants for resistance to tetracycline and streptomycin. The K88/Raf plasmid was mobilized with equal efficiency from RecA$^+$ or RecA$^-$ donors. The percentage of transconjugants containing cointegrate plasmids varied markedly in repeated matings using the same donor and recipient strains. This variability is probably due, at least in part, to the instability of the cointegrates. Storage of strains containing cointegrates usually results in disassociation, but stable cointegrates can be isolated at a low frequency. Nine stable cointegrates have been analyzed by comparison of restriction endonuclease fragment patterns and filter blot hybridization against the cloned K88 determinant. These studies showed that cointegration involves a specific region in each plasmid. Each stable cointegrate had suffered a deletion of sequences from the K88/Raf plasmid. The deletions appear to have a single point of origin and most terminate at one of two sites resulting in loss of all or part of an 8.2 megadalton HindIII fragment containing the K88 determinant. We are currently examining the nature of the sequences involved in cointegration.

STABILITY OF PLASMID R1-19 IN HYPER-RECOMBINANT

Escherichia coli K-12 STRAINS

Haydée K. Torres, and
M. Carmen Gómez-Eichelmann

Departamento de Biología Molecular
Instituto de Investigaciones Biomédicas
Universidad Nacional Autónoma de México
México 20, D. F., MEXICO

The plasmid R1-19 is a composite molecule cointegrated by two components: the RTF and the r-det. The r-det, which carries the drug resistance genes, is flanked by two insertion sequences IS1. In E. coli, R1-19 is a relatively stable composite molecule. In S. typhimurium, the RTF and the r-det, dissociate at a high frequency generating multi-sensitive cells which retain the RTF component. The dissociation involves a recombination (recA-dependent) between the two IS1.

In the present work, the stability of R1-19 in $recA^+$, hyper-rec (polA1 and dam-3), and recA⁻ E. coli strains was analized by subcultivating the cells without selective pressure and by checking for antibiotic resistance markers. In the $recA^+$ strains the plasmid was quite stable, segregating multi-sensitive cells at low frequencies. The plasmid, however, showed great instability in the hyper-rec strains and was completely stable in the recA strain. In addition to the high percent of multi-sensitive cells, a low percentage of segregants Km^s, Km^s Ap^s, and Cm^s Sm^s $-Sp^s$, was found in the hyper-rec strains. Approximately 90 to 95% of the multi-sensitive cells retained the RTF component.

The instability found for R1-19 in E. coli hyper-rec strains is similar to that described for S. typhimurium. Therefore, the different behavior observed for R1-19 in E. coli and S. typhimurium $recA^+$ strains, is probably due to a lower recombination level in E. coli as compared to that of S. typhimurium.

STUDY OF pPK237, A BROAD-HOST RANGE MULTIRESTITANT PLASMID ORIGINATING FROM PSEUDOMONAS AERUGINOSA RESISTANT TO GENATAMICIN

Tzelepi E., Angelatou F., Vomvoyani B. and
Kontomichalou R.

Athens University School of Medicine
Department of Clinical Therapeutics
Alexandra Hospital, Athens, Greece

Plasmid PK237, originating from a Gm-Cb resistant Pseudomonas aeruginosa isolate, is a wide-host range, multiresistant and very stable plasmid, which carries genes for resistance to mercury and eleven antibiotics.

Three variants of it were obtained: PK237-2a, PK237-10 and PK237-16. Molecular weight determinations revealed that the original pPK237 is one molecule of 67 Md and that the variants are deletion mutants of it.

From crude preparation of E.coli K12+pPK237 two Gm-modifying enzymes were detected, which were characterized after purification as AAC(3)I and AAD(2"). On the other hand radioassay results from crude preparations of cultures carrying the variants distinguished them in: a) high or low level activity and b) with both or only one of the two enzymes detected. This variation explained the differences in levels of Gm resistance mediated by these plasmids.

Beta-lactamase detection and characterization showed that a TEM-I b-lactamase is mediated by pPK237 and pPK237-2a, while the variants pPK237-10 and pPK237-16 mediate a PSE-2 b-lactamase.

From the above findings and previous results a tentative mapping is proposed, which suggests the possible evolutionary relationships between the original plasmid and its variants.

HIGH EXPRESSION OF GENES IN E. COLI BY CLONING ON AMPLIFIABLE PLASMID VECTORS

Bernt Eric Uhlin and Alvin J. Clark

Department of Molecular Biology
University of California
Berkeley, California 94720

To increase expression of cloned genes in E. coli we used small derivatives of a "runaway"-replication mutant of plasmid R1[1]. The plasmids show temperature-dependent loss of control of copy number resulting in amplification of plasmid DNA in the cells. Therefore, gene products coded for by the plasmid may be overproduced due to the increased number of plasmid copies to levels as high as 1000-1500 per cell. New plasmid vectors constructed in vitro are shown in Table 1. A derivative of plasmid pBEU1 carrying the E. coli recA gene enabled us to overproduce the recA protein without stimulating its proteolytic activity and to obtain and purify proteins from recA mutants that cannot be derepressed by nalidixic acid or UV light treatment.

Table 1. Plasmid Cloning Vectors.

Plasmid	Kilobases	Single Restriction Sites	Antibiotic Resistance[c]
pBEU1[a]	17.4	BamHI, HindIII, HpaI, SstI	Ap
pBEU27	10.8	BamHI	Sp
pBEU28	9.2	EcoRI	Km
pBEU43	7.7	EcoRI, HpaI	Ap
pBEU50[b]	9.9	BamHI, EcoRI, HindIII, HpaI	Ap, Tc

[a] pBEU1 carries the entire transposon Tn3.
[b] Sites for BamHI and HindIII in region coding for Tc resistance.
[c] Ap, Sp, Km, and Tc denote resistance to ampicillin, spectinomycin, kanamycin, and tetracycline, respectively.

Acknowledgements.
Our work was supported in part by NIH research grant No.AI05371 from the National Institutes of Allergy and Infectious Diseases and in part by American Cancer Society, Inc. research grant No.NP-237. B.E.U. was supported by a Long Term Postdoctoral Fellowship from the European Molecular Biology Organization (EMBO).

Reference.
1. B.E. Uhlin, S. Molin, P. Gustafsson, and K. Nordström, Gene 6:91 (1979).

PLASMID (pKM101)-MEDIATED MUTAGENESIS AND REPAIR

Graham C. Walker, Pamela J. Langer, William G.
Shanabruch, Stephen J. Elledge, and Stephen C. Winans
Biology Department, Massachusetts Institute of
Technology, Cambridge, MA 02139

The 35.4 kb N-incompatibility plasmid pKM101 makes cells more
resistant to killing by agents such as UV and more sensitive to
mutagenesis by these agents. These effects are $recA^+lexA^+$-
dependent (1). E. coli umuC mutants seem to be specifically
deficient in "error-prone repair" and these deficiencies are
suppressed by pKM101 (2). These results are consistent with pKM101
coding for a unique component of "error-prone repair" and probably
explain why pKM101 plays such a key role in the Ames test (3). By
a combination of insertion mutagenesis, deletion mapping and
cloning we have identified a region of at least 1900 bp but less
than 2400 bp which is required for these effects (4). Interestingly the region of pKM101 responsible for mutagenesis/repair is
surrounded by inverted repeats.

In addition we have used insertion and deletion mutants to
localize several genetic regions on the plasmid genome. In
clockwise order on the pKM101 map are: i) the bla gene - coding for
a β-lactamase, ii) the "Slo" region - responsible for retarding
cell growth on minimal medium, iii) the tra genes - enabling
pKM101 to transfer conjugally, iv) sensitivity to IKe phage v) a
single and double strand endonuclease vi) fip - fertility inhibition of P group plasmids (functions iv, v, and vi map within the
tra region), vii) the muc gene(s) - responsible for enhancing UV
and chemically-induced mutagenesis in the cell, and viii) the "Rep"
region - essential for plasmid replication. In addition we have
shown that pKM101 arose from its parental plasmid, R46, by the
deletion of a 14 kb region of DNA.

REFERENCES

1. Walker, G.C., 1977, Molec. Gen. Genet., 152:93.
2. Walker, G.C., and Dobson, P.P., 1979, Molec. Gen. Genet. 172:17.
3. McCann, J., Spingarn, N.E., Kobori, J., and Ames, B.N., 1975,
   Proc. Natl. Acad. Sci., U.S.A., 72:979.
4. Shanabruch, W.G., and Walker, G.C., 1980, Molec. Gen. Genet.
   179:289.

THE CONSTRUCTION OF NOVEL CLONING VEHICLES FOR USE WITHIN STAPHYLOCOCCUS AUREUS AND BACILLUS SUBTILIS

C. Ron Wilson*, Sarah E. Skinner and William V. Shaw
Department of Biochemistry, University of Leicester
Leicester, England LE1 7RH

Cm resistance plasmids pCW7 and pC221 of *Staphylococcus aureus* have been characterized by the construction of detailed restriction maps and by the identification of restriction sites on both plasmids which map within either the structural gene encoding CAT or its controlling elements. The number and order of recognition sites for endonucleases *AluI*, *HinfI*, *MboI* and *TaqI* on pCW7 and pC221 were determined. Circularization of the largest *MboI* fragment (1.8 kb) from pC221 formed a stable replicon (pCW41) which encoded an inducible CAT. To identify sites mapping within the Cm resistance determinant Cm Tc recombinant plasmids were constructed *in vitro* from pCW41 or pCW7 and Tc resistance plasmid pCW3 (Table 1). Then site-specific mutations were introduced by filling in the complementary ends of selected restriction sites present on DNA from pCW7 or pCW41 with *E. coli* polymerase I followed by recircularization of the recombinant plasmid by blunt-end ligation. Pol I treatment of the *BstEII* site on pCW41 DNA and the *BstEII* or *BglII* site present on pCW7 DNA resulted in the loss of both the recognition site and Cm resistance.

Cm Tc recombinant plasmids pCW48 and pCW59 should prove to be useful as molecular cloning vehicles in *S. aureus* and *Bacillus subtilis*. The *BstEII* site on pCW48 and the *BglII* and *BstEII* sites on pCW59 can be used for the insertional inactivation of Cm resistance. The versatility of plasmid pCW59 for cloning is increased by the ability of the *BglII* site (A↓GATCT) to accept restriction fragments produced by digestion with endonucleases *MboI* (↓GATC), *BamHI* (G↓GATCC), *BclI* (T↓GATCA) and *XhoII* (Pu↓GATCPy).

Table 1 – Description of Plasmids

Plasmid Number	Size	Pheno-type[a]	Description
pC221	4.4 kb	Cm	Natural isolate.
pCW3	4.5 kb	Tc	" "
pCW7	4.2 kb	Cm	" "
pCW41	1.8 kb	Cm	*MboI* fragment A from pC221.
pCW48	6.1 kb	CmTc	*HpaII* restricted pCW41 inserted into *HpaII* site of pCW3.
pCW59	5.3 kb	CmTc	*HindIII* fragment A from pCW3 inserted into the *HindIII* site of pCW7. Spontaneous deletion of 1.2 kb of pCW7 DNA.

[a]Phenotype = phenotype of strain carrying the plasmid.

*Present address: Bioproducts Research Laboratory, The Dow Chemical Company, Midland, Michigan 48640.

EXPRESSION OF EUKARYOTIC GLYCOPROTEINS IN BACTERIA

Michael D.Winther & George A.M.Cross

Dept. of Immunochemistry, The Wellcome
Research Laboratories, Langley Court,
Beckenham, Kent BR3 3BS

Sequential expression of variant surface glycoproteins (VSGs) enables the parasitic protozoan Trypanosoma brucei to evade the immune response of its mammalian hosts (Cross 1978). Studies of several isolated VSGs have indicated extensive amino acid diversity and the absence of a hydrophobic segment which might serve to anchor the carboxy-terminus to the membrane. Nucleotide sequence data suggests that the primary translation product of one VSG gene contains a hydrophobic tail at the carboxy-terminus which is not found on the isolated mature glycoprotein (J.C. Boothroyd et al (1980) Nature, 288:624). We are using clones of the VSG gene as a model system for studying the expression of eukaryotic glycoproteins in bacteria.

Complementary DNA (cDNA) molecules corresponding to the VSGs of several variants have been synthesised and cloned in to the Pst I site of pBR322 using G·C tailing (Hoeijmakers et al 1980). Immunological screening of eight cDNA clones for VSG 117 indicates that four clones produce VSG polypeptides at a low level ($\sim 1 - 5 \times 10^2$ molecules/cell). The bacterial synthesis of VSG polypeptide is probably directed from the β-lactamase promoter though not as a fusion product with the β-lactamase protein. The four expressing clones contain only part of the structural gene for the VSG so synthesis of this polypeptide in E.coli may be initiated at an internal methionine.

Boothroyd, J.C., Cross, G.A.M., Hoeijmakers, J.H.J. and Borst, P., 1980, A variant surface glycoprotein of Trypanosoma brucei synthesized with a C-terminal hydrophobic 'tail' absent from purified glycoprotein, Nature, 288:624.

Cross, G.A.M., 1978, Antigenic variation in trypanosomes, Proc. Royal.Soc.London Ser.B, 202:55.

Hoeijmakers, J.H.J., Borst, P., Van den Burg, J., Weissmann, C. and Cross, G.A.M., 1980, The isolation of plasmids containing DNA complementary to messenger RNA for variant surface glycoproteins of Trypanosoma brucei, Gene, 8:391.

PHEROMONE-INDUCED AGGREGATION SUBSTANCE IN STREPTOCOCCUS FAECALUS

Y. Yagi, R. Kessler, B. Brown D. Lopatin and D. Clewell
The University of Michigan
Ann Arbor, Michigan

When exposed to specific sex pheromones excreted by recipient cells, certain plasmid-containing donor strains of S. faecalis modify their surfaces to become adherent, enabling them to aggregate with recipients (see Clewell, this volume). Pheromone-induced donors will also self-aggregate in the absence of recipient cells; this response is inhibited by chloramphenicol or rifampin. Aggregated cells are readily dissociated upon exposure to EDTA; the aggregation of induced cells has been found to require divalent cations as well as phosphate. Exposure of EDTA-dissociated cells to trypsin, SDS (0.05%), or heat prevents reaggregation when the cells are subsequently placed in an optimum environment for aggregation.

An antiserum was prepared against a gluteraldehyde-fixed preparation of an induced strain (39-5) carrying the conjugative plasmid pPD1. Absorption with uninduced cells resulted in an antiserum which, using a fluorescent antibody technique, was reactive only with induced cells. The inducible antigen has been designated aggregation substance (AS) and can be extracted (with 1% Triton X-100) and monitored by immunoelectrophoresis techniques. The absorbed antiserum was also used in combination with electron microscopic analyses using a horse-radish peroxidase immunological stain. The latter revealed an amorphous material present on the surface of induced, but not uninduced, cells.

In addition to pPD1, pheromone-induced aggregation responses are conferred by pAD1, pOB1, pAMγ1, pAMγ2 and pAMγ3. (At least three different compatibility groups are represented here.) By microscopic fluorescent antibody detection, the antiserum prepared against induced cells carrying pPD1 was found, in all cases, to readily cross-react with induced (but not uninduced) strains separately harboring these plasmids. It is not certain yet whether AS is directly determined by these plasmids or by a chromosome-borne determinant under plasmid-control.

A DNA-DIRECTED CELL-FREE SYNTHESIS SYSTEM CAPABLE OF USING LINEAR DNA FRAGMENTS AS TEMPLATE

H.-L. Yang[1], G. Zubay[2], M. Cashel[3]

The Public Health Research Institute of the City of
New York, Inc., N.Y.C., N.Y. 10016[1] Columbia University,
N.Y.C., N.Y. 10025[2] N.I.H., Bethesda, MD. 20205[3]

A new cell-free system (reconstructed cell-free system) has
been recently developed which overcomes two major defects of the
S-30 system. Since the extract is prepared from a recB mutant,
defective in linear DNA specific nuclease, the introduced DNA is
very stable. Contaminated chromosomal DNA which usually creates
background synthesis has been eliminated by modifying the method
of preparation of cell extract. This cell-free synthesis system
has the following unique features; 1) it can use linear DNA or DNA
fragments as templates, 2) it has a high efficiency of synthesis
both at transcriptional and at translational level, 3) it has good
fidelity of gene expression and, 4) it has very little background
synthesis.

This RC system can be applied to identify the gene product to
study the genetic structure and to analyze the regulatory mechanism.

SURVEY OF A CONFERENCE: TURISTA OR NOT TURISTA?

Stuart B. Levy
Tufts University School of Medicine
Boston, Mass.

One of the topics under discussion at the conference was the relationship between plasmids and diarrhea. Since "turista" often afflicts travellers to foreign countries, a survey of the attack rate of gastrointestinal problems in participants was made. Among the more than 200 participants, about 190 were visitors to the Dominican Republic. 114 responded to the questionnaire.

The first reported illness occurred on the second day of the conference. By the end of the five-day meeting, 47 were affected. The post-conference survey showed that 67/114 had suffered some mild or more severe symptoms of "turista." The Figure below records the daily incidence of newly-affected individuals (mild + severe) over the conference and post-conference period. In both mild and severe cases, the incidence peaked at 4-5 days and then dropped off. 41.2% of the those who responded remained unaffected. 18 conferees had mild symptoms (cramps, loose stools) which lasted 1-3 days. The remaining 49, however, developed moderate to severe symptoms which lasted 2-14 days. In two individuals, a multiply-resistant Shigella sonnei was isolated.

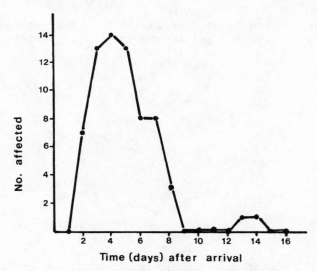

Incidence of gastrointestinal symptoms among conference participants

Of the parameters examined, e.g. food and water consumption, previous travel history, the following conclusions could be made: a)no South or Central American visitor reported any illness; b) the unaffected and mildly-affected groups were highly-represented by persons who had previously travelled to countries in South and Central America or Asia (Table); c) the affected (mild + severe) were more apt to have eaten cold salads at the hotels or other restaurants. There was no correlation between where the salad was eaten and the attack rate.

Group	# of responders	% eating salads	% travelled[+]
Unaffected	34[*]	47.1	85.3
Mild	18	77.8	72.2
Mod–Severe	49	77.5	44.9

[*]excludes 13 responders who did not complete the questionnaire
[+]those with previous travel to Central or South America or Asia

44.4% of the unaffected and 6-12% of the affected had travelled before and ate no salads. Obviously there were lessons learned by some through travel that were not learned by others. In fact, those who had travelled and did not eat salads represented 61% of the unaffected and only 15-17% of the affected groups. Moreover, 63% of the affected group had been sick on prior travels, but only 40% of those in the unaffected group. Only three individuals,who remained unaffected,were taking prophylactic medication: two were taking trimethoprim-sulfonamides; one was taking Keflex.

It appears from this mini-survey that prior travellers who avoided uncooked foods, e.g. cold salads, would be less susceptible to diarrheal disease. Besides food habits, another possibility for the correlation between prior travel and less disease would be if the travellers retained an immunity from previous trips. This possibility my explain why certain salad-eating travellers were less affected than others: a larger proportion of the mild group than the severe group had travelled before.

At the least, the results would suggest that plasmid investigators should travel more and eliminate cold salads from their diets. In what percentage of cases plasmids were involved is still a question.

STATEMENT REGARDING WORLDWIDE ANTIBIOTIC MISUSE

Antibiotics have been developed to treat diseases caused by micro-organisms in humans, animals, and cultivated plants. However, these antimicrobial agents are losing their effectiveness because of the spread and persistence of drug-resistant organisms. Moreover, unless steps are taken to curtail the present situation we may find a time when such agents are no longer useful to combat disease.

We are faced with a worldwide public health problem. It is due in large part to the indiscriminate use of antibiotics, especially in the following practices: a) dispensing antibiotics without prescription; b) using clinically-useful antibiotics as growth promoters in animal feeds and on agricultural crops; c) prescribing antibiotics for ailments for which they are ineffective; d) misleading consumers by advertising antibiotics as "wonder drugs," especially in areas where dispensing is not regulated; e) using different labeling and advertising to sell the same product in different parts of the world.

Let no one suppose that widespread use of antibiotics is in any way a substitute for good sanitation and personal hygiene. Efforts in improving these mainstays of infectious disease prevention and control must be encouraged and strengthened. At the same time, it is imperative to increase awareness of the dangerous consequences of antibiotic misuse at all levels of usage: consumers, prescribers, dispensers, manufacturers, and government regulatory agencies. Only then can we begin to institute measures to curb the unnecessary use and flagrant misuse of these drugs.

We, the undersigned, have drafted this statement to instigate action towards halting this ever-increasing worldwide problem. We would like this communication to serve as the impetus for organizing national and international committees from which directives for prudent antibiotic use can be established. As a first step, we urge that a uniform practice in the prescription and distribution of antibiotics be implemented and enforced in those areas where adequate medical expertise is already available. Furthermore, we urge that proper standards of advertising and dispensing of these drugs be agreed upon and adhered to in all nations of the world.

The above statement evolved from presentations and discussions during the conference on <u>Molecular Biology, Pathogenicity and Ecology of Bacterial Plasmids,</u> held in Santo Domingo, Dominican Republic, January, 1981. All those who signed did so as individuals and not as representatives of their institutions.

Mark Achtman (W. Germany)
Toshihilo Arai (Japan)
Louis S. Baron (USA)
Peter Barth (England)
Peter M. Bennett (England)
Douglas E. Berg (USA)
Matthew Binns (USA)
David Bradley (Canada)
Paul Broda (England)
James Brunton (USA)
Lars Burman (Sweden)
Ted Butler (USA)
Felipe Cabello (USA)
Felicity Carr (USA)
Ananda Chakrabarty (USA)
Bruce Chassey (USA)
Patricia Cherguin (USA)
Ian Chopra (England)
Joanna Clancy (USA)
Don B. Clewell (USA)
Royston Clowes (USA)
John Collins (W. Germany)
Jose Ramiro Cruz (Guatemala)
Joanne Cullinane (USA)
Michael S. Curiale (USA)
Naomi Datta (England)
Julian Davies (Switzerland)
Irving Delappe (USA)
David Dubnau (USA)
Gary Dunny (USA)
Thomas Edlund (Sweden)

Rudolf Eichenlaub (W. Germany)
Lynn Elwell (USA)
Alicia Espinosa-Lara (Mexico)
Stanley Falkow (USA)
W. Edmund Farrar (USA)
Susan Feinman (USA)
David Figurski (USA)
Rudiger Fock (W. Germany)
Timothy J. Foster (Ireland)
F.C.H. Franklin (W. Germany)
Ernst Freese (USA)
Juan Garcia-Lobo (Spain)
Cindy Gawron-Burke (USA)
Walter Gilbert (USA)
Werner Goebel (W. Germany)
Tania Gomes (Brazil)
Carmen Gomez-Eichelman (Mexico)
Joseph Gots (USA)
Robert B. Grant (Canada)
Gary Gray (USA)
Nigel Grindley (USA)
Patricia Guerry-Kopecko (USA)
Walter Guild (USA)
Miguel Guzman (Columbia)
Robert Hallewell (USA)
Norma Harnett (Canada)
Donald Helinski (USA)
Israel Hertman (Israel)
Jane Hogan (USA)
Gregor Hogenauer (Austria)
Thea Horodniceanu (France)

Garret Ihler (USA)
Joseph Inselburg (USA)
Karen Ippen-Ihler (USA)
V. N. Iyer (Canada)
Joseph F. John (USA)
A. W. B. Johnston (England)
Clarence I. Kado (USA)
Sarah Kagan (USA)
Akira Kaji (USA)
Hideko Kaji (USA)
Bruce Kline (USA)
Ellen L. Koenig (Dominican
 Republic)
P. Kontomichalou (Greece)
Dennis Kopecko (USA)
Yankel Kupersztoch (Mexico)
David Laux (USA)
Donald J. LeBlanc (USA)
Esther Lederberg (USA)
Sally Leong (USA)
Morris Levin (USA)
R. Paul Levine (USA)
Jay A. Levy (USA)
Stuart B. Levy (USA)
Paul S. Lovett (USA)
Bonnie Marshall (USA)
Sarah McIntire (USA)
Laura McMurry (USA)
Eugene W. Nester (USA)
H.J.J Nijkamp (Netherlands)
Kurt Nordstrom (Denmark)
Steffan Normark (Sweden)
Richard Novick (USA)
Eiichi Ohtsubo (USA)
Hisako Ohtsubo (USA)
Jorge Olarte (Mexico)
Sunil Palchaudhuri (USA)
J. C. Palomares (Spain)
William Paranchych (USA)
Ciro Peluffo (Uruguay)
Evelio J. Perea (Spain)
Wolfgang Piepersberg
 (W. Germany)
Barry Polisky (USA)
R. H. Pritchard (England)

Gaetano Privitera (Italy)
William Reznikoff (USA)
Carla Pruzzo (Italy)
William Reznikoff (USA)
Vidal Rodriguez-Lemoine
 (Venezuela)
Jack Rosenthal (Dominican
 Republic)
Bernard Rowe (England)
Robert H. Rownd (USA)
R. Bradley Sack (USA)
Bernard Sagik (USA)
Mirja Salkinoha-Salonen
 (Finland)
Joachim Sanchez (Mexico)
Konosuke Sano (Japan)
Diogenes S. Santos (Brazil)
John Sanders (England)
Rudiger Schmitt (W. Germany)
June Scott (USA)
Vittorio Sqaramella (Italy)
Avidgor Shafferman (Israel)
Richard Silver (USA)
Simon Silver (USA)
Frederick Sparling (USA)
Heather Stieglitz (Mexico)
Scott Stibitz (USA)
Gunther Stotsky (USA)
Johan H. Stuy (USA)
Anne O. Summers (USA)
Chikanori Tachibana (Japan)
Diane E. Taylor (Canada)
Grace M. Thorne (USA)
Kenneth Timmis (W. Germany)
John F. Timoney (USA)
Aslihan Tolun (Turkey/USA)
Bernt-Eric Uhlin (Sweden/USA)
Jan van Embden (Netherlands)
Graham Walker (USA)
David Watkins (USA)
William Watkins (USA)
Neil S. Willetts (Scotland)
C. Ron Wilson (USA)
Huey Lang Yang (USA)
M. Yoshikawa (Japan)

GLOSSARY

Reference should be made to the following publications; for information on plasmids to R. P. Novick, R. C. Clowes, S. N. Cohen, R. Curtiss, N. Datta, and S. Falkow (1976) Uniform nomenclature for bacterial plasmids: A proposal. Bacteriol. Rev. <u>40</u>, 168-189, and for transposons and insertion sequences to A. Campbell D. Berg, D. Botstein, E. Lederberg, R. Novick, P. Starlinger, and W. Szybalski (1977) Nomenclature of transposable elements in bacteria. In "DNA insertion elements, plasmids and episomes". Eds. Bukhari, A. I., J. A. Shapiro and S. L. Adhya, Cold Spring Harbor Laboratory, New York.

The following items are particularly important.

<u>Cointegrate</u> – a genetic element composed of two or more complete replicons in covalent linear continuity where the component replicons are known to be capable of physically independent replication. Cointegrates may be formed by recombination, transposition, <u>in vitro</u> construction or other mechanisms (see Clowes, 1972).

<u>Complementary DNA (cDNA)</u> – a single or double-stranded sequence of DNA in which the sequence on one strand is complementary to that of a messenger RNA. Usually derived by <u>in vivo</u> or <u>in vitro</u> synthesis using a DNA polymerase (reverse tran-scriptase) from a retrovirus such as avian myeloblastosis virus (see Rougeon <u>et al</u>, 1975).

<u>Conjugation (bacterial)</u> – the process of genetic exchange between bacteria dependent upon cellular contact, in which genetic material is transferred from one organism (the <u>donor</u>) to another (the <u>recipient</u>).

<u>Copy-number mutant</u> – a plasmid in which the copy number (the number of molecules of a specific plasmid per genome equi-valent or per host cell) has been changed by mutation.

683

Cosmid - a plasmid containing the sequence of and around the
    cohesive (cos) terminus of λ phage. The remaining sequences
    are usually those required for plasmid replication and for
    antibiotic resistance (see Collins & Brunning, 1978).

Direct repeat - two identical base sequences in a double-stranded
    DNA molecule.

Enterotoxin - a toxin synthesized by an enteric microorganism,
    usually Escherichia coli.

Hfr - the state of harboring a conjugative plasmid that is inte-
    grated into the chromosome and consequently is able to
    promote oriented chromosomal transfer to suitable recipients.

Insertion sequence (IS) element - a DNA segment, generally
    shorter than 2kb, which contains no known genes unrelated
    to insertion function, and which can insert into several
    sites in a genome. Symbols IS1, IS2, IS3, IS4, IS5, etc.

Inverse repeat (inverted repeat) - two DNA sequences (up to
    several hundred nucleotides in length) in a double-stranded
    DNA, one sequence of bases being repeated with the same
    polarity in the complementary strand.

    e.g.   5' —— ACAAACT----------------AGTTTGT—— 3'
            3' —— TGTTTGA----------------TCAAACA—— 5'

The two sequences are separated by other bases. If they are
continuous or separated by only one base, they are termed a
palindromic sequence.

K-antigen - a surface antigen of a bacterial cell that permits
    the cell to adhere to the cells of the intestinal mucosa of
    the alimentary tract.

Leader region - a sequence of DNA from which a messenger RNA is
    transcribed, which may be either terminated near the 3' end
    of this region, or may continue through the sequence of the
    adjacent structural gene(s). A mechanism of regulating
    certain enzymes.

Marker rescue - a recombination experiment in which the presence
    of certain genetic regions determining phenotypic properties
    can be detected by recombination of these regions into a
    replicon defective for these properties.

Maxicells - cells heavily irradiated by ultraviolet light to
    extensively damage chromosomal DNA which is consequently
    unable to produce active messenger RNA and protein. If
    plasmids are present in these cells, there is a lower
    probability that the plasmid DNA (due to its smaller size)

will be damaged, and can in consequence be used to detect
plasmid-specific messenger RNAs and proteins (see Sancar
et al, 1979).

Minicells - the product of cell division of a mutant bacterial
    strain. At each cell division, one normal cell and one
    cell (minicell) without chromosomal DNA result. Many
    plasmid DNAs are transferred into minicells, which when
    separated from normal cells by centrifugation, can be used
    to determine plasmid-specific messenger RNAs and proteins.

Mobilization - the process by which a conjugative plasmid brings
    about the transfer of DNA to which it is not stably and
    covalently linked.(see N. Willetts, 1980).

Nick translation - a method to prepare highly radioactive DNA,
    resulting from treatment with DNA polymerase I, in which
    the $3' \rightarrow 5'$ exonuclease activity removes base sequences
    adjacent to a single-stranded 'nick' and in which the $5' \rightarrow 3'$
    polymerizing activity replaces them with radioactive deoxy-
    ribonucleotides.

Northern blot - see Southern blot

Plasmid - a replicon that is stably inherited (i.e. readily
    maintained without specific selection, in an extrachromo-
    somal state. Naturally occurring plasmids in prokaryotes
    are generally dispensable.

    colicin - 'Col' plasmid, any plasmid that carries genetic
    information for the production of a colicin.

    conjugative - a plasmid that can bring about the transfer
    of DNA by conjugation.

    F - the prototype "fertility factor" responsible for conju-
    gation in the E. coli K12 strain of Cavalli-Sforza et al
    (1953) and by Hayes (1953) in their early studies of
    bacterial mating.

    F' - an F derivative incorporating a segment of the bacte-
    rial chromosome.

    non-conjugative - a plasmid that cannot bring about the
    transfer of DNA by conjugation.

    resistance (R) - a plasmid that carries genetic information
    for resistance to antibiotics and/or other antibacterial
    drugs.

Pribnow box - a DNA sequence of approximately seven bases
     situated approximately five bases in the 5' direction
     from the first base of a promoter, involved in the initia-
     tion of transcription (see Promoter).

Promoter - the site at which RNA transcription is initiated on
     the DNA template (see Rosenberg & Court, 1979).

R-loop - a segment of double-stranded DNA, in which one of the
     DNA strands has been displaced by homologous RNA, and there-
     by produces a structure visible by electron microscopy (see
     Thomas et al, 1976).

Replication origin - the DNA site (or sites) on a replicon from
     which the replication of DNA is initiated.

Southern blot - a method of DNA:RNA hybridization, by which a
     DNA preparation is cleaved into fragments with one or more
     restriction enzymes, the fragments are separated on an
     agarose gel, then denatured and transferred by capillarity
     to a sheet of cellulose nitrate paper, which is saturated
     with a radioactive labelled messenger RNA preparation,
     thereby identifying by autoradiography those DNA fragment(s)
     which have homology with the mRNA. The method has been
     modified for DNA:DNA and RNA:DNA hybridization, which are
     sometimes loosely referred to 'Northern' blots (see E. M.
     Southern, 1975).

Transfer (tra) genes - those genes carried on a conjugative
     plasmid that are responsible for the donor phenotype.

Translocation - see Transposition

Transconjugant - a bacterial cell that has received genetic
     material from another bacterium by conjugation.

Transposition element or sequence (or transposon) - a well-defined
     genetic element usually of constant size which contains genes
     unrelated to insertion function, and that transposes intact
     from one genetic locus to another. Transposition (Tn)
     elements are generally larger than 2kb, and a number (e.g.
     Tn1, Tn2, Tn3, etc.) is allocated to each independent
     isolate from nature, even if it is apparently identical to
     some previous isolate.

Transcription - the synthesis of a single-stranded RNA molecule
     by an RNA polymerase enzyme, from a double-stranded DNA
     molecule, the sequence of bases on the RNA molecule being
     complementary to those on one of the strands of the DNA
     molecule being transcribed.

References

Cavalli, L. L., J. Lederberg and E. M. Lederberg (1953) J. gen.
    Microbiol. 8, 89–103.
Clowes, R. C. (1972) Bacteriol. Rev. 36, 361–405.
Collins, J. and H. J. Bruning (1978) Gene 4, 85–92.
Hayes, W. (1953) J. gen. Microbiol. 8, 72.
Oxender, D. L., G. Zurawski and C. Yanofsky (1975) Proc. Nat.
    Acad. Sci. USA 76, 5524–5528.
Rosenberg, M. and D. Court (1979) Ann. Rev. Genet. 13, 319–353.
Rougeon, F., P. Kourilsky and B. Mach (1975) Nucl. Acids Res. 2,
    2365–2378.
Sancar, A., A. M. Hack and W. D. Rupp (1979) J. Bacteriol. 137,
    692.
Southern, E. M. (1975) J. Mol. Biol. 98, 503.
Thomas, M., R. L. White and R. W. Davis (1976) Proc. Nat. Acad.
    Sci. USA 73, 2294–2298.
Willetts, N. (1980) Mol. Gen. Genet. 180, 213–217.

CONFERENCE PARTICIPANTS

ACHTMAN, MARK, Max Planck Institut, Berlin, West Germany
ALFARO, GUILLERMO. Instituto Investigaciones Biomedicas, Mexico
ARAI, TOSHIHIKO. Keio University, Tokyo, Japan
BAQUERO, F. Cetrao Especial, Madrid, Spain
BARON, LOUIS S. Walter Reed Army Institute, Washington, D.C.
BARTH, PETER T. Imperial Chemical Industries, Cheshire, England
BARUA, DHIMAN. World Health Organization, Geneva, Switzerland
BENNETT, PETER M. University of Bristol, Bristol, England
BERG, DOUGLAS E. Washington Univ. Med. Schoo, St. Louis, MO
BERTRAND, KEVIN. University of California, Irvine, CA
BINNS, MATTHEW. Washington Univ. Med. School, St. Louis, MO
BRADLEY, DAVID. Univ. of Newfoundland, St. John's, Newfoundland
BRODA, PAUL. University of Manchester, Manchester, England
BRUNTON, JAMES. Univ. of Alberta, Edmonton, Alberta
BURCHALL, JAMES. Wellcome Research Labs, Research Triangle Pk., NC
BURMAN, LARS G. Tufts Univ. Medical School, Boston, MA
BUTLER, TED. Tufts-New England Medical Center Hospital, Boston, MA
BUU-HOI, ANNIE. Centre Hopital Universitaire, Paris, France
CABELLO, FELIPE. New York Medical College, Valhalla, NY
CAVAZZA, MARIA E. Acta Cientifica Venezolana, Caracas, Venezuela
CARLTON, BRUCE C. University of Georgia, Athens, GA
CARR, FELICITY P.A. Washington Univ. Med. School, St. Louis, MO
CHAKRABARTY, ANANDA M. University of Illinois, Chicago, IL
CHASSY, BRUCE. N.I.D.R., N.I.H., Bethesda, MD
CHERGUIN, PATRICIA. Washington Univ. Med. School, St. Louis, MO
CHOPRA, IAN. University of Bristol, Bristol, England
CLANCY, Joanna. University of Illinois, Urbana, IL
CLEWELL, DON B. Unviersity of Michigan, Ann Arbor, MI
CLOWES, ROYSTON C. University of Texas, Richardson, TX
COHA GONZALES, JUANA M. Universidad Nacional San Marcos, Lima, Peru
COLLINS, JOHN. Biotech, Inst., Braunschweig-Stockheim, W. Germany
CRUZ, JOSE. Instituto de Nutricion, Guatemala, Guatemala
CULLINANE, JOANNE. Tufts Univ. School of Medicine, Boston, MA
CURIALE, MICHAEL. Tufts Univ. School of Medicine, Boston, MA
DATTA, NAOMI. Royal Postgraduate Medical School, London, England
DELAPPE, IRVING P. NIAID, NIH, Bethesda, MD
DOUGAN, GORDAN. Moyne Institute, Trinity College, Dublin, Ireland

DUBNAU, DAVID.   N.Y. Public Health Research Institute, New York, NY
DUNNY, GARY M.   NYS Veterinary College, Cornell Univ., Ithaca, NY
EDLUND, THOMAS.   University of Umea, Umea, Sweden
EICHENLAUB, RUDOLF.   Ruhr-Universitat Bochum, Bochum, West Germany
ELWELL, LYNN P.   Wellcome Research Labs, Research Triangle Park, NC
ESPINOSA-LARA, ALICIA.   Escuela National Ciencias, Mexico D.F.
FALKOW, STANLEY,   Stanford Univ. Med. School, Stanford, CA
FARRAR, W. EDMUND,   Medical University of S.C., Charleston, SC
FEINMAN, SUSAN E.   Consumer Product Safety, Bethesda, MD
FIGURSKI, DAVID H.   College of Phys. & Surg., Columbia Univ., NY, NY
FOCK, RUDIGER.   University of Hamburg, Hamburg, West Germany
FOSTER, TIM J.   Univ. of Dublin, Trinity College, Dublin, Ireland
FRANKLIN, F.C. Max Planck Inst.-Molek. Genetik, Berlin, W. Germany
FREESE, ERNST.   National Institutes of Health, Bethesda, MD
FROST, LAURA.   University of Alberta, Edmonton, Alberta
GARCIA LOBO, JUAN M.   University of Santander, Santander, Spain
GAWRON-BURKE, CYNTHIA.   University of Michigan, Ann Arbor, MI
GILBERT, WALTER,   Harvard University, Cambridge, MA
GOEBEL, WERNER.   Unviersitat Wurzburg, Wurzburg, West Germany
GOMES, TANIA.   Escola Paulista de Medicale, Sao Paulo, Brazil
GOMEZ-EICHELMAN, M. CARMEN,   Inst. Investig. Biomed., Mexico D.F.
GOTS, JOSEPH S.   Univ. of Penn. Medical School, Philadelphia, PA
GRANT, ROBERT B.   Hospital for Sick Children, Toronto, Ontario
GRAY, GARY.   University of Wisconsi, Madison, WI
GRINDLEY, NIGEL.   Yale University, New Haven, CT
GRINSTED, JOHN.   University of Bristol, Bristol, England
GUERRY-KOPECKO, PATRICIA.   Genex Laboratories, Rockville, MD
GUILD, WALTER.   Duke University, Durham, NC
GUNSALUS, I.C.   University of Illinois, Urbana, IL
GUZMAN, MIGUEL A.   Instituto Nacional de Salud, Bogota, Colombia
HALLEWELL, ROBERT.   Univ. of California, San Francisco, CA
HARFORD, NIGEL.   Smith-Kline-Rit, Rixensart, Belguim
HARNETT, NORMA M.   University of Guelph, Ontario
HELINSKI, RONALD R.   University of California, La Jolla, CA
HERTMAN, ISRAEL.   Israel Inst. for Biol. Res., Ness Ziona, Israel
HIRSH, DWIGHT.   Univ. of California Vet. School, Davis, CA
HOGAN, JANE.   Tufts University School of Medicine, Boston, MA
HOGENAUER, GREGOR.   Sandoz Research Institute, Vienna, Austria
HORODNICEANU, THEA.   Institut Pasteur, Paris, France
IHLER, GARRET.   Texas A&M College of Med., College Station, TX
INSELBURG, JOSEPH.   Dartmouth Medical School, Hanover, NH
IPPEN-IHLER, KARIN.   Texas A&M College of Med., College Sta., TX
ISTURIZ, TOMAS. Universidad Central de Venezuela, Caracas, Venezuela
IYER, V.N.   Carleton University, Ottawa, Ontario
JACKS, THOMAS M.   Merck, Sharp & Dohme, Rahway, NJ
JOHN, JOSEPH F.   V.A. Medical Center, Charleston, SC
JOHNSTON, ANDREW W.B.   John Innes Institute, Norwich, England
KADO, CLARENCE I.   University of California, Davis CA
KAGAN, SARAH A.   University of Wisconsin, Madison WI
KAJI, AKIRA.   Univ. of Penn. Med. Sch., Philadelphia, PA

KAJI, HIDEKO. Univ. of Penn. Med. Sch., Philadelphia, PA
KLINE, BRUCE. Mayo Clinic Foundation, Rochester, MN
KOENIG, ELLEN L. Univers. Pedro H. Urena, Santo Domingo, D.R.
KONTOMICHALOU, POLYXENI. Univ. of Athens Med. Sch., Athens, Greece
KOPECKO, DENNIS J. Walter Reed Army Hospital, Washington, DC
KUPERSZTOCH, YANKEL M. Dept. de Genetica-C.I.E.H. del I.P.M.,
  Mexico DF
LAIRD, WALTER J. F.D.A., Bureau of Biologics, Bethesda, MD
LAUFS, RAINER. Univ. of Hamburg, Hamburg, W. Germany
LAUX, DAVID. University of Rhode Island, Kingston, RI
LEAL, EGLIS. Hospital Universitario, Maracaibo, Venezuela
LeBLANC, DONALD J. Nat. Inst. of Dental Research, Bethesda, MD
LEDERBERG, ESTHER M. Stanford Univ. Sch. of Med., Stanford, CA
LEONG, SALLY. University of California, La Jolla, CA
LEVIN, MORRIS. U.S. E.P.A., Washington, DC
LEVY, JAY A. Univ. of California Med. Ctr., San Francisco, CA
LEVY, STUART B. Tufts University School of Medicine, Boston, MA
LOVETT, PAUL S. University of Maryland, Catonsville, MD
MACRINA, FRANCIS. Medical College of Virginia, Richmond, VA
MANIS, JACK J. The Upjohn Co., Kalamazoo, MI
de MARIN, CARMEN. Hospital Universitario, Maracaibo, Venezuela
MARIN, NERIO. Hospital Universitario, Maracaibo, Venezuela
MARSHALL, BONNIE. Tufts University School of Medicine, Boston, MA
MARTINEZ, ADA. Hospital Universitario, Maracaibo, Venezuela
McINTIRE, SARAH A. V.A. Medical Center, Dallas, TX
McMURRY, LAURA. Tufts University School of Medicine, Boston, MA
MEDEIROS, ANTONE A. The Miriam Hospital, Providence, RI
MENDOZA, ALEXIS. Universidad Central de Venezuela, Caracas, Venezuela
MOLINA, EMILVA. Hospital Universitario, Maracaibo, Venezuela
MOSELY, STEVE L. Univ. of Washington School of Med., Seattle, WA
NASSER, DELIL. National Science Foundation, Washington, DC
NESTER, EUGENE W. Univ. of Washington Sch. of Med., Seattle, WA
NIJKAMP, H. JOHN J. Vrije Universiteit, Amsterdam, Netherlands
NORDSTROM, KURT. Odense University, Odense, Denmark
NORMARK, STAFFAN. University of Umea, Umea, Sweden
OLARTE, JORGE. Hospital Infantil de Mexico, Mexico, DF
OLIVER, DAPNA R. Oakland University, Rochester, MI
PALCHAUDHURI, SUNIL. Wayne State University, Detroit, MI
PALOMARES, J.C. Universidad de Sevilla, Sevilla, Spain
PELUFFO, CIRO A. Instituto National de Higiene, Montevideo, Uruguay
de PERALTA, VICTORIA. Univ. Catolica Madre y Mestra, Santo Domingo,D.R.
PEREA, EVELIO J. Universidad de Sevilla, Sevilla, Spain
PETERSON, VIRGINIA. University of Missouri, Columbia, MO
PIEPERSBERG, WOLFGANG. University of Wisconsin, Madison, WI
PINEDA, MARITZA. Hospital Universitario, Maracaibo, Venezuela
POLISKY, BARRY. Indiana University, Bloomington, IN
PRIETO, GUSTAVO. Hospital Universitario, Maracaibo, Venezuela
PRITCHARD, ROBERT H. University of Leicester, Leicester, England
PRIVITERA, GAETANO. Ospedale L. Sacco, Milan, Italy
PRUZZO, CARLA. Instituto Microbiologia, Genoa, Italy

RAMIREZ, JOSE L. Universidad Central de Venezuela, Caracas, Venezuela
REED, RANDALL R. Sterling Hall of Med., Yale Univ., New Haven, CT
REIS, HENRIQUETA L. Escola Paulista de Medicina, Sao Paulo, Brazil
REZNIKOFF, WILLIAM. University of Wisconsin, Madison, WI
RODRIGUEZ-LEMOINE, VIDAL. Acta Cientifica Venezolana, Caracas, Venez.
ROSENTHAL, JACK. Universidad Pedro H. Urena, Santo Domingo, D.R.
ROUSSEL, AGNES. Institut Pasteur, Paris, France
ROWE, BERNARD. Central Public Health Lav., London, England
ROWND, ROBERT H. University of Wisconsin, Madison, WI
SACK, R. BRADLEY, Johns Hopkins University, Baltimore, MD
SAGIK, BERNARD. Drexel Institute, Philadelphia, PA
SALKINOJA-SALONEN, MIRJA. Univ. of Helsinki, Helsinki, Finland
SANCHEZ, JOACHIM. University of Bristol, Bristol, England
SANO, KONOSUKE. University of Wisconsin, Madison, WI
SANTOS, DIOGENES S. Escola Paulista de Medicale, Sao Paulo, Brazil
SAUNDERS, JOHN R. University of Liverpool, Liverpool, England
SCHMIDT, FRANCIS J. University of Missouri, Columbia, MO
SCHMITT, RUDIGER. Universitat Regensberg, Regensberg, West Germany
SCOTT, JUNE R. Emory University, Atlanta, GA
SGARAMELLA, VITTORIO. University of Pavia, Pavia, Italy
SHAFFERMAN, AVIGDOR. University of California, La Jolla, CA
SHAPIRO, JAMES A. University of Chicago, Chicago, IL
SHIPLEY, PATRICIA L. Medical College of Virginia, Richmond, VA
SILVER, RICHARD P. Bureau of Biologics, F.D.A., Bethesda, MD
SPARLING, P. FREDERICK. Univ. of N.C. Med. Sch., Chapel Hill, NC
STIBLITZ, E. SCOTT. University of Wisconsin, Madison, WI
STIEGLITZ, HEATHER. G.I.E.H. del I.P.M., Mexico, D.F., Mexico
STOTZKY, GUNTHER. New York University, New York, NY
STUY, JOHAN H. Florida State University, Tallahassee, FL
SUMMERS, ANNE O. University of Georgia, Athens, GA
TACHIBANA, CHIKANORI. Tufts Univ. School of Medicine, Boston, MA
TALLY, FRANCIS P. Tufts-New England Medical Center, Boston, MA
TARDIFF, GINETTE. Hospital for Sick Children, Toronto, Ontario
TAYLOR, DIANE E. Hospital for Sick Children, Toronto, Ontario
THORNE, GRACE M. Tufts-New England Medical Center, Boston, MA
TIMMIS, KENNETH N. Max Planck Institut, Berlin, West Germany
TIMONEY, JOHN F. Cornell Univ. Sch. of Med., Ithaca, NY
TOLUN, ASLIHAN. University of California, La Jolla, CA
UHLIN, BERNT-ERIC. University of California, Berkeley, CA
URDANETA, LARES. Hospital Universitario, Maracaibo, Venezuela
VARGAS, GEANNETTE. Hospital Universitario, Maracaibo, Venezuela
VAN EMBDEN, JAN. Ruks Institut, Bilthoven, Netherlands
VAN MONTAGU, MARC. Rijksuniversieteit Gent, Gent, Belgium
VAPNEK, DANIEL. University of Georgia, Athens, GA
WALKER, GRAHAM C. Mass. Institute of Technology, Cambridge, MA
WATKINS, DAVID R. EPA Industr. Environ. Res. Lab, Cincinnati, OH
WATKINS, WILLIAM. University of Rhode Island, Providence, RI
WESTPHELING, JANET. University of Wisconsin, Madison, WI
WILLETTS, NEIL S. University of Edinburgh, Edinburgh, Scotland
WILLIAMS, PETER H. University of Leicester, Leicester, England

WILSON, C. RON. Dow Chemical Corporation, Midland, MI
WINTHER, MICHAEL D. Wellcome Research Labs, Kent, England
WOLF-WATZ, HANS. National Defence Research Institute, Umea, Sweden
YAGI, YOSHIHIKI. University of Michigan, Ann Arbor, MI
YANG, HUEY-LANG. Public Health Research Institute, New York, NY
YOSHIKAWA, MASANOSUKE. University of Tokyo, Tokyo, Japan

Photos compliments of L. Baron and C. Tachibana

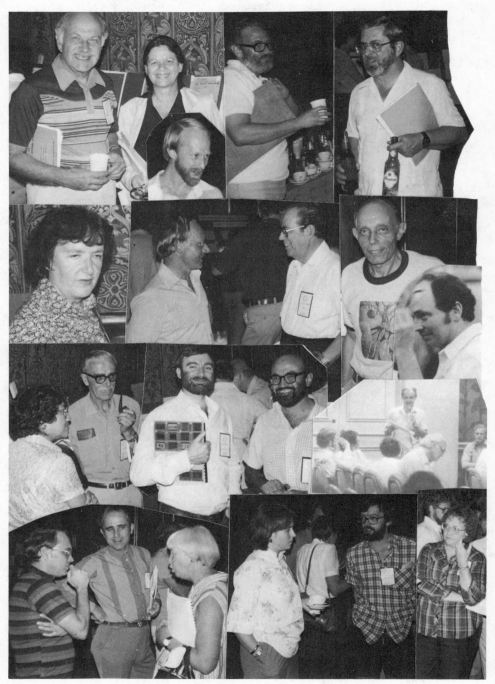

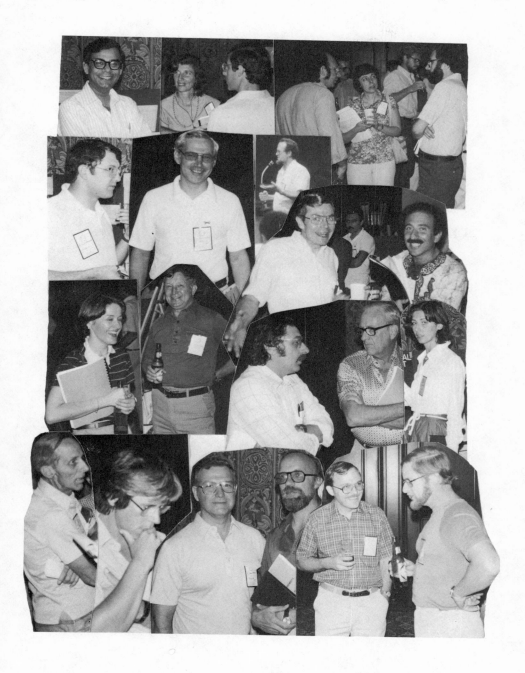

AUTHOR INDEX

Aagaard-Hansen, H. 291
Adsit, J.C.   557
Affonso, M.H.T.   649
Aguero, M.E.   587
Alfaro, G.   575
Ali, S.A.   622
Allen, A.D.   663
Altenbuchner, J.   359
Ando, T.   576
Angelatou, F.   669
Arai, T.   576, 577, 623
Arbuthnott, J.P.   640
Armstrong, K.   279
Assaf, L.M.   539

Bagdasarian, M.   604
Bagdasarian, M.M.   604
Ball, P.R.   592
Baguero, F.   578
Baron, E.S.   557
Baron, L.S.   111, 579
Barth, P.T.   439
Bartlett, J.   586
Barua, D.   580
Bechhofer, D.   602
Bennett, P.M.   581, 654
Berg, D.E.   381
Bergstrom, S.   169
Bertrand, K.   582
Bijlsma, I.G.W.   101
Binns, M.M.   583
Biswas, G.   237
Blackman, E.   237
Bohlander, F.A.   617
Bölin, I.   584

Bradley, D.E.   217
Brewin, N.J.   487
Bricker, J.   603
Broda, P.   511
Brown, B.   674
Burman, L.G.   585
Buswell, J.   653
Butler, T.   586
Buu-Hoi, A.   616

Cabello, F.   587
Cafferkey, M.   588
Cabezon, T.   612
Carlton, B.C.   589
Carr, F.P.A.   583
Carson, G.R.   51
Cashel, M.   675
Cavazza, M.E.   650
Chakrabarty, A.   519
Chassy, B.   590
Chatterjee, D.K.   519
Chiang, S.J.   591
Chifari, F.A.   461
Chopra, I.   592
Christie, P.J.   557
Clancy, J.   593
Clark, A.J.   670
Clewell, D.B.   191, 608, 658,
                             674
Clowes, R.C.   591
Cohen, P.S.   625
Coleman, D.C.   594
Collins, J.   429
Courvalin, P.   624
Cowan, J.A.   661

697

SUBJECT INDEX

Acinetobacter, 520
  calcoaceticus , 441
Actinomycetes, 153, 191, 192
Aerobacter aerogenes, 129, 147
Agarose gels, 8, 52, 54, 77, 86,
        103, 113, 115, 118, 141,
        228, 230, 234, 243, 244,
        432, 441, 445, 462, 468,
        470, 488, 490, 493, 501,
        523, 524, 541, 542, 619,
        636, 644
Agrobacterium tumefaciens, 401-
        410, 467-486, 628
Alcaligenes, 520
  eutrophus, 441
Antibiotic
  resistance
    amikacin, 147-149, 601, 610
    aminocyclitols, 146, 147,
        151-153, 620
    ampicillin, 11, 12, 15, 23-28,
        52, 66-68, 71-78, 237-246,
        357, 382-388, 411, 412,
        440, 441, 457, 459, 525,
        539, 540, 544, 548-550,
        599, 600, 665
    cephalothin, 63, 541, 545
    chloramphenicol, 11-15, 72-78,
        84, 85, 135, 145, 150-153,
        191, 199, 200, 313, 352-
        357, 395, 445-448, 457-
        459, 539, 541, 544, 548,
        551, 569, 588, 652, 672
    erythromycin, 51-60, 64, 81,
        82, 84, 87, 88, 146, 150,

Antibiotic (continued)
  resistance (continued)
    erythromycin (continued)
        151, 153, 157, 191, 197,
        658
    gentamicin, 2-4, 8, 9, 148,
        150, 151, 468, 541, 588,
        623, 645
    kanamycin, 45, 87, 88, 135,
        148, 201, 328, 371-390,
        393-395, 440, 445-447,
        468, 470, 472, 491, 539,
        540, 548, 550, 569, 603,
        664
    MLS, 85, 86, 88, 148, 193,
        200, 227, 234, 647
    neomycin, 371-380, 462, 463
    rifamycin, 135, 136, 139
    streptomycin, 11, 12, 86-88,
        135, 148, 150, 227, 234,
        355-357, 402, 440-446,
        525, 539, 548, 550
    sulfonamide, 21, 27, 135,
        146, 355, 402, 440-446,
        540-542, 544, 568, 569
    tetracycline, 11, 12, 51-56,
        61-88, 104, 145, 146,
        150, 152, 199, 200, 202,
        227, 234, 359-370, 384-
        388, 412, 440, 444, 446,
        457-459, 512, 525, 539,
        541, 548, 550, 568, 569,
        581, 582, 586, 594, 597,
        608
    tobramycin, 2, 4, 148, 150